ESSENTIAL ULTRASOUND ANATOMY

Berhanu Kindu

ALLIED HEALTH PRESS

Essential Ultrasound Anatomy

Author: **Berhanu Kindu**

Allied Health Press
4164 Lakeshore Road
Burlington ON L7L 1A4
Canada
www.alliedhealthpress.com
Email: orders@arclereducation.com

ISBN: 978-1-77956-806-9

ABOUT THE AUTHOR

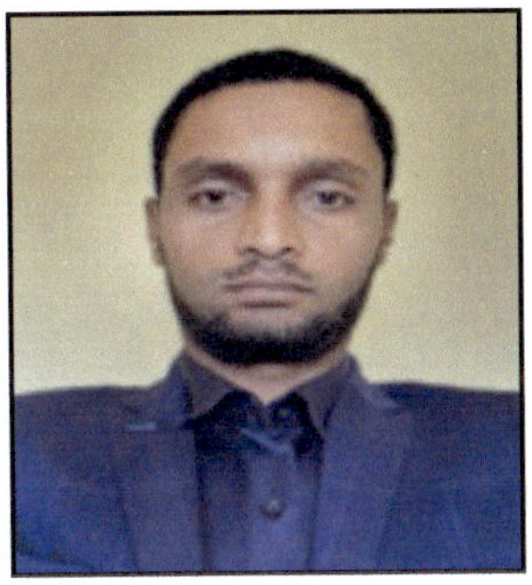

Berhanu Kindu Ashagrie, lecturer and researcher of Human Anatomy at Debre Tabor University, Ethiopia. He has been working in Debre Tabor University since 22 September, 2018 as a lecturer and researcher of Human Anatomy, Histology, Embryology and other related fields of science. Since then, he has been publishing research articles, review manuscripts, and teaching materials in health science and related fields of science.

He graduated with Bachelor's degree from Debre Markos University in Public Health (BSc) and Master's degree from University of Gondar (one of the top legendary universities in Ethiopia) in Human Anatomy (MSc).

Brief Table of Contents

Detailed Table of Contents

CHAPTER 3

Ultrasound Image Interpretation and Terminology 71

CHAPTER 4

Neck and Thyroid Ultrasound 107

CHAPTER 5

CHAPTER 6

CHAPTER 14

Vascular Access and Soft Tissue Imaging Ultrasound 449

CHAPTER 15

Ultrasound in Emergency and Critical Care 481

LIST OF FIGURES

PREFACE

Ultrasound imaging ranks among the most useful of the diagnostic tools of modern clinical practice. Unlike other imaging modalities, ultrasound is real-time imaging, portable, free from ionization, and applicable to a wide range of medical specialties. From patient triage at the initial presentation in emergency departments to therapeutic intervention in the operating room, its usefulness in increasing diagnostic efficiency and accuracy has increased immensely. But without its basis in anatomical understanding and imaging principles, even its ready access cannot be readily mastered. For clinicians, sonographers, and students alike, bridging the gap between anatomical understanding and ultrasound visualization is the pathway to clinical proficiency.

The use of ultrasound for anatomical examination grants dynamic access to physiological processes and pathologies. From assessment of vascular perfusion to estimation of organ size and echotexture to identification of structural abnormalities, the modality's specific strength lies in its direct clinical correlation. Effective sonographic image acquisition and interpretation are based on a solid understanding of the modality's technical parameters and anatomical conditions. Knowledge of standard scanning planes and patient positions, and systematic image interpretation, is also the basis of diagnosis. This makes structured educational materials essential to students and practitioners seeking to acquire confidence and reliability in ultrasound assessments.

Essential Ultrasound Anatomy aims to provide a short and practical review of sonographic anatomy from the angle of actual clinical practice. With a combination of physics fundamentals, technical training, and region-specific anatomy content, the book is an all-round resource for students going into practice as well as practitioners who wish to enhance their skills. The chapters emphasize applied knowledge such that readers can relate anatomical structures to their ultrasonographic appearances. Each section combines lucid explanation with clinical relevance, giving a concise learning experience of sonographic anatomy.

Chapter 1 presents the fundamental concepts of ultrasound physics and equipment. It explains important concepts such as transmission of sound waves, acoustic impedance, image resolution, and the operation of probes and transducers. The aim is to give the reader an impression of how image quality relies on machine controls and anatomical considerations.

Chapter 2 is dedicated to standard scanning maneuvers and patient positioning routines. The chapter emphasizes the significance of probe direction, application of gel, ergonomics, and standardized methods for consistency in image acquisition. It also contains tips for real-life improvement in patient comfort and operator fatigue reduction.

Chapter 3 addresses ultrasound image interpretation and terminology most frequently used. It describes distinguishing between echogenicities, recognizing artifact patterns, and using descriptors like hypoechoic, anechoic, and isoechoic. This chapter assists in setting the stage for accurately interpreting clinical findings.

Chapter 4 is devoted to ultrasound scanning of the neck and thyroid. Emphasis is put on the identification of cervical lymph nodes' normal appearance, vascular markers, isthmus, and lobes of the thyroid. Pathologic presentations, including cysts, nodules, and goiters, are also described in the chapter.

Chapter 5 is dedicated to the chest and pleural space. Techniques for detecting pleural effusions, pneumothorax, and consolidations are described. An overview of the anatomy of the thorax, consisting of rib shadows, lung sliding, and the diaphragm, is provided as context while examining the respiratory system.

Chapter 6 introduces basic cardiac anatomy on transthoracic ultrasound. Key cardiac structures, including chambers, valves, pericardium, and interventricular septum, are introduced. Common views are included in the chapter, like parasternal long axis and apical four-chamber views, to orient the student.

Chapter 7 addresses peritoneal and abdominal wall ultrasound imaging. Hernia assessment, ascites, hematomas, and fascial planes are discussed. Students are able to distinguish between layers of the abdominal wall and peritoneal spaces.

Chapter 8 deals with the liver and biliary tract. Visualization of hepatic segments, intrahepatic and extrahepatic bile ducts, and the gallbladder is addressed. Diagnostic characteristics of hepatomegaly, cholelithiasis, and bile duct dilation are presented.

Chapter 9 focuses on the urinary tract and kidneys. Anatomical orientation of the renal medulla, cortex, pelvis, and collecting system is presented. The detection of hydronephrosis, cysts, stones, and bladder pathology is emphasized by the chapter.

Chapter 10 focuses on ultrasound evaluation of the pancreas and spleen. It addresses scanning planes for spleen size and texture and methods for finding and interpreting the pancreas in spite of its deep and inconstant location.

Chapter 11 covers sonographic imaging of the aorta and inferior vena cava. Transverse and longitudinal scanning are outlined for aortic diameter measurement and assessment of aneurysm, and IVC collapse assessment in volume status estimation.

Chapter 12 covers pelvic anatomy in men and women. The chapter is filled with protocols for the evaluation of the uterus, ovaries, bladder, prostate, and seminal vesicles. The chapter also covers transabdominal and transvaginal scanning techniques.

Chapter 13 introduces musculoskeletal ultrasound with emphasis on tendons, ligaments, joints, and soft tissue structures. Clinical scenarios include evaluation of the rotator cuff, effusions, and muscle tears, with emphasis on alignment of the probe and dynamic scanning.

Chapter 14 deals with soft tissue and vascular access examination. It gives techniques for the identification of veins to cannulate, for the detection of abscesses, and for the characterization of masses or foreign bodies in subcutaneous tissues.

Chapter 15 highlights the utilization of ultrasound in the critical and emergency care environments. It discusses focused assessment with sonography for trauma (FAST), point-of-care cardiac and lung evaluation, and rapid identification of free fluid or tamponade.

This book is written for a general readership that includes undergraduate allied health and medical students, internal medicine and radiology trainees, emergency medicine doctors, critical care medicine physicians, sonographers, and nurse practitioners. It is highly valuable to students new to the learning of ultrasound skills, as well as clinicians who wish to refine more accurate anatomical recognition during point-of-care scanning. Instructors can also utilize it as a teaching supplement for formal ultrasound education.

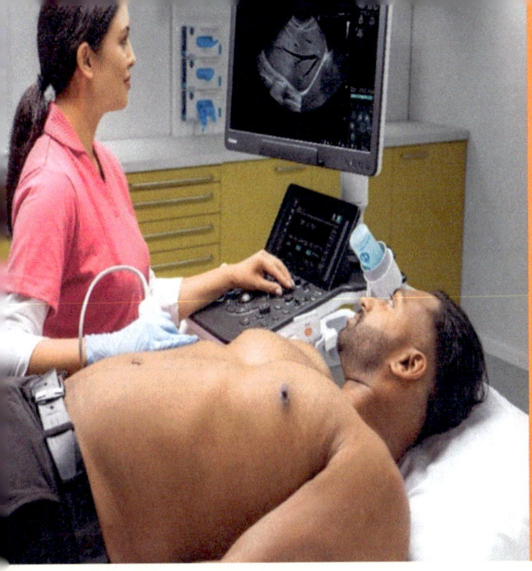

Chapter 1

BASICS OF ULTRASOUND PHYSICS AND INSTRUMENTATION

Contents

Introduction

The use of ultrasound technology has revolutionized the landscape of diagnostics and medical imaging. This non-surgical process employs high-frequency sound waves, which are transmitted through tissues and then reflected back to form images of the inner body. The fundamental physics behind ultrasound depends upon the behavior of sound waves in various tissues of varied densities. Therefore, ultrasound imaging has no problem distinguishing between liquids and soft tissues, enabling the visualization of organs and pathology in the human body. Its ability to record images in real-time makes ultrasound extremely valuable in obstetrics, echocardiography, and musculoskeletal imaging, hence becoming a valuable tool in modern medicine.

Due to technological advancements, various imaging modalities are now available that offer high diagnostic sensitivity. Included among these technologies are color Doppler ultrasound, which provides crucial information about blood flow and vessel integrity, and three-dimensional imaging, which provides a more detailed comprehension of anatomy. Furthermore, the incorporation of ultrasound simulators into training programs has gained momentum, as these simulators provide significant advantages to the training of healthcare professionals. As per the World Federation for Ultrasound in Medicine and Biology (WFUMB), ultrasound simulation enables specialists to acquire expertise in a simulated environment, thus improving clinical performance, along with learner assurance and lowering the workload on healthcare facilities (Dietrich et al., 2023). This new approach proves the importance of simulation in developing expertise in ultrasound imaging, which will ultimately benefit practitioners and patients. While with numerous advantages, ultrasound does have some disadvantages that take the form of the necessity for expert interpretation and potential limitations in some cases. Factors such as operator skill, patient body habitus, and presence of intervening structures can affect image quality and diagnostic consistency. Secondly, there can be a high learning curve in gaining competence in ultrasound skills, with the need for extensive training programs with an emphasis on pragmatic skills. Overcoming these challenges requires continued research and development to refine ultrasound technology and enhance training techniques. The synergy between continued technological innovation and high-quality educational practices will be the key to shaping the future of ultrasound as the cornerstone of medical imaging (Royo et al., 2019). High-quality training and new tools will be essential to realize the full capabilities of this critical imaging modality (Figure 1.1).

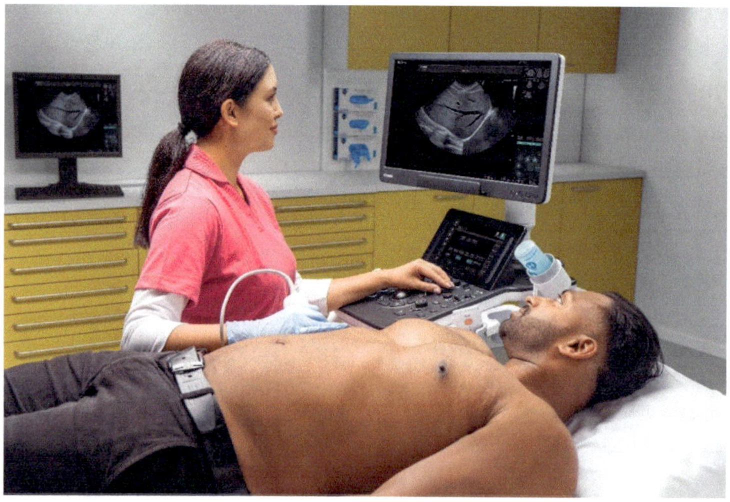

Figure 1.1. Introduction to ultrasound.

Source: uk.medical.canon. https://uk.medical.canon/wp-content/uploads/sites/8/2024/10/Aplio-Me-PR-2.jpg.

Definition of Ultrasound

Ultrasound, which is applied in medical imaging, is a non-invasive diagnostic technique employing high-frequency sound waves to produce images of internal body organs. Contrary to X-rays, which employ ionizing radiation, ultrasound is based on the concept of echoing sound waves and is thus safer for the patient as well as the practitioner. The fundamental operation is the emission of sound waves by a transducer that passes through the body and reflects off various tissues. These echoes are converted by the transducer into images on a screen so that doctors can scan organs, blood vessels, and even fetal development when a woman is pregnant. The ability of ultrasound to provide imaging in real-time increases its usefulness for diagnosis, particularly in soft tissue conditions, and makes it a valuable tool in numerous different clinical settings. The use of ultrasound extends far beyond imaging; it has the ability to be used therapeutically as well. A variety of different modalities, including therapeutic ultrasound, employ sound waves both for treatment and for imaging purposes, for example, to shatter kidney stones or to stimulate tissue healing. Its application in the guidance of procedures, for example, injections and biopsies, is one excellent example of its contribution to current medicine. Moreover, technology has provided portable ultrasound machines, which have made it widely accessible for the first time in various settings, including underserved and remote areas. By combining ultrasound technology with the analysis of real-time data, medical practitioners can make more informed decisions, hence making ultrasound a fundamental component of contemporary medical practice. With further technology development in ultrasound technology, instructional materials, and literature enhance understanding and application throughout disciplines. For instance, the use of sensor-equipped mobile devices to discuss their application shows the innovative way that ultrasound can be used in physics learning spaces to bridge gaps between conceptual understanding and application (Monteiro & Marti , 2022). In addition, studies on the use of bioactivity in ultrasound reflect a greater emphasis on its nutritional and medicinal applications and how it will revolutionize fields of endeavor beyond medical practices (Campos et al., 2021). As technology in ultrasonic applications develops, so too does the understanding of its usage and definition, and with it, the necessity to research its application in both therapy and diagnosis.

Historical Evolution of Ultrasound Technology

The history of ultrasound technology as a medical imaging modality goes back to a series of advances that have transformed medical imaging. The earliest application of ultrasound was primarily during World War II in sonar technology, founded on its underlying principle of reflection of sound waves. Its application in medicine began in the late part of 1940s when researchers such as Dr. Karl Dussik experimented with its ability to image the human body. Dussik's breakthroughs included imagining brain tumors by using ultrasound, a significant milestone in medical imaging. The early uses were limited by the technology because they relied primarily upon single-frequency waves that produced only partial detail. As the 1950s progressed, advancements in electronic technology enabled more sophisticated ultrasound machines, which offered improved image quality and better diagnostics. In the 1970s, there were tremendous developments in the technology of ultrasound with the introduction of real-time imaging that provided a moving image of internal organs. At this point in time, A-mode and B-mode ultrasound systems were established; the former provided details regarding amplitude and the latter translated spatial information into two-dimensional images. This was followed by the innovation of Doppler ultrasound, which allowed quantification of blood flow, further propelling the diagnostic application of ultrasound. Physicians were then able to visualize and assess hemodynamics in various conditions and hence enhance patient outcomes. The surge in research and innovation in ultrasound systems throughout this decade formed the foundation of the myriad applications that can be seen in current medical practice, further substantiating ultrasound's value in medical environments. With continuing improvement in ultrasound technology well into the late 20th and early 21st centuries, the incorporation of computer systems and imaging software enabled drastic enhancements in both effectiveness and efficiency. Current ultrasound scanners feature multidimensional imaging, making it possible to construct three-dimensional reconstructions of body structures. Furthermore, innovation in transducer technology development permitted higher frequency ranges, with enhanced detail and diagnostic accuracy. The implementation of new algorithms and processing also enabled better visualization of complex structures beyond previous constraints of clarity. As ultrasound is utilized to a great extent in all sorts of varied specialties—obstetrics to cardiology—the technology has firmly established itself as a pillar of non-invasive medical imaging. In totality, the evolution of ultrasound technology depicts an astounding journey marked by epochal innovations and interdisciplinary contributions, epitomizing its central role in contemporary healthcare as it continues to evolve (Figure 1.2).

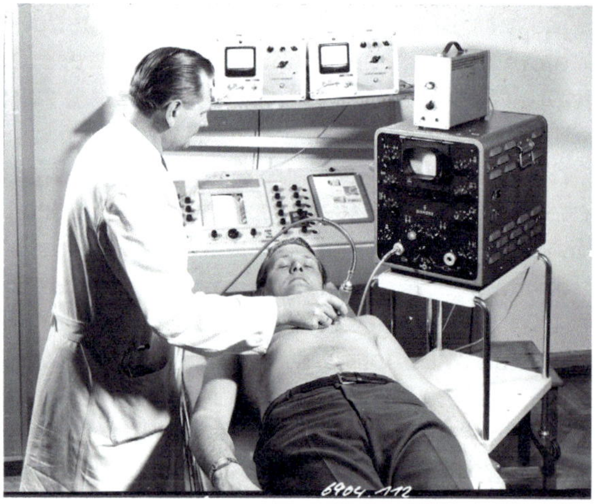

Figure 1.2. Historical development of ultrasound technology.

Source: Siemens Healthineers. https://www.siemens-healthineers.com/en-in/ultrasound/news-stories/history

Importance of Ultrasound in Medical Imaging

The use of ultrasound for clinical imaging cannot be overstated, as it stands out for not using invasive procedures and for having imaging in real-time. The process is founded on wave propagation principles, where it uses high-frequency sound waves to generate images of internal organs within the body. Unlike other imaging techniques, such as X-rays or MRI, the ultrasound does not involve ionizing radiation and is thus safer, particularly in risky groups such as pregnant women and children. Real-time imaging of the organs allows dynamic assessment, which plays an important role in a multitude of clinical situations, from obstetrics to emergency situations. Hence, the safety profile and versatility of ultrasound are major factors that contribute to its universal application in medicine, which enables accurate diagnoses and better patient outcomes. The advancement in ultrasound technology renders it an integral part of diagnostic as well as therapeutic procedures. Moreover, the advancement in ultrasound system with new techniques has widened its applications. Improvements in imaging technology, such as 3D and Doppler ultrasound, have enhanced the quality of diagnostic products. Such developments enable doctors to inspect blood flow, structural abnormalities, and even organ functioning with unprecedented precision. Moreover, ultrasound can penetrate through tissue barriers such as soft and hard bodies to provide accurate intervention and biopsy without the need for more invasive interventions. The merit of ongoing research and development in ultrasound is underscored, with new uses of emerging technology set to enhance and expand further its clinical application, pushing the boundaries of what is achievable in medical imaging. The educational aspect of ultrasound is also important, as medical education continues to add simulation technologies to enhance learning even more. As has been noted in recent literature, simulation using ultrasound offers a clinical education platform that enables practitioners to hone their skills under controlled conditions. Not only does this novel method decrease pressure on overcrowded clinical environments, but it also instills learner confidence as they work through ultrasound applications. The World Federation for Ultrasound in Medicine and Biology has emphasized the key role of simulation when training in ultrasound, outlining its benefits and pitfalls. As technology continues to evolve, the application of simulation in ultrasound education appears to have the potential to transform how healthcare workers and medical students gain their skills, ultimately leading to better outcomes and care for patients (Dietrich et al., 2023) and filling the future demand for skilled practitioners in this significant area of medical imaging.

1.1. Principles of Ultrasound Physics

The physics of ultrasound comprises key concepts that establish the formation of images and the behavior of sound waves as they pass through different body tissues. Central to ultrasound technology is understanding the passing of sound waves through any medium, depending on their frequency, wavelength, and speed. The frequency of the ultrasound waves, typically 1 to 15 megahertz, directly influences penetration and resolution of the imaging process. The higher the frequency, the higher the resolution but with poor penetration, so best suited for superficial structure imaging. By contrast, lower frequencies penetrate deeper with a loss of resolution, pointing to the trade-off clinicians must strike in making transducer settings to optimize diagnostic usefulness and acoustical quality in generating distinguishable images of anatomical structures. Understanding the interaction between ultrasound waves and tissues is important for successful imaging and diagnosis. When the sound waves come across the borders of different tissues, such as fat and muscle or muscle and bone, they reflect, refract, or transmit based on the acoustic properties of the interacting tissues. The acoustic impedance, a measure that depends on medium density and velocity, is a major factor determining the above interactions. Proper interpretation of rebounding echoes allows sonographers to recognize tissue characteristics and detect pathological features such as cysts or tumors. Further, advances in Doppler ultrasound techniques allow the quantification of blood flow, which assists with diagnostic testing by revealing information about hemodynamics that regular imaging does not.

The subtle balance of these ideas allows complete use of ultrasound as an *in-vitro* diagnostic aid. Additionally, emerging advancements in ultrasound technology have fueled innovation in software and instrumentation that enhance image acquisition and interpretation. Artificial intelligence and machine learning are increasingly being applied in the integration of ultrasound systems, enabling enhanced image analysis and processing, which further advances diagnostic accuracy and workflow efficiency. For instance, detection algorithms may assist in identifying abnormalities as adjuncts to human interpretation. In addition, continuous advances in transducer design and the employment of advanced techniques like three-dimensional (3D) and four-dimensional (4D) imaging demonstrate the evolution of ultrasound physics and hardware. This convergence of the most modern technology not only broadens the scope of applications of ultrasound but also unites its position as a core modality of modern medicine, linking its historical roots with the promise for future developments and innovations (Kaysir et al., 2023; Burmeister et al., 2022) (Figure 1.3).

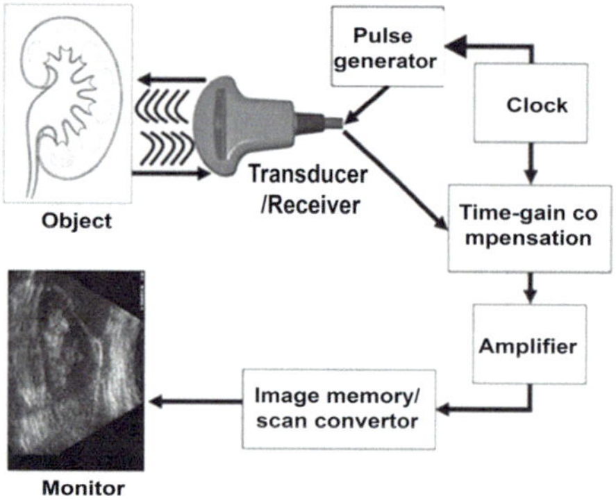

Figure 1.3. Physical principles of ultrasound.

Source: Fulgham, P.F. (2015). The Physics and Technique of Ultrasound. In: Chan, L., Tse, V., the, S., Stewart, P. (eds) Pelvic Floor Ultrasound. Springer, Cham. https://doi.org/10.1007/978-3-319-04310-4_1

1.1.1. Sound Wave Properties

An understanding of the nature of sound waves is essential to appreciate the fundamentals of ultrasound physics and instrumentation. Sound waves are mechanical longitudinal waves that require a medium to propagate, from solids and liquids to gases. Particle oscillations convey energy in these waves and lead to regions of rarefaction and compression. Properties and behaviors of sound waves are regulated by frequency, wavelength, and amplitude. Frequency, measured in hertz, regulates the pitch of the sound, and wavelength regulates the ability to travel; more accurate wavelengths can bend around objects more sharply than longer wavelengths. These simple properties not only regulate sound waves' travel through media but also contribute significantly to their application in ultrasound technologies. In ultrasound, the physical properties of the sound wave have a direct role in the effectiveness and integrity of imaging modalities and therapeutic uses. For instance, the interaction of ultrasound waves with biological tissues is dependent on acoustic impedance, which is derived from the density of the medium and the velocity of sound in the medium. When ultrasound waves cross interfaces between two tissues that are different, some of the sound energy is reflected and the remaining crosses over. The reflection depends on the difference in acoustic impedance, which is crucial when attempting to distinguish between various tissue types during diagnostic imaging.

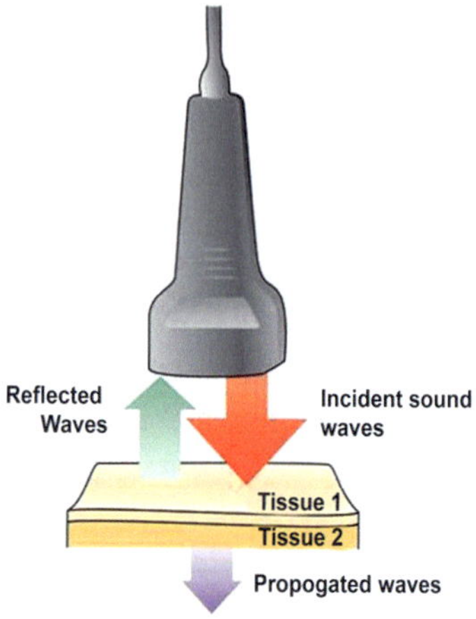

Figure 1.4. Sound wave properties of ultrasound.

Source: https://radiologykey.com/wp-content/uploads/2017/04/c02-fig-005.jpg.

Being aware of these sound wave properties enables experts to maximize ultrasound parameters and enhance image quality, consequently making medical examinations and interventions more convenient. Besides, the application of ultrasound in medicine, particularly High Intensity Focused Ultrasound (HIFU), demonstrates the profound importance of sound wave properties in medicine. HIFU demonstrates the ability to localize deposition of acoustic energy and thus create thermal effects with the potential to target and treat diseased tissue selectively. Through control of parameters such as intensity and exposure duration, researchers have outlined mechanisms for induced controlled tissue changes, which have applications in pain management and cancer treatment. Recent research has shown trends in compound action potential

(CAP) measurements at different intensities, demonstrating that focused interventions can have reversible or irreversible effects on neural tissues, reflecting the precision made possible with an understanding of sound wave properties (Jabbary, 2021). This comingling of physics and medicine underscores the role played by sound wave characteristics in both diagnostic and therapeutic conditions (Figure 1.4).

1.1.2. Interaction of Sound Waves with Tissues

The action of sound waves in interacting with biological tissues is a fundamental principle of ultrasound physics and equipment. As sound waves move through different media, they experience such phenomena as reflection, refraction, and absorption, which are essential to the creation of diagnostic images. This interaction is based on the acoustic characteristics of tissues, that is, their density and compressibility. When sound waves travel from a medium like fluid to a denser medium like muscle or fat, some of the wave is reflected while the remaining portion continues to penetrate deeper, allowing for differentiation between tissues. Understanding these interactions is very important to achieve maximum ultrasound image quality and for beneficial diagnostic applications in clinical practice. Generally, the effective application of these principles to hand-held devices and high-frequency transducers further enhances our ability to visualize internal structures well. Furthermore, the improvement in imaging methods has been driven additionally by signal processing, which significantly enhanced the interpretation of the interaction between tissue and sound waves. In conventional ultrasound imaging, the reconstruction algorithms, which were based on physical principles, were limited in their ability to accurately describe complex tissue structures because of the assumptions made concerning the underlying measurement models. To overcome such limitations, newer methods, which are based on statistical modeling and take advantage of greater model complexity, have been proposed. The latest developments have brought to the fore the evolution of deep learning techniques, which learn dynamically from big data sets to enhance image quality and precision. In blending the old with the new, by merging classic principles with modern data-driven wisdom, the field of ultrasound imaging continues to evolve, with novel methods to respond to complex clinical questions and improve patient outcomes (Luijten et al., 2023). Lastly, the medical uses of greater interactions of sound waves with tissues reach well beyond imaging. A novel use is ultrasound-induced drug delivery, where sound waves offer targeted delivery of treatment agents to make the therapy more effective and targeted. A tremendous potential of the modality exists in hundreds of clinical trials and new applications, highlighting its scope as a non-invasive treatment modality. The behavior of sound waves and the living tissues upon them in this context not only establishes the potential effectiveness of ultrasound technology but also emphasizes its ability to revolutionize treatment protocols. As the science continues to advance, ongoing research on the behavior of these interactions provides opportunities for refining the understanding and use of the possibilities provided by the ultrasound, ushering in more integrated patient treatment modalities (Delaney et al., 2022).

1.1.3. Doppler Effect in Ultrasound

The Doppler effect is a physical phenomenon that is central to the functionality of ultrasound imaging. It is defined as the change in the frequency or wavelength of a wave with respect to a moving observer relative to the source. In medical ultrasound, the Doppler effect can be used by clinicians to assess blood flow and body movement. When the ultrasound waves are insonated into the body, they strike moving red blood cells, which reflect the waves to the transducer. The frequency of reflected waves is altered depending on the direction of blood flow; reflected waves from cells moving toward the transducer have an increased frequency, while those from cells moving away have a decreased frequency. This frequency change is measurable in quantitative terms to produce valuable information concerning the velocity and direction of blood flow, and for this reason, it serves as a main tool in most clinical assessments. The clinical applications of the Doppler effect from ultrasound are valuable, particularly in monitoring cardiovascular conditions. Physicians can employ Doppler ultrasound techniques to accurately diagnose arterial obstructions, venous insufficiency, and congenital heart malformations. For instance, through Doppler examination, the professional practitioner can view the speed of blood flow and detect any abnormalities that may indicate future health complications. The possibility of detecting these abnormalities facilitates early intervention that can fundamentally alter patient outcomes. This is also supplemented by training programs that aim to integrate point-of-care ultrasound (POCUS) into medical training, addressing a substantial lack of enhanced training resources in rural and underserved populations, as highlighted by recent education studies (Johnson et al., 2024). Such advancements ensure future medical practitioners are properly equipped to apply ultrasound technology to the maximum benefit in practice. Other than clinical applications, an understanding of the physics involved in the Doppler effect application in ultrasound imaging is necessary to be able to make accurate diagnoses. Some factors influencing the accuracy of Doppler measurements are the insonation angle, patient movement, and frequency of the ultrasound wave used. Curricula incorporating a focus on clinical practice and real-world applications help to support better comprehension of such concepts, thereby enabling practitioners to enhance their diagnostic skills (Royo et al., 2019). As technology evolves, progress in ultrasound machines also advances Doppler ultrasound capabilities, paving the way for more sophisticated methods of image formation and improved diagnosis. Thus, the study of the Doppler effect not only improves the art of ultrasound but also significantly enhances patient care and clinical results in the practice of medical imaging (Figure 1.5).

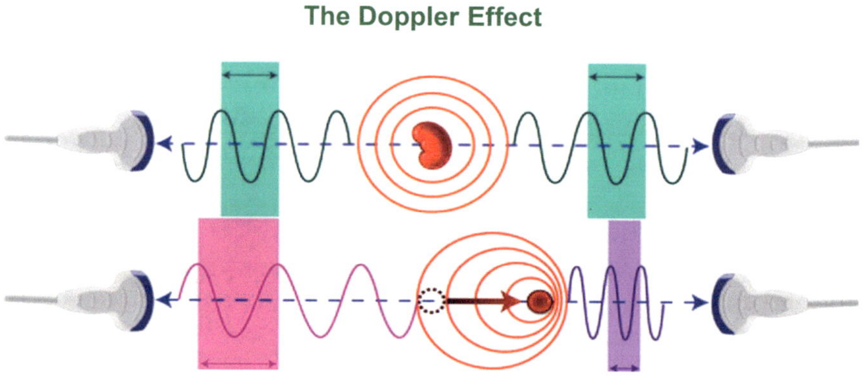

Figure 1.5. Doppler effect in ultrasound.

Source: Kaproth-Joslin, Katherine & Nicola, Refky & Dogra, Vikram. (2015). The History of US: From Bats and Boats to the Bedside and Beyond. Radiographics: a review publication of the Radiological Society of North America, Inc. 35. 140300. 10.1148/rg.2015140300

1.2. Ultrasound Wave Generation

The generation of the ultrasound waves is an essential component in ultrasound technology, whereby electrical energy is transformed into mechanical waves through the use of certain transducers. The transducers include piezoelectric materials, which possess the unique feature of producing electrical charges when subjected to mechanical pressure. An alternating electrical current is supplied to the transducer, and it produces vibration, which results in the emission of ultrasound waves into the surrounding medium. This is elementary in medical imaging, where several modalities of imaging, for example, Doppler and B-mode ultrasound, utilize different frequencies and waveforms. By optimizing these parameters, doctors can obtain extremely accurate images and information regarding soft tissue anatomy, blood flow, and organ motion to enable more effective diagnosis and monitoring of various diseases. Frequency and wavelength are extremely important in wave creation in ultrasound because they directly contribute to penetration depth and resolution. Higher frequencies give greater resolution with shorter wavelengths, but could be more readily absorbed by low penetration depth tissues. Lower frequencies penetrate deeper but with reduced information detail. This is a compromise that is acceptable in selecting an optimum frequency for diagnostic purposes.

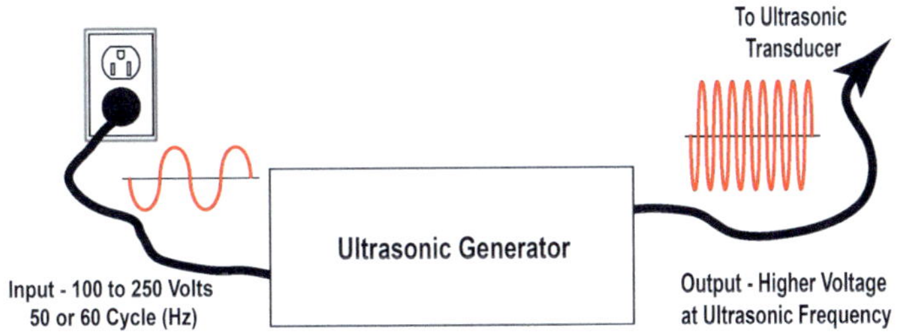

Figure 1.6. Ultrasound wave generation.

Source: https://www.blackstone-ney.com/wp-content/uploads/2024/07/Ultrasonic-Generator-Schematic.jpg.

The frequency decision is particularly important in pediatric and obstetric scanning, where tissue resolution in the soft tissues has to be balanced against the need to visualize deeper structures. Familiarity with these forces is not just of interest to operators, but also to ongoing technical and methodological innovation in ultrasound, which continues to advance with the development of new materials and electronic innovations being introduced into transducer design. Advances in the field, such as the integration of machine learning and sophisticated data analysis algorithms, have also enhanced the effectiveness of ultrasound wave generation. New technologies employ algorithms that optimize image quality, automate anatomical defect detection, and enable real-time data processing. Such technologies are also being modified to enhance non-invasive measurement techniques, like photoacoustic spectroscopy (PAS) techniques for monitoring blood glucose levels, solving issues due to low penetration and the interfering presence of materials in blood. Through the extension of the capabilities of traditional ultrasound applications, such breakthroughs demonstrate the importance of interdisciplinary research combining ultrasound physics with modern computational techniques. This convergence will likely lead to massive patient monitoring and diagnostic improvements, ultimately benefiting healthcare outcomes overall (Monteiro & Marti, 2022; Kaysir et al., 2023) (Figure 1.6).

1.2.1. Piezoelectric Effect

The piezoelectric effect is a fundamental process that is the underlying operation of ultrasound imaging devices employed in medicine for diagnosis. The process is seen when certain materials acquire an electric charge when subjected to mechanical stress. Piezoelectric materials, typically placed in transducers, in ultrasound transfer electrical energy to vibrating mechanically and hence produce sound waves. The sound waves are sent through the body tissues and bounce off various structures. The transducer subsequently records returning echoes and converts them into electrical signals to produce diagnostic images.

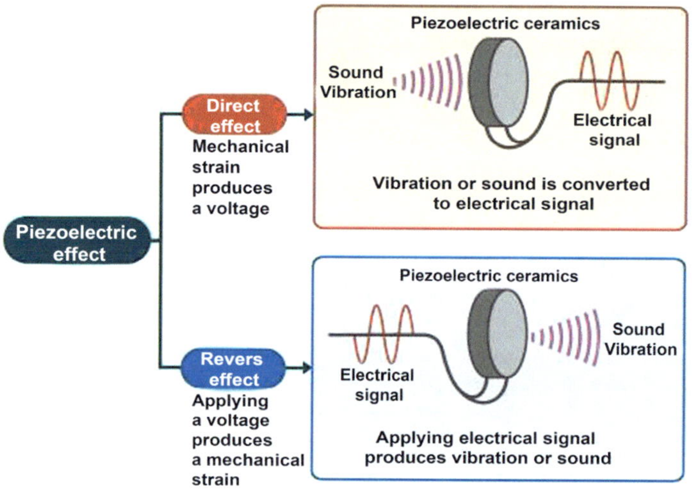

Figure 1.7. Ultrasound piezoelectric effect.

Source: https://www.he-shuai.com/wp-content/uploads/2021/02/piezoelectric-effect-.jpg.

The conversion process shows the direct relationship between electrical phenomena and mechanical energy and points out the most important role piezoelectricity plays in ultrasound technology. The selection of piezoelectric materials in ultrasound equipment has a direct effect on the efficiency of imaging devices. Commonly utilized materials are lead zirconate titanate (PZT) because of its high conversion efficiency and large frequency range. The materials must be engineered precisely in order to optimize their properties for an application, leading to significant gains in imaging sensitivity and resolution. Additionally, as scientists explore new materials and technologies, such as nanostructured piezoelectric films, the potential of enhanced performance in medical imaging devices emerges. Continued innovation in this field not only increases the precision of diagnosis but also provides the means for non-invasive procedures in numerous applications in medicine, thus broadening the applicability of ultrasound technology. The piezoelectric effect is applied in ultrasound physics for purposes that extend far beyond diagnostic imaging; it is also applicable for therapeutic purposes. For instance, focused ultrasound therapy employs piezoelectric transducers to deliver directed energy to targeted tissues to facilitate procedures such as tissue ablation or modification. Therapeutic applications take advantage of the controlled manipulation of sound wave propagation facilitated by piezoelectric materials to maintain integrity in surrounding tissue with minimal damage. Furthermore, the improvements in machine learning techniques and digital signal processing have improved image resolution to be better and treatment to be more accurate, illustrating a revolution in the field. As more studies explore these uses, the piezoelectric effect can be the foundation for innovations in future ultrasound physics and equipment, leading towards enhanced diagnostics as well as therapeutic outcomes (Kaysir et al., 2023; Westerbeek, 2022) (Figure 1.7).

1.2.2. Transducer Design and Function

Transducers are essential components in the ultrasound device that transform mechanical energy into electrical signals and vice versa. The two-way function provides for transmission of the ultrasound waves into the body and reception of the reflected waves. Transducer design is inherently advanced, requiring a subtle balancing of several physical principles, including the piezoelectric effect, where some materials will generate an electric charge when subjected to mechanical stress. The development of new transducer geometries and materials has significantly advanced imaging quality and resolution, enabling greater clinical applications. The development of high-frequency transducers, for instance, has increased spatial resolution at the expense of tissue penetration, and thus the selection has to be made with care based on the need for diagnosis. Transducer design is therefore less of a problem of technology and more of a judicious compromise of physical parameters and clinical needs. Apart from material selection, the use of transducers has expanded with automation and robot development. Robot-assisted medical imaging, for example, optimizes the placement of ultrasound transducers by exact control over positioning. Robot facilitation of such results allows real-time, precise adjustments in imaging trajectories, enhancing image quality and diagnostic sharpness. Merging robot-based systems allows for the attainment of sophisticated imaging regimes that would be challenging through exclusive human operation. Such abilities enable preassembled compound acquisitions, hence increasing preassembled effective apertures of transducers and allowing volumetric imaging. Technology development of transducers in robotic platforms, therefore, not only increases the diagnostic utility of ultrasound but also opens doors to future developments in imaging modalities, as seen in developments in elastography and photoacoustic imaging, where accurate control of trajectory is paramount (Salcudean et al., 2022).

Moreover, recent studies of transducer technology emphasize signal processing techniques optimized for enhancing imaging performance. Recent studies have introduced new deep learning-based algorithms to significantly improve timing analysis in transducer systems, for example, the application of neural networks to enhance time resolution (Ai et al., 2023). This new approach enables data processing of information collected by silicon photomultipliers, a standout example of a transducer. Leveraging inherent time correlations in the signal, such sophisticated models are capable of yielding high resolutions and stability even in noisy experimental environments. With the advancing technology, the combined synergy between transducer development and advanced signal processing will be crucial for developing ultrasound technology capable of meeting the increasing demands for precision and purity in medical imaging equipment (Figure 1.8).

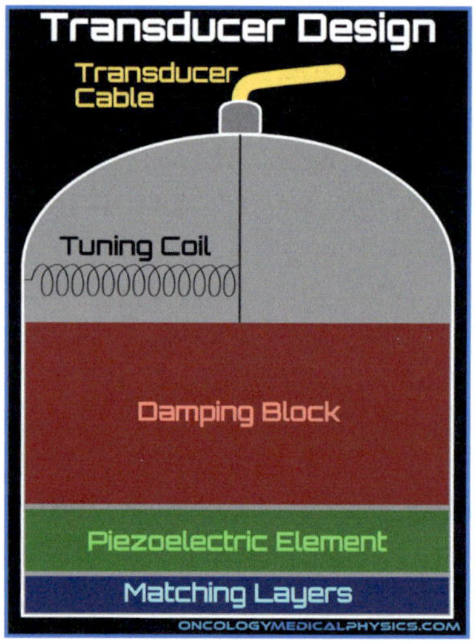

Figure 1.8. Transducer design and function.

Source: https://oncologymedicalphysics.com/wp-content/uploads/2020/07/Ultrasound-transducer-design-OMP.png.

1.2.3. Types of Ultrasound Transducers

Transducers in the field of ultrasound technology are the most critical devices since they possess the ability to convert electrical energy to ultrasound waves as well as vice versa. The two principal types of ultrasound transducers include the continuous wave (CW) and pulsed wave (PW) transducers. The continuous wave transducers can generate a consistent stream of ultrasound waves, which have various applications, such as Doppler ultrasound, where it is essential to measure blood flow. On the other hand, pulsed wave transducers emit brief pulses of ultrasound to identify tissue depth and structure. This difference is important because the kind of transducer employed will affect the quality and specificity of the resulting imaging, which in turn will influence diagnostic outcomes in clinical care. Another form of diversification in ultrasound technology is linear array and convex array transducers. Linear array transducers employ an array of lineal small elements to generate sound waves in a parallel beam. These transducers are employed for high-resolution imaging of surface structures and find application in vascular studies and musculoskeletal studies. Convex array transducers employ a curved array of elements to generate a broader field of view in order to image deeper structures, such as those found in scans of the abdomen. Each transducer has certain merits and demerits, and health care professionals must select the appropriate transducer cautiously as per the specific examination requirements and the patients' factors. Advances in ultrasound technology during recent years have also brought about some high-end transducer designs, such as phased array transducers. The transducers use electronic steering techniques to produce dynamic images, which is particularly beneficial to cardiac imaging when sudden movement is needed. Besides this, developments in ultrasound simulation have also enhanced the training and education of physicians in terms of exposure to real-like environments that mimic challenging clinical cases (Dietrich et al., 2023). This implementation indicates the evolving future of ultrasound equipment, a potential future in which transducer design continues to be refined to meet the growing demands of medical imaging. This evolution turns ultrasound into a valuable member of the diagnostic arsenal of modern medicine (Barua et al., 2022) (Figure 1.9).

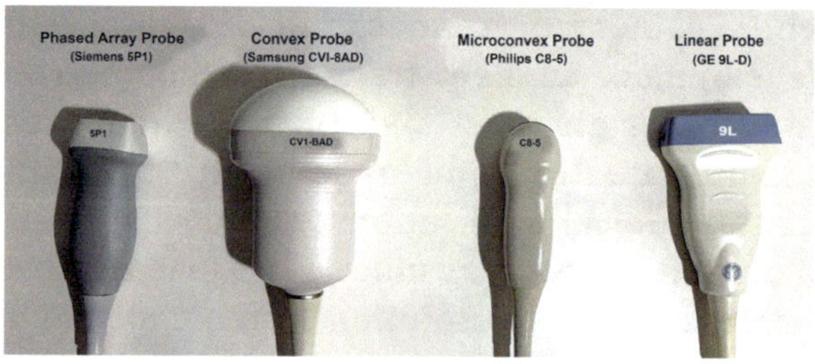

Figure 1.9. Ultrasound transducer types.

Source: https://lbnmedical.com/wp-content/uploads/2024/06/Ultrasound-transducer-types-comparison.png.

1.3. Image Formation in Ultrasound

Ultrasound image formation is based almost wholly on the knowledge of the interaction between tissues and sound waves in the body. The fundamental principle is the emission of high-frequency sound waves, which are produced by a transducer, a device that receives the returning echoes as well. When these sound waves strike different types of biological tissues, they produce echoes based on the acoustic impedance differences. This phenomenon is the principle behind the identification of various tissue types, as various tissues, such as bone, muscle, and fluid, reflect sound waves to different degrees. These echoes are converted to electrical signals, which are processed to create images that provide critical diagnostic information about the internal body structures, thereby qualifying ultrasound as a potent clinical diagnostic tool. To achieve optimal image quality in ultrasound, various factors must be considered, including the choice of frequency and the design of the transducer. Increased frequency provides higher resolution, allowing for better perception of detail; however, it has a lower penetration depth, which may be unsuitable for imaging deeper structures. Conversely, lower frequency penetrates tissue more easily but compromises resolution. The selection of frequency thus becomes a matter of clinical need and anatomical factors. The ability of the ultrasound system to accommodate return echoes via techniques such as time-gain compensation and dynamic range correction also enhances imaging capability. The adjustments enable the operator to control signal amplification at various depths, thus ensuring consistent image quality within the region under examination, allowing clinicians to make appropriate judgments based on images acquired (Weigers et al., 2019). Modern ultrasound imaging utilizes advanced methods such as Doppler ultrasound, which measures the dynamics of blood flow by calculating changes in frequency of reflected sound on the moving red blood cells. The modality is also crucial for vascular and cardiac related diseases diagnosis. In addition, advances in three-dimensional (3D) imaging allow volumetric data to be acquired and more complex anatomical visualization than in two-dimensional images. As technology in ultrasound has improved, it is becoming integrated with other modalities to improve diagnostic accuracy and patient management. Utilization of contrast agents, for instance, maximized further the visualization of perfusion and definition of anatomical boundaries. All in all, these breakthroughs in ultrasound image generation reflect the technology's leading role in today's medical diagnostics, influencing clinical decisions and patient outcomes (Samei & peck, 2019) (Figure 1.10).

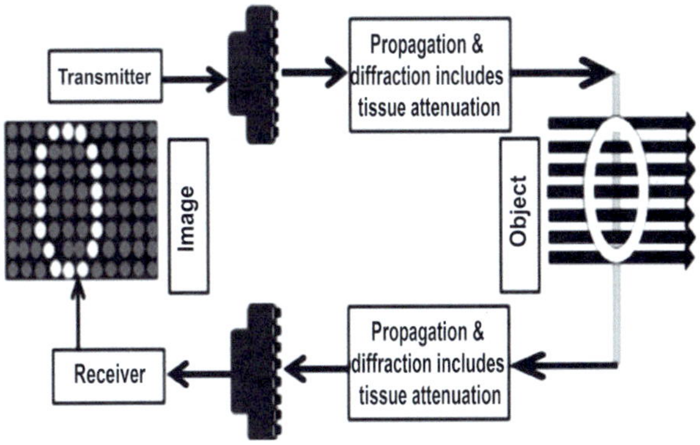

Figure 1.10. Schematic diagram of ultrasound image formation.

Source: Shahin Uddin, Muhammad & Halder, Kalyan & Tahtali, Murat & Lambert, Andrew & Pickering, Mark & Marchese, Margaret & Stuart, Iain. (2016). Intelligent estimation of noise and blur variances using ANN for the restoration of ultrasound images. Applied Optics. 55. 8905-8915. 10.1364/AO.55.008905.

1.3.1. Echoes and Their Role in Image Creation

The action of echoes is critical to the function of ultrasound technology and plays a significant role in creating diagnostic images. When ultrasound waves are sent from a transducer and travel through body tissues, they encounter interfaces between structures—like organs, fluids, or tissues—with different acoustic properties. These interfaces bounce back some of the ultrasound energy towards the transducer, producing echoes. The amount of time it takes for the echoes to return permits the ultrasound system to record the depth at which the interface is, thus making it possible for an image to be formed. The relationship between tissue sound speed and echo delay is critical; it allows for the determination not only of the position of the tissues but also their size, shape, and consistency, thereby making correct diagnosis and treatment planning possible (Bortot et al., 2023).

Formation of an image depends on the ability to manipulate and interpret the reflected echoes. Each echo is an image of information about the tissue properties from which they originate, and these may be different on the basis of density, elasticity, etc. Modern ultrasound systems utilize this echo information, preparing it through signal averaging and filtering, to enhance the sharpness and contrast of the image. The time and amplitude of the echoes can be mapped by these systems into a grayscale image that visually distinguishes among different tissues in the body. Also, technological advances such as Doppler ultrasound use the principles of echoes to provide not only static images but also real-time functional information about the blood flow and motion, thus expanding the medical application of ultrasound technology beyond the visualization of anatomy (Burmeister et al., 2022). Other than the basic principles of echo, nanotechnology's application to ultrasound imaging is turning into a significant advancement in medical physics. Nanoparticles may be employed as targeted contrast agents that enhance the echogenicity of specific tissues for improved imaging studies and visualization of cancerous lesions. This new application demonstrates the potential of echoes and sound wave interactions with engineered materials for the improvement of diagnostic accuracy. With ongoing research, such innovations will transform the function of ultrasound in image-guided surgery and cancer diagnosis on the basis of amplified echo dynamics to minimize positive surgical margins and maximize patient outcomes. This innovation in ultrasound emphasizes the critical synergy between physics, technology, and clinical application in further advancing diagnostic devices (Bortot et al., 2023).

1.3.2. 2D, 3D, and Doppler Imaging Scanning Methods

The investigation of the methods used in ultrasound scanning is at the core of the study of the general subject of ultrasound physics and instrumentation. Two-dimensional (2D) imaging is the foundation of ultrasound technology, providing real-time anatomical structure images to practitioners. The technique uses a linear or curved transducer to transmit and receive sound waves and create images that represent interfaces between different tissues. The convenience and speed of 2D imaging make it an invaluable resource in the majority of medical diagnoses, such as obstetrics and echocardiography. Even though 2D imaging only offers a limited view of the body's spatial relationships, the methodology's efficiency and effectiveness in delivering immediate visual feedback continue to further establish its role in clinics, thereby promoting quick decision-making and interventions. Technical advancement in ultrasound has made it possible to develop three-dimensional (3D) imaging techniques, which raise the ability of regular ultrasound to a new level. 3D ultrasound forms volumetric images with a complete depiction of complex anatomical details by reconstructing a number of 2D slices taken from multiple angles. This technique is particularly beneficial in uses like obstetrics, wherein it enhances visualization of fetal anatomy and growth, allowing clinicians to assess conditions that might be masked in 2D images. Surgical planning is also enabled by 3D imaging through the provision to render intricate maps of anatomy. While 3D imaging offers more detail, it is occasionally accompanied by longer processing time and requires specialized software and hardware.

Therefore, the integration of 3D ultrasound technology is a significant benchmark for ultrasound medicine in reacting to the call for greater sophisticated imaging capabilities. Doppler imaging brings yet another level of sophistication to ultrasound modalities in that it provides information regarding blood flow and motion dynamics.

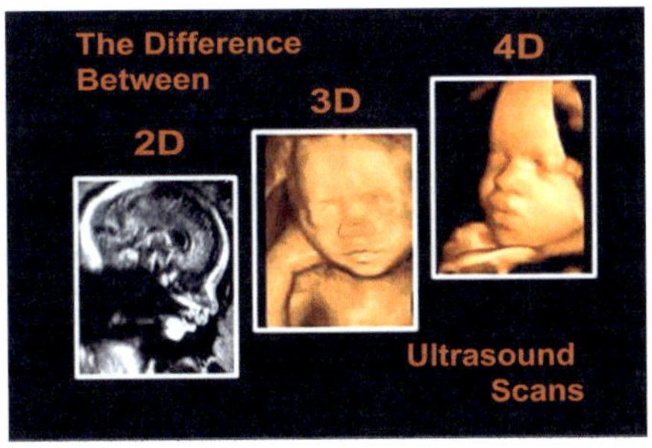

Figure 1.11. Scanning techniques (2D, 3D, and Doppler imaging).

Source: Ambady Scan Centre. https://ambadyscan.com/blog/different-types-of-fetal-scans-during-pregnancy/

The method uses the Doppler effect to measure the frequency change of sound waves reflected from moving blood cells. Thus, Doppler imaging may be employed for the diagnosis of most cardiovascular ailments and can measure parameters like the speed of blood flow as well as direction. Varying forms of Doppler ultrasound are available, from color Doppler to pulsed-wave Doppler, and each is employed to depict as well as measure blood flow in different situations. Doppler imaging finds its use beyond diagnosis because it plays an important part in therapy monitoring and follow-up with surgery. By the incorporation of Doppler strengths and 2D and 3D imaging techniques, medical professionals have a comprehensive approach to evaluating the health of patients and significantly enhancing care provision in multiple facets of practice (Dietrich et al., 2023; IEEE, 2022) (Figure 1.11).

1.3.3. Image Resolution and Quality Factors

With respect to ultrasound imaging, resolution and image quality are of maximum significance to enable proper diagnosis and management of the patient. Image resolution means the detail that is obtainable with the ultrasound image, which in turn contributes to the interpretative capacity of the clinician. Images of higher resolution enable better delineation of anatomical structures and, thus, better identification of pathology. Variables influencing resolution include the intensity of the ultrasound waves, transducer design, and spatial arrangement of the detected signals. Transducers with higher frequencies will provide better resolution but lower penetration by default, and therefore are well-suited to superficial structures. Therefore, the selection of adequate transducer frequencies is important for optimizing image results while effectively addressing clinical applications. Besides resolution, image quality also refers to contrast, dynamic range, and signal-to-noise ratio (SNR). Contrast refers to the capacity to differentiate between various tissue types, and this is necessary in the detection of abnormalities. Dynamic range is necessary when imaging the extremes of tissue densities encountered in tests. High SNR is necessary as well because it minimizes noise presence so that better clarity can be achieved in images. More recent techniques, such as harmonic imaging and adaptive focusing, have entered practice to further enhance image quality. With these technologies, clinicians can better visualize complicated structures, which is necessary to make the proper diagnosis. Surprisingly, the utilization of novel simulation technologies has also been found to improve learning results in ultrasound training and thus equip future professionals with the ability to utilize these high-quality imaging technologies effectively (Dietrich et al., 2023). Finally, the progression of ultrasound technology is symbiotically linked with ongoing research and development that focuses on better image resolution and quality. New methods, such as photoacoustic imaging and ultrasound simulations, spearhead it. Particularly, NIR-SERS (Near-Infrared Surface-Enhanced Raman Spectroscopy) techniques enable detection arrangements and enhancing substrates to be tailored, which facilitate bioanalytical imaging and demonstrate the potential of real-time cellular measurements (Deriu et al., 2023). With advancements in the field, the need for high-quality imaging becomes apparent, especially for point-of-care use, where timely diagnostics can have a great impact on patient management. The intersection of high-resolution imaging with innovative educational strategies guarantees the healthcare professionals' continued ability to apply ultrasound technologies, enhancing the overall health climate through increased diagnostic powers.

1.4. Ultrasound Instrumentation

When looking at ultrasound machines, one should appreciate the vital role played by transducers in the ultrasound machines. Transducers have the capability of converting electrical energy into sound waves, by the piezoelectric effect, so that they can transmit and receive sound waves. These waves, upon hitting varying densities of tissue, get reflected back towards the transducer, which demodulates the returning signals to create images of body structures. The choice of transducer frequency is of utmost importance in deciding the final image quality and penetration depth because higher frequencies yield higher resolution in shallow structures, while lower frequencies penetrate deeper tissue with lower resolution. Proper insight into these dynamics must be understood to optimize imaging findings and make appropriate diagnoses by judicious choice of frequency and transducer type (Burmeister et al., 2022). This fundamental knowledge is the foundation for the efficiency of ultrasound in the majority of clinical uses, leading to technological and technique advancements in the topic. Besides transducers, equipment in ultrasound also requires sophisticated electronic systems to process the signals acquired. These include electronics like amplifiers, analog-to-digital converters, and image processors, all of which work in conjunction to maximize the quality of the ultrasound image. The signals that are fed back to the transducer tend to be weak and need to be amplified prior to their conversion to digital forms amenable to manipulation and display on monitors. Advanced imaging capability includes algorithms for post-processing and image reconstruction that can considerably enhance diagnostic precision. Additionally, modern ultrasound equipment employs Doppler technology to analyze blood flow, another source of information gleaned from a patient's single exam. Clinicians and technicians must know these electronic devices in order to diagnose and adjust the performance of ultrasound during practice (Rath et al., 2020). One of its most powerful advantages is the portability and versatility of ultrasound machine, making it an effective tool in many medical settings. In contrast to other imaging modalities, such as CT and MRI, ultrasound equipment can be easily transported, making it easily employable in the bed setting or field operations. Being cost-effective is further boosted by this portability since ultrasound does not involve ionizing radiation and is therefore safer for both patients and professionals. The advances in software and hardware have made ultrasound technology more accessible, providing real-time imaging that facilitates real-time decision-making in a clinical environment. Furthermore, the application of ultrasound to interventional procedures, such as guided injection and minimally invasive surgery, demonstrates its rising value in modern medicine. This combination of availability, security, and flexibility ensures that ultrasound machinery is always at the forefront of diagnosis and treatment (Rath et al., 2020) (Figure 1.12).

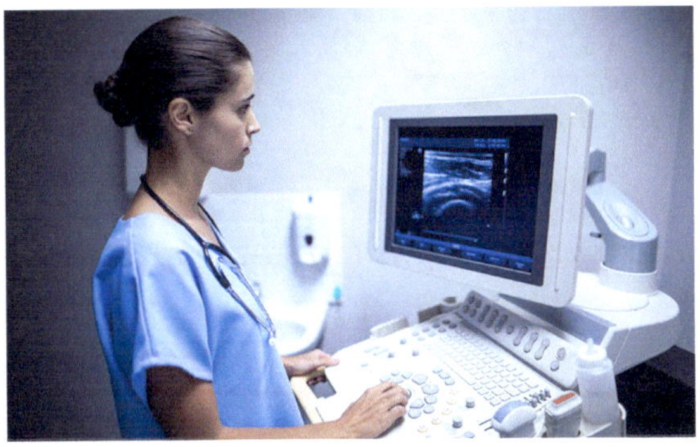

Figure 1.12. Ultrasound instrumentation.

Source: Hannah Murphy (2022) Health Imaging. Ultraound. *https://healthimaging.com/topics/medical-imaging/ultrasound-imaging/how-well-does-o-rads-perform-nonselected-low-risk-cohort*

1.4.1. Components of Ultrasound Machines

The complexity of ultrasound machines is in their fundamental parts, each with a purposefully designed function contributing to the total functionality and efficiency of the machine. The transducer is at the heart of the ultrasound technology, and it serves dual-duty roles as a receiver and transmitter of sound waves. When subjected to electrical energy applied to piezoelectric crystals held within the transducer, they vibrate, generating high-frequency sound waves. These waves pass through the body and reflect off internal tissues to return to the transducer. The process of converting these echoes to an electrical signal is necessary for imaging. The design and function of the transducer play a significant role in the ultrasonographic image quality and thus are an essential component of ultrasound machinery and one worthy of serious consideration in apparatus acquisition as well as in clinical practice. In addition to the transducer, ultrasound equipment features a CPU responsible for deciphering the input sound waves. The processing unit handles complex algorithms in real time to transform electrical signals received from the transducer to diagnostic images on a monitor. The ability of a CPU to execute advanced imaging techniques, such as Doppler imaging and harmonic imaging, allows ultrasound equipment to be more proficient for diagnosis. Moreover, improved computing power allows more precise measurements, leading to more accurate determinations of multiple physiological states. With the medical requirement for reliability in diagnosis, CPU technology development has a direct relationship with complex ultrasound application development, allowing real-time diagnosis and continued learning about patient conditions. Lastly, the integration components of ultrasound machines are display screens, user interfaces, and specialized software that together enhance the machine's usability and functionality. These features allow useful information and facilitate greater user interaction through intuitive configurations that simplify imaging parameter manipulation for clinicians. Moreover, advances in software allow the implementation of features like automated measurement and advanced image manipulation. With advancing technology, ultrasound devices increasingly feature connectivity options that allow data sharing and integration into electronic health records to ultimately improve patient care. Improvements in ultrasound technology, particularly in the development of intuitive interfaces and high-performance data handling systems, underscore the critical interrelationship between instrumentation and efficient clinical practice, a path that medical imaging technology is likely to follow (Figure 1.13).

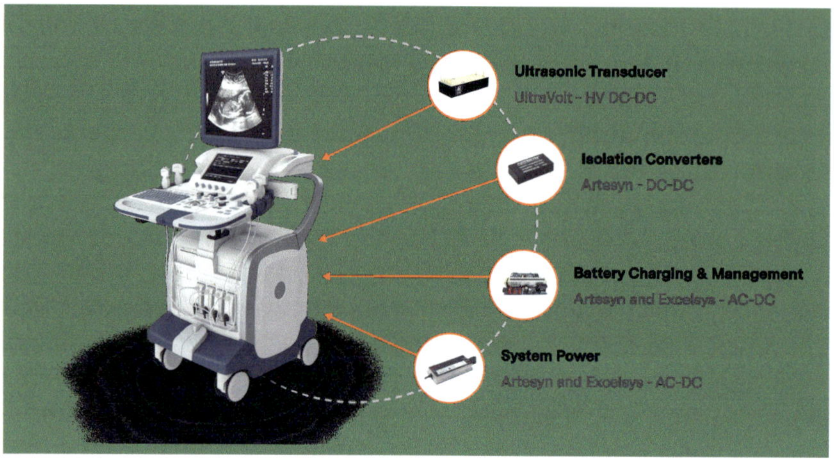

Figure 1.13. Components of ultrasound machines.

Source: Advanced Energy/Ultrasound. https://www.advancedenergy.com/en-us/applications/medical/medical-imaging/ultrasound

1.4.2. Signal Processing in Ultrasound Systems

The role of signal processing in ultrasound equipment is instrumental to the accurate interpretation of image data. Raw data from ultrasound is initially susceptible to noise and artifacts, which easily hide diagnostic details. Appropriate signal processing techniques are thus pivotal to enhancing image quality via filtering of spurious noise while maintaining the integrity of the relevant signals. This is vital to provide medical practitioners with unambiguous and true images necessary for effective diagnoses. Advanced algorithms, such as time-gain compensation, are applied to compensate for amplitude compensation of the signals received from various depths and, therefore, for attenuation. Using these advanced techniques, ultrasound systems are able to receive more trustworthy and interpretable information and hence better clinical outcomes and patient care. To that end, further, the application of technologies like machine learning is changing the process of signal processing in ultrasound devices. Techniques based on artificial intelligence can scan vast amounts of ultrasound data and identify patterns that might not be immediately apparent to clinicians. Not only does this enhance diagnostic accuracy in ultrasound scans, but it also streamlines clinic workflows. For instance, machine learning techniques may be applied to automatically classify and rank ultrasound images, in turn assisting practitioners in managing high volumes of patients efficiently. As this technology evolves, its application to processing ultrasound signals will likely reduce human error and increase diagnostic confidence, to both promote advances in personalized medicine. In addition to machine learning, research into new signal processing techniques is important to overcome the shortcomings of traditional ultrasound. Emerging techniques focus on applying photoacoustic spectroscopy, particularly in the mid-infrared, for better tissue characterization and also disease detection. Conventional ultrasound primarily relies on reflection of sound waves, but photoacoustic techniques have the benefit of using optical properties and thus provide extra contrast that may be useful in imaging specific tissues or pathology. But impediments such as low penetration depth and interference from other blood components have to be navigated carefully to obtain credible results. Through systematic management of these hindrances through enhanced signal processing mechanisms, researchers are bridging the gateway to more robust non-invasive diagnostic tools capable of transforming patient care (Kaysir et al., 2023; Monteiro & Marti, 2022).

1.4.3. Display Technologies Used in Ultrasound

The development of display technology in ultrasound scanning has significantly enhanced the effectiveness of the medical diagnostic equipment. The images used to be displayed on cathode ray tube (CRT) screens, whose absence in recent technology would sometimes weaken visual acuity and depth perception. However, with the introduction of liquid crystal display (LCD) and light-emitting diode (LED) screens, image clarity has taken off. These newer displays have enhanced contrast ratios, color fidelity, and resolution that make the anatomical structures and pathology more visible to health care professionals. Furthermore, the mobility of these displays has been enhanced, making ultrasound applications more versatile in a variety of clinical settings, from hospitals to mobile units. With advancements in display technology, the potential for better diagnostics and patient care becomes increasingly clear, transforming the domain of ultrasound imaging. Apart from advancements in display technologies, the addition of sophisticated software algorithms has further increased the capability of ultrasound imaging. Digital signal processing allows real-time image processing and modification, thus enabling alteration of ultrasound images to meet specific diagnostic needs. For instance, techniques like adaptive filtering eliminate noise and improve the visibility of minute anatomical details. Enhancements to the display software also serve to add depth to image interpretation while streamlining the clinician's workflow. Furthermore, most modern ultrasound machines feature touch-screen displays that make user interaction simple, and practitioners can easily manipulate settings, make adjustments, and markup images. The merging of high-end display technology with enhanced software functionality indicates the groundbreaking impact on diagnostic imaging, emphasizing the critical role of easy-to-use systems in patient management. Moreover, the invention of three-dimensional (3D) and four-dimensional (4D) ultrasound technologies is a groundbreaking advancement in display methods that significantly enhances the visualization of complex structures. Compared to traditional two-dimensional (2D) ultrasound imaging, 3D ultrasound allows clinicians to visualize anatomical structures in different planes and projections, offering greater detail and spatial context. 3D ultrasound is particularly valuable in obstetrics and gynecology, where high-fidelity visualization of fetal anatomy and growth can be an important diagnostic and treatment-planning consideration.

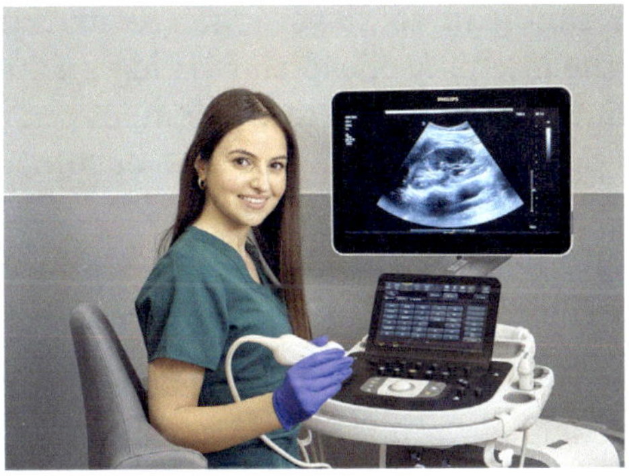

Figure 1.14. Display technologies used in ultrasound.

Source: Maternity Home. Ultrasonography. https://maternity-home.com/ultrasonography/

The application of 4D ultrasound adds the aspect of time, which makes dynamic visualizations possible to allow for continuous observation of movement within the fetal context. Technologies like these advanced displays increase diagnostic precision and pose new challenges for comprehending and evaluating medical diseases, as shown by the extensive influence contemporary imaging has on medical practice (Figure 1.14).

1.5. Safety and Bioeffects of Ultrasound

The safety and bioeffects of ultrasound have attracted considerable attention, particularly because the technology is increasingly becoming common in medical treatment and imaging. Ultrasound is generally regarded as a safe imaging device since it is non-ionizing, and unlike X-rays and CT scans, it does not involve ionizing radiation, which has been found to be hazardous to health. But the potential for bioeffects of ultrasound exposure, especially in susceptible populations such as neonates and pregnant women, needs careful examination. It has been found through research that ultrasound can produce thermal and mechanical effects, which can lead to tissue change or damage when the intensity of exposure is high. Thus, the clinicians are required to implement stringent safety principles for the purposes of controlling risks, which means ultrasound has to be applied prudently and based on the principles of As Low As Reasonably Achievable (ALARA).

Beyond thermal and mechanical impacts, researchers have discovered certain biological reactions to ultrasound that merit close examination. The phenomenon of cavitation, whereby gas bubbles in tissues can be created and destroyed as a result of the action of ultrasound waves, has been the focus of fear about cell and tissue damage. Stable cavitation, although in certain cases may enhance therapeutic action, has the potential to cause inertial cavitation with the generation of free radicals and damage to cells. Understanding these bioeffects requires sensitive insight into the ultrasound parameters utilized, including frequency, intensity, and exposure time. With the advancement of technology in the area of ultrasound, ongoing research is necessary to deconstruct the complexities of ultrasound bioeffects and refine safety measures that function to protect the patient while maximizing diagnostic efficacy. Medical professionals must remain aware of the implications of ultrasound bioeffects in making diagnoses and therapies. The optimum training and expertise about new safety practices are an inherent part of medical education, particularly for professionals who utilize ultrasound frequently. It is also important for manufacturers of ultrasound equipment to ensure high priority on safety measures in their equipment, such as limiting output intensity and incorporating real-time monitoring of exposure rates. Through a collaborative effort on the part of clinicians, researchers, and manufacturers, the process of ultrasound may enhance the safety record without compromising the valuable information that it continues to yield regarding patient health. Such shared responsibility not only lends greater assurance to the use of ultrasound as a diagnostic modality but also public trust in the healthcare system (Hoskins et al., 2010).

1.5.1. Thermal Effects of Ultrasound Exposure

The heat effect of ultrasound exposure is of significant significance in numerous applications, primarily in treatments and medical imaging. Ultrasound waves, as they travel through tissues, generate heat due to energy absorption and scattering by the encountered material. The process can bring about a rise in the tissue temperature, a phenomenon of therapeutic and diagnostic interest. For example, in therapeutic ultrasound, controlled heat can be beneficial to enhance tissue healing and increase blood flow, necessary in physiotherapy and rehabilitation. Excessive thermal effects, on the other hand, can lead to unintended damage to tissues around the focused area, emphasizing the importance of proper monitoring of ultrasound intensity and duration. These subtleties should be well understood by practitioners to be able to take advantage of the benefits of ultrasound and be able to counteract the possible risks involved in thermal exposure. In clinical practice, the management of thermal effects in most cases follows adopted safety guidelines, taking into consideration the intensity of ultrasound exposure and treatment duration. As research has shown, even slight increases in temperature can alter enzymatic functions and influence cellular response, making precision very important when using ultrasound. For example, experiments have shown that certain enzymatic functions can change with spectacular modifications when temperatures are merely slightly increased (Karad Kžić, 2021). This brings up the question of the delicate balance between optimizing therapeutic aims and evading unwanted thermal effects. Therapeutic protocols recommend maintaining the temperature in line with the observation during ultrasound treatment so that it remains within safety limits, thus enabling practitioners to optimize the effects without increasing the risk for complications that arise from excessive thermal loading. Furthermore, the interaction between biological tissue and ultrasound raises issues of safety as well as effectiveness in a broad spectrum of medical applications. The thermal accumulation effect occurs when successive exposure to ultrasound leads to cumulative heating, and this may predispose tissues to injury if not adequately managed. This effect is particularly relevant in treatments such as high-intensity focused ultrasound (HIFU), where significant thermal effects are induced by design for therapeutic purposes. However, precision in these techniques requires a thorough knowledge of tissue characteristics and ultrasound parameters in order to prevent unintentional thermal damage (Stanković et al., 2021). Therefore, ongoing research and innovation in ultrasound technology must continue to optimize safety measures and the therapeutic potential of this modality, leading to improved patient care (Figure 1.15).

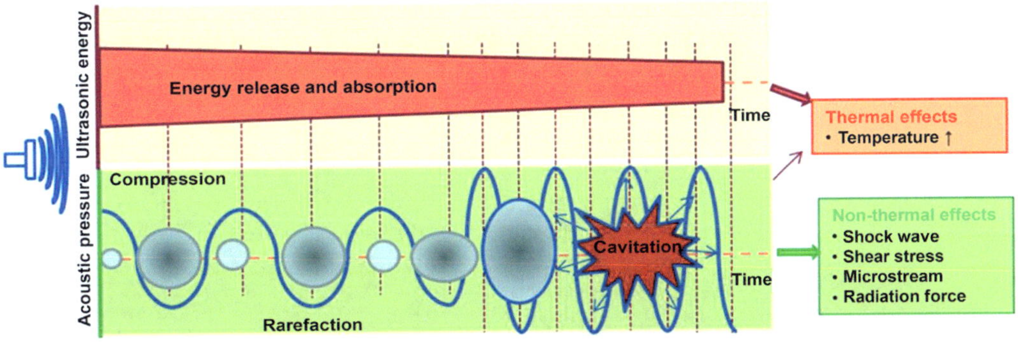

Figure 1.15. Thermal effects of ultrasound exposure.

Source: Wang, Jiwei & Lai, Bin & Nanayakkara. et.al.. (2019). Experimental Data-Mining Analyses Reveal New Roles of Low-Intensity Ultrasound in Differentiating Cell Death Regulatome in Cancer and Non-cancer Cells via Potential Modulation of Chromatin Long-Range Interactions. Frontiers in Oncology. 9. 600. 10.3389/fonc.2019.00600.

1.5.2. Mechanical Effects and Cavitation

The mechanical effects of ultrasound are the focus of the application of this technology to therapy as such, particularly through such effects as cavitation. Cavitation is the production, growth, and implosion of bubbles in a liquid due to its exposure to acoustic energy. The advanced process generates compressional and tension forces, generating shockwaves with local high pressure and temperature. Such mechanical forces can be employed to rupture cellular membranes and enhance drug delivery, making cavitation an essential component of many medical procedures. As an illustration, the energy-rich bubbles generated under ultrasonic cavitation have been shown to penetrate bacterial biofilms so that targeted treatment of infection otherwise resistant to conventional antibiotics is made possible, thus demonstrating the intersection of cavitation and ultrasonic applications in modern medicine. Current studies demonstrate the ability of ultrasound-induced cavitation to enhance the efficacy of antifungal and anticancer therapies. Ultrasound-induced destruction of biofilms with specificity can lead to a significant enhancement in the efficacy of antimicrobial agents, as indicated by the development of $Fe_3O_4/MnCO_3$ microbubbles that utilize the cavitation-induced mechanical force to disrupt methicillin-resistant Staphylococcus aureus (MRSA) biofilm architecture and generate reactive oxygen species through a sonodynamic effect. This new technique shows the potential of mechanical forces from cavitation to induce therapeutic effects greater than those of traditional therapies. Ultrasound's potential to induce mechanical dissociation of biofilms not only improves our knowledge on microbial resistance but also offers new possibilities for the creation of more effective treatment protocols, with the growing involvement of mechanical effects in ultrasound physics and instrumentation being illustrated (Yuwen et al., 2025). Furthermore, the link between mechanical action and drug delivery is highlighted in oncology by ultrasound-stimulated microbubble cavitation (USMC), a method that enhances the therapeutic efficiency of chemotherapy agents. In an examination of therapeutic outcomes of USMC with gefitinib for ovarian cancer treatment, it was demonstrated that this method significantly elevated drug concentration within cancer tissues and resulted in higher inhibition rates of tumors and extended survival times. The mechanical action of cavitation increases the penetration of drugs, with a potentially useful entry point in side-stepping complications of conventional treatment. With its enhancement of drug resistance and poor drug delivery, USMC shows the serious implications of ultrasound-mediated mechanical effects to its use in the treatment protocols for better oncological treatments (Chen et al., 2024) (Figure 1.16).

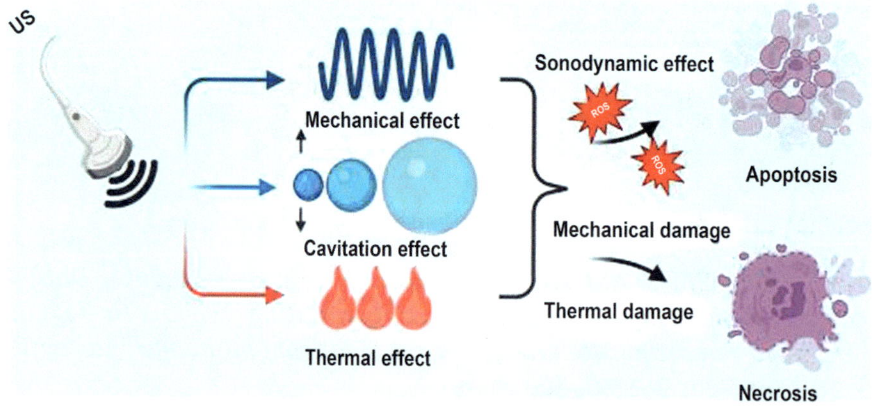

Figure 1.16. Mechanical effects and cavitation ultrasound use.

Source: Maocheng Zuo, Rong Xiao, et.al (2024). Ultrasound-activated mechanochemical reactions for controllable biomedical applications. Smart Materials in Medicine, 5(4); 461-476. https://doi.org/10.1016/j.smaim.2024.09.001.

1.5.3. Guidelines for Safe Ultrasound Use

Ultrasound application safety is a primary concern in therapeutic as well as diagnostic uses. Ultrasound imaging, being physically safe by virtue of its non-ionizing radiation, nonetheless requires appropriate guidelines so as to allow for the minimization of risks associated with its use. Operators are encouraged to follow recommended practices that involve the use of the lowest intensity required and most appropriate contact between transducers and the skin in an attempt to minimize discomfort and tissue damage. Also, operators should be cognizant of patient-specific factors such as age, health status, and pathologies involved that may alter the risk factor for complications in the course of ultrasound procedures. Regular training of the technique and the protocol of the ultrasound operators is required to ensure compliance with such guidelines and ensure patient safety during clinical procedures, emphasizing the critical role played by experienced practitioners in the safe operation of this technology (Ward et al., 2023). In addition to the training of the operators, the equipment employed in ultrasound examinations should also be regularly tested for safety and effectiveness. This entails quality control by frequent quality control assurance and maintenance of ultrasound machines to ensure accurate image formation without compromise on the patient's welfare. These vendors also give guidelines on calibrating and operating their equipment, which need to be adhered to strictly by medical staff. Moreover, any variation in routine procedures—for example, those involving the use of advanced imaging techniques—must rest on the most up-to-date clinical evidence and according to guidelines from the relevant medical physics professional societies. Combining all these considerations leads to achieving the benefits of the use of ultrasound while maintaining an uncompromising commitment to patient safety. As such, it is a harmonious practice among physicists, technologists, and clinical personnel that fosters an atmosphere that supports the safe application of ultrasound technology (Newhauser et al., 2022).

Lastly, including a patient-centered approach when introducing safe ultrasound use guidelines is necessary. Communication among health care providers and patients is effective in decreasing anxiety for ultrasound exams and enhancing patient satisfaction overall. Educating patients about the procedure, indications, potential risks, and benefits can empower them as well as improve compliance with examinations. Similarly, protocols should be adjusted to take into consideration special populations, such as pediatric patients or ambulatory patients with reduced mobility, who may have special issues or heightened risks. Institutionalizing a safety culture that touches on informed consent, pre-procedure screening, and same-day post-procedural follow-up ensures ultrasound practice is not only clinically effective but also ethically sound. Fostering an active safety culture among healthcare professionals decreases the dangers of ultrasound use while maximizing the technology's performance in practice (Ward et al., 2023).

1.6. Clinical Applications of Ultrasound

Ultrasound's medical applications have transformed diagnostic and treatment protocols in the numerous branches of medicine. Ultrasound is used universally in obstetrics to follow the development of the fetus, for which real-time imaging is crucial in establishing the viability and health of the fetus. Both its non-invasive nature of imaging and absence of ionizing radiation make it particularly patient- and clinician-friendly. Beyond obstetrics, ultrasound has also gained widespread use in the examination of abdominal organs, including the liver and kidneys, and heart disease through echocardiography. These applications utilize the fundamental principles of ultrasound physics, such as propagation and reflection of sound waves, through which physicians can diagnose internal structures with great accuracy and make timely decisions for treatment and diagnosis. The utilization of ultrasound in clinics is increasing as studies investigate new approaches and technologies that enhance its diagnostic power (Dietrich et al., 2023). The application extends into therapeutic interventions, for example, guided injections and biopsies. In musculoskeletal medicine, ultrasound diagnoses tendon injury effectively and directs injections into joints, a process that enhances precision and minimizes patient discomfort. This ability to integrate imaging and therapy emphasizes the value of ultrasound technology, enabling real-time imaging that enhances diagnosis and treatment planning. Furthermore, advancements in ultrasound technology, such as three-dimensional imaging and Doppler techniques, have increased the information given to healthcare professionals. These developments highlight the need for robust training courses merging theoretical understanding and practical skills to equip medical professionals with the competencies required for effective use of ultrasound in practice (Burmeister et al., 2022). The increasing variety of indications of ultrasound application has also led to the development of simulation-based educational programs. Simulation offers a low-risk, safe environment in which practitioners can practice and develop their skills and confidence in ultrasound procedures before engaging with real patients. Simulation, in the view of the state-of-the-art document by the World Federation for Ultrasound in Medicine and Biology (WFUMB), can offer a quicker learning curve with patient safety during the period of learning. Incorporating simulation into ultrasound education programs encourages proficiency that is essential for effective clinical practice. With improvements in ultrasound technology, the integration of high-fidelity simulation alongside traditional training methods may be key to revolutionizing the learning paradigm of upcoming medical professionals and equipping them with the demands of modern clinical practice (Dietrich et al., 2023) (Figure 1.17).

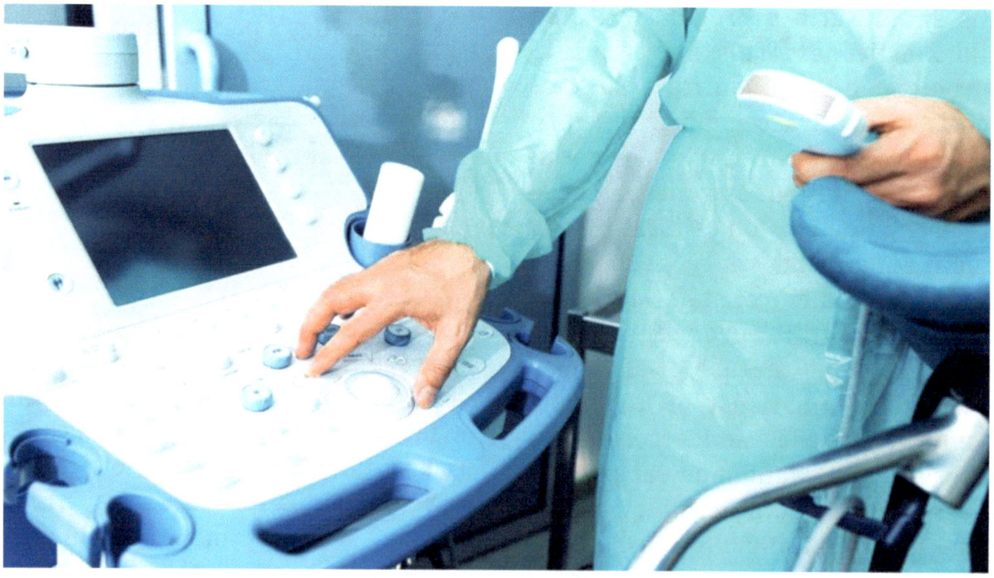

Figure 1.17. Clinical applications of ultrasound.

Source: https://www.uscimaging.com/wp-content/uploads/2022/08/1-min-1024x576.jpg.

1.6.1. Obstetric and Gynecological Ultrasound

In obstetric and gynecologic ultrasound, new imaging technologies have become essential tools for clinicians. The ultrasound methods apply high frequencies of sound waves to produce visual images of the internal reproductive organs and fetal growth, offering important information about normal and disease conditions. As the professionals become skilled at the interpretation of such pictures, they are better equipped to handle patient care efficiently. The role of ultrasound in obstetrics and gynecology is not only to enhance the accuracy of diagnosis but also to facilitate the process of patient management, allowing intervention at a previous stage when necessary. In addition, the evolution in ultrasound equipment technology, including 3D and Doppler imaging, has expanded clinical applications, enabling medical professionals to have richer and more targeted measurements of the mother's and the fetus's physiological state. Moreover, advances in the education of ultrasound, particularly simulation-based education, have reshaped the paradigms for training obstetrics and gynecology practitioners to the core. Ultrasound training programs based on simulation have gained spotlights for their ability to enhance the learning process using real-life, experiential learning without the immediate pressure of a clinical setting. The World Federation for Ultrasound in Medicine and Biology (WFUMB) posits that the integration of simulators—ranging from low-fidelity to high-fidelity—has the potential to significantly improve clinical learning outcomes and confidence among learners. Through the practitioner's capability of refining his or her technical skills within a simulated environment, such learning activities ultimately contribute toward improving patient care and result quality within obstetric and gynecological units. The evolving ultrasound simulation environment opens the door to an even closer integration of imaging science and its applications in clinical medicine into clinical practice (Dietrich et al., 2023). Besides adding more value to training and education, obstetric and gynecological ultrasound has greater implications for the healthcare system in general. By detection and management of complications before viability, such as ectopic pregnancy or fetal anomalies, ultrasound may be indispensable in keeping morbidity and mortality rates to a minimum. This function has not escaped the attention of educational institutions and medical facilities, with training collaborations being established to advance higher competence in ultrasound technology among medical practitioners (Liu et al., 2015). Through investment in robust ultrasound education and simulation, the health profession aims to facilitate high-quality practice standards and reinforce overall healthcare delivery systems. As technology continues to shape practice in obstetric and gynecologic ultrasound, active research and collaboration must be maintained to further improve the efficacy and scope of this essential diagnostic tool (Figure 1.18).

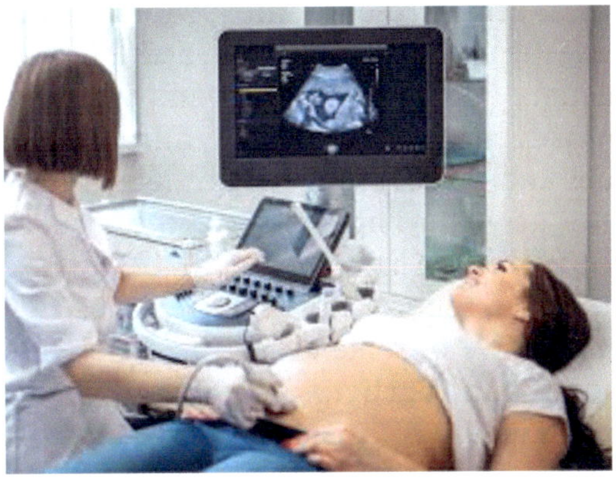

Figure 1.18. Obstetric and gynecological ultrasound.

Source: https://s3.amazonaws.com/static.organiclead.com/Site-f859dd19-b65f-4524-8064-a1aa06f7055d/shutterstock_1485769484.png.

1.6.2. Cardiac Ultrasound (Echocardiography)

Cardiac ultrasound, or echocardiography, is an essential instrument in contemporary cardiovascular diagnosis, offering a non-invasive method of imaging cardiac structures and assessing their functional integrity. Employing high-frequency sound waves to generate dynamic images of the heart, echocardiography allows clinicians to investigate parameters of chamber dimensions, wall motion, and valvular function. With improvement in ultrasound technology, the quality of echocardiographic images has improved over and above to make more accurate diagnoses as well as treatment plans tailor-made to individual patients suffering from heart diseases. The integration of high-technology imaging techniques, including Doppler ultrasound, has further increased the use of echocardiography for assessing blood flow and finding hemodynamic defects, so as to make echocardiography a precious commodity in both the routine clinical practice and the specialized cardiology clinic. The physics behind ultrasound serves as the groundwork for the echocardiographic process, namely for the process of sound wave transmission, reflection, and conduction. Sound waves from a transducer travel through different heart tissues and reflect back to the transducer based on the acoustic impedance of the structures encountered. This process facilitates the creation of echocardiographic images, which are indicative of some determinants of cardiac anatomy and function. Further, the choice of ultrasound uses' frequency is a compromise between resolution and penetration depth, with higher frequencies providing better resolution but at the expense of penetration depth. Understanding these principles not only enhances the expertise of healthcare providers carrying out echocardiograms but also refers to ongoing education and training on ultrasound machines, as highlighted by advancements and concerns raised in recent literature (Dietrich et al., 2023). As a growing demand for cardiac ultrasound occurs, the significance of effective training programs for echocardiography consequently increases. Simulation-based education has emerged as one method of enhancing learning for healthcare professionals using hands-on experience in a controlled environment without endangering the patients. Employing low-fidelity as well as high-fidelity simulators, students can develop skills in image acquisition, interpretation, and clinical decision-making. Current controversies surrounding ultrasound simulation pinpoint its benefits in prepping health professionals for real-world use, emphasizing that proper integration into curricula is important to developing competency in ultrasound practices (Michens, 2017). This shifting educational landscape looks into the centrality of echocardiography as an integral part of cardiac treatment, further emphasizing its significance both in medical education and in optimizing patient care.

1.6.3. Musculoskeletal Ultrasound

Musculoskeletal ultrasound, or MSK ultrasound, is an essential imaging modality for the diagnosis of musculoskeletal illness, offering an affordable and non-invasive means for the assessment of soft tissues, muscles, tendons, and joints. The ability to see real-time movement and dynamics of these structures offers medical professionals detailed diagnostic information that enhances outcomes for patients. Compared to more traditional imaging techniques such as X-rays or MRIs, MSK ultrasound is particularly adept at assessing superficial structures and is thus best suited for the diagnosis of conditions such as tendon rupture, bursitis, and joint effusions. With advancements in technology utilizing ultrasound, the addition of higher frequency transducers and improved imaging algorithms yields higher resolution and improved anatomical detail, thus broadening the clinical application of the technique. Thus, constant advancement of MSK ultrasound is essential to achieve its general acceptance as a norm in regular musculoskeletal assessment and treatment planning. The training component of MSK ultrasound teaching is increasingly being noted as professionals try to enhance proficiency and expertise with this imaging modality. Organizations such as the World Federation for Ultrasound in Medicine and Biology suggest that educational programs incorporate simulation into ultrasound education. Simulation technology provides a new way of training that enables learners to hone their skills in a simulated environment before they are put into practice in clinical environments. Through providing a hands-on learning experience, ultrasound simulators enable the improvement of the confidence and clinical skills of learners while minimizing the workload in busy clinical schedules. With the development of simulators, there is emerging potential for curriculum integration, providing an effective learning environment that equips medical students and practitioners alike with a firm grasp of ultrasound skills. This ensures the next generation of healthcare workers are equipped to utilize MSK ultrasound effectively in clinical practice (Dietrich et al., 2023).

Progress in ultrasound physics and equipment is essential to enhancing the quality and efficacy of MSK ultrasound imaging. The innovation in ultrasound technology, such as the development of portable ultrasound units and the application of advanced imaging techniques, is an innovation that facilitates increased practical and convenient application of MSK ultrasound in various health institutions. Ongoing interaction between practitioners and researchers at platforms such as the SPIE Medical Imaging is a sign of ongoing efforts towards sharing information about new ultrasound technologies. Such forums offer the perfect environment to share new concepts and approaches related to ultrasound physics, opening doors for a brighter future in musculoskeletal imaging. As specialists keep researching and establishing the role of MSK ultrasound in clinical practice, it is hoped that the modality will more and more become an essential part of diagnostic imaging, allowing for improved surgery and therapy in musculoskeletal disease (Wang et al., 2022).

SUMMARY

As the study of ultrasound physics and instrumentation comes to an end, it is realized that it has a central role in contemporary medical diagnosis and therapy. Wave propagation and interpretation of echoes are principles involved in the efficient application of this technology. With improvements in imaging modalities, medical practitioners can ensure greater precision in the diagnosis of diseases, which has beneficial effects on patient treatment. Ongoing improvements in ultrasound technology, ranging from improved image resolution to real-time imaging, are further transforming the medical imaging landscape. Such progress is an excellent example of the necessity of integrating physics principles into clinical practice and, therefore, of having robust training systems that impart theoretical, along with practical knowledge, to clinicians of the future. In addition, recent advances in non-invasive techniques, that is, photoacoustic spectroscopy (PAS), highlight the potential for ultrasound and related technologies to expand their diagnostic capabilities further. The increasing prevalence of diabetes, as noted, necessitates novel ways of tracking blood glucose levels effectively, which can be enabled by ultrasound technologies. Through overcoming challenges such as inadequate penetration depth and interference from other blood components, researchers are moving closer to viable solutions for real-time glucose monitoring. This intersection of ultrasound physics and groundbreaking research is a prime example of the strength of interdisciplinary teamwork in healthcare innovation, ultimately delivering better patient care. And when coupled with machine learning, PAS in the mid-infrared range can enhance detection sensitivity, demonstrating the dynamic development of applications of ultrasound in medicine (Kaysir et al., 2023).

In summary, the integration of physics in ultrasound technology not only enhances diagnostic capacity but also paves the way for new developments that can transform patient care. With the advancement of the discipline, clinicians and physicists both will be required to carry out research alongside each other, interpreting theoretical advancement to clinical practice. The teaching materials for experimental physics through different technologies also have the promise of stimulating generations of scientists and medical practitioners to come. The materials enable improved understanding of how physics theory is applied in practice, enhancing the learning process. In the context of the ongoing trends and demands for ultrasound physics and instrumentation today, ongoing research and education remain essential to continue stimulating innovation that addresses the needs of patients and health practitioners (Monteiro & Marti, 2022).

In our exploration of the physics and instrumentation of ultrasound, there emerge a variety of basic concepts emerge as central to understanding technology as well as application. Ultrasound is based on the propagation of sound waves through various media, such that it is the nature of the tissues that the waves are propagating through that governs their appearance and behavior. The physical principles of reflection, refraction, and attenuation involved in the interaction of sound waves with soft tissues are the basis of diagnostic imaging. Knowledge of these effects allows practitioners to effectively manipulate ultrasound frequency and mode to enhance resolution and depth penetration in clinical use, thus demonstrating how basic physical principles directly determine useful methods in medical imaging. Moreover, new technologies have introduced new methods that improve the performance of imaging, particularly in complex biological media. Among these innovations are wavefront shaping and computational techniques for the manipulation of sound waves in tissue, which open up avenues for diffraction-limited imaging beyond previous depths. The advances point to how ongoing research and advancements are transforming the practice of ultrasound and how they are an ongoing scientific community striving to revolutionize medical imaging. As emphasized in recent literature, these technological advances not only enhance the precision of imaging but also require a full grasp of the physics involved, emphasizing the symbiotic relationship between theoretical knowledge and its application in ultrasound technology (Gigan et al., 2022).

Finally, the operation of ultrasound devices, including transducers and imaging modules, plays a crucial role in rendering the best results under various clinical scenarios. Modern ultrasound devices incorporate high-technology design elements to provide versatile imaging needs, ranging from prenatal diagnosis to sophisticated musculoskeletal assessment. Integration between hardware functionality and software algorithms defines the best image quality and user-friendly operation. With instrumentation development, the necessity to understand its underlying physics is highlighted, demonstrating integration of physics and engineering design. The ongoing dialogue between these disciplines emphasizes the constant need to innovate and adapt within the practice of ultrasound, paving the way for the future production of advances in ultrasound technology and medical applications (Abi et al., 2020).

CLOSER LOOK

DOPPLER ULTRASOUND

Doppler ultrasound is a non-invasive body imaging technique that applies the principle of the Doppler effect to assess and image blood flow in the circulatory vessels in the body. Unlike conventional ultrasound, which primarily identifies stationary anatomical structures using high-frequency sound waves, Doppler ultrasound identifies the change in frequency of back-reflected sound waves because of the movement of red blood cells. As the blood flows towards the transducer, the frequency of the incoming sound wave increases; when it flows away, the frequency decreases. The changing frequency is thus picked up and shown either as color images or waveforms of the spectrum, providing useful information regarding the direction, velocity, and quality of the blood flow. Doppler ultrasound is widely applied in cardiovascular medicine, obstetrics, nephrology, and other surgical specialties to diagnose and monitor diseases such as arterial occlusion, deep vein thrombosis, carotid artery stenosis, varicose veins, peripheral arterial disease, and fetal circulation abnormalities. Four types of Doppler ultrasounds include continuous wave Doppler, pulsed wave Doppler, color Doppler, and power Doppler. Continuous wave Doppler is best for measuring high-velocity flow but lacks depth resolution. Pulsed wave Doppler can measure velocity at a single depth but is limited by aliasing with high velocity. Color Doppler overlaying direction and velocity of flow onto a gray-scale image gives a global image of vascular anatomy and flow dynamics. Power Doppler, as it is less sensitive to the direction of flow, is more sensitive to low-flow states and is used in detecting tissue and organ perfusion. In clinical practice, Doppler ultrasound is essential in the assessment of cardiac valve function through the detection of stenosis or regurgitation patterns of turbulent flow and evaluation of vascular grafts and fistulas. In obstetrics, it is essential in the assessment of fetal well-being through measurement of the umbilical artery, uterine artery, and middle cerebral artery flow in high-risk pregnancies complicated by intrauterine growth restriction or preeclampsia. In renal and hepatic disease, Doppler is indicated to quantify organ perfusion and for the diagnosis of vascular complications such as renal artery stenosis or portal hypertension. One strength of Doppler ultrasound is that it is safe (no ionizing radiation), real-time, repeatable, and relatively low-cost. Accuracy and quality of the study are highly dependent on the operator and can be hampered by patient body habitus, vessel tortuosity, and calcification. Interpretation of Doppler study requires skill in waveform analysis, familiarity with normal and disease patterns of flow, and correlation with the clinical situation. An illustration is a peripheral artery monophasic waveform suggesting downstream obstruction or broadening of the spectrum from turbulence secondary to stenosis. Developments in ultrasound technology, including 3D and contrast-enhanced Doppler, are increasingly expanding its role as a diagnostic imaging tool. Moreover, handheld and portable Doppler devices are increasingly used in bedside and emergency settings to quickly establish perfusion and vessel integrity. Overall, Doppler ultrasound is an important diagnostic tool in modern medicine, offering dynamic, functional information that complements structural imaging and supports timely clinical decision-making.

References

1. Abi, B., Acciarri, R., Acero, M. A., Adamov, G., Adams, D. L., Adinolfi, M., Ahmad, Z., et al. (2020). Volume I. Introduction to DUNE. *Journal of Instrumentation, 15*, T08008. https://doi.org/10.1088/1748-0221/15/08/t08008 (accessed on 12th July 2025).
2. Ai, P., Xiao, L., Deng, Z., Wang, Y., Sun, X., Huang, G., Wang, D., Li, Y., & Ran, X.. (2023). Label-free timing analysis of SiPM-based modularized detectors with physics-constrained deep learning. *Machine Learning: Science and Technology, 4*. https://www.semanticscholar.org/paper/9d4b9befcdbcf0252dc7c7edae00bae88ed87d97 (accessed on 12th July 2025).
3. Barua, A., Achamyeleh, Y. G., & Al Faruque, M. A. (2022). A wolf in sheep's clothing. In *Proceedings of the 2022 ACM SIGSAC Conference on Computer and Communications Security*. https://doi.org/10.1145/3548606.3560643 (accessed on 12th July 2025).
4. Bortot, B., Mangogna, A., Di Lorenzo, G., Stabile, G., Ricci, G., & Biffi, S. (2023). Image-guided cancer surgery: A narrative review on imaging modalities and emerging nanotechnology strategies. *Journal of Nanobiotechnology, 21*. https://doi.org/10.1186/s12951-023-01926-y (accessed on 12th July 2025).
5. Burmeister, J., Busse, N. C., Cetnar, A. J., Howell, R. R., Jeraj, R., Jones, A. K., King, S. H., et al. (2022). Academic program recommendations for graduate degrees in medical physics: AAPM Report No. 365 (Revision of Report No. 197). *Journal of Applied Clinical Medical Physics, 23*. https://doi.org/10.1002/acm2.13792 (accessed on 12th July 2025).
6. Campos, M. G., Anjos, O., Chica, M., Campoy, P., Nôžková, J., Almaráz-Abarca, N., Carelli Barreto, L. M. R., et al. (2021). Standard methods for pollen research. *Journal of Apicultural Research, 60*, 1–109. https://doi.org/10.1080/00218839.2021.1948240 (accessed on 12th July 2025).
7. Chen, J., Wang, J., Yan, X., Zhang, X., Zhang, Z., Li, H., & Wang, Y. (2024). Enhancing the therapeutic efficacy of gefitinib on subcutaneously transplanted SKOV3 ovarian cancer tumors in nude mice via ultrasoundstimulated microbubble cavitation. *Experimental and Therapeutic Medicine, 28*. https://www.semanticscholar.org/paper/82dfa558abc9becdb7b10ac9358ba0098414baaa (accessed on 12th July 2025).
8. Delaney, L. J., Isguven, S., Eisenbrey, J. R., Hickok, N. J., & Forsberg, F. (2022). Making waves: How ultrasound-targeted drug delivery is changing pharmaceutical approaches. *Materials Advances, 3*, 3023–3040. https://doi.org/10.1039/d1ma01197a (accessed on 12th July 2025).
9. Deriu, C., Thakur, S., Tammaro, O., & Fabris, L. (2023). Challenges and opportunities for SERS in the infrared: Materials and methods. *Nanoscale Advances, 5*, 2132–2166. https://doi.org/10.1039/d2na00930g (accessed on 12th July 2025).
10. Dietrich, C. F., Lucius, C., Nielsen, M. B., Burmester, E., Westerway, S. C., Chu, C. Y., Condous, G., et al. (2023). The ultrasound use of simulators, current view, and perspectives: Requirements and technical aspects (WFUMB state of the art paper). *Endoscopic Ultrasound, 12*, 38–49. https://doi.org/10.4103/eus-d-22-00197 (accessed on 12th July 2025).
11. Gigan, S., Katz, O., de Aguiar, H. B., Andresen, E. R., Aubry, A., Bertolotti, J., Bossy, E., et al. (2022). Roadmap on wavefront shaping and deep imaging in complex media. *Journal of Physics Photonics, 4*, 042501. https://doi.org/10.1088/2515-7647/ac76f9 (accessed on 12th July 2025).

12. Hoskins, P. R., Martin, K., & Thrush, A. (2010). *Diagnostic Ultrasound.* Cambridge University Press. https://play.google.com/store/books/details?id=W8LB26lsHjMC&source=gbs_api (accessed on 12th July 2025).

13. IEEE. (2022). Program. *2022 IEEE/MTT-S International Microwave Symposium–IMS 2022.* https://doi.org/10.1109/ims37962.2022.9865554 (accessed on 12th July 2025).

14. Jabbary, S. (2021). Effect of high intensity focused ultrasound on neural compound action potential: an *in vitro* study. Toronto Metropolitan University. https://doi.org/10.32920/ryerson.14647980 (accessed on 12th July 2025).

15. Johnson, J. I., Beasley, H. K., Southwick, D., Lords, A. M., Kessler, R., Vrablik, M., & Baker, R. T. (2024). Development of a hybrid point-of-care ultrasound curriculum for first year medical students in a rural medical education program: A pilot study. *BMC Medical Education, 24.* https://doi.org/10.1186/s12909-023-05005-6 (accessed on 12th July 2025).

16. Karadžić, K. (2021). Radiation monitoring system. *Book of Abstracts.* https://doi.org/10.21175/rad.abstr.book.2021.28.20 (accessed on 12th July 2025).

17. Kaysir, M. R., Song, J., Rassel, S., Aloraynan, A., & Ban, D. (2023). Progress and perspectives of mid-infrared photoacoustic spectroscopy for non-invasive glucose detection. *Biosensors, 13,* 716. https://doi.org/10.3390/bios13070716 (accessed on 12th July 2025).

18. Liu, F., Shi, X., Wilson, C., Pokrajac, D., Bakić, P. R., & Maidment, A. D. A. (2015). Image-based biomarker of breast cancer risk: Analysis of risk disparity among minority populations. https://doi.org/10.21236/ada616763 (accessed on 12th July 2025).

19. Luijten, B., Chennakeshava, N., Eldar, Y. C., Mischi, M., & van Sloun, R. J. G. (2023). Ultrasound signal processing: From models to deep learning. *Ultrasound in Medicine & Biology, 49,* 677–698. https://doi.org/10.1016/j.ultrasmedbio.2022.11.003 (accessed on 12th July 2025).

20. Mickens, R. E. (2017). Nonstandard finite difference schemes. *Notices of the American Mathematical Society, 65,* 17–18. https://doi.org/10.1090/noti1617 (accessed on 12th July 2025).

21. Monteiro, M., & Martí, A. C. (2022). Resource Letter MDS-1: Mobile devices and sensors for physics teaching. *American Journal of Physics, 90,* 328–343. https://doi.org/10.1119/5.0073317 (accessed on 12th July 2025).

22. Newhauser, W., Gress, D. A., Mills, M., Jordan, D. W., Sutlief, S. G., Martin, M., & Jackson, E. F. (2022). Medical physics workforce in the United States. *Journal of Applied Clinical Medical Physics, 23.* https://doi.org/10.1002/acm2.13762 (accessed on 12th July 2025).

23. Pizarro, A., Manfreda, S., & Tubaldi, E. (2020). The science behind scour at bridge foundations: A review. *Water, 12,* 374. https://doi.org/10.3390/w12020374 (accessed on 12th July 2025).

24. Rath, E., Sharfman, Z. T., & Amar, E. (2020). Practical office ultrasound for the hip surgeon: Current concepts. *Journal of ISAKOS: Joint Disorders & Orthopedic Sports Medicine, 5,* 89–97. https://doi.org/10.1136/jisakos-2019-000407 (accessed on 12th July 2025).

25. Royo, S., & Ballesta-Garcia, M. (2019). An overview of lidar imaging systems for autonomous vehicles. *Applied Sciences, 9,* 4093. https://doi.org/10.3390/app9194093 (accessed on 12th July 2025).

26. Salcudean, S., Moradi, H., Black, D., & Navab, N. (2022). Robot-assisted medical imaging: A review. *Proceedings of the IEEE, 110,* 951–967. https://www.semanticscholar.org/paper/81cb99f644d8259adce13efc82b48dc4ee87acb0 (accessed on 12th July 2025).

27. Samei, E., & Peck, D. J. (2019). *Hendee's physics of medical imaging.*

28. Stanković, J., Krajinović, M., Kržanović, N., Živanović, M., Kojić, A., & Božović, P. (2021). TLD-100 post-irradiation fading characteristics according to IEC 62387:2020 standard. *Book of Abstracts.* https://doi.org/10.21175/rad.abstr.book.2021.31.12 (accessed on 12th July 2025).

29. Wang, A., Cunningham, I. A., Danielsson, M., Fahrig, R., Flohr, T., Noo, F., Tingberg, A., et al. (2022). Science and practice of imaging physics through 50 years of SPIE Medical Imaging conferences. *Journal of Medical Imaging, 9*(S1). https://doi.org/10.1117/1.jmi.9.s1.012205 (accessed on 12th July 2025).

30. Ward, P., Athanassoglou, V., & McNarry, A. F. (2023). Safe use of high flow nasal oxygen in apnoeic patients for laryngotracheal surgery. *European Journal of Anesthesiology, 40*, 801–804. https://doi.org/10.1097/eja.0000000000001890 (accessed on 12th July 2025).

31. Westerbeek, E. Y. (2022). *Introducing Vortex Chromatography.* https://doi.org/10.3990/1.9789036554770 (accessed on 12th July 2025).

32. Wiegers, S. E., Ryan, T., Arrighi, J. A., Brown, S. M., Canaday, B., Damp, J. B., Díaz-Gómez, J. L., et al. (2019). 2019 ACC/AHA/ASE advanced training statement on echocardiography (revision of the 2003 ACC/AHA clinical competence statement on echocardiography). *Catheterization and Cardiovascular Interventions, 94*, 481–505. https://doi.org/10.1002/ccd.28313 (accessed on 12th July 2025).

33. Yuwen, L., Liu, Y., Xu, F., Zhang, C., Chen, X., Yin, Z., Liang, B., et al. (2025). $Fe_3O_4/MnCO_3$ microbubbles for efficient elimination of bacterial biofilms by mechanical/sonodynamic effects under ultrasound irradiation and magnetic field targeting. *Biomaterials Science.* https://www.semanticscholar.org/paper/225a38223b542a88cdeff6c1d2eed584b8070df9 (accessed on 12th July 2025).

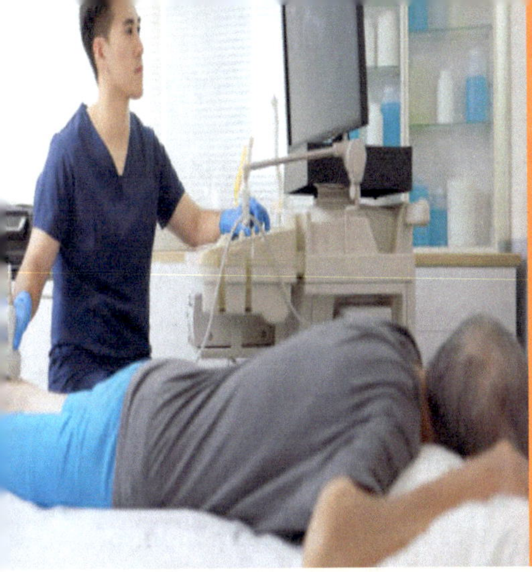

Chapter 2

ULTRASOUND SCANNING TECHNIQUES AND PATIENT POSITIONING

Contents

Introduction

The creation of ultrasound scanning technologies is a significant milestone in medical imaging, emerging as a corner-stone in current diagnostics. Through the utilization of high-frequency sound waves, ultrasound technology facilitates the visualization of organs and soft tissues and offers critical information without using ionizing radiation common with other imaging modalities. As it is a non-invasive and universal instrument, ultrasound has widespread uses in all fields of medicine, including obstetrics, cardiology, and urology. This review will discuss the efficiency of ultrasound scan techniques, looking into how patient positioning can significantly influence diagnosis results. On the basis of technological advancements and integrating artificial intelligence has also improved ultrasound's diagnostic capability to become a part of modern medicine (Ullah et al., 2025). Precise patient placement during ultrasound examinations is essential for optimal image quality as well as facilitating accurate diagnoses. The success of an ultrasound scan does not solely rely on the proficiency of the technician and the advanced technology but mainly on how the patient is placed and positioned. For instance, patient positioning changes can optimize acoustic windows and thus improve visualization of structures. Further, some positions will need to accommodate specific anatomical areas effectively based on the nature of the examination. With recent technology, such as that found in the Apple Vision Pro setup, patient and sonographer ergonomics are greatly improved with features such as multiscreen displays that maximize the procedural environment (Montoro Neto et al., 2025). This synergy depicts commitment to enhancing ultrasound practice by adapting patient positioning practice. As the universe of ultrasound scanning techniques continues to evolve, understanding the interaction between technique and patient positioning is most critical for optimal clinical outcomes. Advances in ultrasound technology, for example, better image resolution and processing speeds, combined with synergistic optimization of support tools, are redefining the paradigm of diagnostic imaging. Patients benefit from not only improved diagnostic accuracy but also minimized procedure time and increased comfort, resulting in an overall increase in satisfaction. Examination will consider how these technological advancements, in addition to strategic patient positioning, are shaping the future of ultrasound diagnostics. The objective remains simple: to utilize such innovations towards greater clinical efficacy in a manner that ensures patient safety and comfort in diverse medical conditions (Ullah et al., 2025) (Figure 2.1).

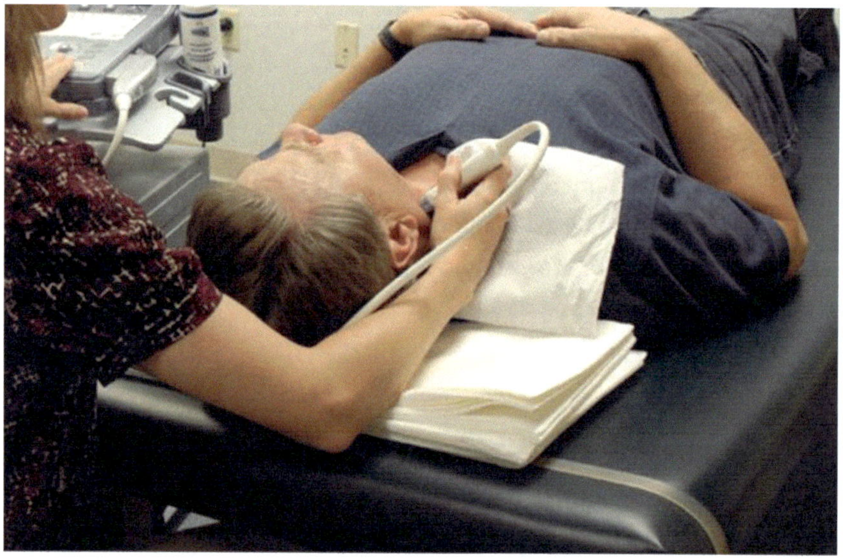

Figure 2.1. Ultrasound scanning techniques and patient positioning.

Source: https://radiologykey.com/wp-content/uploads/2016/12/image00432-1.jpeg.

Definition of Ultrasound Scanning

Ultrasound scanning or sonography is a diagnostic imaging technique involving the use of high-frequency sound waves to visualize internal body structures. The non-invasive technique is particularly useful in medical diagnostics since it has the ability to perform real-time imaging as well as notuse of ionizing radiation, making it the best choice in most clinical applications. The process begins with the application of a gel onto the skin of the patient to enable the transmission of sound waves generated by a transducer. The sound waves engage in interaction with the tissues to give rise to echoes, which are converted to images by a computer. As a result, ultrasound scanning has broad applications in obstetrics, cardiology, and musculoskeletal evaluation, allowing clinicians to gain critical information about organ morphology, blood flow, and even disease states in a limited time frame. The flexibility of one of the characteristics of ultrasound scanning results is largely due to the patient's position during scanning. Appropriate positioning plays a critical role as it can significantly enhance the quality of the images produced and the final diagnostic accuracy. For instance, in obstetric scanning, specific positions can optimize visualization of the fetus and surrounding anatomy. Similarly, in those cases when vascular anatomy needs to be assessed, say in a vascular ultrasound, positioning of patients can be employed to place the blood vessels being examined in alignment with the ultrasound beam, thus achieving improved images. Ultrasound scanning modifications explicitly supplement the increasing need for precise and accurate diagnosis, as seen in cases where proper positioning enabled intervention, emphasizing the importance of merging effective scanning with careful patient positioning in clinical practice. Further, advancements in ultrasound technology have brought innovations addressing the issues faced by traditional scanning practices. Current research has developed adaptive techniques that enhance image quality and security in ultrasound imaging. An example of research points to embracing new force control techniques to maximize patient-ultrasound equipment interaction[s¶vc¥⍰, bypassing the limitations of conventional techniques (Xiao et al., 2025). The adaptive technique not only maximizes the imaging process but also enhances compliance and patient comfort. In addition, research into new techniques, such as ultrasound-guided stellate ganglion blocks, reflects the increasing value of ultrasound use in therapy, affirming the importance of precise ultrasound scanning techniques that, through appropriate positioning of the patient, can lead to improved clinical outcomes (Mo et al., 2024). Through continued innovation of these techniques, the clinical use of ultrasound scanning is set to continue its advancement and spread to broader clinical applications in the treatment of patients.

Importance of Patient Positioning in Ultrasound

In ultrasound technology, ideal patient positioning is critical in optimizing image quality and diagnostic accuracy. Ideal positioning enables sonographers to access desired anatomical structures while avoiding interference from overlying tissues. Various ultrasound exams, differently, demand alternative orientations for patients; for example, the supine, lateral, or upright positions can each be significant in disclosing important information. Identification of anatomical landmarks and the pathophysiologic importance of the position can also help towards improving imaging results. Greater awareness of positioning can reduce repeat scans, and therefore patient exposure to unwarranted procedures, as well as enhance overall workflow in clinical settings. Thus, positioning becomes a key driver to the extent of utilization of ultrasound in medical diagnostics, and it warrants much focus from educators and medical practitioners as well. Moreover, patient comfort and confidence are significantly determined by proper positioning during ultrasound procedures. Discomfort may stem from physical resistance, which ultimately degrades the images obtained. Imagers must create an environment in which patients feel at ease, allowing proper positioning without causing distress or anxiety. Such a patient-centered environment enhances imaging outcomes as well as enhances the patient experience overall. Transparency in communication about the procedure and the significance of positioning can demystify the process, which has been shown to affect patient cooperation positively on scans. By placing priority on comfort as well as clinical effectiveness, healthcare providers are able to optimize the technical quality of the ultrasound procedure as well as the interpersonal dynamics of patient care, reinforcing the necessity for well-thought-out positioning strategies in the clinical setting. Finally, adherence to current guidelines is of utmost significance in reinforcing the function of patient positioning in ultrasound. Evidence-based practice should be included in clinicians' protocols to not only obtain technical success of the exams but also patient safety and satisfaction. Organization recommendations, such as those of the American Thyroid Association and the European Society of Cardiology, emphasize careful consideration of positioning with specific diagnoses, pointing out the point of convergence of clinical evidence and practical applicability in the instance of ultrasound. Such standards are complete manuals that need to be considered by health professionals in an effort to enhance their proficiency, with the emphatic point that correct positioning is not an ancillary matter but the cornerstone of successful ultrasound examinations. Complying with such standards ensures a culture of excellence in ultrasound imaging, which will ultimately lead to improved patient results (Haungen et al., 2015; Members ATF et al., 2014).

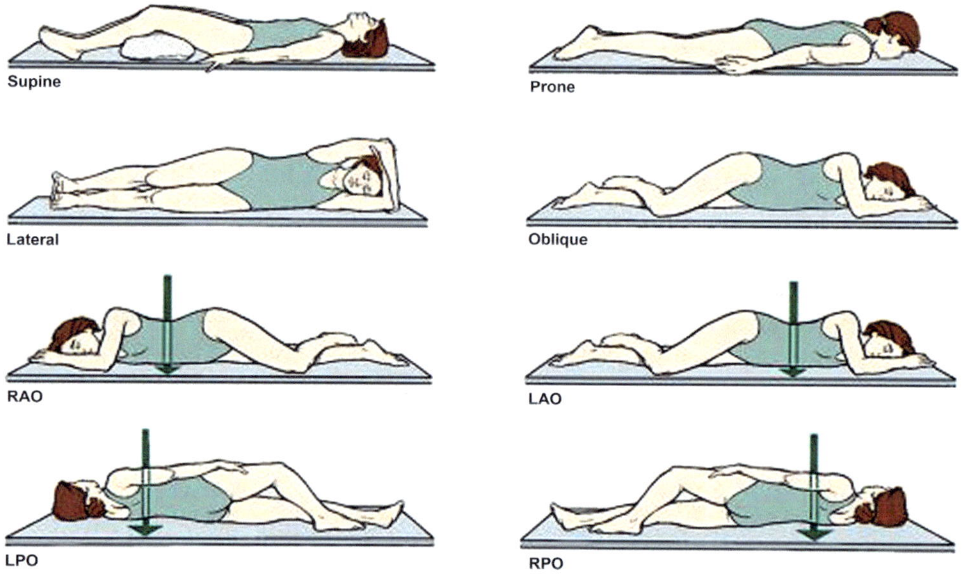

Figure 2.2. Patient positioning in ultrasound.

Source: https://radiologykey.com/wp-content/uploads/2022/12/C2-FF3.gif.

2.1. History of Ultrasound Technology

The history of the technology of ultrasound has seen revolutionary changes from the onset of its development in the early 20th century. It was developed from sonar machines employed in World War I to detect submarines. The principles of sound wave propagation and reflection formed a foundation for developing its medical use, which began to materialize during the 1950s. Pioneering work by researchers such as Dr. Karl Dussik, the earliest to apply ultrasound to neurology, pushed a revolution in diagnostic imaging techniques. This period ushered in the shift from rudimentary apparatus to progressively sophisticated imaging devices, ultimately leading to the first commercial ultrasound scanners in the 1960s. With advances in technology, sonographers can now see organs and tissue in real-time, vastly enhancing diagnostic capability. These advancements placed ultrasound in the limelight of clinical practice, paving the way for further advancements in scanning technology and patient positioning. As technology improved the ultrasound, its applications expanded significantly, and it was applied to other fields of medicine. Ultrasound became a standard procedure in obstetrics and gynecology by the 1970s and 1980s, providing expecting parents with their initial impressions of their future babies. The development of Doppler ultrasound further updated this specialty with the ability to assess circulation and blood flow, most important in both maternal and fetal well-being. Simultaneously, additional advanced imaging technology provided for adequate assessment of abdominal, cardiac, and vascular disease. The active development of ultrasound technology also coincided with a time of increased safety and patient comfort, as physicians began to adopt protocols prioritizing optimal patient positioning and view during scanning. These advancements were not only a sign of technological progress but also reflected the heightened sensitivity toward the patient experience in medical diagnosis. The recent technologies in the field of ultrasound have moved towards the inclusion of three-dimensional imaging as well as portable systems, further revolutionizing its clinical application. Freehand 3D ultrasound systems are a significant step forward, allowing practitioners to take volumetric images independent of the limitations of conventional machines. This ability is especially relevant for emergency care applications where immediate evaluation is critical. For instance, studies have demonstrated the ability of freehand 3D ultrasound to accurately track midline shifts in neurologic patients, overcoming restrictions imposed by conventional imaging modalities such as CT and MRI (Mathur et al., 2025). Furthermore, recent development in ultrasound-guided interventions demonstrates its applicability beyond diagnosis, such as the treatment of insomnia via stellate ganglion blocks (Mo et al., 2024). These developments not only underscore the ultrasound's versatility but also bear out its role as a fundamental tool of contemporary clinical practice, once more emphasizing the ongoing need for professional operator placement and technique refinement to achieve optimal diagnostic accuracy (Figure 2.3).

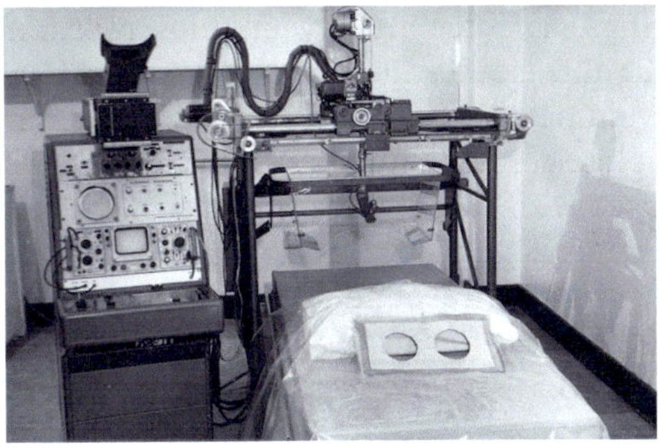

Figure 2.3. History of ultrasound technology.

Source: https://www.asum.com.au/wp-content/uploads/2015/08/117_UI0094-e1592444040300.jpg.

2.1.1. Development of Ultrasound Imaging

Advances in ultrasound imaging technology have revolutionized medical diagnostics by offering real-time imaging of the internal anatomy in a minimally invasive manner. The first ultrasound systems, which were primarily applied for obstetric scanning in the middle of the 20th century, were simple two-dimensional (2D) imaging techniques that provided rudimentary anatomical data. Over the years, advances in transducer technology, signal processing, and image algorithms provided more sophisticated modalities, such as three-dimensional (3D) imaging and elastography. These developments significantly improved diagnostic accuracy and expanded the applications of ultrasound to such fields as cardiology, musculoskeletal sonography, and abdominal examination. The incorporation of computer algorithms and artificial intelligence has further improved image quality, allowing automatic measurement and improved diagnostic efficiency. The history of ultrasound imaging is a classic example of the crossroads of technological development and clinical necessity in the healthcare industry. Additionally, new technologies such as freehand 3D ultrasound have been shown to enhance situational flexibility within intensive care settings. The technology enables rescanning of 2D ultrasound images into comprehensive 3D volumetric presentations, thus providing a complete assessment of anatomy from multiple perspectives. The advances in sensor technology, with electromagnetic tracking, allow for greater accuracy in ultrasound imaging, validating the ability to track critical conditions like midline shift (MLS) in neurocritical patients. The literature indicates that the accuracy of freehand 3D ultrasound is equivalent to conventional imaging modalities such as CT and MRI, with its potential utility for emergency cases. By allowing bedside monitoring without the need for patient transportation, such developments in ultrasound imaging decrease risk exponentially and also enhance patient care during emergency procedures (Mathur et al., 2025). Additionally, the application of machine learning and artificial intelligence to ultrasound imaging not only streamlines the process but enhances scan quality and interpretability as well. Recent advances have been made in the development of sensor-less systems, which estimate contact force based on deep learning algorithms applied to ultrasound image sequences (Choi et al., 2025). These advancements cut across the drawbacks of traditional sensor-based measurements to allow effective control of contact forces during robotic ultrasound scanning. Such developments eliminate the requirement for additional hardware without sacrificing high-resolution imaging, which is crucial in providing maximum diagnostic outcomes. Moreover, improved patient positioning techniques taking into account the differences in anatomy can significantly influence the quality of ultrasound images as well as diagnostic precision. With the advancement of ultrasound technology, the ability of ultrasound to guide and recommend clinical decision-making means that the field needs sustained research and development.

2.1.2. Key Milestones in Ultrasound Technology

The evolution of ultrasound technology has been marked by significant milestones that have transformed its application in medical diagnosis. The origin of ultrasound in the 1920s laid the foundation for its clinical use, especially the development of A-mode (amplitude mode) and B-mode (brightness mode) imaging in the 1950s. These early imaging techniques improved the visualisation of anatomical structures, allowing clinicians to make more informed decisions regarding patient care. Subsequently, the development of Doppler ultrasound technology in the 1960s made possible the analysis of blood flow, further augmenting ultrasound's diagnostic capabilities. This technical breakthrough not only enhanced cardiovascular imaging but also assisted in monitoring fetal health during pregnancy, thus pointing towards a significant leap in safety as well as effectiveness in obstetric practice. The 1980s and the 1990s witnessed a boom in innovation in ultrasound technology, significantly enhancing its scope and versatility. One of the most important advances was the introduction of real-time imaging, which facilitated dynamic viewing of dynamic structures, such as the heart and blood vessels. This feature transformed the manner in which practitioners undertook diagnostics, permitting immediate assessment and intervention. In addition, the introduction of three-dimensional (3D) ultrasound imaging provided another dimension of depth of information to healthcare practitioners, particularly in gynecology and obstetrics. The ability to generate high-resolution volumetric images facilitated better fetal anatomy evaluation and abnormality detection, thereby better prenatal care and outcomes. These advances characterized the importance of ultrasound as a safe, non-invasive imaging method with huge clinical applications. The last decade has seen the integration of artificial intelligence (AI) into ultrasound machines as a game-changer in medical imaging. AIs potential to improve image analysis by using deep learning algorithms has drastically enhanced diagnostic precision and accuracy. Through improved image interpretation and autonomous detection of abnormalities, AI has the potential to decrease human error and improve clinical decision-making. This revolution can be seen especially in uses across multiple domains, such as cardiology and obstetrics, where fast and accurate identification of conditions is crucial. As healthcare becomes more reliant on technology advancement, AI-assisted ultrasound machines can potentially enhance patient care through more customized and timely interventions. With ongoing development and research, the application of AI in ultrasound technology will expand the difference between image diagnosis and effective patient management, lending credence to the dynamic nature of the practice (Varnosfaderani & Forouzanfar, 2024; Coelho, 2023) (Figure 2.4).

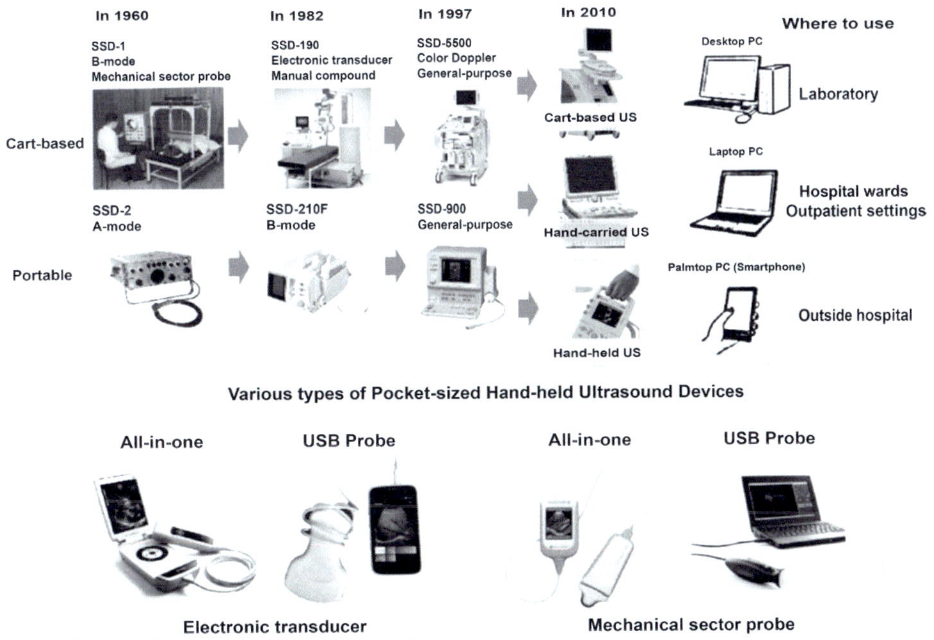

Figure 2.4. Key milestones in ultrasound technology.

Source: Kobayashi, Tadashi & Kato, Hiroyuki. (2016). Development of Pocket-sized Hand-held Ultrasound Devices Enhancing People's Abilities and Need for Education on Them. Journal of General and Family Medicine. 17. 276-288. 10.14442/jgfm.17.4_276.

2.1.3. Evolution of Scanning Techniques

The advancement of scanning technology has been one of the biggest revolutions in medical imaging, both in diagnostics and patient safety. Ultrasound technology has itself experienced tremendous advancements since it was discovered. In the past used in the form of rudimentary assessments, the technology has evolved to encompass sophisticated modalities that can create real-time images of internal structures, leading to precise diagnostic imaging. With the application of contrast-enhanced ultrasound with three-dimensional (3D) imaging, the capability of ultrasound has been enhanced further so that more accurate assessments of complex pathologies can be carried out. In procedures such as urology, where precise location assessment of the disease is important, ultrasound-guided procedures have become essential components of planning and executing minimally invasive procedures, exhibiting a shift toward personalized patient treatment methods (Dobruch, 2013). A turning point within the history of ultrasound scanning techniques is the integration of ultrasound guidance within invasive procedure to enhance precision and safety. The use of ultrasound during liver biopsies is one such model for this development; it has been found through research that ultrasound-guided tissue sampling is superior to blind conventional techniques, thereby limiting complications (Ghent, 2009). This move is part of a larger trend in the medical profession towards patient-centered care through greater diagnostic accuracy and reduction of procedural risks. The increasing use of ultrasound as an adjunct to interventional procedures has revolutionized several specialties, not just highlighting the technical advances but also altering the philosophy of minimally invasive operations with a focus on the patient's well-being. Thus, the employment of novel ultrasound methods is proof of overall progression of healthcare practice with a preference for accuracy in treatment and diagnosis. Nevertheless, the transition from traditional to novel modes of scanning has evoked ongoing debate regarding the most appropriate way of utilizing them in practice. Critics have argued that certain newer machines lack sufficient evidence of improved safety or efficacy over established procedures. Moreover, the financial implications associated with introducing ultrasound-guided procedures, that is, increased spending and training requirements, challenge their accessibility in different healthcare environments (Ghent, 2009). It is important to scrutinize these factors closely, as the introduction of new scanning techniques needs to be justified on technological merits as well as consider the systemic implications. As the technology evolves, a balanced approach promoting empirical intensity along with inventiveness will be essential in determining optimal scanning practices in the ever-evolving landscape of medical imaging.

2.2. Principles of Ultrasound Imaging

The principles of ultrasound imaging are the interaction of sound with biological tissue, relying on high-frequency acoustic waves to produce diagnostic images. The transducer sends out the sound waves, which move through the body and reflect off different tissues, returning echoes detected by the transducer. Tissues reflect sound waves in varying ways depending on their densities, enabling one to differentiate between structures such as muscles, organs, and fluids. This technique can yield real-time images, enabling medical professionals to see the anatomical structures in motion, thus making ultrasound a precious tool in medical practice. Moreover, improving imaging techniques, such as 3D reconstruction, has also increased the accuracy of interpreting ultrasound images, further justifying the modality's place in contemporary diagnostics. It is imperative to learn these basic principles to use them efficiently and ensure patient safety when conducting an ultrasound procedure. Patient positioning plays a central role in optimizing ultrasound imaging outcomes, as it largely dictates the quality and reliability of images obtained. Choice of position can facilitate or hinder access to the target anatomical structure, which influences accuracy in diagnosis. For instance, specific positions, such as supine or lateral position, may enhance visualization of specific organs or vascular structures so that pathologies are better imaged. Additionally, correct positioning diminishes distress and anxiety in the patient during the procedure, thus facilitating greater cooperation and image quality. Intentional patient positioning is not merely a comfort issue but contributes to the diagnostic value of ultrasound scans. By synchronizing patient positioning with the inherent principles of ultrasound imaging, the clinician can enhance diagnostic precision and patient outcomes significantly. New technologies in the guise of freehand 3D ultrasound and ultrafast Doppler imaging demonstrate the ingenuity of this diagnostic modality and its integration into clinical practice. These new modalities enable enhanced visualization and measurement of complicated anatomy, allowing more precise assessment during procedures. To illustrate, freehand 3D ultrasound enables operators to construct volumetric images from 2D scans, improving visualization of anatomical details and allowing surgical planning and interventions. Similarly, ultrafast Doppler imaging provides real-time information on blood flow dynamics, enabling clinicians to visualize complex vascular networks during neurosurgery and other complex procedures. These advancements not only enhance the diagnostic potential of ultrasound but also propel a shift toward more personalized and dynamic patient care guidelines. As the field advances, it is necessary for professionals to keep themselves abreast with the principles and development concerning ultrasound imaging in order to provide appropriate patient care (Figure 2.5).

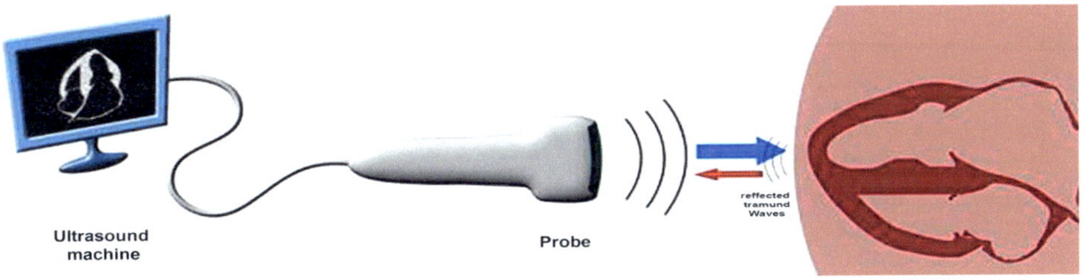

Figure 2.5. Principles of ultrasound imaging.

Source: https://external-content.duckduckgo.com/iu/?u=https%3A%2F%2Fwww.medicalworkseg.com%2Fvirtualecho%2Fhelp%2FUltrasound%2520principles_files%2Fimage002.jpg&f=1&nofb=1&ipt=a5657198fde6760b2286548a7458fe1464b89c04ef44aabde8b5065cad75626e.

2.2.1. Basic Physics of Ultrasound Waves

The physics underlying ultrasound waves is crucial to the success of methods of ultrasound scanning, particularly medical imaging. Ultrasound waves are high-frequency sound waves of frequency between 1 and 15 MHz, which travel through body tissues. When an ultrasound transducer emits these waves, they travel through the body until they strike interfaces of varying tissues, reflecting and refracting. Acoustic impedance changes at these interfaces generate echoes that are picked up by the transducer. This send-and-receive capability makes it possible to produce sonographic images so that healthcare providers can view internal structures non-invasively. Understanding this physics is important in simplifying ultrasound protocols and improving diagnostic findings since different tissues reflect and absorb the ultrasound waves in unique manners, and may affect the image detail and quality of the final images produced. In addition, the behavior of the ultrasound waves in interacting with biological tissue also determines the patient's position to be adopted in scanning procedures. Each position can change the angles at which the ultrasound waves impinge upon different tissues and thereby enhance the quality of the images. For example, in musculoskeletal ultrasound, angulation of the transducer on the joint can enable the examination of structures that might be obscured by bone or other tissues. This patient positioning importance arises directly from the basic physics of ultrasound propagation since good imaging is frequently facilitated by an appreciation of how ultrasound waves propagate and behave within the body. Furthermore, in these advanced uses, such as shear wave elastography, understanding these behaviors of waves yields valuable assessments of tissue stiffness and wellness, ultimately showing the uses of these fundamental physical principles in healthcare (Sedano &Sedano, 2023). With ultrasound imaging, wave propagation principles are likewise pivotal when considering the limitations present with the technology. Such parameters as the dispersion of ultrasound waves when passing through tissues can reduce the effectiveness of imaging, particularly in deeper structures within the tissues. Furthermore, resolution and penetration are determined by frequency; high-frequency waves have greater resolution but less penetration, while low-frequency waves have less resolution but more penetration. Hence, achieving that equilibrium is key to diagnostic clarity. While practitioners use these physics principles to drive real-world situations, they acquire knowledge of how to effectively modify scanning parameters to suit particular patient conditions, and ultimately improve patient care. Additionally, ultrasound techniques advance further by incorporating these fundamental principles, illustrating how comprehensive knowledge of ultrasound physics continues to play a critical role in clinical application today (Peterson & Fenech, 2021) (Figure 2.6).

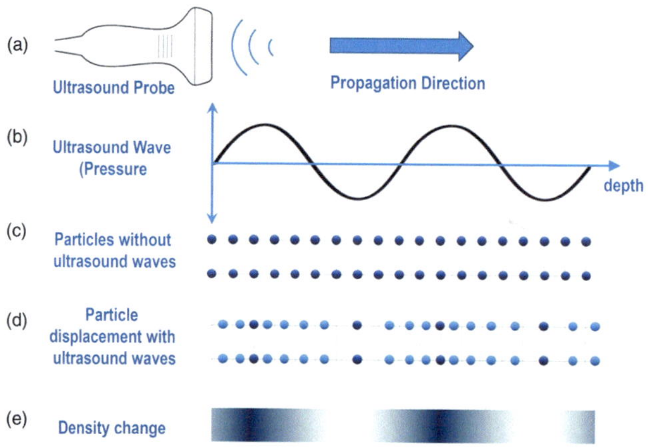

Figure 2.6. Basic physics of ultrasound waves.

Source: https://external-content.duckduckgo.com/iu/?u=https%3A%2F%2Fradiologykey.com%2Fwp-content%2Fuploads%2F2024%2F02%2Fc01f001.jpg&f=1&nofb=1&ipt=7a86a87c57d295c7de045a45b5090cc3552da77a3419308ce0ceb73f184ac8db.

2.2.2. Interaction of Ultrasound with Body Tissues

The way ultrasound behaves when interacting with body tissues forms a fundamental principle upon which the effectiveness of ultrasound scanning techniques relies. Upon emitting high-frequency sound waves from a transducer, these sound waves travel through body tissues that vary in acoustic impedance. The contrast in impedance creates reflection, refraction, and attenuation effects, essentially impacting the quality of the formed ultrasound images. For instance, denser tissues like bone exhibit high reflection and so create bright areas in the resultant images, while softer tissues like fluids exhibit low reflection and hence become dark. This information enhances the skill of clinicians in positioning patients so as to have optimal angles and scanning depths for obtaining the most informative images towards precise diagnosis. Further, the utilitarian and economic uses of ultrasound technology are broader in therapy compared to diagnostic imaging. The properties of ultrasound are also usable for therapy, for example, in the cavitation phenomena within the tissues. With the application of ultrasound waves, they can produce microbubbles that collapse, creating localized heat and shattering of diseased tissues by methods such as High-Intensity Focused Ultrasound (HIFU). This highlights the versatility of ultrasound, both as a diagnostic and a therapeutic tool. The capacity to take into account how various tissues in the body respond in a distinct manner to ultrasound provides the possibility of directed patient positioning to provide optimal therapeutic gain, a multiaxial synergy in which technology meets clinical practice. Further, the use of machine learning techniques on ultrasound scanning is also revolutionizing tissue interaction principles. Algorithms from computers analyzing the complex relationship between ultrasound wave patterns and tissue characteristics can potentially enhance image reading and consequently deliver more accurate diagnoses and assessments. For instance, convolutional neural networks analyze scans to seek patterns not easily visible to the human eye. As this technology develops in conjunction with ultrasound technology, it can potentially offer vastly improved diagnostic accuracy with less dependence on human interpretation. This partnership of advanced imaging techniques and machine learning systems represents not only an advance in the effectiveness of imaging but also advances in patient-specific positioning techniques that avail themselves of such advancements to produce for more understandable and informative scans, which ultimately contribute further toward patient health (Doyle & Wang, 2019; Ker et al., 2017) (Figure 2.7).

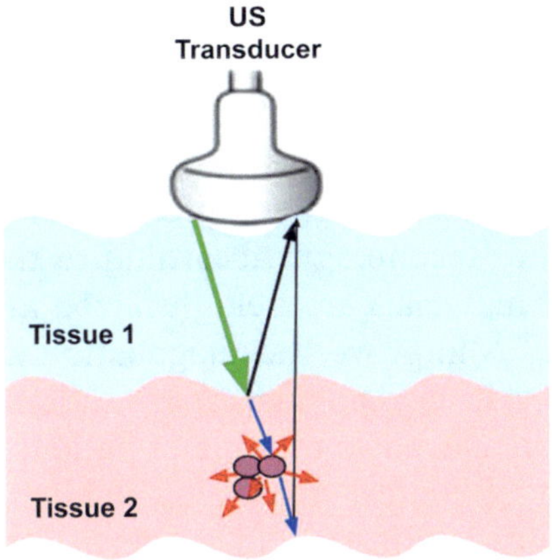

Figure 2.7. Interaction of ultrasound with body tissues.

Source: Almahfouz Nasser, Sahar & Sethi, Amit. (2023). Simulating Ultrasound images from CT Scans. 10.1101/2023.01.16.23284615.

2.2.3. Image Formation and Interpretation

Ultrasound scanning image formation is closely tied to the physics of the sound wave and how it interacts with the tissues of living organisms. The high-frequency sound waves emitted by the ultrasound transducer traverse through the body tissues and reflect back after hitting interfaces between different tissues of different densities. This returning echo is processed to create visual images. The quality of formed images relies upon several variables, including the frequency of the ultrasound waves, machine gain levels, and the directionality at which the emitted waves are projected. High-frequency sound waves obtain a higher resolution at the cost of penetration depth, which in most instances necessitates careful attention to patient positioning for best image quality and diagnostic effectiveness, especially in problematic anatomical regions. Ultrasound image interpretation relies considerably on the experience of the clinicians and the circumstances of the examination. The sonographic and radiologic interpreters must be familiar with the normal vs. abnormal findings, as well as the anatomy visible on the ultrasound. The dynamic nature of ultrasound imaging presents a few unique challenges and requires real-time evaluation that tends to be correlated with patient positioning. By angulating the patient position, practitioners can maximize the visualization of particular organs or lesions. As an example, having the patient positioned in left lateral decubitus can be advantageous for imaging the heart since it brings the heart closer to the transducer and provides improved visualization of the left ventricular wall motion, thus maximizing diagnostic yield and patient safety during the process. Furthermore, the action of ultrasound contrast agents has advanced the power of ultrasound imaging, particularly for non-hepatic applications. Increased image generation in the use of microbubble ultrasound contrast enhances blood or tissue echogenicity, which facilitates better comprehension of more detailed anatomy that cannot be seen using standard ultrasound technology. According to the updated guidelines, for instance, of EFSUMB, these new contrast materials are being utilized more in various applications, including cardiac and vascular imaging, to improve the diagnostic outcome. The possibility of better characterizing pathology, especially in challenging cases, underscores the value of understanding the principles of image formation as well as the role of patient positioning in optimizing ultrasound scanning methods for a variety of clinical situations, highlighting the mutual dependence of technological advancement and clinical utilization in modern ultrasound diagnostics (Sidhu et al., 2018; Alexander et al., 2017) (Figure 2.8).

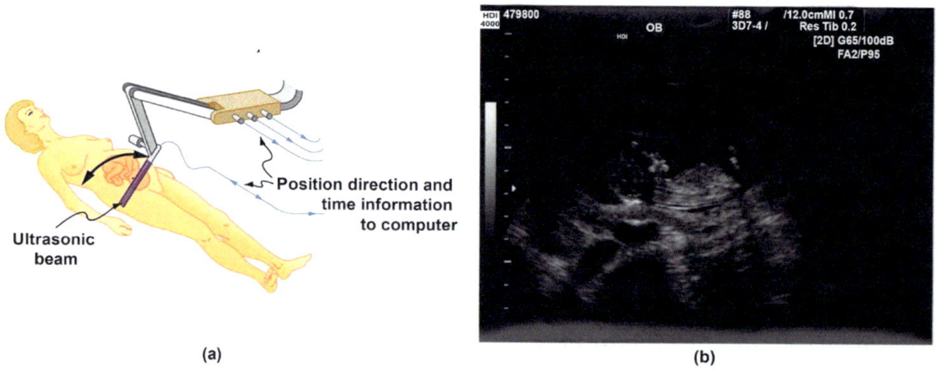

Figure 2.8. Image formation and interpretation in ultrasound scanning.

Source: https://s3-us-west-2.amazonaws.com/courses-images-archive-read-only/wp-content/uploads/sites/222/2016/01/20112957/Figure_18_07_04a.jpg.

2.3. Types of Ultrasound Scanning Techniques

The variability of ultrasound scanning techniques is invaluable in the pursuit of greater diagnostic accuracy and the best patient outcomes. Traditional B-mode ultrasound is unique among other techniques and popular for its ability to visualize real-time images of soft tissues, a life-saving equipment in obstetrics, cardiology, and routine sonography. The technique relies on sound waves that reflect off tissue boundaries to form cross-sectional images, allowing clinicians to study structural defects. Moreover, advancements in Doppler ultrasound technology enable practitioners to measure blood flow and vascular status and view arterial as well as venous systems in real-time. These capabilities emphasize the importance of employing the appropriate scanning method depending on clinical requirements and patient-related aspects, hence optimizing the efficiency of diagnostic imaging. In addition to B-mode and Doppler techniques, 3D and 4D ultrasound scanning is an emerging technology that has come to play a critical role in imaging. Three-dimensional ultrasound scanning allows volumetric data to be gathered, providing a better representation of anatomical structures. Obstetric imaging is particularly favored by this technique, and the possibility of examining fetal development is improved compared to 2D imaging. Although 4D ultrasound adds this concept by bringing in the time dimension, it can visualize the dynamic motion of structures like fetal movement. These sophisticated techniques demand very exact patient positioning in order to achieve optimal image quality and proper diagnostic interpretation, as the sonographer will have to move the transducer to get the required anatomical planes effectively. The integration of these modalities illustrates the ongoing evolution of ultrasound technology in addressing diverse clinical demands. Furthermore, the technique of ultrasound-guided intervention has been popular in the clinic, showing the direction toward more precise and less invasive interventions. For instance, in stellate ganglion blocks for insomnia, identification of vascular anatomy using ultrasound scanning increases safety and efficacy, particularly with anatomical variations creating risk in standard procedures. In methods such as the lateral paravein out-of-plane approach, very high accuracy is attainable when targeting neural structures with fewer complications. This personalized approach puts focus on proper patient positioning, which is crucial for the success of such procedures. As the field of ultrasound continues to expand, research and innovation will be at the forefront to streamline these approaches, potentially leading to novel applications and improved patient management algorithms in clinical practice (Tai et al., 2025; Mo et al., 2024) (Figure 2.9).

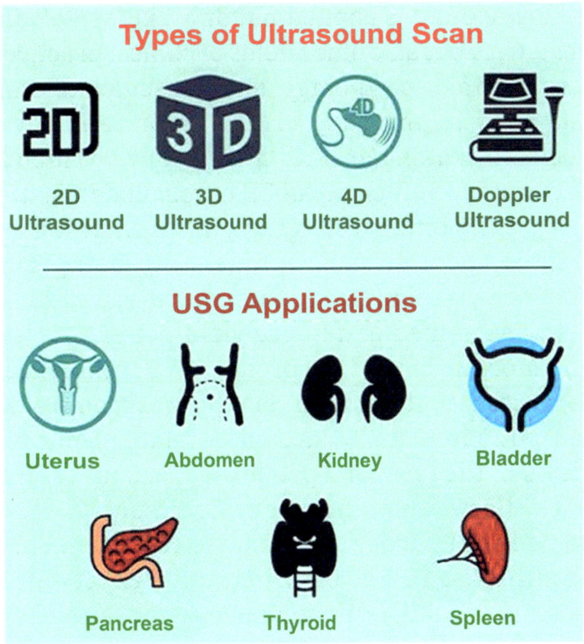

Figure 2.9. Types of ultrasound scanning techniques.

Source: https://external-content.duckduckgo.com/iu/?u=https%3A%2F%2Ftse4.mm.bing.net%2Fth%2Fid%2FOIP.xavLcGnVGel9RQMgR-ryqQHaIB%3Fr%3D0%26pid%3DApi&f=1&ipt=56f3f437d16597a402dea2ba074e4dd7dd6438ae733571dedd585d2c420ce6b7.

2.3.1. 2D Ultrasound Imaging

Ultrasound imaging is currently the focal point of modern medicine, primarily the application of two-dimensional (2D) ultrasound that creates real-time images of soft tissue structures. The process involves high-frequency sound waves transmitted into the body, where they reflect off internal organs and tissues. The reflections are picked up by a transducer, which converts them into visual displays on a monitor. Compared with other imaging modalities such as computed tomography (CT) or magnetic resonance imaging (MRI), 2D ultrasound is non-invasive, ionising-radiation-free, and particularly optimally suited to trace dynamic physiological processes such as fetal development in pregnancy. Consequently, 2D ultrasound is applied not only extensively in obstetrics but also other fields of clinical practice, for example, cardiology and musculoskeletal diagnostics, providing critical information for decision-making in the clinical environment. Accuracy and efficiency of 2D ultrasound imaging are greatly influenced by patient positioning as well as operator skill. Optimal positioning can enhance visualization of the structural anatomy being examined and hence yield better images and more accurate interpretations. For instance, in obstetric ultrasound, supine positioning of the patients usually aids in obtaining optimal views of the fetus and pelvic organs. Conversely, in cardiac examination, specific tilt angles may be needed in order to obtain views of the heart chambers and valves. Operators' experience is also of similar importance; good operator skill will have its comparative improvement in diagnostic accuracy. In addition, standardization of examination protocols, particularly in 2D ultrasound, eliminates variability and makes interpretation more reliable and, ultimately, with a beneficial effect on patient outcome as it ensures consistency between various operators and facilities. Though 2D ultrasound scanning is an important diagnostic tool, it also has limitations. The skill-biasing feature can lead to inconsistencies in image quality and thus create problems in the proper identification of pathological entities. For example, even though 2D scanning can pick up large lesions, it is less effective with small or subtle lesions. This shortcoming points to a trend in favor of greater focus on the integration of more sophisticated approaches, such as Automated Breast Volume Scan (ABVS) and ultrasound elastography (UE), that enhance diagnostic potential through improved reproducibility and reduced operator dependence. As emphasized in current research, the incorporation of such techniques with traditional 2D ultrasound can yield more accurate characterization of lesions, as evidenced by findings demonstrating enhanced diagnostic performance with complementing imaging modalities (Zhang et al., 2025). These advancements underscore the need for ongoing innovation in ultrasound technology to further optimize patient positioning and approaches toward optimizing the diagnostic utility of 2D ultrasound imaging (Mathur et al., 2025) (Figure 2.10).

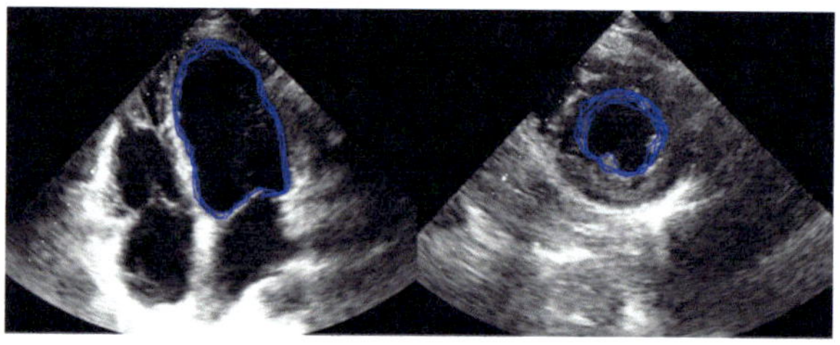

Figure 2.10. 2D ultrasound images of left ventricle.

Source: Sarebani, Maghsoud & Shiran, Mohammad & Bitarafan Rajabi, Ahmad & Rastgoo, Fereidoon & Ojaghihaghighi, Seyedehzahra M & Abbasian Ardakani, Ali. (2020). The impact of frame numbers on cardiac ECG-gated SPECT images with interpolated extra frames using echocardiography. Medical Journal of the Islamic Republic of Iran. 10.47176/mjiri.34.57.

2.3.2. 3D and 4D Ultrasound Imaging

Development in ultrasound technology has seen the introduction of three-dimensional (3D) and four-dimensional (4D) imaging as part of a normal prenatal checkup, with a revolutionized approach to fetal assessment. Unlike the two-dimensional imaging used in the past, 3D ultrasound produces a volumetric image, allowing clinicians to better visualize the complicated anatomical structures. The technology facilitates a more comprehensive study of fetal morphology so that any potential abnormality can be identified. Further, 4D imaging introduces real-time visualization, making it possible for clinicians and parents to actually see fetal behavior and movement. This is an interactive process that can help enhance the emotional connection between parents and the unborn baby. Their application in obstetrics has changed the way obstetricians perform prenatal testing, with better diagnostics that are essential to early intervention and planning, particularly in cases of abnormalities diagnosed in the first trimester (Bilardo et al., 2023).

Positioning of patients during ultrasound imaging is important in ensuring maximum effectiveness of both 3D and 4D imaging. Proper positioning of the patient not only enhances image quality but also enables exhaustive assessment of fetal anatomy. Supine is usually the preferred position since it provides maximum access to the abdominal cavity with minimal patient discomfort. In certain situations, adjustments are necessary, such as the use of lateral positioning to avoid compressions of major abdominal vessels towards the later stages of pregnancy. Appropriate use of transabdominal and transvaginal modalities is very important in the acquisition of high-quality images, especially when dealing with maternal anatomic variation or increased body mass index. As the horizontal plane of the ultrasound beam must intersect target structures accurately, positional adjustments must be strictly managed by the clinicians, whose actions impact the quality of images obtained, especially with advanced 3D and 4D imaging modalities (Panayides et al., 2020). While helpful, 3D and 4D ultrasound imaging application has its challenges. Currently, such technologies are generally reserved for cases necessitating close anatomical assessment and are not standard practice in first-trimester screening. Clinical policy makes strict adherence to accepted practice the priority, with ultrasound study adhering to established viability, proper dating, and assessment of large structural defects within the setting of early prenatal care. In addition, although 3D and 4D imaging possess a high potential to enhance diagnostic capability, they need specialized training and knowledge for handling volumetric data efficiently. This necessity for expert skill sets supports the need for continuous education among ultrasound sonologists and technicians to maintain high-quality practices in using such new technologies. With advancing ultrasound imaging technology, the healthcare industry will have to be vigilant in striking a balance between innovation and guidelines to produce optimal patient outcomes in prenatal care (Bilardo et al., 2023) (Figure 2.11).

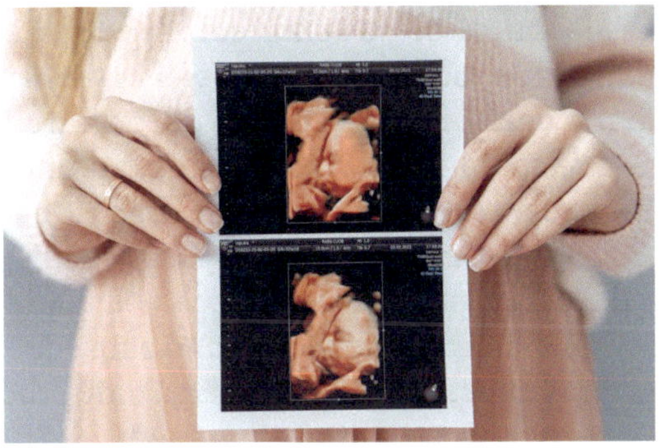

Figure 2.11. 3D and 4D ultrasound imaging.

Source: https://www.pexels.com/photo/a-pregnant-woman-holding-an-ultrasound-picture-7055918/

2.3.3. Doppler Ultrasound Techniques

Doppler ultrasonic techniques have greatly increased the ability to study blood flow in the body, yielding unprecedented data for medical purposes. The techniques take advantage of the Doppler phenomenon, which translates shifts of frequency in backscattered ultrasonic waves off of moving blood cells. Translating such frequency shifts into visual and sound information enables practitioners to effectively measure hemodynamics in real time. This application of Doppler ultrasound extends beyond screening imaging, as it provides information on flow velocity and direction, thereby contributing to diagnosis. The technique is widely applied in cardiology and vascular studies, where information regarding the dynamics of blood flow can inform treatment and predict the course of disease. Hence, the incorporation of Doppler ultrasound into practice enhances diagnostic sensitivity and patient management significantly. The effectiveness of Doppler ultrasound techniques is further enhanced by optimal patient positioning during scanning. Optimal positioning not only helps achieve the best image but also aids in keeping patients comfortable during the procedure. For instance, in assessing vascular conditions, supine with mild elevation of patients could offer better visualization of blood vessels. Furthermore, patient comfort has been determined to influence compliance, a key in the attainment of high-quality results and images (Brasier-Lutz et al., 2023). As observed in comparative imaging mode studies, patient preference will guide the selection of ultrasound modes and subsequently the overall effectiveness of the diagnostic process. By prioritizing patient-centered methods, medical professionals are able to establish a more interactive environment that allows for the optimal use of Doppler ultrasound applications. The incorporation of Doppler techniques into the practice of ultrasound scanning requires a working understanding of both technology and spatial anatomy. Ultrasound, for example, has been used to navigate complex anatomical landmarks, such as the inferior epigastric artery, in laparoscopic procedures such as catheter insertions. Implementation of this technique not only minimizes the chances of complications but also ensures proper device placement within the patient's body (Janež et al., 2023). With the development of Doppler ultrasound, implementation of better imaging modalities, and careful patient positioning will most likely guide the future of new practice in minimally invasive techniques. This technology-technique complementarity reflects the pivotal role of Doppler ultrasound in bridging diagnostic and therapeutic outcomes, thus establishing a critical component of modern ultrasound scanning techniques (Figure 2.12).

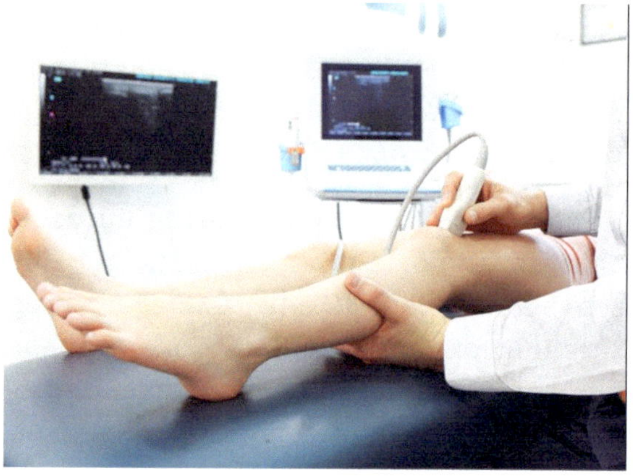

Figure 2.12. Doppler ultrasound techniques.

Source: https://external-content.duckduckgo.com/iu/?u=https%3A%2F%2Fmedia.post.rvohealth.io%2Fwp-content%2Fuploads%2F2020%2F08%2Fdoppler-ultrasound-exam-of-an-arm-or-leg_thumb.jpg&f=1&nofb=1&ipt=ca11a3538dc4066b2a992b1095969342b45570d1bd3436946bf16108439b0d33.

2.4. Patient Positioning Techniques

Proper patient positioning is critical to enhance the maximum results of ultrasound scanning. Not only does proper positioning enhance the quality obtained, but proper positioning also plays a significant role in patient comfort and safety during the process. Some of the most crucial ones include supine, lateral decubitus, and prone positions, with each being appropriate for specific diagnostic needs and anatomical considerations. For instance, the supine position is generally most convenient for scanning the abdomen using ultrasound, since it provides easy access to the anterior abdominal wall and an adequate base for scanning. Similarly, the lateral decubitus position may be useful for imaging structures of the thorax, providing improved exposure of the heart and lungs. In conclusion, understanding these positioning techniques enhances diagnostic quality and patient comfort during ultrasound scanning. Patient positioning is necessary to achieve optimal visualization of the desired anatomy in the course of an ultrasound examination. The use of pillows, wedges, or altering examination table height can significantly enhance patient comfort while affording sonographers greater access to areas of interest. For example, for obstetric ultrasound, proper positioning provides the best views of the baby while keeping the pregnant woman in minimal discomfort. Incorporating adjustable features into ultrasound examination rooms, including tilt features, can facilitate the adjustments for better alignment with the sonographer's line of sight, enhancing both image quality and diagnostic potential. Furthermore, the same techniques may be employed to support patients with mobility issues or other illnesses, showcasing the requirement for tailored techniques among diverse demographic populations.

Technological advancements also accompany patient positioning techniques, as reflected in ongoing research into autonomous initial probe positioning systems. These systems make use of augmented reality markers combined with computer vision algorithms based on AI to deliver higher positioning precision and lower operator dependency, particularly in complex instances such as patient movement. These technologies provide live real-time adjustment and optimize probe placement since they can be observed to achieve a mean depth and xy-plane error that was greater than traditional methods (Zheng et al., 2024). Additionally, the newly acquired capacity to produce strong 3D electrical activation maps resonates with the importance of precise positioning in the context of providing efficient interventions, particularly in cardiological pacing interventions (Fruelund et al., 2022). All these developments foretell higher efficacies and dependabilities in ultrasound scanning operations, thereby resonating the crux of including innovative positioning procedures in routine practice (Figure 2.13).

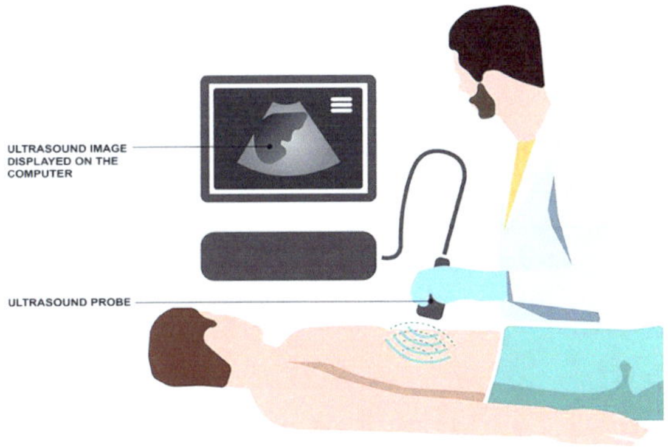

Figure 2.13. Patient positioning techniques in ultrasound scanning.

Source: https://external-content.duckduckgo.com/iu/?u=https%3A%2F%2Fwww.frontiersin.org%2Ffiles%2FArticles%2F516633%2Ffrym-08-00066-HTML-r1%2Fimage_m%2Ffigure-2.jpg&f=1&nofb=1&ipt=849ff28e85cad6a880d68f6d37c8f57aa16e46db26f308e852ebeccd52e1f870.

2.4.1. Common Positions for Abdominal Ultrasound

Patient positioning is of paramount value in the domain of ultrasound imaging, especially for conducting abdominal ultrasounds. Proper positions taken during the procedure are of significance for optimal visibility and attainment of correct diagnostic information. The supine position is most commonly used with easy access to many abdominal organs, like the liver, spleen, and kidneys. Here, patients recline on their back, a position that allows sonographers to take advantage of the natural air-filled structure of the intestines and gives direct access to solid organs. The supine position is also convenient for easy manipulation of the ultrasound probe for thorough scanning along various anatomical planes. This baseline positioning allows for the effectiveness of prompt screening protocols and aids in the accurate diagnosis of conditions such as appendicitis and abdominal masses, which points to the importance of accurate patient positioning in ultrasound scanning protocols. Another standard position that is used during the abdominal ultrasound is the left lateral decubitus position, ideally suited for the investigation of certain conditions. This is the side position where the patient is supine on the left, and this enhances visual inspection of organs in the right abdomen, such as the liver and the gallbladder.

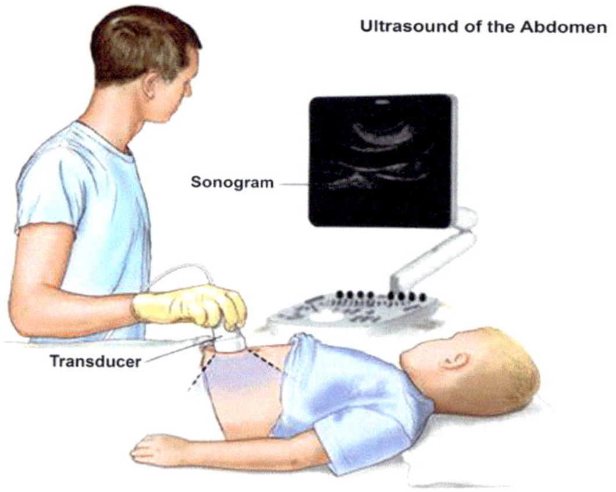

Figure 2.14. Common positions for abdominal ultrasound.

Source: Terese Winslow (2015). Ultrasound, Abdominal, Child. National Cancer Institute.

The left lateral position can also help to evaluate the splenic area, reducing the interference that can be brought about by the stomach's gas-filled contents. This technique is especially important in the assessment of presumptive gallstone or cholecystitis because it may allow for increased visualization of gallbladder distension. Moreover, the left lateral decubitus position becomes widely recommended when assessing obese patients or those with excess abdominal fat because this allows for accommodation to the consequent anatomical changes of excess body mass and maintains optimal image clarity and diagnostic result (Zhang et al., 2025). Lastly, the erect position can also be essential in abdominal ultrasound examinations, particularly in patients with gastrointestinal conditions. With patients in the erect position, one is able to efficiently assess fluid-related conditions such as ascites, utilizing gravity to repose contents in the abdomen. The position enables efficient assessment of some pathologies, enhancing diagnostic sensitivity when assessing fluid levels or other masses intrabdominally. While less common than supine or left lateral decubitus positions, the upright position can significantly improve ultrasonographic findings when diagnosing disorders like intestinal obstruction, for which real-time imaging techniques are employed to quantify peristalsis and bowel motility. Through planned application, patient position remains indispensable in fulfilling the success of abdominal ultrasound scans, ultimately leading to improved diagnostic findings and patient management (Albishare et al., 2025) (Figure 2.14).

2.4.2. Positions for Obstetric Ultrasound

Patient positioning is crucial in obstetric ultrasonography in obtaining precise and clear images while avoiding discomfort and injury. The most commonly applied position is the supine position, and this gives access to the abdomen. The patient will, however, have complications, such as hypotension due to compression of the inferior vena cava by the pregnant uterus, when placed in such a position for long periods. To avoid this risk as much as possible, the left lateral tilt position is generally recommended, particularly in higher pregnancy. The left lateral tilt position is among the positioning techniques that facilitate optimal blood flow with minimal effort as sonographers obtain needed fetal views and measurements. Good patient positioning is not only essential for the quality of imaging results but also for the facilitation of maternal and fetal comfort during the procedure. In addition, specialized positioning techniques can be employed in accordance with clinical situations. For instance, the lateral decubitus position can be helpful in the imaging of specific fetal anatomy and in cases where the mother prefers not to stay in the supine position. Additionally, in specific instances, the comfort level and stability throughout the scan can be improved with aids such as wedges or pillows. Further, when there is a need for pelvic ultrasound scanning, for instance, in screening for ectopic pregnancies or in assessing the health of the ovaries, the positioning of the patients must be rearranged accordingly. These positioning methods must be learned and perfected by the sonographers to ensure that the procedure is made effective and even enhances the patient's comfort throughout the process. More significantly, technology also affects patient positioning protocols in obstetric ultrasound. Technological innovations in hand-carried ultrasound devices now permit use outside the traditional clinical setting, and this calls for adaptability in patient placement. It makes practice change, and practitioners have to be challenged to practice, enhancing their capabilities to support many environments without compromising on diagnostic quality. A good case in point is performing ultrasounds in field settings or within rural areas, where health professionals have to consider the resources available as well as the unique conditions of each patient. As emphasized in contemporary discourse around obstetric ultrasound, adequate knowledge of various positions is crucial for obtaining maximum imaging quality, as well as for ensuring the safety of maternal and fetal health during the scanning process (Tsvetkov et al., 2024; Parker et al., 2022) (Figure 2.15).

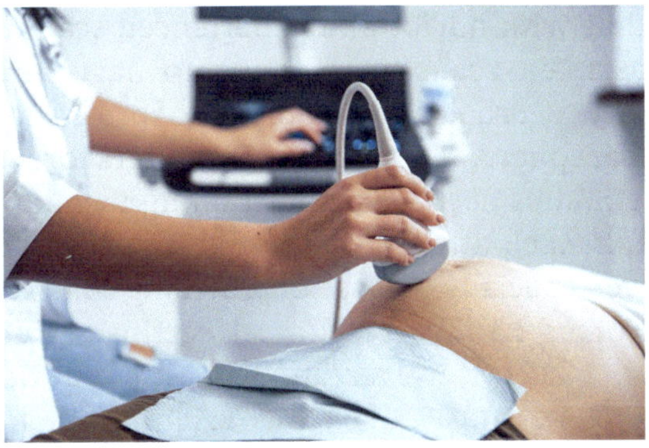

Figure 2.15. Positions for obstetric ultrasound.

Source: Standret/stock.adobe.com. https://t4.ftcdn.net/jpg/03/02/47/55/240_F_302475551_lveqXWf4bdyKBmxC7rY3i8FeJgnaeCjF.jpg

2.4.3. Specialized Positions for Cardiac Ultrasound

In cardiac ultrasound, patient position during scanning is of utmost importance in assisting to obtain accurate diagnoses. Special positions not only ensure optimal quality of images but also assist in assessing cardiac structures and function. For instance, left lateral decubitus is a frequent position utilized for improved visibility of the heart because it enables gravity to assist in straightening cardiac anatomy. This positioning is particularly valuable when imaging in obese or other anatomically varying patients obscuring the standard view. Position selection ultimately can play a substantial role in the ability to obtain satisfactory quality images, often making or breaking the echocardiographic assessment in complex cases. The technology keeps evolving and continues to influence the approach to developing and employing specialized positions in cardiac ultrasound. The FDA-approved Caption Echocardiography system is an example of this advancement, employing artificial intelligence to lead novice practitioners to optimal scanning positions. By leading users step by step through positioning and automatically capturing images, the device reduces the range of human inconsistency. In studies with novice and experienced scanners, AI-assisted scans were found to have image quality regarded as equal to that of professional sonographers. These findings underscore the potential of new tools and training techniques to enhance patient care through the assurance of even specialty personnel providing consistent outcomes in diverse clinical settings (Burke et al., 2022). However, application of specialty positions and advanced technologies in cardiac ultrasound requires a comprehensive understanding of the intrinsic anatomical challenges that clinicians face. For example, as regional anesthesia literature explains, clinicians need to adapt technique based on the individual physiologies of patients, particularly those who are obese with potentially altered anatomical landmarks (De Cassai et al., 2025). Positioning modifications can significantly improve ultrasound guidance and, by default, ensure accurate and effective examinations. Thus, all the patient positioning, operator skill, and technology support need to be brought into alignment to obtain the best outcome in echocardiography, particularly in complicated cases that need customized techniques.

2.5. Factors Affecting Patient Positioning

In ultrasound scanning, patient positioning is a critical factor in the quality of imaging diagnostics and therefore influences procedural success. Anatomical patient consideration is one such significant factor, as certain positions enhance better visualization of targeted organs or structures. Variation in patient body habitus, such as obesity or scarring from earlier surgery, can complicate routine techniques of positioning, necessitating alterations to acquire optimum imaging results. For instance, the side position can be used when the normal supine position hinders access to some anatomical sites. The comfort of the person performing the procedure is also a concern because pain from improper positioning makes the patient shift and affect image quality. Understanding thus comes with the fine balance between patient anatomy and positioning is key to successful ultrasound applications. Also, the physiological and psychological state of the patients is a determinant in establishing proper positioning when there is ultrasound imaging. Pain or anxiety causes unintended tightening of muscles, further complicating the process of imaging and in the process hiding diagnostic accuracy. Position adjustments when stabilizing patients not only make it easier to get good quality images but also influence the patient experience in a clinical setting. A nice illustration is the use of cervical ultrasound scanning during procedures such as stellate ganglion blocks, in which accurate positional accommodations must be made in order to allow space for patients' anatomical differences, particularly those with untypical vertebral artery patterns. This is an illustration of how the collaboration between knowledge of patient anatomy and emotional state will help healthcare workers in delivering effective imaging services. Lastly, the choice of ultrasound scanning technique profoundly affects the strategy of positioning in practice. Studies have shown differing scanning techniques—for example, radial breast ultrasound (r-US) vs. meander-like ultrasound (m-US)—in patient comfort and levels of self-reported satisfaction, thereby creating implications for positioning protocols. With patients reporting higher comfort levels with r-US that can readily be facilitated with some positioning, there is a need for clinicians to consider patient preferences when embracing scanning techniques. Such flexibility not only ensures increased levels of compliance but also promotes a culture of effective communication between providers and patients, ultimately yielding improved imaging outcomes. The evolving understanding of variables influencing patient positioning highlights the importance of synthesizing technical expertise with compassionate care in the ultrasound scanning process.

2.5.1. Patient Comfort and Safety

Patient comfort is a key point in the field of ultrasound scanning techniques and patient positioning. Keeping patients comfortable does not merely make them more satisfied with their visit but also enhances the quality of the imaging result. Improper positioning can lead to discomfort, which can cause the patient to tense up or shift while undergoing the procedure, eventually compromising the quality of the ultrasound images obtained. Providers must maintain patient comfort as a priority by employing supportive methods such as soft cushions, positionally adjustable tables, and open communication about the procedure. Through the creation of an atmosphere that minimizes patient anxiety and discomfort, providers can enhance patient cooperation and participation, essential in providing accurate diagnosis and treatment planning.

Patient safety during ultrasound procedures is also associated with proper positioning and the use of advanced ultrasound scanning technologies. Improper positioning can cause dangers such as falls or unnecessary stress to vulnerable parts of the body, especially among critically ill patients. Adaptive variable admittance control methods used in ultrasound procedures will significantly enhance both comfort and safety. The method ensures precise force tracking, thereby preventing sensitive contact between the patient and the ultrasound transducer. By alleviating possible discomfort and avoiding the risk of injury associated with traditional approaches, these new technologies place emphasis on the integration of technological advances in clinical practice as a way of enhancing patient safety during ultrasound scanning (Xiao et al., 2025). Secondly, the use of new imaging techniques, such as freehand 3D ultrasound systems, presents possibilities for patient safety and comfort improvement during scanning. These systems allow bedside monitoring without the need to move patients to imaging rooms, eliminating the inherent movement and handling risks in critically ill patients. This capability is vital to ongoing monitoring of conditions such as midline shift in neurocritical care settings, where timely decision-making can make or break outcomes for patients. The precision of ultrasound systems and the built-in minimal invasiveness diminish discomfort, further leading to an overall enhanced patient experience. As this technology continues to develop, it is important that medical practitioners remain proficient in utilizing these new technologies to improve patient comfort and safety while maintaining a commitment to high-quality care (Mathur et al., 2025) (Figure 2.15).

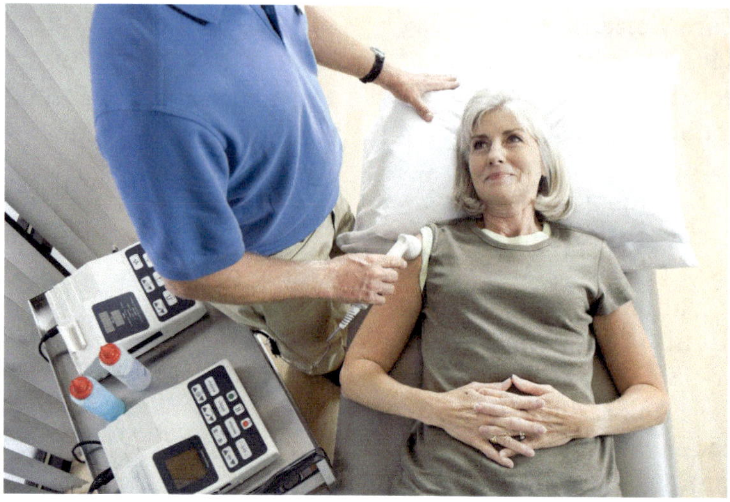

Figure 2.15. Patient comfort and safety in ultrasound.

Source: https://www.verywellhealth.com/thmb/1GTYwN05yg_sYwojUlx_OymN4rM=/1500x0/filters:no_upscale():max_bytes(150000):strip_icc()/image-56a72aff3df78cf77292f423.jpg.

2.5.2. Anatomical Considerations

In the work of ultrasound scanning, anatomical considerations are paramount in patient positioning and the quality of diagnostic imaging attained. Ultrasound results are heavily reliant on the sonographer's skill in identifying anatomical landmarks, whose variability is patient-dependent and hence influenced by factors like body mass index and gestational age. The International Society of Ultrasound in Obstetrics and Gynecology (ISUOG) emphasizes the use of an organized examination protocol that enables proper assessments of fetal anatomy at crucial stages of gestation, from 11 + 0 to 14 + 0 weeks. This period is critical in determining viability, gestational age, and screening for congenital anomalies, and therefore, correct patient positioning becomes central to the attainment of corresponding anatomical planes (Bilardo et al., 2023). Through a thorough understanding of normal anatomy in such procedures, early identification of potential abnormalities is enabled, thereby allowing for essential intervention and management where necessary. Sufficient patient positioning enhances imaging of vital anatomical structures throughout the examination course of ultrasound. The ideal position can significantly improve image quality, reducing the likelihood of suboptimal images from overlaying tissues or inadequate acoustic windows. As an illustration, a transabdominal study could be warranted in patients presenting with a lower body mass index because visualization of fetal anatomy is superior. But in patient cases of increased abdominal girth, a transvaginal scan may offer better resolution and contrast (Malinger et al., 2020). Since active positioning methods are handled directly by sonographers, they can offer a full examination of anatomical structures such as the fetal head, spine, and vital organs, which are essential for diagnosing conditions like neural tube defects or cardiac defects. Thus, having some understanding of how patient posture and anatomical access interrelate is key to optimizing ultrasound outcomes. In addition to positioning the patient, sonographers must be proficient at employing techniques that are adaptable to anatomical variations between gestational ages. A constantly changing fetal anatomy between the first two trimesters requires a dynamic scanning method. Specific anatomical landmarks, such as the crown-rump length and nuchal translucency, must be accurately measured during the early gestation phase to guide clinical decision-making for further referral or assessment (Bilardo et al., 2023). Additionally, sonographic skill in obtaining and interpreting anatomical planes is an important consideration in the identification of structural anomalies because some are more visible at specific time periods. Therefore, rigorous training and adherence to prescriptive standards, as provided by ISUOG, enable sonographers to more effectively handle the complexities of fetal anatomy, both raising the precision of diagnoses and the quality of patient care in obstetric imaging (Figure 2.16).

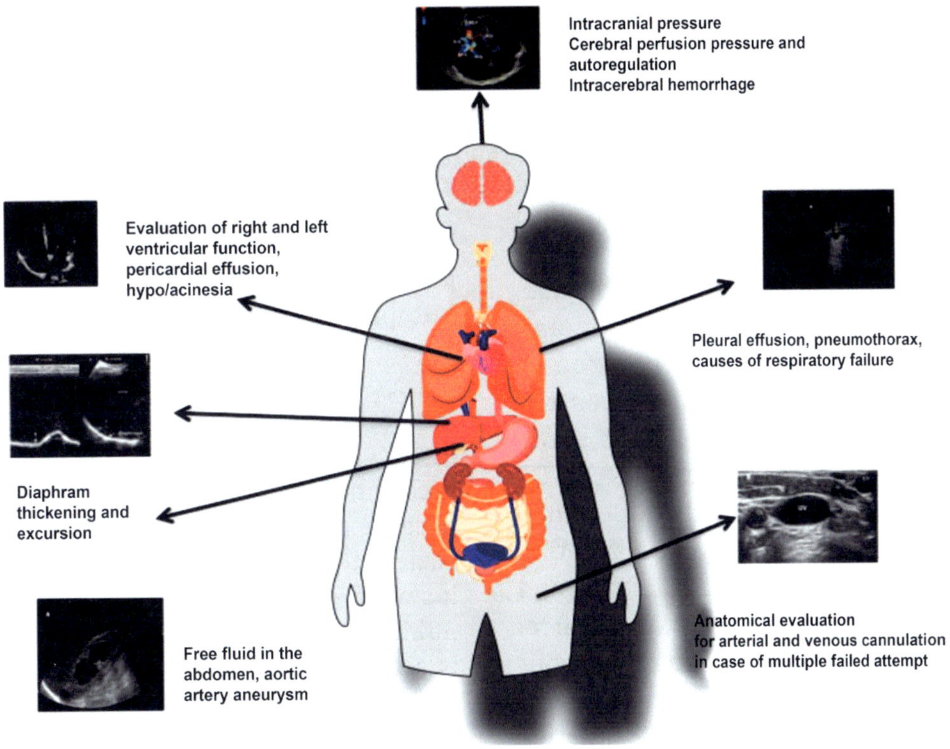

Figure 2.16. Anatomical considerations in ultrasound.

Source: Messina, A., Robba, C., Bertuetti, R. et al. (2022). Head to toe ultrasound: a narrative review of experts' recommendations of methodological approaches. J Anesth Analg Crit Care 2, 44. https://doi.org/10.1186/s44158-022-00072-5 .

2.5.3. Specific Diagnostic Requirements

In ultrasound scanning, some diagnostic needs are imperative to achieve for the delivery of maximum patient care and sound medical assessment. As ultrasound technology has developed, its application for diagnosing various medical conditions increasingly requires accurate patient placement and tailored scanning techniques. For instance, anatomical and pathological considerations in the patient dictate the optimal placement of the transducer for the best image quality. Research on the viability of freehand 3D ultrasound systems for serious purposes, such as measuring midline shifts in brain trauma patients, points to the importance of certain diagnostic measures.

Not only do these types of procedures offer bedside monitoring, but they also bypass serious limitations associated with traditional imaging modalities. With optimization of these diagnostic criteria, patients can be assisted with improved results through early intervention without the hazards of moving critically ill patients to imaging rooms (Mathur et al., 2025).

Differences in patient status, such as age and physiological conditions, also contribute to the difficulty of looking for improved ultrasound diagnostics. A recent study investigated the role of age, sex, and smoking status in the visualization of the vocal cords in patients with thyroid disease and emphasizes the necessity for the diagnostic adjustment that is needed. As indicated by the study, advanced age and lifestyle factors are related to ossification of the thyroid cartilage, which complicates the usefulness of ultrasound scanning. The study indicates that in patients over the age of 57 years, ultrasound procedures may be suboptimal due to this ossification, thereby necessitating other types of tests or alternative ultrasound techniques for accurate diagnosis. Hence, adjusting the protocols of ultrasound to suit the profiles of patients remain imperative for achieving diagnostic success in practice (Subbotina et al., 2024). Finally, compliance with established guidelines for ultrasound scanning is essential to meet certain requirements for diagnosis. Specialized training in color Doppler imaging and 3D reconstructions augments sonographers' skills for accurate evaluation of structural and functional parameters across varying clinical settings. The integration of guidelines, such as guidelines for the evaluation of midline shift by the Brain Trauma Foundation, establishes uniform practices on which to base confidence in ultrasound diagnosis across a range of conditions. Through concentration on systematic approaches to patient positioning and imaging, healthcare professionals can significantly enhance the standardization of ultrasound results. Thus, a concerted effort toward achieving these diagnostic requirements through rigorous training, ongoing research, and adherence to best practices ultimately leads to improved healthcare for ultrasound technology-reliant patients (Mathur et al., 2025).

2.6. Ultrasound Scanning and Positioning Issues

The application of ultrasound scanning is the pivotal focus in most diagnostic applications, but providers have numerous challenges in implementing it. Of importance is the challenge related to patient positioning because this can impact the quality of images attained directly. Effective positioning is important in order to access the target anatomy accurately, particularly in cases involving anatomy difficult to visualize, such as the testes or retroperitoneal organs. For instance, according to (Belfield & Findlay-Line , 2022), proper attention to patients' positioning is required to acquire a quality scan for initial imaging examination of a testicular tumor. Poor or incorrect positioning produces poor-quality images that do not provide definite diagnostic information, and these images might need repeat examination, resulting in patient discomfort and anxiety. In addition to patient positioning, the technical aspect of conducting the ultrasound scan presents its own set of difficulties.

The operator must masterfully glide the transducer over the skin in an attempt to produce quality images, as pointed out by Goel et al. (2022). Coordination is particularly difficult with acute injury patients or in patients requiring urgent assessment within field conditions. The need to maintain constant acoustic coupling with motion over varied surfaces contributes to the procedure's complexity. All these contribute to leading an operator to fatigue, ultimately affecting the reliability and efficacy of the ultrasound scan. Moreover, acquiring a true characterization of the abnormalities may be hindered, especially by the capacity limitations of routine ultrasound imaging techniques in complex cases. Finally, the interpretation of ultrasound findings becomes challenging when diagnostic characteristics overlap between conditions. For instance, the appearance of a testicular tumor can be mimicked by pathologies such as orchitis, posing challenges in diagnosis as indicated in Belfield & Findlay-Line (2022). Furthermore, small testicular lesions hinder visual detection on ultrasound, leading to false positives or false negatives. As the demand for precision in imaging increased, the implementation of newer technologies—such as automated ultrasound systems—stood as a potential solution to overcome these challenges. Through the utilization of new methods, including robotic assistance and advanced imaging algorithms, practitioners are able to optimize scanning efficiency, diagnostic precision, and ultimately patient care in the medical field of ultrasound (Figure 2.17).

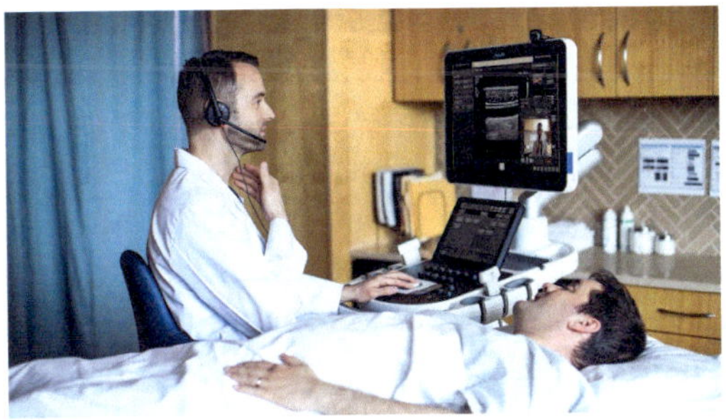

Figure 2.17. Challenges in ultrasound scanning and positioning.

Source: https://www.philips.com/c-dam/corporate/innovation-and-you/global/dec-2021/hero-blog-ultrasound.jpg.

2.6.1 Technical Limitations of Ultrasound

The technical limitations of ultrasound are the supreme considerations when it comes to ultrasound scanning techniques and patient positioning. Despite its advantages, that is, non-invasive, real-time imaging, ultrasound is susceptible to a number of technical problems that can compromise diagnostic accuracy. For instance, the quality of images obtained can be significantly affected by the patient's body mass index (BMI), the occurrence of gas in the intestines, and the selection of transducer frequency. A high BMI tends to cause more attenuation of the ultrasound waves, thus poor image resolution. Besides, artifacts caused by overlying structures or bone can obscure critical diagnostic information, thus making anatomical features difficult to correctly assess. Understanding these aspects will enable healthcare providers to maximize the performance of the ultrasound imaging and attain optimal patient positioning for improved visualization. Another major drawback of ultrasound machines is their operator dependence. Image quality and, more so, interpretation are significantly based on the proficiency and expertise of the ultrasound technician or clinician. Variability in operator technique can lead to inconsistency in image acquisition and interpretation, further impacting patient care. Additionally, the learning curve of gaining expertise in conducting ultrasound techniques can prove a heavy load on inexperienced operators. They can also have difficulty maintaining the proper orientations and angles when positioning the transducer, resulting in misinterpretation of what they are observing. Cautious training and application of standardized protocols are, therefore, needed to overcome the issues of operator dependency and enhance the reliability of ultrasound as a diagnostic method. In addition, standardization is not merely an issue of operator skill but also technology applied in ultrasound scanning. Quality and setting differences in equipment can cause differences in output image and measurement accuracy. Moreover, poor standardization of ultrasound protocols and guidelines can bring about interpretation differences, which can affect clinical outcomes. For example, the lack of clearly stated imaging criteria can lead to misdiagnosis, particularly in complex cases where precise measurement is important. In addition, as technology such as 3D and Doppler ultrasound continues to get better, there is still an urgent need for new protocols to incorporate these technologies into enhancing diagnostics while overcoming existing limitations. Merging well-tested guidelines with trustworthy technologies is important for maximizing ultrasounds' overall efficiency in clinical practice, as attested to by institutions such as ISUOG (Coutinho et al., 2022) and the rising demand for exosomal research in optimizing diagnostic routines (Doyle & Wang, 2019).

2.6.2. Patient-Related Problems

The efficiency of the utilization of ultrasound scanning techniques depends largely on several patient-related challenges, which could negatively affect both the accuracy of the scans and the patient's experience overall. Of primary concern is the distress and discomfort felt by patients during procedures, particularly when scanning sensitive areas. For instance, patients undergoing cervical ultrasound examinations may worry about what will be discovered or the invasiveness of the test. Such anxiety causes them difficulty in being able to maintain the necessary position, leading to suboptimal imaging results. Methods of minimizing anxiety, including making explicit explanations concerning what is to be done and the use of comfort-oriented patient positioning, can contribute to greater cooperation from patients and better outcomes. Thus, dealing with psychological and physical discomfort is crucial in the effective application of ultrasound in clinical practice. Other than emotional complications, the specific individual anatomical features of each patient form challenges during scanning with ultrasound. The difference in anatomy makes the standard scanning protocol difficult, and hence, visualization and interpretation of results become troublesome. For example, in cervical ultrasound, anatomical variations such as variant vertebral artery patterns can be dangerous during procedures aimed at interventions like stellate ganglion blocks, as recommended in recent literature. Very careful patient positioning is required to avoid complications from such variation. As observed in clinical reports, ultrasound-guided approaches could be modified in patients with uncommon anatomical features. Therefore, understanding the individual anatomy of the patient not only facilitates improved imaging but also enhances safety and efficiency with ultrasound exams, emphasizing the necessity of individualized approaches to patient positioning. Technical limitations inherent in the ultrasound machine can also impact imaging and diagnostic quality, representing a significant patient-related issue. Traditional imaging modalities are usually reliant on advanced configurations and susceptible to artefacts, and can complicate the examination of joint movement or soft tissue anatomy. For instance, when it comes to imaging of the patellofemoral joint using traditional imaging, metal artefacts may cover valuable diagnostic information. Advances in technology in the use of ultrasound, such as the combination of 2D ultrasound with advanced motion tracking techniques for three-dimensional reconstruction, offer solutions that are highly promising against such challenges. These advances promise to improve significantly the accuracy of joint evaluation but bring along the responsibility of ensuring proper patient positioning and comfort during scanning. With increasing technology, it is important to continue optimizing procedures in ultrasound scanning so as to effectively address these patient-complexity concerns optimally, as noted in recent research methods like integrating the VIO methodology towards better utilization of ultrasound-based assessments (Mo et al., 2024; Buchanan et al., 2024) (Figure 2.18).

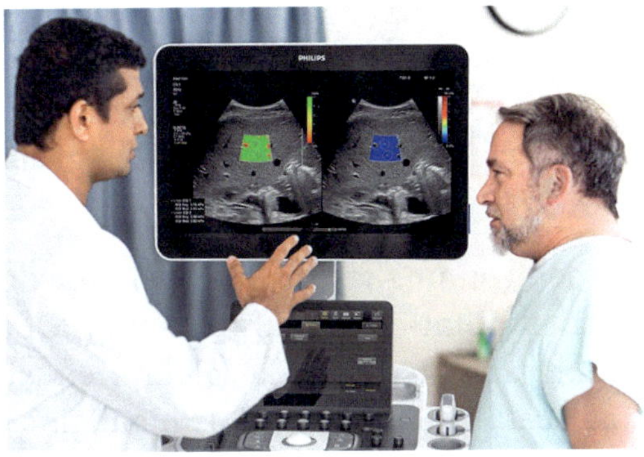

Figure 2.18. Patient-related challenges.

Source: https://www.philips.com/c-dam/corporate/innovation-and-you/global/dec-2021/02-image-blog-ultrasound-lfq.jpg.

2.6.3. Solutions to Common Positioning Issues

Resolving prevalent positioning issues in ultrasound scanning is of basic significance in achieving optimum diagnostic images, which subsequently enhances patient safety and comfort. A popular solution amongst these is the utilization of support equipment, such as foam wedges or cushions, to align a patient's position, particularly in challenging areas like the abdominal area or pulmonary regions. The gadgets help minimize movement, thus allowing better visualization of anatomical features. Moreover, the use of tiltable and rotatable exam tables ensures that patients can be placed in appropriately for specific scans such as echocardiograms or abdominal ultrasounds. Such flexibility not only assists in gaining quality images but also suits the varied body sizes and conditions of patients, which indicates a patient-centered element in sonography practice. A second effective method of avoiding positioning challenges is the use of guided ultrasound. For instance, utilitarian application of real-time ultrasound during procedures can enhance positioning and accuracy. This method has been proven to be effective in vascular access and regional anesthesia, where correct anatomical visualization is essential to avoid complications like nerve damage or vessel puncture. Along with this, the application of advanced imaging modalities, that is, three-dimensional ultrasound, can potentially aid in improved understanding of complex anatomical relationships so that positioning can be adjusted accordingly. This integrative strategy focuses on training sonographers and physicians in advanced ultrasound techniques so that future positioning pitfalls are eliminated during scanning. Last but not least, promoting patient communication during the ultrasound procedure is an essential solution to preventing positioning challenges. Instructing patients on the positioning process and movement involved can remove anxiety, facilitating cooperation and tranquility during exams. Providing direct instructions not only reassures patients but also forms a part of their overall active involvement in the process. Additionally, having feedback channels through which discomfort is communicated allows healthcare professionals to take prompt action in adjusting positioning. This interactive communication allows for a harmonious environment that significantly enhances diagnostic reliability while ensuring that patient safety and comfort are adequately addressed, a necessity in the provision of quality healthcare (Tayler et al., 2020; Doyle & Wang, 2019).

SUMMARY

Advances in ultrasound scanning techniques have transformed diagnostic practice in a number of fields of clinical practice. The shift not only emphasizes the importance of technological change but also the utmost importance of correct patient positioning to enhance imaging outcomes. Familiarity with a variety of ultrasound techniques and optimal positioning approaches can lead to more accurate diagnoses and enhanced patient care. As shown by numerous meta-analyses, ranging from those comparing ultrasound-guided procedures with traditional procedures, the accuracy of ultrasound can minimize complications and increase success rates and thus aid healthcare professionals in making the right clinical decisions (Huang et al., 2025).

Moreover, contrast of different imaging modalities is a determining factor in decision-making for patient treatment. For instance, current studies indicate that point-of-care ultrasound (POCUS) is of greater diagnostic utility compared to chest radiography for diseases like pleural effusion, especially in the aspect of patient positioning during testing (Zaki et al., 2024). This highlights the importance of medical practitioners having skills in ultrasound techniques because their integration into routine assessments can enhance diagnostic capabilities and patient care, particularly in emergency departments or resource-limited environments. In synthesizing the learning from the review of ultrasound scanning technology and patient positioning, it is evident that research and training are needed to maximize these benefits. Critical analysis of existing practices reveals an imperative need to standardize procedures and upgrade educational systems to provide healthcare professionals with the required skills in ultrasound use and patient positioning. Through the establishment of a culture of continuous learning and the adaptation of best practices, the health care industry can achieve improved patient outcomes, improved delivery efficiency, and increased alignment of ultrasound technologies with clinical needs in the future.

Precise patient positioning is a critical aspect of integrating ultrasound scanning methods into clinical practice. The quality of images obtained during ultrasound scans depends directly on careful attention to the patient's posture, and to obtain optimal results from ultrasound scans, such details are carefully observed. Several positions, including supine, lateral, or prone, are utilized, each serving a diagnostic purpose. For example, particular conditions will demand positional modifications to achieve optimal visibility of anatomical structures, thereby enhancing the diagnostic rate. Furthermore, proper patient positioning minimizes discomfort and facilitates cooperation during the procedure, critical for the effective achievement of high-quality images. The relationship between effective positioning and ultrasound technique emphasizes the need for health care clinicians to be competent in both the technology and patient-focused strategies that account for individual anatomy and clinical conditions. In evaluating the advances in ultrasound technologies, an intensified emphasis is being placed on the need for standard operating procedures (SOPs) that have patient positioning guidelines. The development of SOPs is necessary to enhance the consistency of image quality among operators and environments. The protocols are not just a template for conducting ultrasound scanning procedures but also a guide ensuring compliance with best practice. For example, variations in ultrasound machines and transducer models can require tailored positioning techniques to optimize imaging. Consequently, the development of comprehensive training programs representing the most up-to-date knowledge in ultrasound technology and patient positioning is a necessity for sonographers and radiologists. The programs would enhance practice excellence as well as intimate familiarity with the physiological implications of positioning on imaging findings. As technology progresses in ultrasounds, the role of patient involvement in positioning should not be underestimated. The patients must be educated on the value of cooperation during scanning, as their compliance may play an important role in the quality of ultrasound images obtained. The use of open communication regarding the requirement for some positions and reassurance on the procedure can enhance compliance and minimize anxiety. Patient involvement facilitates cooperation and enhances the experience and result of ultrasound scans. The convergence of these key points highlights not only the technical aspects of ultrasound scanning but also the profound interplay of human variables dictating diagnostic effectiveness. As underscored in recent guidelines, emphasizing both the technological and experiential aspects of ultrasound procedures will powerfully advance patient care in practice (Mathijssen, 2020; Percie et al., 2020).

CLOSER LOOK

SONOGRAPHY

Sonography, ultrasonography, or diagnostic medical ultrasound is a widely used imaging method that employs high-frequency sound waves to produce real-time images of internal body structures. It is non-invasive, radiation-free, and relatively low-cost, and thus a diagnostic tool of first choice in numerous specialties. Sonography achieves this by emitting the sound waves into the body through a handheld device called a transducer. These sound waves bounce off liquid and organs and tissues, and the returning echoes are picked up by the transducer and converted to visual forms by the ultrasound equipment. The operator's experience, the frequency of the sound waves, and the acoustic properties of tissues to be examined have a significant impact on the quality and interpretation of such images. The higher frequency waves are more resolved but less penetrating, so they are reserved for superficial structures, whereas lower frequencies penetrate more poorly but more clearly. Sonography is also used extensively in obstetrics to monitor fetal growth, estimate gestational age, diagnose congenital malformations, and perform amniocentesis. In gynecology, it is used to evaluate the uterus, ovaries, and adnexa for abnormalities such as fibroids, cysts, or pregnancy outside the uterus. Sonography of the abdomen is necessary for assessment of organs like the liver, gallbladder, kidneys, spleen, pancreas, and bladder, and for the detection of gallstones, hydronephrosis, liver masses, and other diseases. Cardiac sonography, or echocardiography, assesses heart structure and function, valve integrity, chamber size, and ejection fraction, which are critical in the diagnosis of heart failure and valve disease. In vascular studies, Doppler sonography measures arterial and venous blood flow, which helps diagnose such conditions as DVT, arterial stenosis, and aneurysm. Sonography of the musculoskeletal system yields dynamic images of tendons, ligaments, joints, and soft tissue masses and is frequently used in orthopedics and sports medicine. Moreover, point-of-care ultrasound (POCUS) is increasingly used by emergency and critical care physicians to conduct rapid bedside ultrasounds for the evaluation of free fluid, directing fluid resuscitation, or monitoring cardiac activity in resuscitation. Sonography complements mammography by differentiating cystic and solid masses and assisting biopsies. Sonography is an online real-time guidance modality for aspirations, biopsies, catheter placements, and injections in interventional procedures, increasing accuracy and reducing complications. Even though sonography has many advantages, it also has certain limitations, such as dependency on the operator, less penetration in obese patients, and difficult imaging of gas-filled or bone-covered structures. Artifacts such as shadowing or enhancement must be recognized and interpreted correctly. New technological developments, including 3D and 4D imaging, contrast-enhanced ultrasound, elastography, and embedding with artificial intelligence, are rapidly enhancing the diagnostic capability of sonography. Despite the advent of other high-resolution imaging technologies like CT and MRI, sonography remains essential due to its portability, safety, and ability to generate images in real time. It is particularly important where there is radiation risk involved, such as in pregnancy or pediatric patients. Being a central tool in both interventional and diagnostic medicine, sonography evolves by expanding the breadth of the detection of disease, management, and procedural direction in many different clinical applications.

References

1. Albishare, E. A., Bushaala, N. M., Radwan, M. A., Elfergani, M. A., & Ben Amer, H. M. (2025). The diagnostic value of abdominal ultrasound in children with acute abdominal pain. *SAS Journal of Medicine*. https://www.semanticscholar.org/paper/46825a00a3a0278cc1f43d62584427ebcc5f6c9d (accessed on 12th July 2025).
2. Alexander, E. K., Pearce, E. N., Brent, G. A., Brown, R. S., Chen, H., Dosiou, C., Grobman, W. A., et al. (2017). 2017 Guidelines of the American Thyroid Association for the diagnosis and management of thyroid disease during pregnancy and the postpartum. *Thyroid, 27*, 315–389. https://doi.org/10.1089/thy.2016.0457 (accessed on 12th July 2025).
3. Authors/Task Force Members, Erbel, R., Aboyans, V., Boileau, C., Bossone, E., Di Bartolomeo, R., Eggebrecht, H., et al. (2014). 2014 ESC Guidelines on the diagnosis and treatment of aortic diseases. *European Heart Journal, 35*, 2873–2926. https://doi.org/10.1093/eurheartj/ehu281 (accessed on 12th July 2025).
4. Belfield, J., & Findlay-Line, C. (2022). Testicular germ cell tumors—The role of conventional ultrasound. *Cancers, 14*, 3882. https://doi.org/10.3390/cancers14163882 (accessed on 12th July 2025).
5. Bilardo, C. M., Chaoui, R., Hyett, J., Kagan, K. O., Karim, J., Papageorghiou, A. T., Poon, L. C., et al. (2023). ISUOG Practice Guidelines (updated): Performance of 11–14-week ultrasound scan. *Ultrasound in Obstetrics and Gynecology, 61*, 127–143. https://doi.org/10.1002/uog.26106 (accessed on 12th July 2025).
6. Brasier-Lutz, P., Jäggi-Wickes, C., Schädelin, S., Burian, R., Schoenenberger, C., & Zanetti-Dällenbach, R. (2023). Patient perception of meander-like versus radial breast ultrasound. *Ultrasound International Open, 10*. https://www.semanticscholar.org/paper/482664abf04d3c55aac239bc98647702b31fc45b (accessed on 12th July 2025).
7. Buchanan, R., Tu, S. J., Camurri, M., Mellon, S. J., & Fallon, M. (2024). 3D freehand ultrasound using visual inertial and deep inertial odometry for measuring patellar tracking. In *2024 IEEE International Symposium on Medical Measurements and Applications (MeMeA)*. https://www.semanticscholar.org/paper/a093c86804deda3ffad752bdcafe2af3638a1c38 (accessed on 12th July 2025).
8. Burke, D., Corrigan, N., Herlihy, M., Nasaj, O., Dickson, J., Delaney, D., & Westrup, J. (2022). Real world evaluation of artificial intelligence echocardiography image guidance and acquisition with novice scanners in multiple clinical settings. *European Heart Journal–Cardiovascular Imaging*. https://www.semanticscholar.org/paper/18a27d1a1e520e043589c927fc87a1d62ed0d035 (accessed on 12th July 2025).
9. Choi, E., Qian, L., & Park, S. (2025). Sensor-free contact force guidance for ultrasound imaging. *Proceedings of SPIE, 13412*, 1341207–1341207-5. https://www.semanticscholar.org/paper/6ad4c5691ea07413d7d9de4d3c8224ed4ab6efb9 (accessed on 12th July 2025).
10. Coelho, L. (2023). How artificial intelligence is shaping medical imaging technology: A survey of innovations and applications. *Bioengineering, 10*, 1435. https://doi.org/10.3390/bioengineering10121435 (accessed on 12th July 2025).

11. Coutinho, C. M., Sotiriadis, A., Odibo, A., Khalil, A., D'Antonio, F., Feltovich, H., Salomon, L., et al. (2022). ISUOG Practice Guidelines: Role of ultrasound in the prediction of spontaneous preterm birth. *Ultrasound in Obstetrics and Gynecology, 60*, 435–456. https://doi.org/10.1002/uog.26020 (accessed on 12th July 2025).

12. De Cassai, A., Zarantonello, F., Pistollato, E., Pettenuzzo, T., Busetto, V., Sella, N., & Boscolo, A. (2025). Regional anesthesia in obese patients: Challenges, considerations, and solutions. *Saudi Journal of Anaesthesia, 19*, 221–226. https://www.semanticscholar.org/paper/2a27c02fb5b29766439c1b5d923af1a646b10566 (accessed on 12th July 2025).

13. Dobruch, J. (2013). Virtual guidance of urologic surgery. *Central European Journal of Urology, 66*, 453. https://www.semanticscholar.org/paper/0a0fa84acb2d2089e60098cd15e6987434628d8e (accessed on 12th July 2025).

14. Doyle, L. M., & Wang, M. Z. (2019). Overview of extracellular vesicles, their origin, composition, purpose, and methods for exosome isolation and analysis. *Cells, 8*, 727. https://doi.org/10.3390/cells8070727 (accessed on 12th July 2025).

15. Fruelund, P., van Dam, P. V., Melgaard, J., Soegaard, P., Sommer, A., Lundbye-Christensen, S., Riahi, S., et al. (2022). Novel non-invasive 12-lead ECG-based imaging method with potential to guide and optimize right ventricular lead implantation. *EP Europace*. https://www.semanticscholar.org/paper/954a90472ca2fb1a913919eae8fdf3d411c2d53a (accessed on 12th July 2025).

16. Ghent, C. (2009). Who should be performing liver biopsies? *Canadian Journal of Gastroenterology = Journal Canadien de Gastroenterology, 23*(6), 437–438. https://www.semanticscholar.org/paper/58a20915694a529b228fd86a1062a668aecb8b5b (accessed on 12th July 2025).

17. Goel, R., Abhimanyu, F., Patel, K., Galeotti, J., & Choset, H. (2022). Autonomous ultrasound scanning using Bayesian optimization and hybrid force control. In *2022 International Conference on Robotics and Automation (ICRA)*. https://doi.org/10.1109/icra46639.2022.9812410 (accessed on 12th July 2025).

18. Haugen, B. R., Alexander, E. K., Bible, K. C., Doherty, G. M., Mandel, S. J., Nikiforov, Y. E., Pacini, F., et al. (2015). 2015 American Thyroid Association management guidelines for adult patients with thyroid nodules and differentiated thyroid cancer: The American Thyroid Association Guidelines Task Force on Thyroid Nodules and Differentiated Thyroid Cancer. *Thyroid, 26*, 1–133. https://doi.org/10.1089/thy.2015.0020 (accessed on 12th July 2025).

19. Huang, Y. C., Lu, Y. H., & Ting, W. Y. (2025). Ultrasound-guided vs. non-ultrasound-guided femoral artery puncture techniques: A comprehensive systematic review and meta-analysis. *The Ultrasound Journal, 17*. https://www.semanticscholar.org/paper/e191ba43532be19cf952cacd2d125c1c63edb44d (accessed on 12th July 2025).

20. Janež, J., & Grosek, J. (2023). Minimally invasive peritoneal dialysis catheter insertion with intraoperative ultrasound-Doppler measurement of rectus muscle width and inferior epigastric artery localization. *Surgical Techniques Development*. https://www.semanticscholar.org/paper/1434aa70952392c2e29e7cb8c2bace5f356c28da (accessed on 12th July 2025).

21. Ker, J., Wang, L., Rao, J. P., & Lim, C. C. T. (2017). Deep learning applications in medical image analysis. *IEEE Access, 6*, 9375–9389. https://doi.org/10.1109/access.2017.2788044 (accessed on 12th July 2025).

22. Malinger, G., Paladini, D., Krajden Haratz, K., Monteagudo, A., Pilu, G., & Timor-Tritsch, I. E. (2020). ISUOG Practice Guidelines (updated): Sonographic examination of the fetal central nervous system. Part 1: Performance of screening examination and indications for targeted neurosonography. *Ultrasound in Obstetrics and Gynecology, 56*, 476–484. https://doi.org/10.1002/uog.22145 (accessed on 12th July 2025).

23. Mathijssen, I. M. J. (2020). Updated guideline on treatment and management of craniosynostosis. *Journal of Craniofacial Surgery, 32*, 371–450. https://doi.org/10.1097/scs.0000000000007035 (accessed on 12th July 2025).

24. Mathur, B., Patel, R. U., Ferry, M. Z., Saber, H., Sarwal, A., & Majewicz Fey, A. (2025). A feasibility study: Freehand 3D volumetric reconstruction ultrasound scanning for midline measurement in adults. *Proceedings of SPIE, 13412*, 134120A–134120A-9. https://www.semanticscholar.org/paper/9f1ca7c50f50aec38def2e700c248363accc51dc (accessed on 12th July 2025).

25. Mo, K., Qian, L., Tian, J., Liao, J., Tan, F., Kong, W., Yu, X., et al. (2024). Ultrasound-guided stellate ganglion blockade–Patient positioning is everything: A case report demonstrating the efficacy of a modified out-of-plane approach. *Frontiers in Neuroscience, 17*. https://www.semanticscholar.org/paper/c22a957266c6843a43410ec8d0a78b6dd1553dae (accessed on 12th July 2025).

26. Montoro Neto, R., Vicentini, F., Ugino, R. T. S., Danilovic, A., Marchini, G., Torricelli, F., Batagello, C., et al. (2025). Mixed reality ultrasound-guided mini-ECIRS with Apple Vision Pro™–First case report. *International Brazilian Journal of Urology: Official Journal of the Brazilian Society of Urology, 51*. https://www.semanticscholar.org/paper/38bb3b0f9d798cbef555a65cf5d99ba3925238f8 (accessed on 12th July 2025).

27. Panayides, A. S., Amini, A. A., Filipović, N., Sharma, A., Tsaftaris, S. A., Young, A. A., Foran, D. J., et al. (2020). AI in medical imaging informatics: Current challenges and future directions. *IEEE Journal of Biomedical and Health Informatics, 24*, 1837–1857. https://doi.org/10.1109/jbhi.2020.2991043 (accessed on 12th July 2025).

28. Parker, P., Pynn, H., Haldane, A., Ballard, M., König, T., & Johnston, A. M. (2022). UK field medical care 2032: One military vision. *BMJ Military Health*. https://www.semanticscholar.org/paper/ebec8ab97cdfb6290e7d8b9b76d2658cfba166e3 (accessed on 12th July 2025).

29. Percie du Sert, N., Ahluwalia, A., Alam, S., Avey, M. T., Baker, M., Browne, W. J., Clark, A., et al. (2020). Reporting animal research: Explanation and elaboration for the ARRIVE guidelines 2.0. *PLoS Biology, 18*, e3000411. https://doi.org/10.1371/journal.pbio.3000411 (accessed on 12th July 2025).

30. Peterson, M., & Fenech, M. (2021). Workshop presentations. *Sonography, 8*. https://www.semanticscholar.org/paper/1e0f87ec41e9fc123f60682aa4eb670ecc7dbf70 (accessed on 12th July 2025).

31. Sedano, O., & Sedano, J. (2023). AB1547 shear-wave elastography ultrasound of second metacarpophalangeal in synovium of rheumatoid arthritis. *Annals of the Rheumatic Diseases*. https://www.semanticscholar.org/paper/f19177a027cabd996fd05356eaf6ed98c9dbe7e3 (accessed on 12th July 2025).

32. Sidhu, P. S., Cantisani, V., Dietrich, C. F., Gilja, O. H., Săftoiu, A., Bartels, E., Bertolotto, M., et al. (2018). The EFSUMB Guidelines and Recommendations for the Clinical Practice of Contrast-Enhanced Ultrasound (CEUS) in non-hepatic applications: Update 2017 (Long

version). *Ultraschall in der Medizin–European Journal of Ultrasound, 39*, e2–e44. https://doi.org/10.1055/a-0586-1107 (accessed on 12th July 2025).

33. Subbotina, M. V., Besednova, D. O., & Ishenko, A. A. (2024). Possibilities of ultrasound scanning for assessment of vocal fold mobility in patients with thyroid disease. *Head and neck. Russian Journal*. https://www.semanticscholar.org/paper/377aa7f8c80a73d75b81353a061ff19a6cc7767f (accessed on 12th July 2025).

34. Tai, D., Phat, L. T., Kien, T. T., Anh, N. N., Hai, N. X., Sandwall, P., Bradley, D., et al. (2025). Enhancing patient positioning accuracy: Evaluating daily cone beam computed tomography in the Halcyon system. *Japanese Journal of Clinical Oncology*. https://www.semanticscholar.org/paper/febc9e18788179c8ecdf054fab0248354e908764 (accessed on 12th July 2025).

35. Taylor Wild, K., Rintoul, N. E., Kattan, J., & Gray, B. W. (2020). Extracorporeal Life Support Organization (ELSO): Guidelines for neonatal respiratory failure. *ASAIO Journal, 66*, 463–470. https://doi.org/10.1097/mat.0000000000001153 (accessed on 12th July 2025).

36. Tsvetkov, V. G., Lakhin, R., Polezhankin, E. V., Chartorizhsky, E. V., & Tsygankov, K. (2024). Optimization of ultrasound navigation techniques for brachial plexus block using proximal subclavian access. *Regional Anesthesia and Acute Pain Management*. https://www.semanticscholar.org/paper/147784118c60ddcc9bda24433a9750b380d6a078 (accessed on 12th July 2025).

37. Ullah, F., Rehman, A. U., Khan, R. D., & Khan, A. (2025). The future of cardiac imaging: Innovations in MRI, CT, and ultrasound technologies. *Indus Journal of Bioscience Research*. https://www.semanticscholar.org/paper/1d06d5bfdc048606a809da00f139bf02915a02a3 (accessed on 12th July 2025).

38. Varnosfaderani, S. M., & Forouzanfar, M. (2024). The role of AI in hospitals and clinics: Transforming healthcare in the 21st century. *Bioengineering, 11*, 337. https://doi.org/10.3390/bioengineering11040337 (accessed on 12th July 2025).

39. Verhoef, L., Soloukey, S., Mastik, F., Generowicz, B. S., Bos, E. M., Schouten, J., Koekkoek, S., et al. (2025). Freehand ultrafast Doppler ultrasound imaging with optical tracking allows for detailed 3D reconstruction of blood flow in the human brain. *IEEE Transactions on Medical Imaging, PP*. https://www.semanticscholar.org/paper/87a348d9bc57c87e90e81c30d3ff93c30d7d8145 (accessed on 12th July 2025).

40. Xiao, S., Wang, T., Long, Y., & Yang, L. (2025). Optimizing variable admittance control for remote ultrasound scanning under uncertain environment. *IEEE Access, 13*, 83274–83284. https://www.semanticscholar.org/paper/ccb0a8fbe98b73815f47269734271de721189996 (accessed on 12th July 2025).

41. Zaki, H. A., Albaroudi, B., Shaban, E. E., Shaban, A., Elgassim, M., Almarri, N. D., Basharat, K., et al. (2024). Advancement in pleura effusion diagnosis: A systematic review and meta-analysis of point-of-care ultrasound versus radiographic thoracic imaging. *The Ultrasound Journal, 16*. https://www.semanticscholar.org/paper/417494a1ca87600b8fe20bc8a5984354a69f35c8 (accessed on 12th July 2025).

42. Zhang, F. Y., Wang, F. J., Wang, Z. F., & Qi, X. Q. (2025). Enhancing pediatric abdominal pain diagnosis: The role of ultrasound layered scanning technique. *Quantitative Imaging in Medicine and Surgery, 15*, 4039–4046. https://www.semanticscholar.org/paper/2a350df3aebb3f2957

18462ceec9b8793c552025 (accessed on 12th July 2025).

43. Zhang, L., Peng, Y., He, Y., Wei, Z., Gan, L., & Zhang, J. (2025). Innovative integration of automated breast volume scan and ultrasound elastography for enhanced differentiation of benign and malignant breast lesions. *Scientific Reports, 15.* https://www.semanticscholar.org/paper/9fd751c50bcdd2073cf545c9fe14b1ea039723ce (accessed on 12th July 2025).

44. Zheng, Y., Wang, W., Ferhusoglu, H., Subramaniyam, T., Xu, Z., Rhode, K., & Housden, R. (2024). Fiducial marker-based patient-to-robot registration and target tracking for automatic extra-body ultrasound imaging. In *2024 IEEE 20th International Conference on Automation Science and Engineering (CASE).* https://www.semanticscholar.org/paper/8f4c98f01f7ae349d5390091e2ac7a6467917c79 (accessed on 12th July 2025).

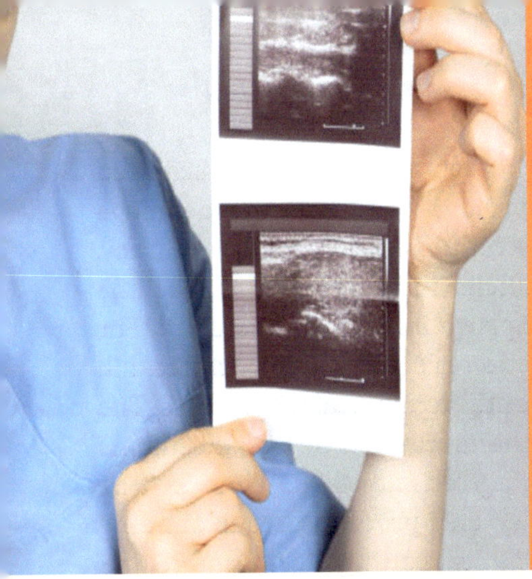

Chapter 3

ULTRASOUND IMAGE INTERPRETATION AND TERMINOLOGY

Contents

Introduction

In medical diagnosis, the use of ultrasound imaging has been of significant interest due to its non-invasive nature, as well as providing real-time imaging. The technology is of prime importance in most medical specialties, particularly in emergency medicine and obstetrics. For instance, in the evaluation of abdominal pain, ultrasound is essential in diagnosing gallstones and acute cholecystitis, among others. An ordered interpretation of ultrasound images is imperative since it can affect clinical decisions as well as patient outcomes. While procedures on ultrasound are deemed significant, there is a gap concerning comprehension of the influence of clinical context on image interpretation. This void necessitates further study to explain the capability of contextual information to enhance diagnosis and enhance diagnostic performance during analysis of ultrasound images, as noted by Rodrigues et al. (2025).

Also, the complexity of ultrasound images necessitates a deeper understanding of some specialized vocabulary for handling ultrasound interpretation. Terminology has various facets that include image quality, acoustic properties, and patient positioning, all of which influence diagnostic accuracy. Emerging technical advancements, such as the application of artificial intelligence and machine learning in ultrasound evaluation, introduce new paradigms that improve image interpretation. For example, sophisticated algorithms can potentially improve the recognition of significant structures and abnormalities, thereby elevating the level at which ultrasound contributes to medical diagnostics. The impact of these advancements can be seen through an example of the discussion on enhancements to images, such as those made available through dual-energy imaging techniques, as discussed in. It is important that doctors remain current with shifting vocabulary and procedures surrounding ultrasound in order to ensure optimal use of technology within the clinical setting. Furthermore, the advent of sophisticated imaging techniques alongside traditional ultrasound routines puts emphasis on the active role of ultrasound image interpretation. With advances in new imaging modalities such as contrast-enhanced ultrasound and Doppler imaging, they enhance conventional ultrasound capabilities by facilitating more accurate assessments of anatomical and pathological features. Each modality possesses unique ultrasound signatures that require familiarity with local anatomy and the mechanism of disease. The description of ultrasound images based on their properties, like vascular patterns and echogenicity, informs clinicians about the potential condition underneath. Research indicates that such sophisticated interpretations increase reliance on ultrasound diagnostics, as indicated by studies entailing varying imaging modalities and environments, as explained in Zhang et al. (2024). Both the uninterrupted innovation in the world of interpreting ultrasound images and its vocabulary convey the opportunities as well as obstacles of the profession, necessitating that experts be trained to learn continuously and grow (Figure 3.1).

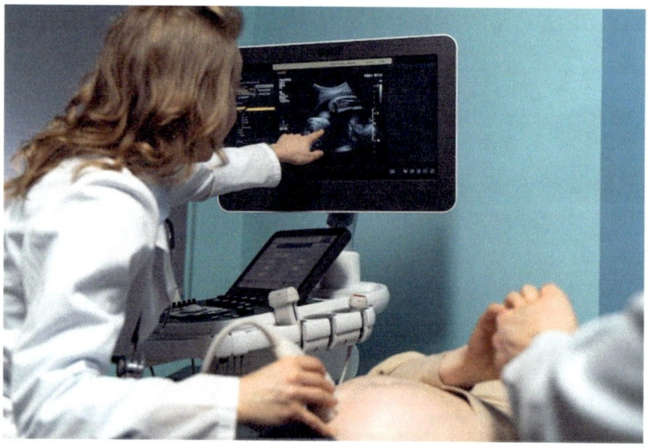

Figure 3.1. Ultrasound image interpretation and terminology.

Source: https://img.freepik.com/free-photo/gynecologist-performing-ultrasound-consultation_23-2149353023.jpg?semt=ais_hybrid&w=740

Definition of Ultrasound Imaging

Ultrasound diagnosis is a non-invasive imaging technique that utilizes high-frequency sound waves to produce real-time images of organs and structures of the body. It employs the emission of ultrasound waves, which reflect off tissues, to create echoes that are translated into visual images in order to be able to see anatomical and physiological conditions in many medical scenarios. It is a significant obstetric aid utilized to monitor fetal development and placental well-being. Furthermore, ultrasound is useful for the examination of soft tissues, vascular routes, and organs by providing exact data on their morphology and function. Visualization of blood flow, as in the case of color Doppler imaging techniques, enhances the study of circulatory dynamics in organs and adds richness to clinical diagnosis and treatment strategies. Overall, ultrasound imaging is a cornerstone in diagnostic medicine, which continues to shed light on complex biological systems. The name ultrasound imaging transcends methodological description. It encompasses the various terminologies radiologists and clinicians use to report ultrasound findings. The Ovarian-Adnexal Reporting and Data System (O-RADS) and the Thyroid Imaging Reporting and Data System (TI-RADS) are reporting systems that were developed to improve communication and the accuracy of diagnoses in specific anatomical areas (Yadav et al., 2024; Verde & Ponsiglione, 2022). These systems categorize ultrasound findings based on given criteria and risk assessments, minimizing ambiguity in interpreting lesions or abnormalities. An instance is the O-RADS system based on a simple lexical structure that helps clinicians to report adnexal lesions, thus allowing for optimal management stratification. Such standardized terminologies facilitate improved clarity in ultrasound reporting, ensuring that a shared understanding is reached among medical professionals while maintaining maximum patient care pathways. Moreover, awareness of the working principles and limitations of the technology is essential for an understanding of the nuances in ultrasound imaging. An ultrasound image quality is decided by numerous factors, including the equipment used, the skill of the operator, and the acoustic properties of tissues being examined. For instance, echogenicity differences, that is, tissue's ability to reflect ultrasonic waves, result in different gray-scale representation on images. The availability of advanced imaging modalities, such as contrast-enhanced ultrasound, also assists with diagnosis by more clearly imaging subtle pathology. Additionally, knowledge of artifacts—unwanted echoes or irregularities in imaging—is important for correct interpretation. Physicians must be vigilant in being able to differentiate between these artifacts and actual pathological findings, a reminder of the necessity for continued education and hands-on practice in proficiency in ultrasound imaging.

Significance of Ultrasound in Medical Diagnosis

Ultrasound technology occupies the focal point in medical diagnosis, with its non-invasive, safe imaging. Its ability to image soft tissues and organs in real time allows clinicians to make good decisions about patient care. For instance, the dual imaging technique utilization, as in, enhances the diagnostic purpose by emphasizing diverse views of vascular health and uncovering potential pathologies. This two-modedicity is not only used to measure blood flow dynamics but also to evaluate soft tissue structures. Practitioners are thus able to diagnose conditions, such as organ malformation or vascular disease, effectively by interpreting ultrasound images that reveal significant anatomical information. Such developments solidify the position of ultrasound at the forefront of diagnostic imaging, noting its utility in modern medical practice. Besides, the educational role of ultrasound use cannot be ruled out. According to data like that referred to in Alshalahi et al. (2025), there is a huge knowledge gap among the population on when, why, and what ultrasound is able to do in prenatal diagnosis. Patients readily acknowledge that ultrasound is necessary in tracking fetal development, but they continue to have misconceptions about its application. For example, although it is certain that most pregnant women believe that ultrasound can detect any fetal malformation, evidence reveals that it is limited in detecting some of them. Therefore, the incorporation of education on ultrasound into practice is necessary if patient expectations are to be equated to facts about medical imaging. Attaining these educational needs can improve patient outcomes and engender a better appreciation of ultrasound's role in obtaining maternal and fetal well-being. Finally, the versatility of ultrasounds in different medical fields is the reason why it is crucial in diagnostic testing, particularly because other technologies like artificial intelligence (AI) are being integrated into its practice. According to Gusev (2025), the integration of AI in ultrasound image analysis can enhance the precision of diagnosis by automating routine processes and identifying subtle patterns in ultrasound data. This synergy between ultrasound and AI paints a picture of an innovative approach to medical imaging that has the potential to accelerate diagnosis and develop tailored treatment plans. As medicine increasingly moves toward precision medicine, the inclusion of the newest technologies in ultrasound marks the beginning of improved healthcare quality. Hence, the future of ultrasound holds not just its traditional uses but wider scopes in predictive analysis as well as customized therapeutic approaches, further justifying its relevance in contemporary medical diagnosis (Figure 3.2).

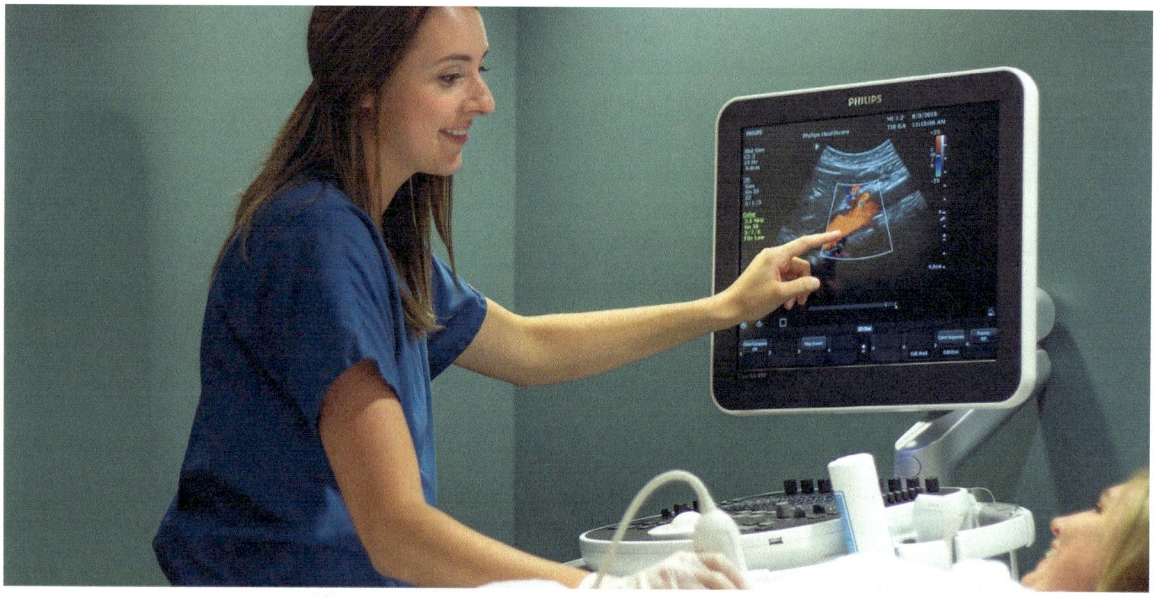

Figure 3.2. Ultrasound in medical diagnostics.

Source: https://www.unmc.edu/alliedhealth/_images/programs/dms-scans-5254-1600x800.jpg.

3.1. Basics of Ultrasound Technology

In the study of ultrasound technology basics, one needs to learn the basic principles of sound wave generation and propagation. Ultrasound machines operate by emitting high-frequency sound waves that are produced by piezoelectric crystals, which convert electrical energy into mechanical energy. When they meet other tissues in the body, these sound waves bounce back to the transducer with varying intensities, thus creating an image based on the variable acoustic characteristics of the tissues. This is demonstrated in, where a clear display of the piezoelectric effect reveals how the ultrasound machine both sends and receives sound waves. The skill to interpret such echoes enables medical practitioners to visualize anatomical structures non-invasively, and thus ultrasound is a critical tool in medical imaging, especially in obstetrics and cardiology. When addressing ultrasound technology, one needs to take into consideration the different imaging modalities and their unique applications. Two of the main types of ultrasound are the conventional grayscale ultrasound and the Doppler ultrasound. The grayscale ultrasound provides a 2D image of internal anatomy, which is critical in detecting soft tissue and organ abnormalities, while the Doppler ultrasound, in particular, quantifies blood flow dynamics and vascular status. This is evident in, which presents grayscale as well as color Doppler images to provide a comparative assessment between static anatomy and dynamic quantitation of blood flow. These modalities allow the detailed evaluation of pathologies such as vascular disease, tumors, and developmental anomalies, buttressing their ordering role within the clinical decision-making process. Further, advancement in ultrasound technology, in terms of the integration of artificial intelligence (AI), is transforming image interpretation and making diagnosis more precise. AI holds the potential to increase the efficiency of image analysis by automating functions such as image segmentation and abnormality detection, which can reduce interpretation time and increase uniformity in diagnosing illnesses. As cited in Gordon et al. (2024), a detailed understanding of the influence of AIs on medical education is essential owing to its implications in the imaging subspecialties. Also, ultrasound technologies such as contrast-enhanced ultrasound and three-dimensional imaging expand the range of capability beyond traditional ultrasound, offering dynamic information regarding anatomical and physiological states. With these advancements, ultrasound technology continues to evolve, cementing its irreplaceable application in today's healthcare diagnostics and driving improved patient outcomes and clinical effectiveness, as posited in the argument of better techniques considered in Akinci et al. (2023).

3.1.1. Principles of Ultrasound Wave Propagation

During the propagation of ultrasound waves, an understanding of how waves react upon encountering various media is crucial to effective imaging interpretation. Ultrasound waves propagate through various tissues, and they rely on tissue density and elasticity for their propagation. These aspects cause the waves to reflect, refract, or scatter, leading to different contrasts in images on the resultant ultrasound scans. Reflection occurs when waves bounce off surfaces between tissues of varying acoustic impedances, and this is employed purposefully to image objects like organs and blood vessels. The applicability of such considerations can be further increased by the incorporation of visual aids illustrating ultrasound principles; for example, the description of ultrasound scans in images, such as and facilitates demonstrating such principles, how varying tissue density creates varying imaging effects and diagnostic information. The rate of ultrasound wave propagation, as well as image quality, also depends on the frequency of ultrasound waves. Higher frequency waves provide better resolution because their wavelengths are shorter, and finer detail in tissues can be detected. But there is a trade-off: higher frequencies contribute to higher attenuation as waves travel into deeper tissues. This property tends to limit imaging of deeper structures, where lower frequency waves are better because they have less attenuation. Thus, the practitioner will be required to harmoniously balance frequency selection based on the clinical case and anatomical region of interest. Its contribution to the echogenicity of ultrasound images is illustrated via images such as and, which depict the capability of different frequencies in delineating anatomical structures and pathologies and highlighting its critical importance in ultrasound imaging. In addition, the behavior of ultrasound waves when they encounter tissues in living tissues is capable of providing valuable information regarding many clinical conditions. For instance, Doppler ultrasound exploits wave propagation theory to assess blood flow dynamics, allowing measurement of vascular status. When the moving blood cells interact with the ultrasound waves, the frequency of back-scattered waves changes, thus allowing for the computation of the flow parameters and any pathology. This principle of frequency shift is central to the evaluation of cardiovascular health and conditions like thrombosis or vessel blockage. Clinical applications, as in and, show the application of these principles in vascular pathway ultrasound imaging, showing how the application of ultrasound technology exceeds structural diagnostic purposes, penetrating into functional tissue function, thereby leading to more effective application of ultrasound in medical diagnosis (Figure 3.3).

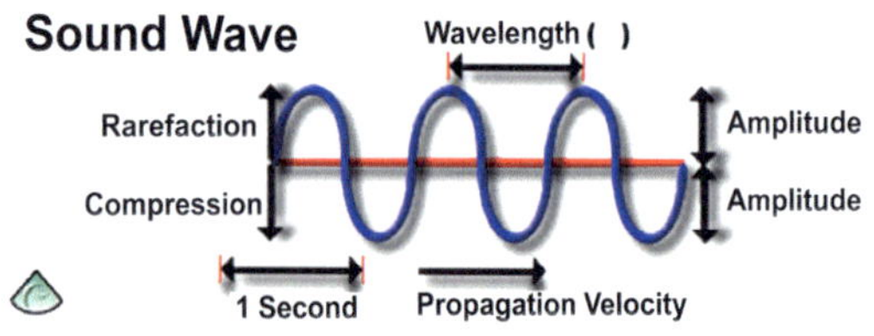

Figure 3.3. Principles of ultrasound wave propagation.

Source: https://eecho.s3.us-east-2.amazonaws.com/loops/20300/soundwave.gif.

3.1.2. Types of Ultrasound Machines

The ultrasound technology environment comprises varied models of equipment appropriate to various clinical applications and imaging requirements. Conventional ultrasound equipment, alternatively referred to as cart-based or console systems, possesses high computing power along with high-resolution imaging. These machines support multiple transducer options to facilitate a range of imaging modalities including 2D, 3D, and Doppler imaging. The capability of such systems to make images of moving organs and flowing blood in real time makes them essential in cardiology, obstetrics, and emergency care. The technology has also given rise to portable and handheld ultrasound equipment that maintains a level of imaging quality that is on par with traditional systems. The size of these systems allows them to be used in point-of-care applications, thereby finding it useful in environments where immediate diagnostics are a necessity. With advancing technology in ultrasound, having knowledge of the operations and applications of such equipment is very important to be able to advance patient care in clinical diagnosis of conditions such as chronic kidney disease and transplantation (Singla et al., 2022).

In addition to the portable and standard type of ultrasound scanners, there are also specialized systems aimed at further enhancing diagnostic capabilities. High-frequency ultrasound equipment, for instance, utilize waves of up to 100 MHz, enabling higher resolution imaging of shallow tissues such as skin and subcutaneous tissue. CEUS has been used more and more in dermatology and aesthetic medicine, where high-resolution imaging can influence treatment planning and monitoring (Mlosek et al., 2020). Contrast-enhanced ultrasound (CEUS) is another significant advancement utilizing microbubble contrast agents for vascular imaging and perfusion analysis in organs. This technique offers a more precise description of tissue characteristics, particularly useful in the evaluation of renal masses or in judging conditions such as renal ischemia. The technologies of ultrasound have not only facilitated easier higher-quality imaging but have also placed higher-quality diagnostics within reach in various healthcare environments, stressing the important role of these specialized machines. Moreover, the importance of new ultrasound technology is amplified by being merged with artificial intelligence (AI) for image interpretation. The software of machine learning can analyze ultrasound images to optimize diagnostic accuracy and build predictive models for patient outcomes. These systems can offer assistance to healthcare workers by recognizing subtle patterns in images in imaging data that might not be recognized on a visual inspection. The coupling of AI with traditional ultrasound modalities paves the way for improved accuracy in the diagnosis of conditions such as chronic kidney disease and monitoring transplant viability, transforming patient management protocols at its very foundation. By filling the medical gap between disparate ultrasound machines and advanced analysis tools, such an advancement not only streamlines clinical decision-making but also becomes in tune with the leading trend towards personalized medicine (Singla et al., 2022). With the evolution of healthcare, knowledge of the nature of ultrasound machines and functionalities has become essential for practitioners who aim at minimizing patient outcomes through effective imaging processes, thereby solidifying ultrasounds place in modern diagnostics (Figure 3.4).

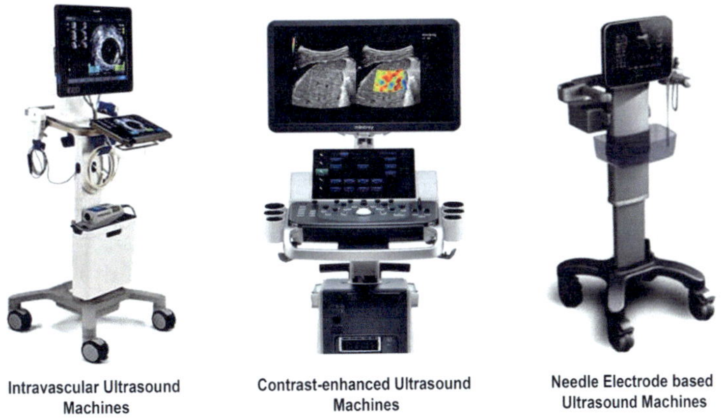

Figure 3.4. Types of ultrasound machines.

Source: https://i.ytimg.com/vi/nCeiLRuaSoc/maxresdefault.jpg.

3.1.3. Role of Transducers in Image Acquisition

The role of transducers in the formation of ultrasound images is the foundation for success in diagnostic imaging. Transducers also act as a transmitter and receiver of the sound waves, with electric energy converted into sound waves that penetrate the body and then are reflected back to the transducer by the various tissues. The piezoelectric effect is crucial; it enables one to obtain high-quality images that clinicians use to make accurate diagnoses. The efficiency of this process relies on several technical factors, including the frequency of the transducer, which has a specific correspondence with penetration depth and resolution in an image. Low-frequency transducers allow deeper structures to be imaged at the expense of resolution. Higher-frequency transducers offer more detail but with reduced penetration, with ramifications for their suitability depending on the clinical situation presented. An appreciation and application of the same principles are crucial to making efficient use of ultrasound imaging, as captured in guidelines documented by relevant associations, for instance, ISUOGs clinical standards (Carvalho et al., 2023). Transducers need to be selected and applied with utmost caution and attention to clinical requirements and the particular characteristics of the patient to be scanned. The variety of transducer shapes, linear, curved, and phased array, also contributes to the difficulty of this choice because each shape possesses different strengths in visualization and application. Linear transducers, for instance, are better for shallow imaging, while phased array transducers can image cardiac structures more effectively due to their ability to steer ultrasound beams from small footprints. Flexibility in transducer technology allows doctors to tailor ultrasound scans based on the specific needs of their patients for better diagnostic outcomes. Tailoring ranges from the use of diverse imaging modalities, from Doppler ultrasound, which assesses blood perfusion and circulatory health, to illustrate the direct influence of transducer technology on clinical outcomes (Singla et al., 2022). Furthermore, the application of state-of-the-art imaging technologies, for example, contrast-enhanced and 3D ultrasound, has revolutionized the role of transducers in medical practice. These technologies offer increased volume imaging and tissue characterization, improving diagnostic assurance in various specialties of medicine, such as nephrology and obstetrics. For example, contrast-enhanced ultrasound allows for imaging of vasculature and perfusion patterns, critical in situations involving assessment of kidney function or tumor detection. Besides efficient training and implementation of standard protocols, the technical advancements of modern transducers offer superior imaging and are a critical element of patient management. The connection of the choice of transducer and clinical application to the ultimate benefit underscores the constant evolution of ultrasound technology with its final product proving its value in optimizing patient care and outcomes in several areas of medical specialties.

3.2. Ultrasound Image Formation

Ultrasound image formation is based largely on the concepts of propagation and echo reflection of sound. Image formation begins with the transducer that emits high-frequency sound waves into the body. As these sound waves interact with tissues, they bounce back to the transducer based on the acoustic impedance of the interacting tissues. The reflected echoes are then converted into electrical signals that construct an image on the screen. The quality of the ultrasound images may entirely be dependent on the frequency of sound waves being used; higher frequencies offer higher resolution but have limited depth of penetration, while lower frequencies have deeper penetration but offer lower image quality. This interaction underscores the importance of selecting the correct transducer frequency for optimal diagnostic imaging in the clinical setting. An understanding of these dynamics is crucial for accurate interpretation of ultrasound and helps to enhance the modality's diagnostic utility, as illustrated in. Ultrasound imaging capability also improves through the application of sophisticated technology such as Doppler ultrasound and contrast-enhanced ultrasound (CEUS). Doppler ultrasound uses the Doppler effect to assess blood flow and vascular illness by measuring differences in frequency of backscattered sound waves as they interact with moving red blood cells. Not only does the procedure image immobile anatomical structures but also provides dynamic information on physiological phenomena such as patterns of blood flow, important in cardiovascular disease diagnosis. Similarly, CEUS employs contrast microbubble agents that improve the visualization of blood vessels and perfusion of tissues. They markedly enhance the diagnostic capabilities of ultrasound to allow more precise evaluations of conditions such as tumors or trauma. As is apparent in contrast methods are capable of producing significant image quality and diagnostic confidence gains in the treatment of most medical disorders.

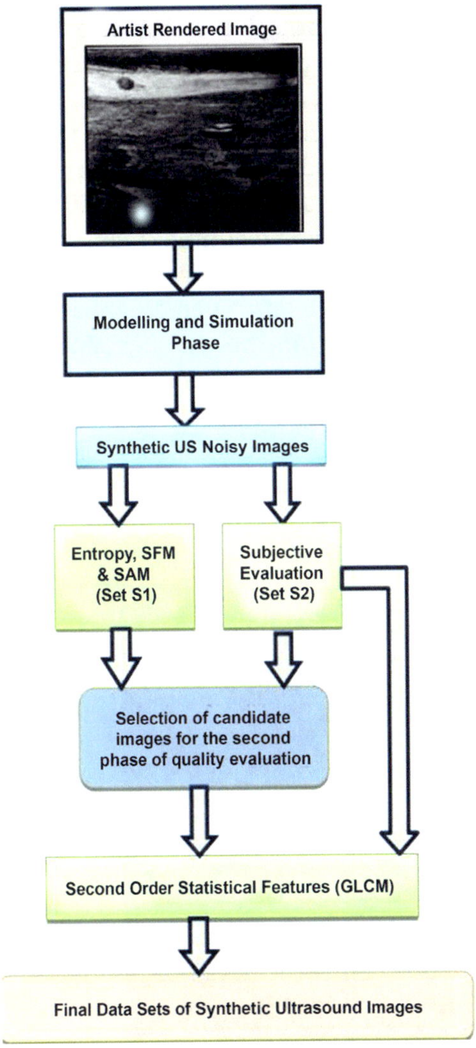

Figure 3.5. Ultrasound image formation.

Source: Singh, Prerna & Mukundan, Ramakrishnan & de Ryke, Rex. (2017). Quality analysis of synthetic ultrasound images using co-occurrence texture statistics. 1-6. 10.1109/IVCNZ.2017.8402511. .

In addition, the application of advanced computational techniques, including machine learning and artificial intelligence, is revolutionizing ultrasound image analysis and interpretation. Such tools can assist radiologists in identifying patterns and abnormalities in imaging data that are not readily discernible, resulting in enhanced diagnostic accuracy. For example, a critical evaluation of the existing literature highlights the ability of Generative Adversarial Networks (GANs) to improve image segmentation within ultrasound imaging, thus leading to better identification of diseased areas and enhanced visualization of critical anatomical structures. Furthermore, incorporating AI has the ability to automate workflows and assist clinicians in making prompt and informed decisions using evidence from ultrasound. This technology is promising because it not only provides backup to existing clinical practice daily but also provides new avenues for research in ultrasound-augmented diagnosis. Utilization of the advance serves to underscore the continuous evolution of ultrasound imaging and its advance in medicine today (Figure 3.5).

3.2.1. Mechanism of Image Creation

In the case of ultrasound imaging, the process of creating images is the conversion of reflections of sound waves to visual images of anatomical structures. The process starts with the emission of high-frequency sound waves produced by piezoelectric crystals in the transducer into the body. These waves are reflected back at varying percentages upon hitting other tissues based on the density and acoustic properties of the surfaces that they hit. The same transducer receives the returned echoes, which are converted from mechanical waves to electrical signals in order to yield a coherent image on a monitor screen. The differing shades of gray on ultrasound images correspond to tissues' relative densities, denser tissues reflecting more sound waves and thus appearing lighter. This fundamental knowledge of how ultrasound images are formed is critical to interpreting images effectively and accurately in practice, as seen in. Beyond simple reflection of sound waves, advanced techniques such as Doppler ultrasound contribute to the diagnostic utility of ultrasound imaging. Doppler ultrasound scans the frequency shift of the returns and echoes from moving targets, such as red blood cells. They are converted to a color image of blood flow, providing information about vessel health and heart function. Color Doppler images, for instance, can identify arteries and veins and quantify the speed and direction of blood in them. This technology not only aids in the detection of abnormalities like thrombosis or stenosis but also optically enhances the diagnostic capability of ultrasound. The mechanism behind this application is an example of the necessity to understand the physics behind the sound waves in medical imaging and highlights the contribution of such next-generation modalities to the care of patients, as evidenced in. Rising AI technologies, including the use of Artificial Intelligence for ultrasound imaging, also show the image construction and interpretation processes. Ultrasound images can be processed by AI algorithms to detect patterns and anomalies that the human eye cannot see. For example, machine learning algorithms can read enormous amounts of ultrasound scans and detect features of conditions like hypoxic-ischemic encephalopathy (HIE) or thyroid cancers to facilitate improved diagnostic accuracy and workflow optimization. The use of AI is a revolutionary strategy in the way ultrasound images are generated and utilized, allowing for improved patient outcomes through increased analytical capabilities. As this technology continues to develop, knowledge of the mechanisms behind image formation, for example, as shown in its use for a range of medical conditions, will be fundamental in realizing its full potential in healthcare settings. The use of AI in ultrasound scan interpretation fits perfectly alongside conventional imaging methods, piling a holistic approach to diagnosis and patient management as shown in (Figure 3.6).

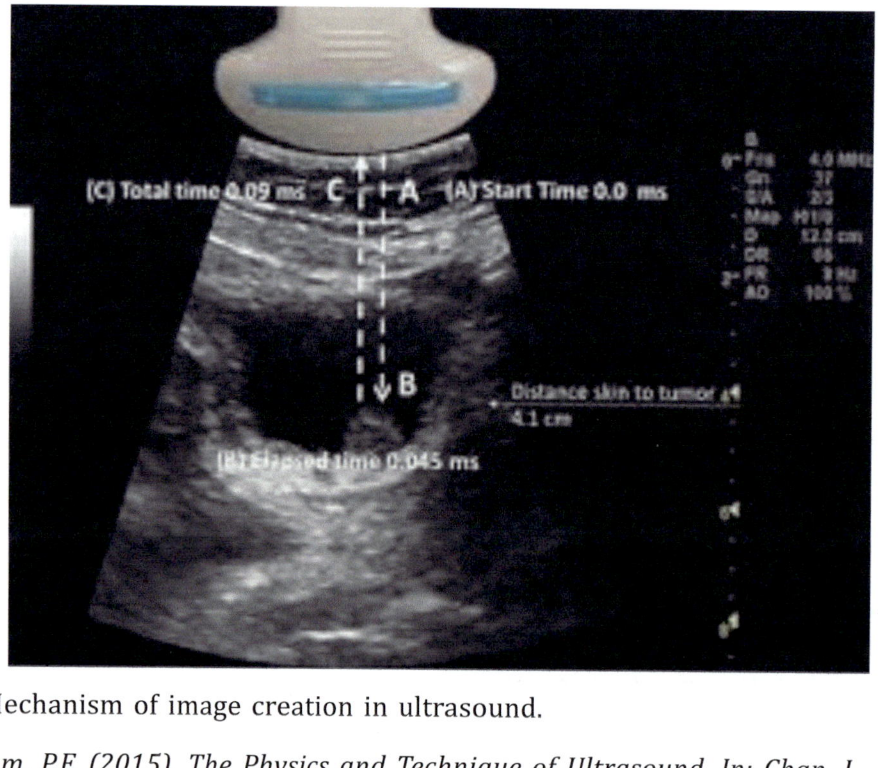

Figure 3.6. Mechanism of image creation in ultrasound.

Source: Fulgham, P.F. (2015). The Physics and Technique of Ultrasound. In: Chan, L., Tse, V., The, S., Stewart, P. (eds) Pelvic Floor Ultrasound. Springer, Cham. https://doi.org/10.1007/978-3-319-04310-4_1

3.2.2. Factors Affecting Image Quality

The accuracy of ultrasound scanning has a close relation with technical parameters that regulate resolution and image clarity acquired. The frequency of the ultrasound waves applied during scanning is among the prime determinants. Greater frequencies are preferable for greater resolution and detail, which is required more importantly for accurate diagnoses, particularly for imaging soft tissues. But it does so at the expense of penetration depth, and therefore is less appropriate to image deeper structures. Conversely, lower frequencies have greater penetration but perhaps at the expense of reduced visibility of detail. Achieving this balance of selection of frequency is important in the modificationof ultrasound examinations for particular clinical needs, for example, in vascular imaging, where exac detail is needed. These factors are evident when images, for example, with varying anatomy , are compared, where frequency selection influences diagnostic performance.

The proficiency of the operator is the second key factor in determining image quality and encompasses both sonographer competency and equipment calibration. An experienced operator can optimize settings, scan at appropriate angles, and select appropriate imaging modalities that maximize image findings. For instance, in the cases observed in and, technical imaging manipulation is directly proportional to the degree of quality visual information offered. Calibration of equipment also affects the quality of emitted and received ultrasound waves, such that images reflect the actual anatomical representation. Maintenance of ultrasound machines and regular software updating equate to consistent performance, lessening equipment-related artifacts that get in the way of diagnostic clarity. Thus, the operator skill and well-maintained technology become the most critical factor in achieving high-quality ultrasound images. Also, the patient-related factors become critical towards delivering ultrasound image quality. Such factors include body habitus, air or gas present in the body, and movement of the patient, which may significantly affect the resultant images. For example, increased body mass index (BMI) can attenuate ultrasound waves and therefore lead to suboptimal image quality, particularly in peripheral organ imaging,as demonstrated in. Similarly, patient cooperation, for example, remaining still during the scan, is required in order not to create motion artifacts that can significantly degrade images. Conditions like the patient's hydration level also influence the echogenicity of tissues and, therefore, visibility. Correction of these patient-related factors is essential in clinical settings to ensure that the images closely represent underlying anatomy, providing a reliable data set for interpretation and ensuing clinical decision.

3.2.3. Interpretation of Grayscale and Color Doppler Images

The interpretation of the gray-scale ultrasound image forms the core of delivering accurate diagnoses in various fields of medicine. Gray-scale imaging utilizes echoes in different shades of echogenicity to identify anatomical structures so that clinicians are able to view organs, tissues, and potential pathologies. In obstetrics, for example, a gray-scale image is capable of showing some features such as the position and size of the fetus's heart, which are important when assessing congenital heart defects. An ultrasound scan may include specific abnormalities presented in grayscale, thus aiding the diagnosis of such abnormalities as developmental anomalies or fluid accumulation. The technique is more effective when used in conjunction with the examination of Doppler images illustrating blood flow patterns of these structures. The worth of quality imaging systems cannot be exaggerated, as they significantly enhance the resolution and quality of the grayscale images and thereby play a role in clinical decision-making and patient management. A good quality grayscale ultrasound image is provided, augmenting this discussion.

Color Doppler ultrasound is a dynamic input into clinical image interpretation by offering details of blood flow and its character. This modality utilizes color coding of images to describe the speed and direction of blood flow and, therefore, proves useful in vascular exams and cardiology studies. In this way, for instance, color Doppler imaging is used to distinguish between normal and abnormal patterns of flow in vessels so that diseases such as vascular occlusions or valvular dysfunction may be identified early. Furthermore, Doppler imaging is essential in obstetrics, as it provides critical information on placental blood supply and fetal circulation. Color Doppler aids in the diagnosis of congenital heart disease through the visualization of the flow dynamics inside the heart and thus informs potential treatment protocols. The image showing color Doppler findings, such as enhances understanding of how this technology collaborates with grayscale imaging to inform clinical practice. The integrated application of grayscale and color Doppler imaging enables thorough assessments of physiological as well as pathological conditions. Successful, comprehensive interpretation requires practitioners to synthesize results from various imaging modalities into a coherent understanding of the state of health of the patient. For instance, fusion of grayscale images that exhibit structural abnormality with Doppler data showing ensuing blood flow changes can be very informative concerning the severity of a disease and its complications. Providers must also be well-versed in the interpretation of these modalities and should also be aware of the professional standards of practice recommended by various professional organizations. Continuing education in ultrasound technique, underpinned by awareness of recommendations from bodies like ISUOG, can significantly enhance the quality of examinations, leading ultimately to better patient outcomes. Such layered diagnostic capability is valuable in today's healthcare, as demonstrated by the ultrasound images, which are a demonstration of the value of broad coverage imaging analysis (Figure 3.7).

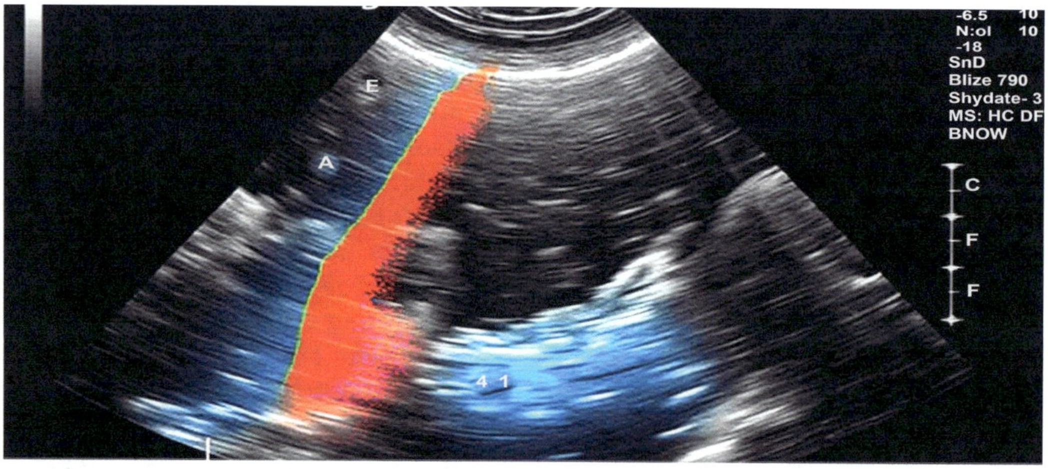

Figure 3.7. Interpretation of grayscale (A) and color Doppler (B) images in ultrasound.

Source:Cho, Jeong & Moon, Kyong & Kim, Hyun & Kang, Jeong & Yoo, Tag & Lee, Seung. (2009). Intratesticular Varicocele Associated with Ipsilateral Extratesticular Varicocele. Korean Journal of Urology. 50. 10.4111/kju.2009.50.8.822.

3.3. Common Ultrasound Terminology

In the clinical application of ultrasound scanning, radiologists and practitioners must share a common terminology. It is basic to learn that a term such as echogenicity is employed to characterize the reflectivity quality of tissues to ultrasound waves. Such an attribute is utilized to differentiate among various types of tissues, for instance, between cystic and solid lesions. Additionally, the tissue composition and the surrounding structures influence echogenicity to aid in diagnosis. A hypoechoic region, for instance, appears darker on the ultrasound monitor compared to surrounding tissues and can show a pathological condition. The significance of echogenicity can also be further illustrated by demonstration of ultrasound images, for example, with various echogenic characteristics of thyroid nodules, pointing to the significance of accurate terminology in everyday practice.

Besides echogenicity, the Doppler ultrasound concept is another vital element of the terminology. Doppler imaging assesses blood flow within vessels and provides valuable insight into vascular pathology and health. The Doppler effect is the change in frequency of ultrasound waves upon reflection from moving targets, such as red blood cells. By observing patterns of blood flow, clinicians can identify diseases such as occlusions or stenosis. The ultrasound pictures, such as in are utilized to demonstrate the application of color Doppler, outlining areas of increased or decreased blood flow. This serves to highlight the integration of Doppler vocabulary into practice and its utility in the accurate diagnosis of cardiovascular disease. Furthermore, familiarity with the different imaging modalities, for example, grayscale versus color Doppler, is key to effective interpretation of ultrasound. Grayscale images provide subtle anatomical detail and are required in the assessment of the morphology of lesions. In contrast, color Doppler images show blood flow, which helps in assessing vascular structures' function. This concurrent process allows clinicians to attain a full description of both idiosyncratic structures and respective blood flow parameters. Images like those in can reveal significant information about vascular pathologies while demonstrating the necessity of learning pervasive ultrasound terminology. It is mandatory to have an efficient line of communication among doctors and improve diagnosis accuracy, ultimately leading to improving the patient's care and treatment (Figure 3.8).

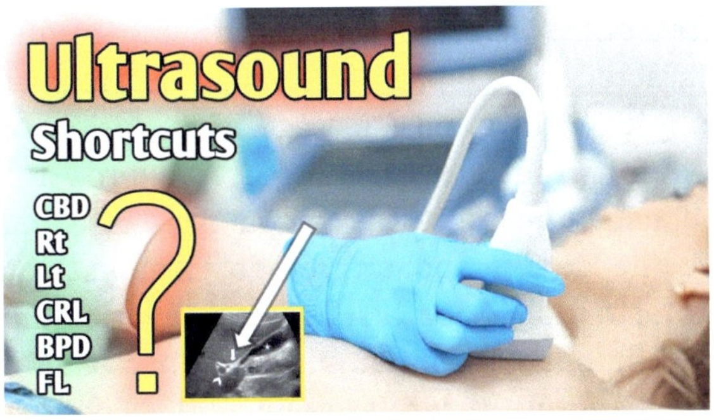

Figure 3.8. Common ultrasound terminology.

Source: https://external-content.duckduckgo.com/iu/?u=https%3A%2F%2Fi.ytimg.com%2Fvi%2FWt9Euxim8Js%2Fmaxresdefault.jpg&f=1&nofb=1&ipt=865943437d7c2e830e128442318c3789463a2165dbd9c9176482b901697a9731.

3.3.1. Key Terms Used in Ultrasound Reports

The languages adopted in the ultrasonography report are significant in conveying messages effectively between medical physicians and making appropriate diagnoses. Terminologies such as echogenic, isoechoic, and hypoechoic describe the tissue density and reflecting properties of tissues as detected by the ultrasonic waves. Echogenic structures appear bright in the image due to higher tissue density, whereas hypoechoic areas indicate low density and less reflection; hence, images will appear darker. Isoechoic areas imply similarity in echogenicity between the suspected tissue and surrounding tissues, which complicates diagnosis. These variations contain vital information regarding the composition of different tissues and can indicate normal or abnormal conditions. For instance, hypoechoic nodules in the liver are suspicious for malignancies, and additional imaging or biopsy is warranted, especially in chronic liver disease patients (Pezzilli, 2021). The precise understanding of such terms enables clinicians to design an appropriate evaluation from ultrasound findings.

Finally, the interpretation of images on ultrasound involves recognition of vascular characteristics, typically reported by means of Doppler ultrasound language. Vascularity and waveform patterns are required words that are used to assess the blood flow and may provide details about thrombosis or vascular malformations. For instance, vascularity may be enhanced by inflammatory processes or tumor activity, while abnormal waveform patterns may suggest venous obstruction or arterial insufficiency. The blending of Doppler ultrasound aptly supplements cardiovascular structural and functional assessment, as evidenced in deep vein thrombosis disease scans. Use of brief yet precise nomenclature in reports allows differentiation between normal physiology and pathological changes and thereby leads to timely and proper management of the patient. Thus, the Doppler ultrasound technique and terminology knowledge remains a significant part in the clinical application of such imaging modalities in various areas of medicine. In pediatric settings, tailored ultrasound terminology demonstrates the necessity for tracking growth and development. Terms such as hyperechoic and anatomical landmarks are regularly employed when describing ultrasound images of pediatric patients. For example, when evaluating a child's kidneys or brain, detection of echogenicity changes could be suggestive of altered growth patterns or developmental abnormalities such as hypoxic-ischemic encephalopathy (HIE). Further, incorporating observations about anatomical landmarks could also comfort clinicians about the development of structures or guide interventional procedures directly. Overall, clear definitions and consistent use of these descriptors in ultrasound reports facilitate effective communication among pediatric experts, finally leading to better patient outcomes and care. Because reports are quite crucial in serving as evidence for follow-up and treatment, good language is an asset, especially in the multidisciplinary management of pediatric rheumatology and other subspecialties (Jenabi et al., 2020).

3.3.2. Understanding Echogenicity and Acoustic Shadowing

Understanding of echogenicity is fundamental to ultrasound image interpretation because it refers to the ability of tissues to reflect ultrasound waves. Tissue structure can be described in relation to echogenicity as hyperechoic (bright), hypoechoic (darker), and anechoic (no echo). The various echogenic characteristics help physicians to differentiate between different tissues, lesions, and fluids. For instance, an anechoic area on a picture of an ultrasound can indicate a cyst or fluid collection, while a hyperechoic area can be indicative of calcifications or solid tumors. Clinically important distinctions defined by echogenicity may play a considerable role in clinical management. A proper understanding of these entities is value-added to diagnostic accuracy and decision-making regarding treatments. Therefore, radiologists must develop expertise in recognizing the echogenic properties of tissues in a way that guarantees the diagnostic potential of ultrasound technology is maximized in most clinical settings.

Another fundamental phenomenon encountered in ultrasound imaging is acoustic shadowing, which occurs when ultrasound waves strike a heavy object that reflects or absorbs the waves and results in a shadow behind the object. This shadowing may obscure beneath its underlying tissues and may conceal important diagnostic detail. As an example, in imaging structures such as gallstones or calcified organs, the acoustic shadow formed may interfere with the accurate assessment of adjacent tissues. Nevertheless, knowledge of the patterns of acoustic shadowing allows practitioners to make intelligent judgments as to which follow-up imaging modality is needed for adequate evaluation. Thus, the experts must not only detect shadowing effects but also understand how they relate to the patient's clinical presentation in order to avoid misinterpretation, and this underscores the importance of better knowledge regarding both echogenicity as well as acoustic shadowing in ultrasound examination. The use of new technologies in ultrasound, such as quantitative ultrasound (QUS), also strengthens knowledge regarding echogenicity and acoustic shadowing. QUS employs advanced imaging techniques to quantify interactions of ultrasound waves with biological tissues and reveal information that is not accessible through traditional B-mode imaging. By characterizing the subtle fluctuations in tissue microstructure, QUS can supply in-depth information on tissue stiffness, composition, and elasticity, which directs the understanding of pathological conditions (Demi et al., 2022; Cloutier et al., 2021). As such, in liver fibrosis evaluation, QUS is able to reveal echogenicity level changes and provide a new avenue to investigate acoustic shadowing effects. This convergence of traditional and new ultrasound techniques is a breakthrough towards increased diagnostic accuracy and broader clinical application in patient management, particularly in difficult cases where echogenicity and shadowing are determinants (Figure 3.9).

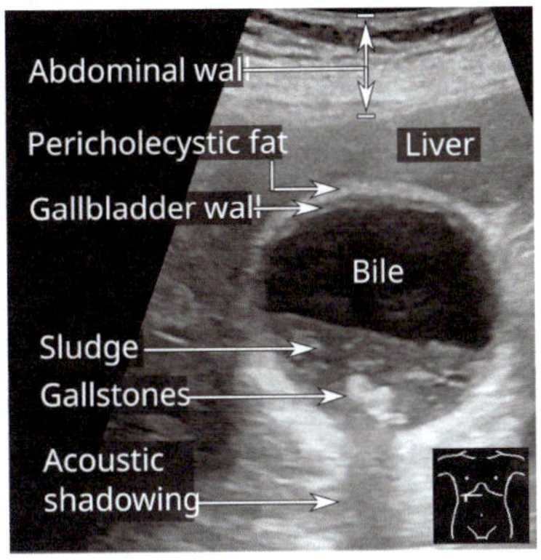

Figure 3.9. Acoustic shadowing.

Source: https://upload.wikimedia.org/wikipedia/commons/c/cc/Ultrasonography_of_sludge_and_gallstones%2C_annotated.svg

3.3.3. Terminology Related to Anatomical Structures

Understanding anatomical structure terminologies is crucial in correct ultrasound image interpretation. Accurate definitions and consistent use of such terms as superficial fascia, deep fascia, and subcutaneous layers support clear communication among health providers, allowing accurate diagnoses and plans of treatment. As emphasized by recent studies, the superficial fascia comprises membranous and fatty elements that vary across different regions of the body, requiring a common definition of such terms to avert clinical misdiagnosis (Pirri et al., 2022). Ultrasound imaging is most crucial in demarcating these anatomical layers, as evidenced by research demonstrating the superficial fascia's typical echogenicity in contrast to surrounding adipose tissue. The regular application and understanding of these terminologies can be authenticated by ultrasound pictures, such as a picture showing the bilaminated feature of superficial fascia, which visually depicts the text's contextual definition. Moreover, enhancing the clarity of terminologies is of most significance for specialist purposes in various domains of medical settings, such as musculoskeletal diseases. Appropriate communication of such terms as anatomical planes, muscle layers, and tendon insertions enhances clinical assessments and speaks a universal language between practitioners. Existing standards emphasize the importance of standardized terms when reporting about musculoskeletal pain and other conditions, ensuring that healthcare workers screen for red flag signs consistently (Lin et al., 2019).

In this regard, ultrasound technology serves as a bridge, offering visual confirmation of anatomical forms difficult to convey otherwise, that is, networks of blood vessels in the musculoskeletal system. Adding ultrasound images, discretely outlining muscle layers and tendon relationships, for example , helps practitioners map anatomical language to concurrent imaging data, thereby maximizing diagnostic acuity. Further, term coordination ensures improved patient outcomes by maintaining improved educational materials for medical students and physicians. Knowledge of the core terms is crucial for those who interpret ultrasound findings during diagnosis. Interdisciplinary cooperation, particularly among sonographers, radiologists, and surgeons, is dependent on a common language when it comes to anatomical locations. For example, in interpreting scans presenting possible pathologies in the thyroid or kidney, clear words ensure clinicians make an informed decision on time. With the aid of ultrasound images that provide unambiguous information regarding structures such as thyroid nodules or renal anatomy, the importance of precise terms in practice is justified. The best example is provided by images that show variations of thyroid nodules, integrating terminological systems with visual data and thereby creating the pedagogical strength needed in both academic and clinical practice (Figure 3.10).

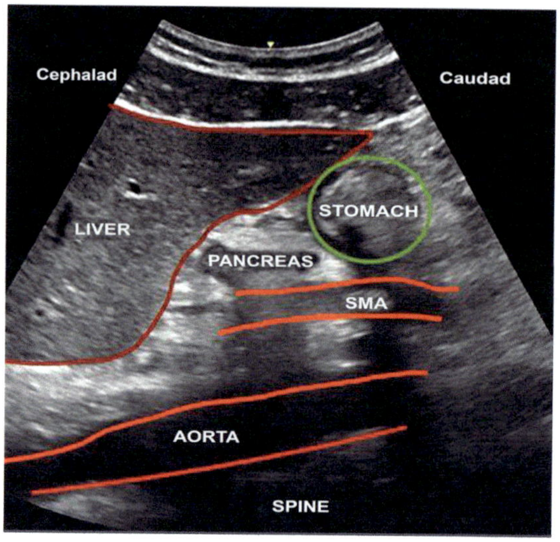

Figure 3.10. Terminology related to anatomical structures in ultrasound.

Source: Flynn DN, Doyal A, Schoenherr JW (2023). Gastric Ultrasound. In: StatPearls [Internet]. [Figure, Gastric Ultrasound, Anatomy. The ultrasound image...] Available from: https://www.ncbi.nlm.nih.gov/books/NBK580524/figure/article-143404.image.f2/

3.4. Clinical Applications of Ultrasound

The clinical applications of ultrasound are diverse and cross medical specialties, with the most well-known applications being in obstetrics and cardiology. In obstetrics, ultrasound is an essential tool for diagnosis to monitor fetal development, and it allows the physician to assess anatomical features, growth patterns, and possible congenital anomalies. The ability of ultrasound to produce dynamic images allows real-time imaging, and this is critical in assessing fetal well-being. This capability is well illustrated in the medical visualizations of the ultrasound scans defining the physiological features of the fetus, as in. In cardiology, echocardiography applies ultrasound technology to visualize cardiac structures, allowing for the assessment of heart function, valvular disease, and hemodynamic status, thus establishing its crucial role in diagnosing cardiovascular disease. In addition, applications of ultrasounds also extend beyond obstetrics and cardiology to assess other pathologies. The modality is useful in the detection and characterization of liver, kidney, and other intrabdominal organ tumors and provides valuable information needed for diagnosis and treatment planning. The use of ultrasound contrast agents enhances image quality and thus allows the assessment of more subtle vascular dynamics and lesions, particularly in differentiating between benign and malignant masses. Uses like hyperenhanced ultrasound highlight ultrasound's role in guiding interventional therapies, as embodied by the renal imaging case studies reported in. These innovations highlight the importance of ultrasound not only as an imaging modality for diagnosis but also in planning treatments. Moreover, the emergence of newer technologies such as high-frequency optical coherence tomography (OCT) also illustrates the continuing evolution of ultrasound technology in the clinic. OCT has been found to be useful for neurointerventional surgery, making it possible to image deep cerebrovascular structures and device deployment assessment during interventional procedures. The combination of OCT with traditional ultrasound imaging enhances visualization, with the potential of millimeter analysis of vascular diseases and therapy outcomes. This unification reflects a significant improvement in the use of ultrasound imaging, as demonstrated by applications described in the current corpus of research publications (Gounis et al., 2018). Ultrasound's ability to develop and integrate with other imaging modalities further characterizes its clinical significance, affirming ultrasound's role as a cornerstone in modern-day diagnostic imaging procedures, particularly in advanced uses like those described in Chernyak et al. (2018) (Figure 3.11).

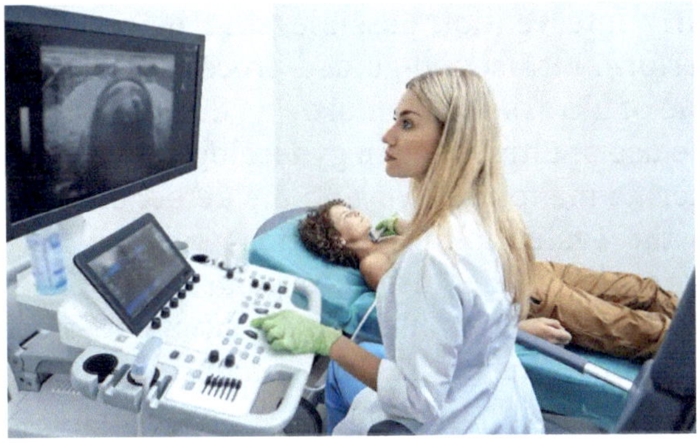

Figure 3.11. Clinical applications of ultrasound.

Source: https://4dmedica.ai/wp-content/uploads/2025/05/como-funciona-un-ecografo-origen-y-proceso.webp.

3.4.1. Use in Obstetrics and Gynecology

In gynecology and obstetrics, ultrasound scanning is a highly useful assistant to prenatal diagnosis and gynecological checks. The non-invasive technique allows visualization of the in-utero fetus, providing critical information regarding fetal growth, anatomical formation, and detection of anomalies. In addition, ultrasound occupies a pivotal position in the assessment of maternal well-being and the diagnosis of conditions such as ectopic pregnancies and ovarian cysts. The resolution and definition of the ultrasound images enable doctors to make informed management decisions throughout treatment planning and pregnancy, as well as for gynecological conditions. As displayed in this ultrasound scan demonstrates the power of the technology in bringing out significant anatomical structures, thereby making the diagnostic process even more thorough. The integration of ultrasound tests into clinical assessments enhances the quality of obstetric and gynecologic care as a whole and results in improved maternal and fetal outcomes. Improved technology in ultrasound, principally the creation of sophisticated techniques such as Doppler ultrasound, has significantly increased the accuracy of diagnosis. Doppler ultrasound assists in assessing the patterns of blood flow in the fetus, placenta, and uterine vessels, providing information about potential complications such as fetal distress or placental insufficiency. It also has application beyond baseline assessment, as seen in, where color Doppler imaging aids in the diagnosis of abnormalities in blood flow patterns that would represent poor pregnancy outcomes. This makes early intervention possible, thus being a key element of prenatal care. Moreover, the ability to perform ultrasound-guided procedures, that is, genetic counseling amniocentesis, underscores the role of ultrasound in improving diagnosis and treatment in obstetrics and gynecology. Furthermore, the use of ultrasound in gynecological practice exceeds reproductive illness evaluation, for example, uterine malformations and the detection of cancer at an early stage. It allows a standard approach to the evaluation of conditions such as fibroids, polycystic ovarian syndrome, and endometrial hyperplasia and therefore guides treatment. Real-time imaging of internal structures ensures proper follow-up of disease course and treatment response. Reference to images, such as those that illustrate the insidious nature of changes in ultrasonographic appearances of gynecologic conditions with time, underscores this. The combination of ultrasound findings with clinical history and other imaging modalities encourages a holistic approach to women's health. Consequently, this means that ultrasound is therefore, a cornerstone of contemporary obstetric and gynecologic practice that provides an important role in enabling effective management and optimizing patient outcomes in a range of scenarios (Figure 3.12).

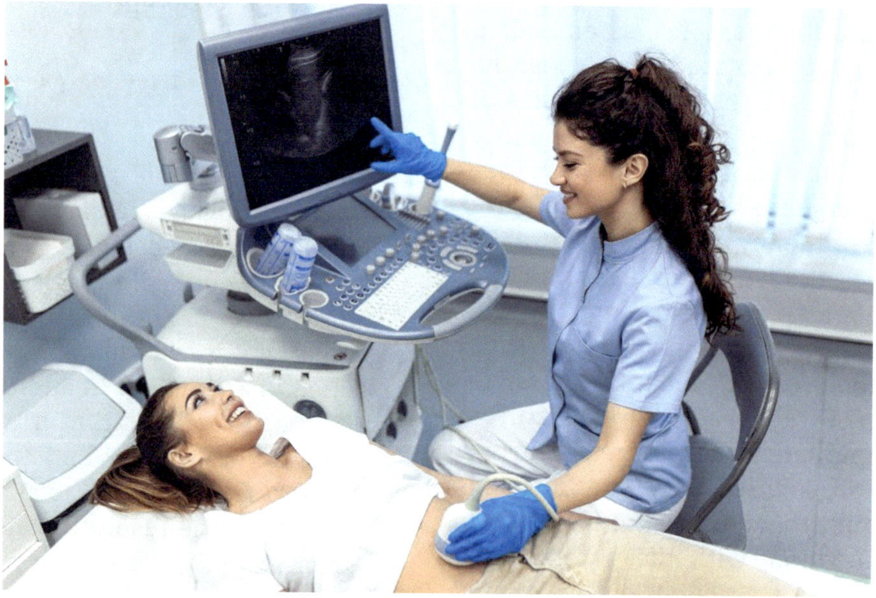

Figure 3.12. Ultrasound use in obstetrics and gynecology.

Source: https://lasvegasobgyncenter.com/wp-content/uploads/2023/11/Ultrasound-Services.jpg.

3.4.2. Applications in Cardiology

Cardiology has significantly progressed due to advances in ultrasound technology, particularly in using echocardiography. Echocardiography is a non-invasive imaging modality that provides significant information regarding cardiac anatomy and function, allowing clinicians to effectively diagnose left ventricular ejection fraction (LVEF). Transthoracic echocardiography may be applied by physicians to image patients with heart failure and other cardiovascular diseases, providing a comprehensive report of left ventricular function and structural alterations. It is, nonetheless, intriguing to note that the integration of artificial intelligence (AI) into echocardiography has revolutionized the diagnostic tool, enabling real-time data analysis and enhancing the accuracy of LVEF estimates. The advent of hand-held ultrasound scanners also enables point-of-care testing, which shows the trend towards more easily accessible and efficient cardiac imaging (Sachpekidis et al., 2022). The importance of echocardiography in cardiology illustrates its fundamental contribution towards diagnosis as well as ongoing management, cementing its role in contemporary practice. In addition, the application of AI-enabled ultrasound machines serves to standardize measurement and reduce operator-dependent variability, a long-standing problem in imaging (Akkus et al., 2021). This innovation is particularly significant in cardiology, where dependence on accurate and reproducible measurements can determine therapy and patient outcomes. Studies have shown that AI algorithms allow the identification of anatomical structures automatically, such as the left ventricular endocardium, with greater efficiency and diagnostic accuracy. In hospitals, these technologies not only streamline the procedure of echocardiography but also facilitate cardiologists in making better-informed decisions by availing themselves of authentic information for complicated cardiovascular ailments. These technologies bring to the fore the fact that the most recent technology needs to be coupled with traditional imaging techniques, giving a glimpse of tomorrow's cardiology medicine. In addition, the applications of ultrasound imaging are also used in other cardiology diagnostic interventions like the assessment of valvular diseases of the heart and the surveillance of cardiac masses or lesions. Visualization of blood flow patterns by Doppler ultrasound further enhances its application towards diagnosis, identifying defects such as stenosis or regurgitation. The essential application of ultrasound imaging is also present in pediatric cardiology, where doctors utilize echocardiograms to monitor congenital heart defects. The comprehensive assessment provided by ultrasound allows for timely intervention along with continuous monitoring, leading to improved patient outcomes. The flexibility of ultrasound technology, as well as its user-friendly nature, positions it at the forefront of cardiology as an indispensable tool, significantly influencing both diagnosis and therapy planning. The current revolution in ultrasound technology—and with it its far-reaching potential—promises to continue to drive cardiovascular care forward as medical practice strives for excellence in patient care (Figure 3.13).

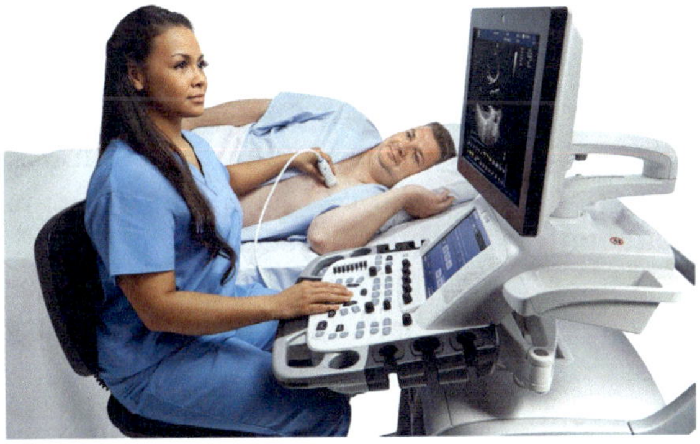

Figure 3.13. Ultrasound applications in cardiology.

Source: https://www.itnonline.com/sites/default/files/field/image/X0000_GE_Vivid%20E9%20with%20XDclear%20Adult%20Echo.jpg.

3.4.3. Role in Musculoskeletal Imaging

Ultrasound is an invaluable tool in the diagnosis and treatment of musculoskeletal diseases of bones, joints, and soft tissues in musculoskeletal imaging. Its real-time imaging capability allows clinicians to analyze dynamic motion such as joint movement and muscle contractions that are typically a prerequisite for measuring functional impairments. Ultrasound imaging flexibility enhances the examination of many anatomical structures, such as tendons, ligaments, and muscles. For instance, the comparison between traditional ultrasound and Doppler ultrasound techniques illustrates the careful assessment of the blood circulation through such tissues, thereby enabling the detection of such pathologies as tendon rupture or joint effusion. This facility is particularly relevant within sports medicine, where rapid diagnosis and intervention are crucial in order to achieve maximal rehabilitation and performance. Moreover, ultrasound is heavily employed in the guidance of interventional procedures in the musculoskeletal system. Its ability to produce real-time images enables precise needle placement for injections, aspirations, or biopsies, significantly improving their effectiveness and safety. For example, in cases where corticosteroid injections are administered for conditions like bursitis or tendinitis, ultrasound allows targeted delivery of drugs to the point of action with fewer opportunities for complications that could be encountered in blind injections. Further, the use of ultrasound in monitoring post-procedure outcomes has enhanced patient care. The success of this imaging modality in the realm of intervention proves the growing place of the modality in clinical practice, solidifying its place as an integral part of musculoskeletal imaging. The advancement of ultrasound technology, including the improvements in 3D imaging and contrast-enhanced ultrasound, also expands its application in musculoskeletal assessment. High-resolution imaging modalities provide greater sensitivity to visualize some pathologies, like hematomas or septic joint effusions and, eventually, assist the clinician in making better decisions regarding patient management. These developments are particularly noted in traumatic injury evaluation, where rapid and accurate diagnosis is paramount. In addition, the application of artificial intelligence to interpret ultrasound scans can revolutionize musculoskeletal imaging through improved diagnostic accuracy and tailored treatment plans, as evidenced in the literature (Najjar, 2023). With the development of ultrasound technology, the role of ultrasound in musculoskeletal imaging is likely to become even more integral to the clinical workflow, reshaping the process of diagnostics in this field (Panayides et al., 2020) (Figure 3.14).

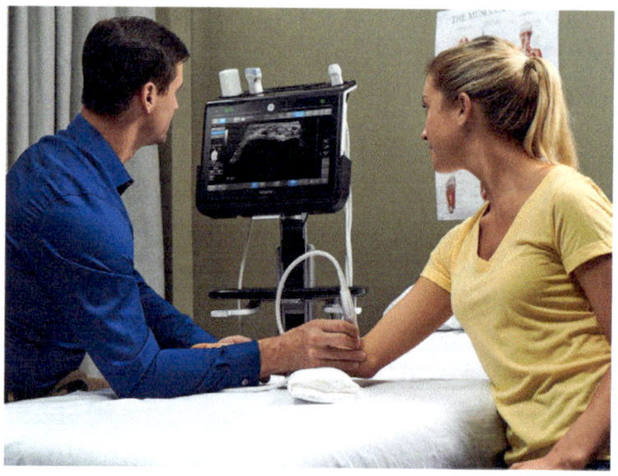

Figure 3.14. Musculoskeletal ultrasound.

Source: https://images-cdn.welcomesoftware.com/Zz04ZTc4YTBjOGNjNDcxMWVkODBmZDEyNmQxYmFmOWI1OQ==/venue-muskuloskeletal.webp.

3.5. Challenges in Ultrasound Interpretation

The interpretation of ultrasound scans is full of pitfalls that can exert a significant influence on outcome. One of the greatest issues is that ultrasound technology is operator dependent; the quality of the interpretation will rest largely with the skill and experience of the sonographer. Variations in technique—transducer position, angle of insonation, and patient anatomy—can result in variable imaging, and it is difficult to make conclusions based on the information gained. In addition, the built-in subjectivity of interpreting ultrasound, as evidenced by comparison of structures that are both normal and abnormal, can lead to variation between practitioners. For instance, in the assessment of tumors using ultrasound, the evaluation will be based on issues like the use of standardized terms such as LI-RADS and classification systems such as the ones mentioned above to reduce interpretative variation (Chernyak et al., 2018). This points to the dire need for frequent training and formulation of strict interpretive guidelines in the field of clinical practice. Another significant challenge lies in the intrinsic limitations of ultrasound technology itself, like problems with the resolution of images and penetration depth. Certain anatomical structures, particularly those deep within the body or engulfed in overlying tissue, cannot be effectively imaged and hence create doubt in the diagnosis. For example, the distinction between cystic and solid lesions can be complex, so careful evaluation of grayscale images and Doppler flow patterns must be undertaken in an effort to avoid the risk of misinterpretation. The impact of these technical limitations is especially observed in diseases like hypoxic-ischemic encephalopathy, where accuracy and timing of interpretation become essential to patient care. The application of technological innovation, such as contrast-enhanced ultrasound, can potentially solve some of these issues, but it also raises other factors that the users must control with caution. Furthermore, there is an urgent need for consistency in terminology and reporting guidelines for ultrasound interpretation. Lack of consistency in the description of how ultrasound findings are reported can lead to glaring differences in patient management and follow-up care. For instance, the evolving role of Artificial Intelligence (AI) in imaging analysis can assist in standardizing interpretation but raises ethical concerns of patient data mismanagement and technical error (Ricco et al., 2017). In conditions like cardiovascular disease, the incorporation of diverse biomarkers in ultrasound analysis can enhance patient specificity but adds more complexity to interpretation and communication among healthcare professionals. Therefore, enhancing terms and category clarity is critical, whereby ultrasound findings are universally understood and responded to.

3.5.1. The Constraints of Ultrasound Technology

Ultrasound technology, while being widely applied in medical imaging, possesses a number of intrinsic limitations that may influence diagnosis as well as patient outcomes. The foremost limitation is that it depends upon the experience and training of operators, and the quality and accuracy of the ultrasound images are significantly varied across operators. This may have implications in interpreting images and even cause missed diagnoses or misdiagnoses. Besides, the variable detection rates of structural anomalies even by experienced operators reflect the manner in which ultrasound's effectiveness is not always a given in any setting or equipment. One of these inconsistencies is evident in the results on anatomical evaluation during mid-trimester scans, where significant inconsistencies in detection rates were noted between facilities and healthcare providers, thereby highlighting that practitioners need to adhere to set guidelines in order to attain optimal results in prenatal evaluations (Salomon et al., 2022). Another significant limitation of ultrasound technology is its limited depth penetration ability for some tissues, which may conceal vital diagnostic information. As an instance, while ultrasound is great at imaging soft tissue, it may not be able to make good images of structures deeper within the body or surrounded by bone or air. It holds particularly for abdominal imaging, in which overlying tissues or gas-filled structures compromise the quality of the ultrasound images. In addition, pathologies such as obesity distort image quality even more seriously through increased tissue thickness. High-resolution imaging techniques, such as those depicted in some cases, can transcend such limitations, but are not universally available for all ultrasonographic examinations and cannot be substituted with other modalities for some cases of definitive diagnosis (Roncato et al., 2020).

Lastly, the interpretation of ultrasound is not faultless and can lead to challenges in clinical decision-making. These include artifacts, operator bias, and the subjective nature of image analysis. For example, artifacts generated by the ultrasound equipment or patient movement may lead to misleading images that appear anomalous, triggering unnecessary examinations or patient alarms. Moreover, the potential for operator bias—whereby a doctor's expectations contort their reading of an image—can compromise objectivity when making a diagnosis. Therefore, strict training and adherence to standardized procedures are necessary to reduce such biases and improve the precision of diagnosis. It is necessary to understand such limitations of ultrasound technology while evaluating its application in practice, as emphasized in images like, which refer to maintaining quality control in imaging practices.

3.5.2. Common Pitfalls in Image Interpretation

Successful interpretation of ultrasound images is full of numerous pitfalls, the most obvious being observer variability. Different operators will bring different levels of knowledge, experience, and ability to the process of interpretation and hence differences in diagnostic findings. This has been amply demonstrated in studies, and the reason for instituting formal training programs for sonographers is therefore enhanced. For instance, the variation in ultrasound images and their interpretation by software and even by experienced sonographers reveals drastic differences in results, indicative of the inherent challenges of subjective image analysis (Xu et al., 2025). The clinical significance of this variation extends to clinical practice, where misdiagnosis and inappropriate management of patients are possible. This built-in risk leans toward the need for frequent measurement calibrations and the implementation of complementary interpretative technology, such as cutting-edge imaging software, to balance errors identified in standard ultrasound protocols. Another common trap in ultrasound image interpretation involves a lack of detection for artifacts. Ultrasound technology is susceptible to various artifacts that can conceal true anatomical information or mimic conditions of disease. For instance, shadowing, enhancement, and ringing artifacts can complicate the clarity of the images, and thus misinterpretation. Clearly illustrates a range of imaging results, in which artifacts may be superimposed on anatomy. It is necessary to understand how these artifacts behave in demarcating actual structures from misleading signals, and sonographers must be instructed to learn to identify and account for such discrepancies. Furthermore, misclassification of artifacts has the potential to result in misdiagnosis due to clinicians being confused by benign and malignant findings. Through enhancing training on the ability to differentiate between these types of imaging abnormalities, professionals can significantly eliminate diagnostic error and enhance patient safety. Incorporating artificial intelligence (AI) into ultrasound imaging has promise but also poses its own interpretative issues. While AI systems can provide improved efficiency and reduced human error by offering second opinions, they are not infallible. Over-reliance by them without proper clinical judgment can result in false conclusions. For example, the AI software's diagnosis of thyroid nodules, as per various studies, shows high agreement with expert sonographer's assessments

(Xu et al., 2025). However, the nuance of biological systems renders context non-reducible. As AI learns from sets of established data, incorrect interpretations could arise from incomplete or biased data. Proper integration of AI should thus ensure that clinical expertise is kept in the forefront to avoid technology assistance replacing but rather complementing human expertise in interpreting ultrasound images (Figure 3.15).

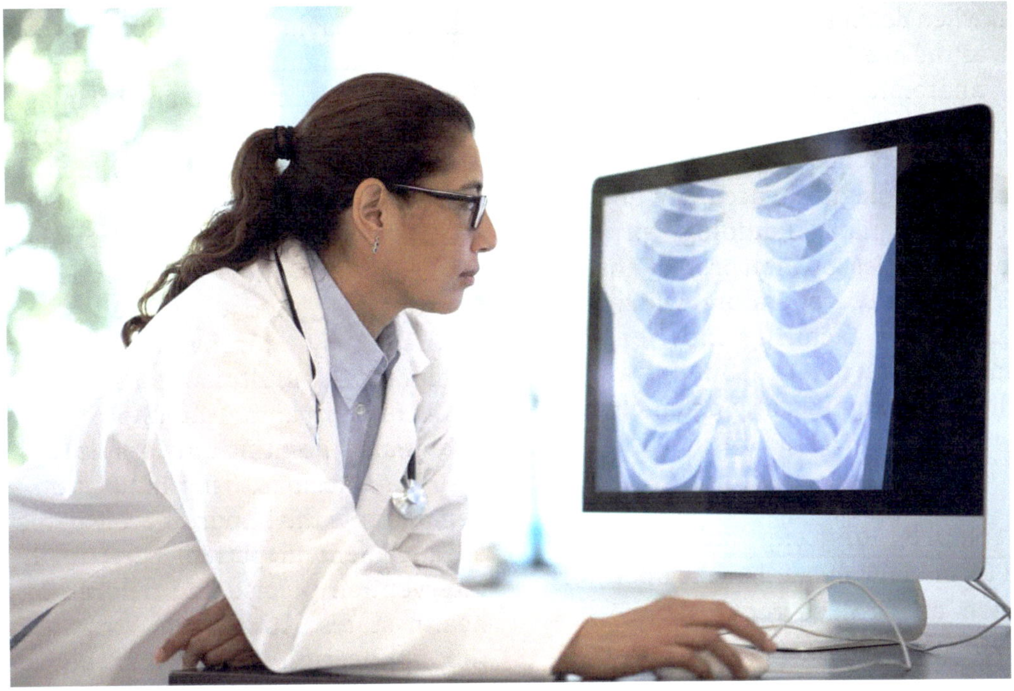

Figure 3.15. Top pitfalls in interpreting common diagnostic images.

Source: https://www.fhea.com/wp-content/uploads/2021/07/Clinical-iStock-1169769901-scaled.jpg.

3.5.3. Importance of Operator Skill and Experience

The proficiency of the ultrasound operator plays a vital role in the evaluation of good and informative image interpretation. A good operator possesses the ability to handle the ultrasound machine with precision and the best imaging parameters to adapt in order to capture the target anatomical structures. Variations in the operator's skill affect image quality and diagnostic outcomes immensely. For instance, the correct procedure of using transducer selection and placement determines the image quality captured. As shown in, the nuanced interaction among different modalities can furnish important information for clinical assessment. Furthermore, operators' experience plays a role in differentiating normal from pathological findings, impacting clinical decision-making and patient management. The operators should receive more advanced training and continuous professional development to enhance their competence and to embrace the technological innovations in the specialty. This emphasis on operator expertise underscores the value of continuing education to achieve excellence in ultrasound imaging. Experience is also paramount in the interpretation of ultrasound images. Experienced operators possess the ability to recognize subtle details that are potentially indicative of underlying pathology, one which arises from experience with extensive numbers of clinical cases. As the subject of Hung et al. (2024) explains, the complexities in interpreting musculoskeletal ultrasound images are high. The need for skill is also re-emphasized when dealing with interpreting lung ultrasound, as the need for operator knowledge of various anatomic patterns and potential anomalies, as discussed in Muñoz et al. (2023). Therefore, the experience level of an operator directly influences diagnosis accuracy and the related treatment plans. Radiology practice reveals the difficulties of interpreting images among less-experienced operators, which lead to misdiagnoses. By factoring experience as an important aspect of ultrasound training, health facilities can significantly enhance their diagnostic function as well as maintain patient safety.

Furthermore, ongoing advances in ultrasound technology mean that the operators need to keep up with current practice and innovations. The application of artificial intelligence to support the interpretation of images, as seen in the case of lung ultrasound and musculoskeletal diagnosis, is reflective of one way in which the operator's skills are needed to change. Although AI can provide assistance, it is vital that clinicians are cautious when looking at the results generated by the systems. Operator competence is not only in the execution of procedures but also in understanding AI-generated information in the overall clinical context. The images presented, for example , reaffirm the significance of operator competence in maximizing the benefit of these technologies. Through the development of a lifelong learning and resilience culture, the medical community can ensure that ultrasound imaging remains a safe, effective, and reliable diagnostic modality in patient management.

3.6. Development of Ultrasound Technology

The evolution of ultrasound technology has completely revolutionized the history of medical diagnosis, paving the way for improved imaging technologies and more precise interpretation. Technologies such as 3D and 4D imaging provide dynamic images of structures, particularly in obstetrics and gynecology, which were never achievable with plain 2D ultrasound. Through the real-time observation of fetal development, clinicians can follow up on fetal health more appropriately and diagnose anomalies early in pregnancy. Moreover, the intersection of dissimilarity on ultrasound scans, as indicated in, is further aimed at improving diagnostic potential by pointing out variance in benign and malignant lesions. This innovation is used to demonstrate the important role of technological advancement in patient care, further making intervention precise and tailored to individual health states. Apart from structural imaging, the application of Doppler ultrasound has revolutionized blood flow measurement and the integrity of the vessels. Doppler technology enables doctors to visualize the movement of blood flow, illustrating heart valve action and identifying potential blockages, as illustrated in. This capability extends beyond diagnosis to guide therapeutic decisions in numerous fields of clinical practice, including vascular medicine and cardiology. Earlier therapeutic intervention, facilitated by the non-invasive capability to assess vascular conditions, has dramatically enhanced patient outcomes, demonstrating the transformative power of high-tech ultrasound technology. These developments are a testament to how ultrasound technology develops further to meet the evolving needs of clinical practice in order to effectively monitor and manage cardiovascular diseases. Another critical component of today's ultrasound developments is the incorporation of artificial intelligence (AI) into image interpretation, enhancing diagnostic accuracy with enhanced workflow efficiencies. AI applications have been promising in automating image analysis, from detecting anomalies to supporting organ and tissue segmentation (Najjar, 2023). This combination provides improved coverage for studying complicated cases, where traditional approaches may fail. Secondly, improved risk stratification and classification algorithms, according to Panayides et al. (2020), allow clinicians to offer tailored treatment plans following more precise prognostic estimation. Since AI continues to advance in the field of ultrasound imaging, it has the potential to change not only the process of image analysis but also the patient experience in general with improved diagnostic capabilities and efficient management protocols (Figure 3.16).

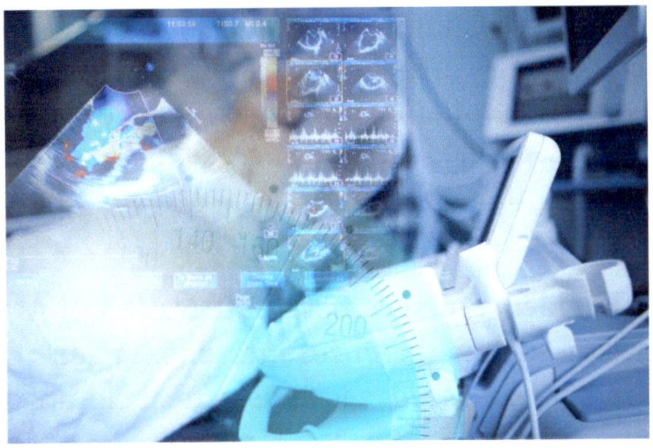

Figure 3.16. Advances in ultrasound technology.

Source: https://external-content.duckduckgo.com/iu/?u=https%3A%2F%2Facertaralabs.com%2Fwp-content%2Fuploads%2F2023%2F04%2Fshutterstock_2156852885.jpg&f=1&nofb=1&ipt=1cf90018cc85b382ac07b1416dfbda40f2ab64c2dee3ede2d3f1461ed20abaec.

3.6.1. Innovations in Imaging Techniques

The evolution of imaging technologies in the ultrasonography domain has brought forth a new era of diagnostic competence and accuracy. Tools such as contrast-enhanced ultrasound (CEUS) have revolutionized the evaluation of all categories of conditions, particularly in nephrology. CEUS's ability to enhance the visualization of renal structures enables clinicians to effectively distinguish between solid and cystic renal masses, thereby providing accurate treatment protocols. Panel (d) clearly demonstrates the relative merits of CEUS over routine ultrasound for renal imaging, highlighting the significant advances in diagnostic precision. Improved risk stratification of renal masses is now possible with this technology, facilitating early intervention in acute processes and management of chronic renal disease. These advances not only improve clinical outcomes but also increase the interpretative capability of ultrasound, in line with the future trends of individualized medicine and individualized therapeutic strategy.

Other advances in ultrasound imaging are reviewed in terms of the integration of artificial intelligence (AI) into the radiological practice. Machine learning and deep learning techniques allow for computerized image analysis, which promises accuracy and efficiency improvements in image interpretation. According to the findings in (Najjar, 2023), AI is not merely a supporting tool but a force of revolution that enables enhanced workflow optimization and predictive analytics in diagnostic imaging. For instance, AI algorithms can assist radiologists in detecting anomalies that do not necessarily stand out to the naked eye, thereby complementing the diagnostic process with empirical evidence. As radiology moves to adopt AI-driven technologies, the impacts carry over into other fields, such as adding depth and richness to diagnostic imaging across a variety of clinical specialties, for example, emergency medicine and chronic disease management. Another important innovation in imaging techniques is the development of shape-morphing sensors. As outlined in Luo et al. (2023), the flexibility of these sensors goes beyond the inherent limitations of rigid counterparts to enable ubiquitous sensing applications in the field of medical diagnostics. Integration in ultrasound imaging enables a wider range of anatomical assessments, particularly in patient-centered examinations where flexibility and comfort are considerations. The transition from rigid conventional imaging to flexible sensors represents a paradigm shift in diagnostic practice that enhances both patient experience and outcomes. By facilitating real-time data capture and paving the way for seamless integration with clinical practice, advanced imaging technologies such as flexible sensors reaffirm the role of flexibility and precision in modern diagnostics. These innovations collectively assist in refining the interpretative horizon of ultrasound scans, highlighting again the cogent imperative of continued investigation and interdisciplinarity within the medical arts.

3.6.2. Integration of Artificial Intelligence in Ultrasound

The incorporation of artificial intelligence (AI) in ultrasound imaging is a revolutionary step in medical diagnosis that improves both efficiency and reliability of image interpretation. AI, through its advanced algorithms, can interpret ultrasound images with a level of accuracy that is usually higher than conventional methods. These algorithms employ deep learning methodologies to identify patterns and abnormalities in ultrasound images that could not be appreciated by human professionals. Thus, this technology allows for earlier diagnosis of tumors and other pathological abnormalities and, in the long run, leads to improved patient outcomes. In this context, the use of AI not only streamlines the work pattern of medical professionals but also ensures that early and accurate diagnoses are made accessible to patients, demonstrating technology's ability to redefine the way medical imaging is managed. This use of AI is adequately demonstrated in the contrast-enhanced ultrasound images that help differentiate benign from malignant lesions, like in. Further, AI-based applications for ultrasound imaging are underpinned by generative AI capabilities that allow a more interactive and intuitive mode of human-computer interaction. With generative models, such as in the guise of OpenAI's ChatGPT, ultrasound equipment can assist with instant contextual answers and diagnostic suggestions as real-time data inputs from medical professionals. Not only does this enhance the user experience, but it also allows for the possibility of personalized approaches in patient treatment. A case in point is information from higher-end imaging that results in tailored treatment options, which cater specifically to a patient's health needs. Utilization of such generative AI tools is a significant movement towards more comprehensive and interactive diagnostic modalities in ultrasound imaging, heralding a future where AI becomes a permanent collaborator in clinical decision-making pipelines, in turn increasing diagnostic accuracy and confidence in various medical specialties (Zhang et al., 2023).

Besides, the successful integration of AI in ultrasound imaging presents challenges that must be addressed cautiously to facilitate its full potential. These challenges involve data quality, the "black box" problem associated with AI models, and ethical concerns of patient data confidentiality. As more AI systems are exposed to advanced datasets, data quality and volume disparities may lead to biased results, which could impair patient care. Second, there is insufficient transparency of AI algorithm, which can generate distrust on the part of radiologists and prevent its widespread use. Overcoming all these requires a many-sided approach through collaboration between radiologists, AI developers, and regulatory bodies to ensure not only efficacy but also ethical usage of AI in practice. The exploration of these challenges forms a critical aspect of understanding AI's trajectory within ultrasound imaging and the broader medical field, indicating the importance of ethical frameworks in shaping future initiatives (Najjar, 2023).

3.6.3. Future Trends in Ultrasound Diagnostics

As advances in ultrasound technology continue, future developments in diagnostics are significantly centered on enhancing image quality and diagnostic accuracy. Developments like three-dimensional (3D) and four-dimensional (4D) ultrasound scanning will provide richer anatomical images compared to two-dimensional imaging. This advancement allows for better visualization of complex structures, particularly in obstetrics, where accurate fetal assessment is paramount. In addition, imaging informatics advances, especially those involving artificial intelligence (AI), promise to transform ultrasound image interpretations to enable more accurate and faster diagnoses. The use of AI in the diagnosis of ultrasound helps identify abnormalities in real time and ensures a much smaller margin of human error and enables personalized medicine strategies. This new paradigm not only maximizes clinical outcomes but also complies with the current trends in medicine that promote patient-centered treatment. Simultaneously evolving progress of technology and informatics constitutes a shining future for ultrasound diagnosis. Moreover, the use of contrast-enhanced ultrasound (CEUS) is going to revolutionize diagnostic techniques, particularly in the evaluation of vascular disease and tumors. CEUS uses microbubble contrast agents to enhance blood flow and tissue characterization visualization, thus assisting in the differentiation between malignant and benign lesions as well as improving treatment planning. The technique surpasses standard ultrasound imaging since it provides dynamic information on perfusion, which ultimately leads to better patient outcomes. As attested to by images of CEUS applications, its efficiency in real-time evaluation of renal masses speaks to its potential in many diagnostic applications. As it continues to improve, it can be a decisive tool in oncology, nephrology, and vascular medicine, complementing traditional imaging methods with an integrated ultrasound diagnosis strategy. The future of CEUS is towards more sensitivity and specificity, which are necessary for making timely and accurate clinical decisions.

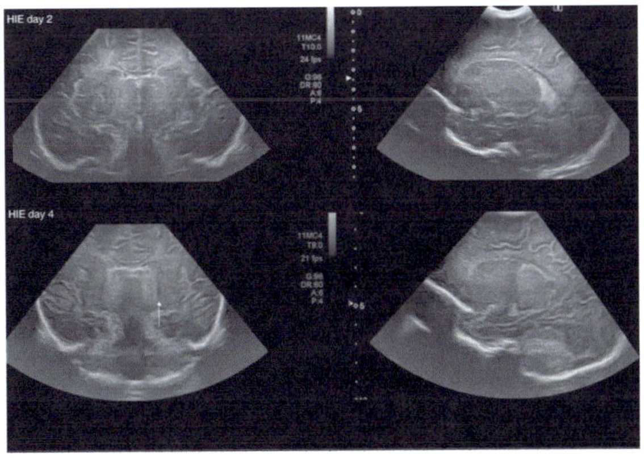

Figure 3.17. Ultrasound scans of hypoxic-ischemic encephalopathy over several days.

Source: Dudink, J., Jeanne Steggerda, S., Horsch, S. et al. (2020) State-of-the-art neonatal cerebral ultrasound: technique and reporting. Pediatr Res 87 (Suppl 1), 3–12. https://doi.org/10.1038/s41390-020-0776-y

The application of interventional ultrasound also promises to expand significantly as more healthcare professionals find its benefits. The technique allows for minimally invasive procedures such as biopsies and drainage under real-time imaging guidance, which can significantly reduce patient recovery time and complications. Ultrasound technology history, including advancements like portable and handheld devices, brings high-level diagnostic capability within reach, so that non-traditional practitioners in places like rural and underserved areas can make required evaluations without the need for massive infrastructure. Portable ultrasound machines highlight a trend toward more ease and efficiency in medicine to complement clinical demands for real-time diagnosis. As can be observed in the series of ultrasound images, ranging from traditional methods to advanced techniques like those presented in and, this shift demonstrates an increased concern for bettering the care of patients by using newer ultrasound technology, paving the way towards an enhanced and fair health care system (Figure 3.17).

SUMMARY

An evaluation of sonographic assessment and ultrasound image interpretation highlights the critical importance of combining clinical context with sonographic evaluations. As indicated in research, such as that correlating clinical context to gallbladder ultrasound interpretation, a subtle understanding derived from clinical context maximizes decisiveness, particularly in complex conditions such as acute cholecystitis. This is significant because it reminds radiologists and clinicians to remember clinical presentations as well as sonographic appearances. Such practices not only improve diagnostic specificity and sensitivity but also deliver focused management strategies, a sign of the shift towards a more unified comprehension of patient care and diagnosis in ultrasound imaging (Rodrigues et al., 2025). Moreover, advances in imaging technology, as reflected in ultrasound images having well-defined anatomical structures, emphasize the growing complexity of ultrasound reports. For instance, images such as and permit ease in pathology differentiation and convey vascular and anatomical information critical for precise assessment. These advances in imaging enable improved understanding of the condition of the patients, thereby promoting evidence-based decision-making within the clinical setting. Further, the expanding use of artificial intelligence in the analysis of ultrasound brings into the process a certain level of complexity and potential (Tmenova et al., 2024). In general, the future of ultrasound image nomenclature and interpretation promises to evolve with the continued explosion in technology and methods. As presented, adding in clinical context maximally improves diagnostic performance, supporting the initial mandate for continuing education and training for the practitioner. Moreover, visual illustrations of contemporary ultrasound practice mirror the evolving landscape of medical imaging in which technology, beyond providing valuable information, also listens to clinical need so that patient care is enhanced. Thus, this convergence of clinical skill and technological innovation has the potential to refine ultrasound practice so that medical practitioners can be optimally equipped to handle the subtleties of diagnostic imaging in every branch of medicine.

In summing up the important points made in the context of ultrasound image interpretation and nomenclature, there is a need to underscore the revolutionary impact of ultrasound technology in medical diagnostics. As shown in several studies, ultrasound imaging technologies like Thoracic point-of-care ultrasound (T-POCUS) have been crucial in diagnosing a range of pulmonary diseases in veterinary medicine. This non-invasiveness, in combination with the ability to image in real time, allows practitioners to make timely and informed decisions regarding patient management, as evidenced by its application in diagnosing diseases such as pleural effusion and pneumothorax (Armenise, 2025). The expectation of reproducible ultrasound findings such as B-lines and the sheared sign also serves to emphasize the contribution made by the use of standardized terminology and interpretation to the achievement of successful diagnoses. Overall, the technological development in ultrasound enhances both patient outcomes and quality of care across many specialty areas in medicine. Apart from its established applications in veterinary and obstetric care, ultrasound imaging finds more and more applications in orthopedics and musculoskeletal testing. Advances like AI-assisted techniques to diagnose rotator cuff tears show the technology's expanding versatility. By applying sophisticated algorithms, the duration required for the evaluation of injuries has reduced considerably, emphasizing how ultrasound reporting is evolving alongside advancements in artificial intelligence and machine learning (Chamundeswari et al., 2025). The rapid analysis aids in early detection, which is critical to facilitate better patient outcomes. The use of AI not only optimizes interpretive accuracy but also efficient workflow in clinical practice, enabling clinicians to pay greater attention to patient care. All such developments require continued investment in training and education to further enhance ultrasound image interpretation and terminology. Furthermore, the key features of ultrasound image assessment need to be familiar with both visual and contextual cues. Images such as those demonstrating the piezoelectric effect and renal ultrasound techniques contribute to the richness of educational discussion of ultrasound jargon and interpretation. Not only do they demonstrate anatomical structures, but they also help in a better understanding of disease processes and imaging modalities. The inclusion of comparative panels and multiple imaging modalities makes the discussion more robust with a clear demonstration of the various strategies being employed in contemporary ultrasound interpretations. It is evident that arming practitioners with these tools and information will enhance their abilities in the evolving science of ultrasound diagnostics, contributing to a culture of excellence in patient care and clinical outcomes.

CLOSER LOOK

CONTRAST-ENHANCED ULTRASOUND

Contrast-enhanced ultrasound (CEUS) is an advanced imaging technique that enhances standard ultrasonography through the use of microbubble contrast agents to visualize blood flow and tissue vascularity in real time. Unlike standard contrast agents used in CT or MRI, CEUS utilizes gas-filled microbubbles (typically produced with inert gases like perfluorocarbon or sulfur hexafluoride) covered by a lipid or protein shell. These microbubbles are trapped intravascularly and small enough to be arterially pumped via the pulmonary vasculature but large enough not to diffuse into the interstitium, making them ideal for imaging vascular structures and perfusion without diffusion in the systemic circulation. Upon intravenous injection, these microbubbles oscillate on encountering ultrasound waves and produce high-intensity echoes, thus significantly enhancing the echogenicity of blood, thus more effectively detecting vascular flow, tissue perfusion, and lesion characterization. CEUS has revolutionized diagnostic imaging, particularly in the evaluation of focal liver lesions, since it can differentiate benign from malignant tumors based on enhancement patterns during arterial, portal venous, and delayed phases. Hemangiomas, hepatocellular carcinoma (HCC), metastases, and focal nodular hyperplasia (FNH) are specific for certain enhancement patterns that can be identified with CEUS without radiation. CEUS is also most useful in the assessment of renal, pancreatic, splenic, and thyroid masses and in the diagnosis of testicular torsion, intestinal ischemia, and trauma-related organ injuries, especially in pediatrics and emergencies. One of its most valuable advantages is CEUS's safety profile. Unlike iodinated or gadolinium agents, ultrasound contrast agents are non-nephrotoxic and rarely cause allergic reactions; thus, CEUS is safe in patients with compromised renal function or contrast media allergies. Additionally, as it uses no ionizing radiation, it can be used repeatedly and safely in sensitive patient groups, for example, children and pregnant women (in well-selected cases). In vascular diagnosis, CEUS can visualize microvascular movement in real-time, assisting in diagnosing aortic aneurysms endoleaks after endovascular repair, and peripheral artery disease. It also plays a critical role in guiding interventional procedures such as biopsies, tumor ablations, and drainage placements by delineating lesion margins and response to treatment more accurately than conventional B-mode ultrasound. Despite all its advantages, CEUS has its drawbacks. Operator dependence, reduced field of view, and failure to image deep structures in obese patients can be limiting factors. Also, it functions less optimally in the presence of calcification or bowel gas. Advances in technology like high-frame-rate ultrasound, harmonic imaging, and fusion imaging are further enhancing the performance of CEUS. As more regulatory approvals of applications of CEUS come in globally, its integration into routine clinical practice is gradually on the rise. Current guidelines from organizations such as the American College of Radiology and European Federation of Societies for Ultrasound in Medicine and Biology (EFSUMB) suggest its use in all hepatic and non-hepatic indications. Lastly, contrast-enhanced ultrasound is a powerful, patient-friendly, and interactive imaging tool that bridges the gap between routine sonography and more invasive or risk-prone imaging techniques to give the clinician an effective, affordable, and real-time diagnostic, monitoring, and interventional guide tool.

References

1. Aggarwal, A., Mittal, M., & Battineni, G. (2021). Generative adversarial network: An overview of theory and applications. *International Journal of Information Management Data Insights, 1*, 100004. https://doi.org/10.1016/j.jjimei.2020.100004 (accessed on 12th July 2025).
2. Akinci D'Antonoli, T., Stanzione, A., Bluethgen, C., Vernuccio, F., Ugga, L., Klontzas, M. E., Cuocolo, R., et al. (2023). Large language models in radiology: Fundamentals, applications, ethical considerations, risks, and future directions. *Diagnostic and Interventional Radiology, 30*, 80–90. https://doi.org/10.4274/dir.2023.232417 (accessed on 12th July 2025).
3. Akkus, Z., Aly, Y. H., Attia, I., Lopez-Jimenez, F., Arruda-Olson, A. M., Pellikka, P., Pislaru, S., et al. (2021). Artificial intelligence (AI)-empowered echocardiography interpretation: A state-of-the-art review. *Journal of Clinical Medicine, 10*. https://www.semanticscholar.org/paper/e6c812388b7e00358cfc38f7923cd879b42aedfa (accessed on 12th July 2025).
4. Alshalahi, S., Alguizzani, N., Alqarni, D., Korkoman, S., Almassari, M., Alotayban, R., & Tehsin, F. (2025). Pregnant women's perceptions and knowledge of obstetric ultrasound in Central Region, Saudi Arabia. *International Journal of Medicine in Developing Countries*. https://www.semanticscholar.org/paper/3f7215c4897b33c290d7189e8ba097b76222f6cc (accessed on 12th July 2025).
5. Alyami, A. S., Majrashi, N., & Shubayr, N. (2021). Radiologists' and radiographers' perspectives on artificial intelligence in medical imaging in Saudi Arabia (Preprint). https://www.semanticscholar.org/paper/17ddc79c59b6ba5aef96c2e0d8b89048a79bfdf3 (accessed on 12th July 2025).
6. Armenise, A. (2025). Point-of-care lung ultrasound in small animal emergency and critical care medicine: A clinical review. *Animals: An Open Access Journal from MDPI, 15*. https://www.semanticscholar.org/paper/31d23dfd32491c3ab0d6d24a29d1c38bc4a5eb14 (accessed on 12th July 2025).
7. Becker, C. M., Bokor, A., Heikinheimo, O., Horne, A. W., Jansen, F., Kiesel, L., King, K., et al. (2022). ESHRE guideline: Endometriosis. *Human Reproduction Open, 2022*. https://doi.org/10.1093/hropen/hoac009 (accessed on 12th July 2025).
8. Bilardo, C. M., Chaoui, R., Hyett, J., Kagan, K. O., Karim, J., Papageorghiou, A. T., Poon, L. C., et al. (2023). ISUOG practice guidelines (updated): Performance of 11–14-week ultrasound scan. *Ultrasound in Obstetrics and Gynecology, 61*, 127–143. https://doi.org/10.1002/uog.26106 (accessed on 12th July 2025).
9. Carvalho, J. S., Axt-Fliedner, R., Chaoui, R., Copel, J. A., Cuneo, B. F., Goff, D. A., Gordin Kopylov, L., et al. (2023). *ISUOG* Practice Guidelines (updated): Fetal cardiac screening. *Ultrasound in Obstetrics and Gynecology, 61*, 788–803. https://doi.org/10.1002/uog.26224 (accessed on 12th July 2025).
10. Chamundeswari, Y. S., Anusha, V., Lakshmi, Y., Sri, S., Deepika, A., Boora, L. K., Sri, Y., et al. (2025). AutoRCuff: CNN-autoencoder-based intelligent detection of rotator cuff tendon tears from ultrasound imaging. *International Journal of Scientific Research and Engineering Trends*. https://www.semanticscholar.org/paper/f0cde4b128169c714af193b7538b13e78090e5a2 (accessed on 12th July 2025).

11. Chernyak, V., Fowler, K. J., Kamaya, A., Kielar, A. Z., Elsayes, K. M., Bashir, M. R., Kono, Y., et al. (2018). Liver Imaging Reporting and Data System (LI-RADS) Version 2018: Imaging of hepatocellular carcinoma in at-risk patients. *Radiology, 289*, 816–830. https://doi.org/10.1148/radiol.2018181494 (accessed on 12th July 2025).

12. Cloutier, G., Destrempes, F., Yu, F. T. H., & Tang, A. (2021). Quantitative ultrasound imaging of soft biological tissues: A primer for radiologists and medical physicists. *Insights into Imaging, 12*. https://doi.org/10.1186/s13244-021-01071-w (accessed on 12th July 2025).

13. .Critchley, H., Babayev, E., Bulun, S. E., Clark, S., Garcia-Grau, I., Gregersen, P. K., Kilcoyne, A., et al. (2020). Menstruation: Science and society. *American Journal of Obstetrics and Gynecology, 223*, 624–664. https://doi.org/10.1016/j.ajog.2020.06.004 (accessed on 12th July 2025).

14. De Santis Santiago, R. R., Xin, Y., Gaulton, T., Alcala, G., León Bueno de Camargo, E. D., Cereda, M., Amato, M. B. P., et al. (2023). Lung imaging acquisition with electrical impedance tomography: Tackling common pitfalls. *Anesthesiology, 139*, 329–341. https://www.semanticscholar.org/paper/9d5f8c2def58caa8e9455c3e3c91f30bb8533d5c (accessed on 12th July 2025).

15. Demi, L., Wolfram, F., Klersy, C., De Silvestri, A., Ferretti, V. V., Müller, M., Miller, D. L., et al. (2022). New international guidelines and consensus on the use of lung ultrasound. *Journal of Ultrasound in Medicine, 42*, 309–344. https://doi.org/10.1002/jum.16088 (accessed on 12th July 2025).

16. Fleming, K. A., Horton, S., Wilson, M. L., Atun, R., DeStigter, K., Flanigan, J., Sayed, S., et al. (2021). The Lancet Commission on diagnostics: Transforming access to diagnostics. *The Lancet, 398*, 1997–2050. https://doi.org/10.1016/s0140-6736(21)00673-5 (accessed on 12th July 2025).

17. Gargano, M., Matentzoglu, N., Coleman, B., Addo-Lartey, E. B., Anagnostopoulos, A. V., Anderton, J., Avillach, P., et al. (2023). The Human Phenotype Ontology in 2024: Phenotypes around the world. *Nucleic Acids Research, 52*, D1333–D1346. https://doi.org/10.1093/nar/gkad1005 (accessed on 12th July 2025).

18. Gordon, M., Daniel, M., Ajiboye, A., Uraiby, H., Xu, N. Y., Bartlett, R., Hanson, J. L., et al. (2024). A scoping review of artificial intelligence in medical education: BEME Guide No. 84. *Medical Teacher, 46*, 446–470. https://doi.org/10.1080/0142159x.2024.2314198 (accessed on 12th July 2025).

19. Gounis, M. J., Ughi, G. J., Marosföi, M., Lopes, D. K., Fiorella, D., Bezerra, H. G., Liang, C. W., et al. (2018). Intravascular optical coherence tomography for neurointerventional surgery. *Stroke, 50*, 218–223. https://doi.org/10.1161/strokeaha.118.022315 (accessed on 12th July 2025).

20. Guillén-Grima, F., Guillén-Aguinaga, S., Guillén-Aguinaga, L., Alas-Brun, R., Onambele, L., Ortega, W., Montejo, R., et al. (2023). Evaluating the efficacy of ChatGPT in navigating the Spanish medical residency entrance examination (MIR): Promising horizons for AI in clinical medicine. *Clinics and Practice, 13*, 1460–1487. https://doi.org/10.3390/clinpract13060130 (accessed on 12th July 2025).

21. Gusev, A. A. (2025). What neural networks and how a urologist can utilize in his routine tasks: Practical tips. *Urology Herald*. https://www.semanticscholar.org/paper/1337547052cd865554cde90fd309979f0d5f2cca (accessed on 12th July 2025).

22. Hung, H. Y., Kao, J. P., Chu, H. Y., Chen, C. P., & Chen, W. S. (2024). Real time musculoskeletal ultrasound image annotations. *Proceedings of SPIE, 13487*, 134870B–134870B-5. https://

www.semanticscholar.org/paper/24548db4fb1ed88f8a70bb0d1a856c41e46c412b (accessed on 12th July 2025).

23. Jenabi, F., Mageean, K. S., Leahy, A., Davidson, B., & de Graaf, H. (2020). EP37 A need to train pediatric rheumatologists in musculoskeletal ultrasound scanning. How do we move forward? *Rheumatology Advances in Practice, 4*. https://www.semanticscholar.org/paper/72d353f029f0b90fb3ebb31353ef12da28341bc0 (accessed on 12th July 2025).

24. Lin, C. H., Lee, M. C., Pan, S., & Lu, C. Y. (2006). Wavelet compression algorithm applied to abdominal ultrasound images. *53*, 11–17. https://www.semanticscholar.org/paper/7d34978f7e2b9822b260444ca7f7afd7da8b2b82 (accessed on 12th July 2025).

25. Lin, I., Wiles, L., Waller, R., Goucke, R., Nagree, Y., Gibberd, M., Straker, L., et al. (2019). What does best practice care for musculoskeletal pain look like? Eleven consistent recommendations from high-quality clinical practice guidelines: Systematic review. *British Journal of Sports Medicine, 54*, 79–86. https://doi.org/10.1136/bjsports-2018-099878 (accessed on 12th July 2025).

26. Luo, Y., Abidian, M. R., Ahn, J. H., Akinwande, D., Andrews, A. M., Antonietti, M., Bao, Z., et al. (2023). Technology roadmap for flexible sensors. *ACS Nano, 17*, 5211–5295. https://doi.org/10.1021/acsnano.2c12606 (accessed on 12th July 2025).

27. Medical imaging techniques: MRI and ultrasound scans [Figure]. (2025). https://assets.cureus.com/uploads/figure/file/1024545/article_river_78934270108b11ef99ffa3ff91ec0b65-fig-1-ok.png (accessed on 12th July 2025).

28. Mlosek, K., Migda, B., & Migda, M. (2020). High-frequency ultrasound in the 21st century. *Journal of Ultrasonography, 20*, 233–241. https://doi.org/10.15557/jou.2020.0042 (accessed on 12th July 2025).

29. Möller, K., Ntovas, S., Hocke, M., On, W., Everett, S. M., Braden, B., Jenssen, C., et al. (2024). Comments and illustrations of the European Federation of Societies for Ultrasound in Medicine guidelines: Rare pancreatic tumors, ultrasound and contrast-enhanced ultrasound features—Malignant mesenchymal tumors. *Endoscopic Ultrasound, 13*, 55–64. https://www.semanticscholar.org/paper/f446b86a81c981dd2505924128a1c5b4b2fed799 (accessed on 12th July 2025).

30. Muñoz, M., Cosarinsky, G., Cruza, J., & Camacho, J. (2023). Deep learning-based lung ultrasound image segmentation for real-time analysis. In *2023 IEEE International Ultrasonics Symposium (IUS)*. https://www.semanticscholar.org/paper/59a2d11e022ebf2c02b9240ec33a20d39d6d0762 (accessed on 12th July 2025).

31. Najjar, R. (2023). Redefining radiology: A review of artificial intelligence integration in medical imaging. *Diagnostics, 13*, 2760. https://doi.org/10.3390/diagnostics13172760 (accessed on 12th July 2025).

32. Panayides, A. S., Amini, A. A., Filipović, N., Sharma, A., Tsaftaris, S. A., Young, A. A., Foran, D. J., et al. (2020). AI in medical imaging informatics: Current challenges and future directions. *IEEE Journal of Biomedical and Health Informatics, 24*, 1837–1857. https://doi.org/10.1109/jbhi.2020.2991043 (accessed on 12th July 2025).

33. Pezzilli, R. (2021). Editorial for "Does training in LI-RADS Version 2018 improve readers' agreement with the expert consensus and inter-reader agreement in MRI interpretation?."

Journal of Magnetic Resonance Imaging, 54. https://www.semanticscholar.org/paper/aa16824ef81c734e5301e1fe79e8033200f33f63 (accessed on 12th July 2025).

34. Pirri, C., Stecco, C., Petrelli, L., De, R., & Özçakar, L. (2022). Reappraisal on the superficial fascia in the subcutaneous tissue: Ultrasound and histological images speaking louder than words. *Plastic & Reconstructive Surgery, 150*, 244e–245e. https://doi.org/10.1097/prs.0000000000009224 (accessed on 12th July 2025).

35. Ricco, J. B., Bartelink, M. L., Björck, M., Brodmann, M., Cohnert, T., Czerny, M., De Carlo, M., et al. (2017). 2017 ESC Guidelines on the diagnosis and treatment of peripheral arterial diseases, in collaboration with the European Society for Vascular Surgery (ESVS). *European Heart Journal, 39*, 763–816. https://doi.org/10.1093/eurheartj/ehx095 (accessed on 12th July 2025).

36. Rodrigues de Castro, B., Bayraktar, H. N., Rodrigues de Castro, J., Poletti, C., Collard, A., & Dupriez, F. (2025). Influence of clinical context on emergency medicine residents' interpretation of gallbladder ultrasound images: A pilot analysis. *Journal of Clinical Ultrasound: JCU*. https://www.semanticscholar.org/paper/379799d9ab7d85643d386c32a1163675150a94a6 (accessed on 12th July 2025).

37. Roncato, C., Perez, L., Brochet-Guégan, A., Allix-Béguec, C., Raimbeau, A., Gautier, G., Agard, C., et al. (2020). Color Doppler ultrasound of temporal arteries for the diagnosis of giant cell arteritis: A multicenter deep learning study. *HAL (Le Centre Pour La Communication Scientifique Directed, 38* Suppl 124), 120–125. https://www.semanticscholar.org/paper/b418b13f3a0e88289c47459c59b9e9a7c684d9e6 (accessed on 12th July 2025).

38. Sachpekidis, V., Papadopoulou, S., Kantartzi, V., Styliadis, I., & Nihoyannopoulos, P. (2022). Use of artificial intelligence for real-time automatic quantification of left ventricular ejection fraction by a novel handheld ultrasound device. *European Heart Journal–Cardiovascular Imaging*. https://www.semanticscholar.org/paper/a20ddebc35990f618bb3cba015d623f22755b767 (accessed on 12th July 2025).

39. Salomon, L., Alfirević, Ž., Berghella, V., Bilardo, C. M., Chalouhi, G. E., da Silva Costa, F., Hernández-Andrade, E., et al. (2022). *ISUOG* Practice Guidelines (updated): Performance of the routine mid-trimester fetal ultrasound scan. *Ultrasound in Obstetrics and Gynecology, 59*, 840–856. https://doi.org/10.1002/uog.24888 (accessed on 12th July 2025).

40. Sesyuk, A., Ioannou, S., & Raspopoulos, M. (2022). A survey of 3D indoor localization systems and technologies. *Sensors, 22*, 9380. https://doi.org/10.3390/s22239380 (accessed on 12th July 2025).

41. Singla, R., Kadatz, M., Rohling, R., & Nguan, C. (2022). Kidney ultrasound for nephrologists: A review. *Kidney Medicine, 4*, 100464–100464. https://doi.org/10.1016/j.xkme.2022.100464 (accessed on 12th July 2025).

42. Stowell, D. (2022). Computational bioacoustics with deep learning: A review and roadmap. *PeerJ, 10*, e13152. https://doi.org/10.7717/peerj.13152 (accessed on 12th July 2025).

43. Tmenova, O., Velikova, Y., Saleh, M., & Navab, N. (2024). Deep spectral methods for unsupervised ultrasound image interpretation. *ArXiv, abs/2408.02043*. https://www.semanticscholar.org/paper/2a3fd79fcaee04a5521f83c206c665c58bb22fe5 (accessed on 12th July 2025).

44. Verde, F., & Ponsiglione, A. (2022). Untangling the ultrasound conundrum of microcalcifications in papillary thyroid cancer. *Journal of Clinical Ultrasound, 50*, 58–59. https://www.

semanticscholar.org/paper/cd4424874409d2f5739e7a37591cc982a76fbde1 (accessed on 12th July 2025).

45. Xu, C., Wang, Z., Zhou, J., Hu, F., Wang, Y., Xu, Z., & Cai, Y. (2025). Application research of artificial intelligence software in the analysis of thyroid nodule ultrasound image characteristics. *PLOS One, 20*. https://www.semanticscholar.org/paper/4ab0681819bc2a3ea4457638fe914ca01e1d88b4 (accessed on 12th July 2025).

46. Yadav, U., Sarawagi, R., Patel, A., Rahul, S., & Malik, R. (2024). Ultrasound assessment of ovarian lesions: O-RADS approach. *Future Health*. https://www.semanticscholar.org/paper/44f5150f34156f253151cf9aa2c0f8529d684806 (accessed on 12th July 2025).

47. Zhang, C., Wang, L., Wei, G., Kong, Z., & Qiu, M. (2024). A dual-branch and dual attention transformer and CNN hybrid network for ultrasound image segmentation. *Frontiers in Physiology, 15*. https://www.semanticscholar.org/paper/6f405d00a754e90d4b603fc4108a1c21dc64dd75 (accessed on 12th July 2025).

48. Zhang, P., & Boulos, M. N. K. (2023). Generative AI in medicine and healthcare: Promises, opportunities and challenges. *Future Internet, 15*, 286. https://doi.org/10.3390/fi15090286 (accessed on 12th July 2025).

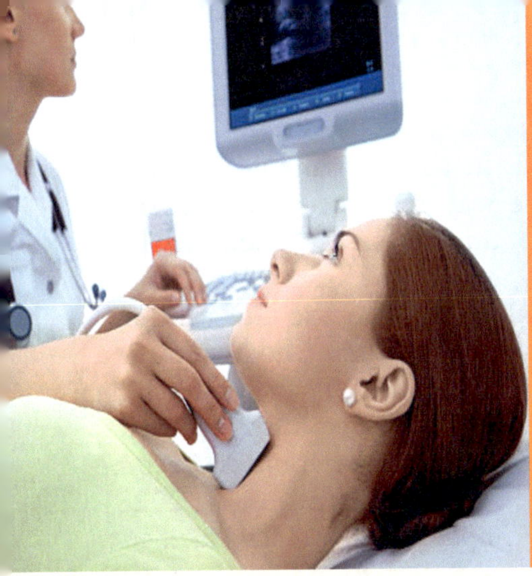

Chapter 4

NECK AND THYROID ULTRASOUND

Contents

Introduction

The advent of new generation imaging machines has revolutionized medicine's diagnostic age, particularly for the diagnosis of thyroid and neck diseases. Thyroid and neck ultrasound is a vital tool for non-surgical assessment of thyroid tissues, lymph nodes, and surrounding tissues. It is an imaging machine through which the physicians can visualize the anatomical structures with precise accuracy, thereby aiding in detecting the pathologies such as nodules, cysts, and tumors. Besides, ultrasound has become increasingly important with its safety profile, lack of ionizing radiation, and low cost, and thus it is the first choice for screening and diagnostic evaluations. The value of this modality is well-established with the rising prevalence of thyroid diseases, which necessitate effective diagnostic algorithms to yield timely and appropriate clinical intervention. Correspondingly, ultrasound is a pillar in the current diagnostic process of neck and thyroid pathology (Complementary E-B and Medicine A, 2023). In the understanding of the clinical use of neck and thyroid ultrasound, it is essential to value its use in primary care with current evidence that investigates its usability and acceptability. Results of a multicentre pilot cross-sectional study point out the way point-of-care ultrasound (POCUS) is becoming more embedded in family practice. To date, this has been beneficial since ultrasound results play a key role in diagnostic efficiency and management decisions. Doctors are able to quickly spot abnormalities and decide on follow-up referrals or therapeutic interventions, hence improving patient care with quick turnaround times. In particular, studies demonstrate a prevalent occurrence of ultrasound changes, proving the effectiveness of POCUS in establishing conditions that require treatment or further examination. Evidence such as this emphasizes growing reliance on ultrasound technology in clinical practices, which means that it has the ability to become indispensable in improving healthcare delivery for thyroid and neck issues (Lesende et al., 2023). As the specialty continues to evolve, it is essential to look at the impact of these advancements on education and training in medicine. Incorporating neck and thyroid ultrasound into curricula ensures that future healthcare providers are well-trained to best use this modality. With diagnostic imaging now becoming part of patient care, understanding its use and interpretation will be a significant factor in decision-making therapy. Besides, ongoing research and practice in ultrasound techniques can foster a culture of continuous learning, ultimately leading to enhanced diagnostic skills in various medical specialties. The implementation of the practices shows an overarching trend towards evidence-based medicine, facilitating continuous improvement in equipment that enables accurate and effective patient assessment in thyroid and neck pathology (Complementary E-B and Medicine A, 2023) (Figure 4.1).

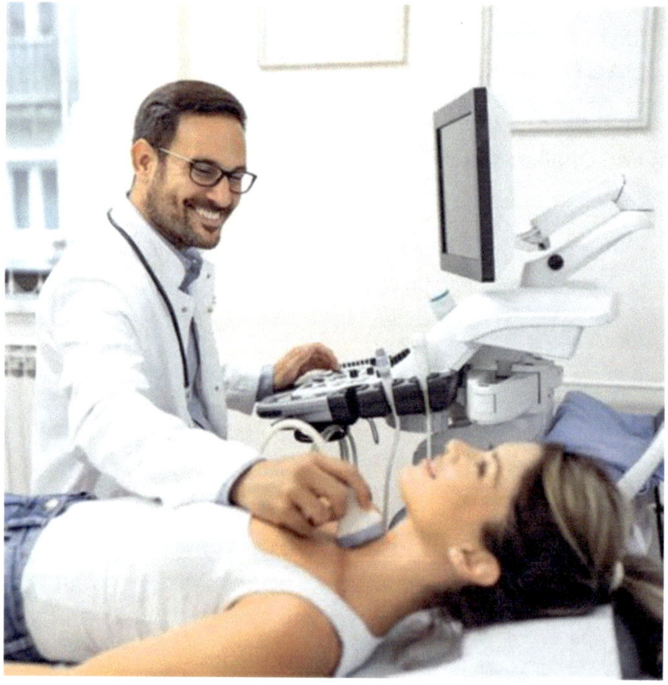

Figure 4.1. Neck and thyroid ultrasound.

Source: https://external-content.duckduckgo.com/iu/?u= https%3A%2 F%2Ftse2.mm.bing.net%2Fth%2Fid% 2FOIP.giDYPvO0KLSnsDDJFkwNwwHaHc% 3Fr%3D0%26pid%3DApi&f= 1&ipt= 4ae77a9d059f3fa51 26661f292b4bc040a472ac2408c08b93ab078d1aef835d1.

Definition of Neck and Thyroid Ultrasound

The definition of neck and thyroid ultrasound is a medical imaging technique that employs high-frequency sound waves to generate high-resolution images of the structures in the neck, with particular focus on the thyroid gland. It is an outpatient examination that is very important in the evaluation of many thyroid disorders, including nodules, inflammation, and cancers. Through the use of ultrasound technology, clinicians can collect information about the morphology and function of the thyroid gland, which can aid diagnosis of conditions that cannot be determined from physical examination alone. Besides, neck ultrasound can visualize surrounding anatomical structures such as lymph nodes and trachea and enable an overall evaluation that aids in treatment planning. This initial imaging machine is widely regarded as safe, efficient, and able to guide interventions like fine needle aspiration biopsy of thyroid nodules, and hence it is a cornerstone in the management process of thyroid diseases. In clinical practice, the application of neck and thyroid ultrasound not only serves as a means of diagnosis but also plays a significant role in the follow up of patients with pre-existing thyroid ailments. The ability to assess the size and character of thyroid nodules over time allows for early intervention should a change be noted that indicates possible malignancy. Furthermore, ultrasound evaluation is necessary in the planning for follow-up treatment, thereby improving patient outcomes. More sophisticated techniques, such as Doppler ultrasound, can further improve the assessment through measurement of blood flow to the thyroid gland and provide additional diagnostic information for hyperthyroidism or inflammation. Therefore, the addition of thyroid and neck ultrasound to routine clinical evaluation is tantamount to a modern, evidence-based practice of endocrine wellness. While there are numerous advantages to it, diagnostic challenge for thyroid lesions often occurs due to the presence of indeterminate nodules, where ultrasound findings cannot definitively indicate malignancy or benignancy. Under such circumstances, the addition of advanced molecular tests, along with routine ultrasound, can improve clinical decision-making. Multiple test methods have been found, for example, Gene Expression Classifier (GEC) and BRAF mutation analysis that enhance malignancy accuracy in indeterminate nodules, as evidenced in corresponding systematic reviews and meta-analyses. Although neck and thyroid ultrasound remain an anchor for initial evaluation, the complementarity of ultrasound imaging and molecular techniques, that is, GAL-3-ICC, is ready to add more depth to the diagnostic framework for thyroid nodules, ultimately impacting surgical intervention and patient prognosis (AIOM-AIRTUM et al., 2017). Ongoing development in such diagnostic steps indicates a step-by-step progression towards precision medicine in endocrinology.

Importance of Ultrasound in Medical Diagnostics

The application of ultrasound in clinical diagnosis, in thyroid and neck studies, has significantly enhanced clinical evaluation protocols. The imaging technology offers several advantages, like being non-invasive, having real-time imaging, and not using ionizing radiation, making the method suitable for various categories of patients, that is, pregnant women and pediatric patients. Ultrasound is particularly useful in thyroid nodule characterization, cervical lymphadenopathy assessment, and fine-needle aspirations (FNA) for cytopathology. As demonstrated in clinical cases, such as the diagnosis of papillary thyroid carcinoma (PTC) in patients with presenting concurrent Kikuchi-Fujimoto Disease, the precise imaging that ultrasound provides is critical for correct diagnoses (Abdullah et al., 2025). Furthermore, ultrasound's capability to facilitate dynamic assessment allows clinicians to track changes in the pathologies of the thyroid over time so that malignancy is addressed early (Kim et al., 2024). In the management of thyroid disease, ultrasound is a useful application in evaluating structural abnormalities and organ shape. The thyroid gland can display different kinds of conditions, including nodules, goiters, and malignancies, which need to be well-evaluated. By the use of ultrasound, medical practitioners are able to diagnose and distinguish benign from potentially malignant nodules, thereby increasing treatment possibilities for patients. The qualitative characteristics of ultrasound, such as echogenicity, nodule margins, and flow of vessels, are incorporated within a complete evaluation that informs clinical decision-making. Further, as in the supportive management of disease conditions such as Kikuchi-Fujimoto Disease using PTC, ultrasound is instrumental in observing lymphadenopathy and assessing long-term response to treatment, testifying to its value in the management of difficult cases (Abdullah et al., 2025; Kim et al., 2024). Furthermore, the cost-effectiveness and accessibility of ultrasound enhance its role in medical diagnosis. Compared with other imaging modalities that can require advanced facilities and more financial resources, ultrasound equipment is more readily available in various healthcare settings, such as outpatient clinics and primary care. This aspect makes it feasible to provide more screening and early diagnosis for thyroid and neck pathologies, particularly for populations at risk for thyroid cancer. The absence of dependence on high-end imaging modalities is that even with limited resources, lifesaving diagnostics can still be provided with impact. Bottom line, the diversified benefits of ultrasound, from its diagnostic accuracy to accessibility, solidify its essential application in the evaluation of neck and thyroid disorders, merging very broad clinical practice without sacrificing patient outcomes (Kim et al., 2024) (Figure 4.2).

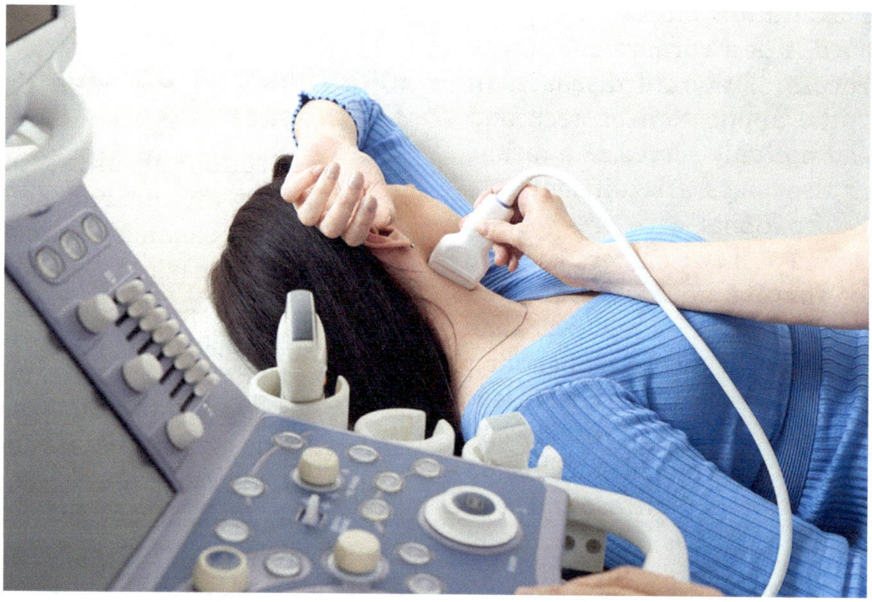

Figure 4.2. Ultrasound in medical diagnostics for the neck and thyroid.

Source: https://cdn.prod.website-files.com/65ee904fcafa8822ef5c61df/67b461d12781888a8c816636_woman-lying-floor-neck-ultrasound-preparation.png.

4.1. Anatomy of the Neck and Thyroid

Neck anatomy comprises various structures that play a critical role in physiological function and pathosis. Comprising life-sustaining organs, muscles, and vascular structures, the region is categorized into distinct zones to enable clinical diagnosis as well as therapeutic interventions. The significant structures are the hyoid bone, trachea, and esophagus, which play a critical role in respiration and digestion. Furthermore, the thyroid gland situated in the anterior part of the neck produces hormones regulating metabolism and endocrine general well-being. Proper understanding of such anatomical landmarks is crucial for physicians, particularly during thyroid and neck ultrasound scanning. Accurate localization enables the detection of abnormalities such as neoplasms or cystic lesions, which may result in successful clinical decision-making regarding the treatment of various neck and thyroid conditions. The anatomical structure of thyroid glands is particularly intriguing, in that two lobes are connected by an isthmus, positioned directly under the larynx.

This butterfly gland is responsible for making and secreting hormones, which are essential in regulating much of the body's functions, including metabolism, heart rate, and body temperature. Detailed knowledge of the blood supply of the thyroids, primarily from the superior and inferior thyroid arteries, is also extremely crucial for clinicians in ultrasound scan procedures. Scans can reveal multiple pathologies like goiters, nodules, and malignancies. An understanding of the gland anatomy improves the accuracy of diagnosis in ultrasound reports and patient outcomes in diagnosis and follow-up treatment intervention, as evidenced by evidence regarding the management of incidental findings in this anatomic site. Furthermore, the anatomical structure of the neck extends to its implications for surgical intervention and disease progression. The pattern of lymphatic drainage of the thyroid is most significant, especially in the context of differentiated thyroid cancer, which has a propensity to metastasize to lymph nodes in the cervical nodes. Papillary thyroid cancer is demonstrated to be the most frequent type to arise, and it becomes imperative to know the various lymphatic compartments of the neck in order to conduct successful surgery. The degree of neck dissection for thyroid cancer treatment is controversial; however, well-selected patients will not incur added morbidity if operations are performed at high-volume institutions where understanding of anatomy plays a pivotal role. This reinforces the paramount importance of well-developed knowledge of neck anatomy among surgeons who manage conditions that benefit from surgical interventions, which results in enhanced patient care and outcomes (Adrian et al., 2018) (Figure 4.3).

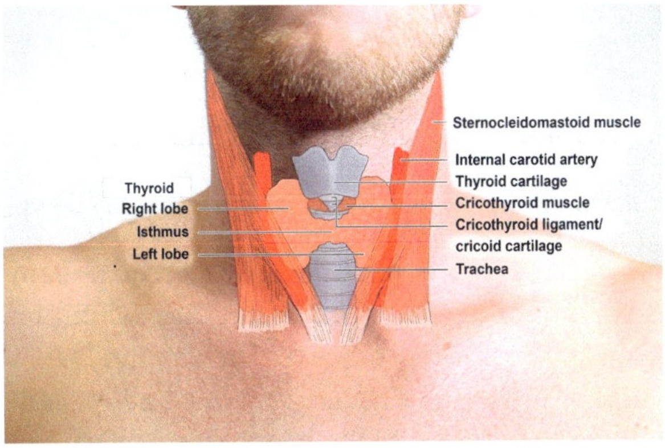

Figure 4.3. Anatomy of the neck and thyroid.

Source: https://external-content.duckduckgo.com/iu/?u=https%3A%2F%2Fmedia-us.amboss.com%2Fmedia%2Fthumbs%2Fbig_58eca1cfbced9.jpg&f=1&nofb=1&ipt=45015861d54ddce02b5371cdfd80d60da93e9d2e79403248873af887cf0bf498.

4.1.1. Major Structures in the Neck

The neck is a significant anatomical region with a variety of important structures that are involved in respiration and endocrine function. The thyroid gland is mostly situated in the front of the neck and has a vital role in metabolism regulation by the secretion of hormones. The gland in the shape of a butterfly surrounds the trachea and has a high level of vascularity, which is particularly pertinent to ultrasound evaluation. Understanding the anatomical relationships between the thyroid gland and neighboring structures, such as carotid arteries and jugular veins, becomes important while interpreting imaging results. Adequate ultrasound techniques can put these relationships into focus, enhancing the assessment of most thyroid conditions, such as goiter and thyroid nodules. The importance of the location of thyroids also reinforces the need for precise imaging modalities that can differentiate normal physiological status and disease conditions so as to guide clinical decisions and patient management. Besides the thyroid gland, there are many cervical lymph nodes that constitute another critical part of the large structures of the neck.

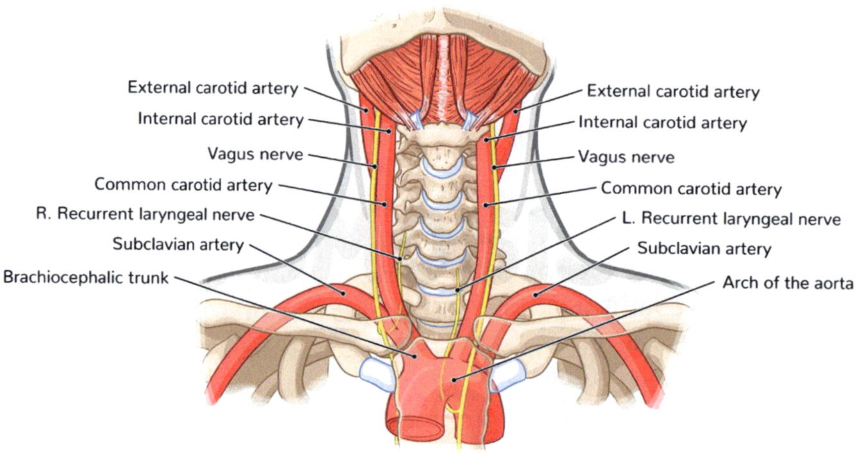

Figure 4.4. Deep structures of the neck.

Source: https://www.osmosis.org/learn/Deep_structures_of_the_neck:_Root_of_the_neck

These lymph nodes are a critical component of the immune system's function and act as an infection filter, and thus are of clinical significance in the diagnosis of a wide array of diseases, including cancers. Ultrasound has also emerged as an important modality for cervical lymphadenopathy evaluation, which allows one to see lymph node size, morphology, and vascularity without invading the patient. In particular, pathology in the guise of abnormalities seen on ultrasound may represent underlying disease, such as infection or metastatic disease from thyroid carcinoma or other head and neck cancers. The use of advanced techniques, such as Doppler ultrasound, also enhances diagnostic specificity by providing additional information on the nature of blood flow within lymphoid tissues. This technology is instrumental in guiding management planning for patients suspected of having lymphatic involvement, thereby having an active role in treatment planning. Of all the neck structures, the great vascular structures, that is, the carotid arteries and internal jugular veins, need special mention in ultrasound examinations. They share a close association with the thyroid and lymphoid tissues, creating a complex anatomy that can be problematic for clinicians. The carotid arteries provide vital perfusion to the neck and head, and are balanced by the internal jugular veins, controlling venous return.

Changes in either structure, either as a result of pathology or anatomical variation, have significant implications. Application of ultrasound for evaluation of these vessels allows detection of diseases such as carotid artery stenosis, thrombosis, or other vascular disease. Moreover, ultrasound can also provide real-time imaging that becomes useful in the course of interventional procedures, thus becoming a crucial modality in both diagnosis and therapy of the neck area (Haddad et al., 2022; Steinberg et al., 2019) (Figure 4.4).

4.1.2. Thyroid Gland Location and Function

The thyroid gland is strategically located in the front portion of the neck, inferior to the Adam's apple, across the trachea. The bilateral, butterfly-shaped organ consists of two lobes connected by an isthmus, enabling it to play several critical roles in physiological function. The fact that the thyroid is in close proximity to other significant structures, for example, the larynx and major blood vessels, makes its location significant both for endocrine function and clinical examination. The thyroid gland secretes and releases hormones, such as thyroxine (T4) and triiodothyronine (T3) that are responsible for regulating metabolism, heart rate, and overall growth and development. Being in this anatomical position allows doctors to use diagnostic methods, such as ultrasound, to monitor the shape of the glands and diagnose possible faults (Cantisani et al., 2018). The role of the thyroid gland goes beyond simply secreting hormones; it is also responsible for regulating the body's metabolism. The thyroid hormones are responsible for keeping the body's metabolic rate—the impact isn't just on energy, but also on weight and temperature regulation. Reduced secretion of the aforementioned hormones results in hypothyroidism, which is characterized by fatigue, weight gain, and intolerance to cold, while excess production results in hyperthyroidism, which may result in restlessness, weight loss, and tachycardia. Definitive imaging techniques, particularly ultrasound, play a vital role in thyroid pathology and focal lesion evaluation. Thyroid ultrasound assesses nodule characteristics, guiding clinical decisions for potential malignancy, thus underlining the gland's impact on overall health (Daminet et al., 2016). The application of ultrasound technology has transformed thyroid practice through the provision of a non-surgical, high-utility method for thyroid imaging. Improved spatial resolution of ultrasound allows clinicians to detect fine structure detail, which is of great value in the diagnosis of the thyroid. In addition, advancements in ultrasound technology enable the standardization of reporting templates for better reproducibility of results across different operators. For instance, characterization of malignancy by ultrasound patterns aids risk stratification and guides investigation and management (Cantisani et al., 2018). Because thyroid conditions may cause multifaceted systemic complications, the anatomical and functional significance identified by specialized imaging only further speaks to including ultrasound as a matter of course in routine neck scans, optimizing patient results and allowing for early intervention where necessary.

4.1.3. Relationship of the Thyroid Gland with Surrounding Tissues

The relationship of the thyroid gland with its surrounding tissues is complex and relevant to understanding both normal physiology and pathologic conditions. The thyroid gland in the anterior neck comes into contact with several anatomical structures, including blood vessels, nerves, and adjacent muscles. This close association increases the risk of surgical complications when undergoing thyroidectomies. Most notably, nerves like the recurrent laryngeal nerve and the external branch of the superior laryngeal nerve are near the thyroid and susceptible to damage in procedures (Man &Chau, 2018). Further, blood supply through the inferior and superior thyroid arteries is behind the functioning of the glands and plays a role in hematogenous dissemination of thyroid neoplasms. This interdependence enhances the need for precise imaging techniques such as ultrasound to assess not only the thyroid gland itself but also adjacent tissues. Ultrasound is an important modality to assess the thyroid relationship to adjacent structures, particularly in thyroid disease diagnosis. CEUS allows clinicians to monitor blood flow and microvascular characteristics of the thyroid and surrounding structures. Recent studies show that parameters such as peak intensity and area under the curve can differentiate thyroid carcinoma from surrounding normal tissues, reflecting vascular dynamics of thyroid disease (Chong et al., 2017).

These results are important in assisting in the acquisition of a broader comprehension of the thyroid's vascular milieu, which subsequently can influence treatment plans. Moreover, CEUS has also been shown to detect microvessel density (MVD) and thereby relate angiogenesis to thyroid cancer even more. Pathological correlations between the thyroid and neighboring structures can lead to diagnostic challenges, such as in cases of misdiagnosis. As a case in point, schwannomas, although they are uncommon, can present as masses near the thyroid and may be inaccurately diagnosed as goiters in ultrasound imaging. This corroborates the requirement for radiologists to be in continuous mind of the anatomical complexities of the cervicothoracic junction (Man & Chau, 2018). Misdiagnosis not only affects patient care but can potentially lead to increased morbidity. Thus, there is a need for clinicians to use clinical evidence with advanced imaging techniques to effectively assess and diagnose thyroid and surrounding tissue-related disorders so as to provide appropriate patient care and optimal surgical outcomes (Figure 4.5).

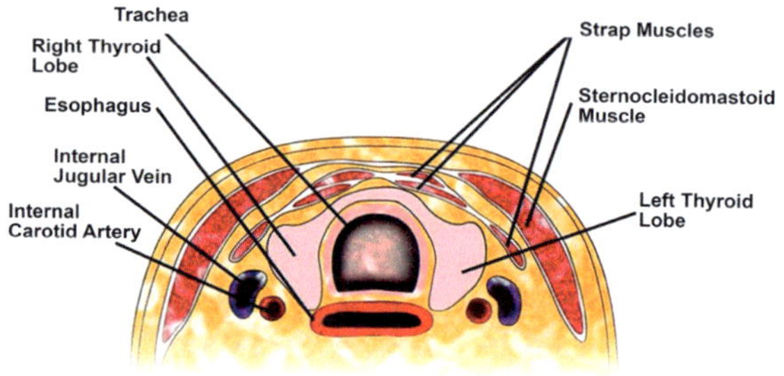

Figure 4.5. Relationship between the thyroid and surrounding tissues.

Source: Nachiappan, Arun & Metwalli, Zeyad & Hailey, Brian & Patel, Rishi & Ostrowski, Mary & Wynne, David. (2014). The Thyroid: Review of Imaging Features and Biopsy Techniques with Radiologic-Pathologic Correlation. Radiographics: a review publication of the Radiological Society of North America, Inc. 34. 276-93. 10.1148/rg. 342135067. .

4.2. Principles of Ultrasound Technology

The fundamental concepts of ultrasound technology are based on the generation of images of internal organs using sound waves. In neck and thyroid ultrasound, the transducer emits high-frequency sound waves into the tissues and receives them back to the device. It is significant as it facilitates images to be created depending on tissue densities encountered. When the sound waves travel through several media such as fluid, muscle, or fat, the ultrasound machine interprets the echoes in order to create a full two-dimensional or three-dimensional picture of the thyroid gland and related anatomical structures. The success of ultrasound imaging relies heavily on the frequency of the ultrasonic sound waves, whereby increasing frequencies give better resolution but lower penetration, an aspect to be put into consideration during assessment of the different pathologies in the neck, including thyroid nodules and other masses (Focal Spot, 2007).

In addition, the transition from traditional modalities toultrasound makes it unique in having some inherent advantages, most notably in terms of safety and diagnostic accuracy. Ultrasound is a non-invasive method that avoids the ionizing radiation associated with techniques such as X-rays and CT scans, making it a less dangerous means of diagnostic imaging, especially in sensitive groups such as pregnant women and children. As applied to thyroid evaluation, this non-invasive nature is coupled with real-time imaging capabilities, enabling practitioners to target interventions such as fine-needle aspiration biopsies in real time. As recent studies report, the advanced diagnostic potential of ultrasound technology has facilitated better clinical outcomes in the diagnosis of benign and malignant thyroid disorders, highlighting its role in everyday clinical practice (Lo Baido et al., 2019).

Recognizing the nuances of ultrasound imaging implies knowledge of the impact of various parameters on diagnostic performance. The quality of the image may be influenced by several factors, such as the expertise of the operators, patient anatomy, and environmental factors when the procedure is performed. For maximum imaging quality, proper scanning techniques, such as optimal positioning of the patient and gain setting adjustments on the ultrasound machine, need to be employed. New ultrasound technology, such as Doppler imaging and elastography, enhances vascular flow assessment and tissue stiffness measurement, respectively. These technologies are crucial in the assessment of thyroid diseases and enable clinicians to discern between benign nodules and malignancies. Incorporating these ideas into the routine practices of neck ultrasound allows it to tackle the diagnosis and treatment of thyroid disease in an effective manner.

4.2.1. Basics of Ultrasound Imaging

Ultrasound imaging is a major diagnostic modality within the realm of neck and thyroid evaluation, which employs high-frequency sound waves to generate images of structures that reside within. At its core, ultrasound relies on piezoelectric principles, whereby transducers convert electrical energy into sound waves that propagate through tissue. As these sound waves encounter different interfaces—tissue borders or fluids—they are rebounced back towards the transducer. This interaction is then translated by advanced computer programs into visual images, allowing clinicians not only to assess the anatomy but also potential pathological changes within the thyroid and adjacent tissues. The lack of use of ionizing radiation makes ultrasound very well adapted to serial examinations, thereby further boosting its application in monitoring conditions over time. Thus, its lack of invasiveness and the capacity to provide real-time imaging position ultrasound at the forefront of diagnostic practice in head and neck pathology (Focal Spot, 2007). One of the key features that defines the efficiency of neck and thyroid ultrasound is the possibility to differentiate between cystic and solid lesions, which is something that is challenging for clinicians to achieve. Offering diagnostic methods like manual palpation can generate uncertainty, particularly in distinguishing subtle differences between types of lesions. This built-in limitation can quite possibly introduce uncertainty in diagnosis and adversely influence treatment planning. Ultrasonography eliminates such barriers through the application of dynamic, high-resolution images to distinguish lesions depending on their acoustic properties. Lesions such as vascular or solid nodules have varying echogenicity, which aids in their classification.

Besides, small-parts ultrasound transducer technology has improved images to be more accurate so that experts can evaluate superficial neck tissues efficiently (Baatenburg de Jong & Rongen, 1990). Thus, ultrasounds supplement traditional diagnosis techniques with a better anatomical perspective without decreasing the risks associated with invasive therapy.

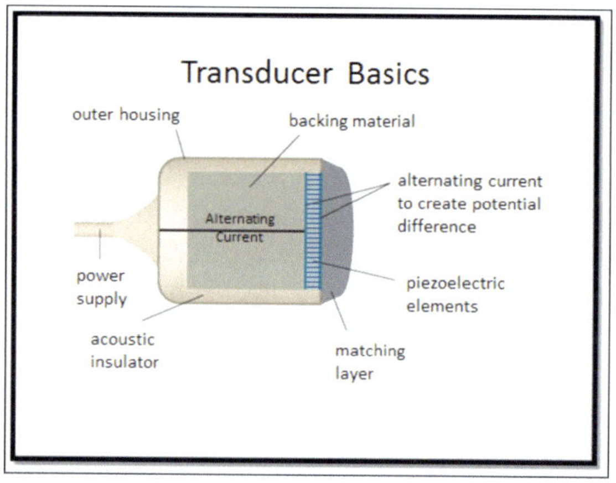

Figure 4.6. Basic principles of ultrasound imaging.

Source: https://www.ukessays.com/essays/physics/ultrasound-imaging-systems-5273.php

The addition of ultrasound to the diagnostic workup for head and neck evaluation also potentially enhances patient safety and comfort. Emerging as a serious challenger to more conventional modalities—like CT or MRI, utilizing ionizing radiation or contrast media—ultrasound emerges as an extremely attractive option. With increasing concern about the cost-effectiveness and availability of existing advanced imaging, the usefulness of a non-invasive, universally accessible diagnostic examination is even further emphasized. The fact that ultrasound can facilitate methods such as ultrasound-guided fine needle aspiration biopsy further establishes its place in the clinic. This method not only enhances the diagnosis but also minimizes the patient's morbidity, as it allows for tissue sampling without extensive surgery. With the era of personalized medicine and individualized treatment regimens being the very essence of healthcare at the moment, utilization of such advanced imaging modalities for the evaluation of thyroid and neck pathology has never been more common (Baatenburg de Jong & Rongen, 1990) (Figure 4.6).

4.2.2. Types of Ultrasound Used in Neck and Thyroid Examinations

Various ultrasound modalities are employed in thyroid and neck examinations, all of which have a specific contribution to management and diagnosis. High-frequency ultrasound is perhaps the most significant of these, as it offers detailed imaging of the superficial tissues like the thyroid gland and lymph nodes in the region. The modality is ideally suited to identify solid versus cystic masses, thus making it easier for clinicians to make accurate diagnoses without having to perform invasive tests. In addition, ultrasound can be supplemented with a Doppler flow study to yield vascularity information that can be absolutely vital in deciding the character of thyroid nodules or lymphatic involvement. The union of these techniques provides an economically feasible, non-invasive way of measuring pathological changes in the area of the neck, useful due to the shortcomings of physical examinations and other imaging techniques like CT and MRI, specifically concerning specificity and associated morbidity (Baatenburg de Jong & Rongen, 1990). Ultrasound use within a clinical environment extends past initial diagnosis; its effectiveness also exists within the follow-up assessment of such conditions as differentiated thyroid cancers (DTCs). With the nature of DTCs tending to become ever more dynamic with more small, localized, and asymptomatic cases, ultrasound has been indispensable in disease follow-up as well as in recurrence risk assessment. Regular cervical ultrasound examinations not only evaluate the baseline status of the disease but also provide dynamic feedback on nodular alterations or lymphadenopathy over time. Technology makes this advancement in management possible, bringing forth more sophisticated methods of ultrasound. Consequently, the follow-up care of patients is largely based on the utility of ultrasound imaging, which plays a pivotal role in the determination of the best course of treatment and hence underpins the established practice of conservative treatment modalities of DTCs (Deandreis et al., 2016).

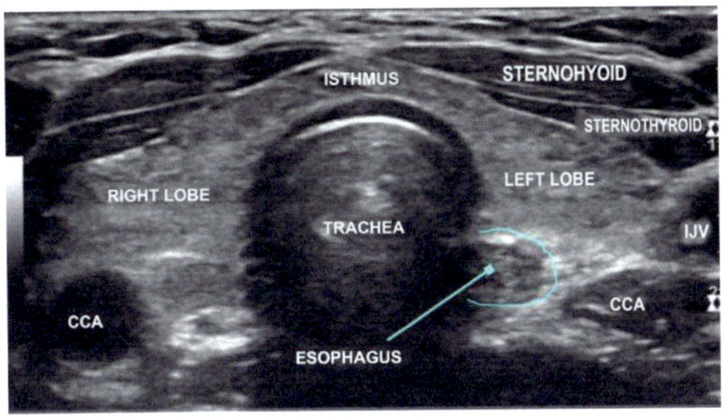

Figure 4.7. Types of ultrasound used in neck and thyroid examinations.

Source: https://external-content.duckduckgo.com/iu/?u=https%3A%2F%2Fendoconsult.b-cdn.net%2Fwp-content%2Fuploads%2Fthyroidusgfig3-624x348.jpg&f=1&nofb=1&ipt=ee12d2de311b9be752d35263b42493a2d86e090c0cfbd3db3e6d47ad801c37f1.

Aside from conventional ultrasound, other modalities such as elastography have proven to be valuable adjuncts to thyroid and neck evaluation. Elastography quantifies tissue stiffness, and its diagnostic value is particularly important in thyroid nodule classification. Elastography is an ancillary tool that can distinguish between benign and malignant lesions and reduce unnecessary biopsies and surgery. Furthermore, the addition of elastography to routine sonographic examinations adds more diagnostic sensitivity, particularly when conventional imaging yields indeterminate results. With the continued evolution of ultrasound technology, these multimodal methods offer an expanded platform for evaluating neck and thyroid pathology. The continued expansion of ultrasound use is needed not only to improve diagnostic returns but also to foster a more delicate understanding of head and neck disease, and it reflects the need for ongoing research and development within the medical community (Baatenburg de Jong & Rongen, 1990) (Figure 4.7).

4.2.3. Advantages of Ultrasound over Other Imaging Modalities

The application of ultrasound in thyroid and neck pathology diagnosis has several significant advantages over other modalities. One primary benefit is cost-effectiveness compared to more advanced imaging modalities such as magnetic resonance imaging (MRI) or computed tomography (CT). Ultrasound equipment is generally less expensive, both in the initial capital outlays and operational expenditures, which makes it more accessible in most clinical environments. Moreover, ultrasound can be performed extremely quickly and in a convenient way in outpatient clinics without irradiation exposure, which is a major risk of CT imaging. This aspect makes it even more relevant in the assessment of sensitive groups that are traditionally screened for thyroid, such as pregnant women and children. In cost-minimizing and risk-reducing aspects, ultrasound is a cornerstone instrument for regular assessments in thyroidology and neck scans. A second critical advantage of ultrasound is its ability to obtain real-time imaging and dynamic evaluation of structures. Unlike static imaging equipment, ultrasound allows for the assessment of vascularity and motion in real time, which is especially critical in imaging thyroid nodules and cervical masses in depth. This real-time capability enhances the potential for guided procedures such as fine-needle aspiration biopsies, allowing clinicians to aspirate tissue specimens from suspected areas with high precision. Additionally, advances in the technology of Doppler ultrasound allowed improved detection of vascular patterns associated with different thyroid diseases, owing to the evolving management protocols for conditions such as differentiated thyroid cancer (DTC) (Deandreis et al., 2016). Through offering minute details of anatomy and physiology, ultrasound has turned out to be an excellent imaging device in the comprehensive examination of thyroid diseases. Lastly, the portability of ultrasound machines also adds to their advantages in being able to deploy them in various clinical environments. Unlike larger imaging machines that require specialized spaces and significant infrastructure, portable ultrasound machines are easily transported to diverse environments, including bedside exams in hospital settings and point-of-care. Such flexibility comes extremely useful during emergencies or in patients with mobility impairments and potentially may not be able to access traditional imaging suites. Also, the absence of ionizing radiation makes ultrasound a safer modality for patients requiring multiple scans, addressing an ever-growing issue of cumulative radiation exposure, particularly for long-term thyroid cancer monitoring (Ahmadi et al., 2016). In brief, the many benefits of ultrasound, including cost, real-time imaging, and portability, make it an essential tool in neck and thyroid imaging, offering the highest quality patient care (Figure 4.8).

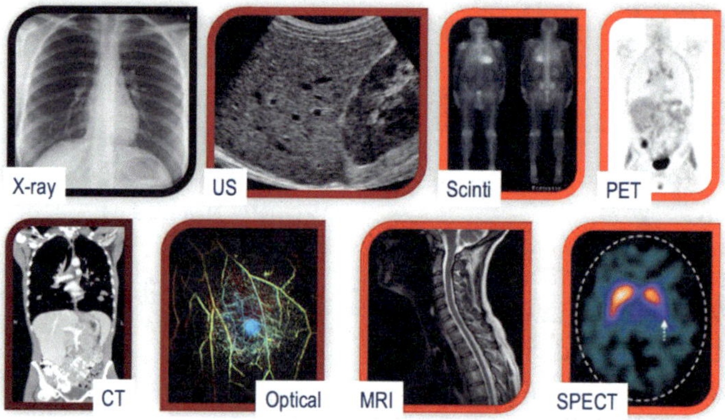

Figure 4.8. Imaging modalities.

Source: Beyer, T., Bidaut, L., Dickson, J. et al. What scans we will read: imaging instrumentation trends in clinical oncology. Cancer Imaging 20, 38 (2020). https://doi.org/10.1186/s40644-020-00312-3

4.3. Indications for Neck and Thyroid Ultrasound

The application of thyroid and neck ultrasound is significant in the initial evaluation of thyroid nodules, often incidentally discovered on imaging performed for other purposes or self-prompted by patients on the basis of palpable masses. Ultrasound is the preferred imaging study due to its non-invasive nature and ability to provide accurate information on the thyroid gland anatomy. Through sonographic evaluation, clinicians are able to define the character of thyroid nodules, including size, content, and vascularity, all of which are of paramount concern in deciding what course of treatment to pursue. Thus, ultrasound not only serves to differentiate benign from malignant nodules but also to provide ongoing observation for changes in nodular features over time, thus playing a significant role in the early detection of clinically significant thyroid pathology. Other than nodular evaluation, ultrasound is useful to uncover parathyroid gland pathologies that may exist in conjunction with thyroid illness. High-resolution ultrasound has enhanced the detection of parathyroid glands, especially in secondary hyperparathyroidism related to chronic renal failure. The feasibility of viewing these glands with ultrasound has been explored and demonstrated to have correlations between parathyroid gland enlargement and elevation of parathyroid hormone levels, observed in more than 40% of patients examined (, Anari et al., 2011). This is an indication of how sonography, apart from providing anatomical information, is diagnostic as well to determine the extent of conditions that affect parathyroid function and thereby decide clinical management and treatment for the affected. Also, ultrasound-guided procedures such as percutaneous radiofrequency thermal ablation show the therapeutic value of neck and thyroid ultrasound.

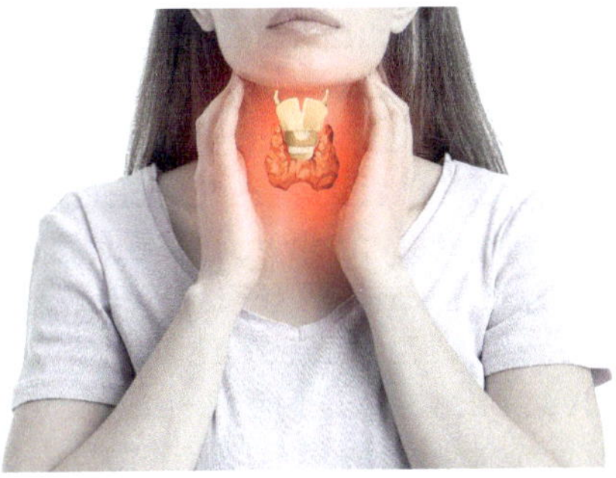

Figure 4.9. Indications for neck and thyroid ultrasound.

Source: https://external-content.duckduckgo.com/iu/?u=https%3A%2F%2Fassets-global.website-files.com%2F5e0143c66e14efc18c6f469d%2F644fe5bf8f79f6a0c8925975_sing%2520(8).jpg&f=1&nofb=1&ipt=c1c179a2f7fa4c63d8e770816c0b67dc74b3973a7483bd81035ce240ca3d631a.

This less-invasive technique offers a valuable way to manage thyroid nodules that meet specific criteria, primarily symptomatic or enlarging rapidly. By employing the use of ultrasound guidance, doctors can specifically target nodules for ablation with less risk of unnecessary destruction of tissues in the surrounding area. A clinical study confirmed that radiofrequency thermal ablation is safe in inducing favorable outcomes in thyroid nodule management, suggesting its incorporation in the overall trend of ultrasound indications in the therapy of thyroid disease (Assanti et al., 2012). The multipurpose use of thyroid and neck ultrasound denotes its pivotal role in both diagnosis and therapy of thyroid and parathyroid disease (Figure 4.9).

4.3.1. Evaluation of Thyroid Nodules

The US is an indispensable tool in the assessment of thyroid nodules and provides vital information that is necessary for diagnosis and treatment. The imaging modality stands out because it offers high spatial resolution, low cost, and the absence of ionizing radiation, making it the gold standard for thyroid pathology assessment. Thyroid ultrasound not only aids in evaluating nodule size and echogenicity but also plays a pivotal role in malignancy risk stratification of the nodules. The most significant findings on ultrasound, such as microcalcifications, irregular margins, and hypervascularity, are instrumental in determining the classification of the risk of thyroid nodules. These parameters assist clinicians in making referral decisions for additional diagnostic workup or treatment plans. Overall, the efficiency of ultrasound detection of suspicious nodules on proven by its essential role in thyroid cancer early detection and resultant clinical management procedures applied in clinical practice (Cantisani et al., 2018).

Notwithstanding the wide advantages of thyroid ultrasound, it has some problems, particularly those attendant upon operator dependence and variability of imaging quality. Proper interpretation of ultrasound findings is subject to the technologist's level of experience and the equipment used, leading to inconsistency in diagnosis. In attempts to overcome these limitations, there has been a drive for standardized reporting guidelines of thyroid ultrasound to enhance reproducibility and accuracy in diagnoses. Recent consensus recommendations have proposed the use of standard terms and criteria to be applied globally in conveying the findings of ultrasound. This standardization includes a documented scoring system of ultrasound signs of malignancy that, aside from enhancing communication between healthcare practitioners, makes it easier for patient management algorithms. By advancing the use of a uniform approach, these programs aim to reduce variability and improve the consistency of ultrasound assessments in clinical practice (Cantisani et al., 2018). The inclusion of fine needle aspiration cytology (FNAC) in the evaluation process further advances ultrasound results and assists in the workup of thyroid nodules. Even though FNAC is globally regarded as the yardstick for obtaining cytological samples, the process is linked with non-diagnostic results as the primary setback. Data reveal that the first trial of FNAC can yield non-diagnostic results in a significant percentage of cases and multiple procedures might be required in some cases to establish definitive results. Surprisingly, factors such as ultrasound guidance significantly increase the likelihood of diagnostic sample procurement, particularly when performed by experienced radiologists. The rate of malignancy in the setting of non-diagnostic FNAC results is still low, but the cumulative hazard drops with repeated sampling attempts, thus emphasizing the significance of proper patient management methods in such a scenario. Thus, the combination of FNAC and ultrasound is central in offering a comprehensive evaluation of thyroid nodules and guiding clinical procedures.

4.3.2. Assessment of Neck Masses and Lymphadenopathy

The assessment of neck masses and lymphadenopathy is important in their identification as possible malignancies and directing their treatment. Physicians are prone to employ the traditional tools of palpation and imaging modalities in the evaluation of these conditions. Despite their popularity, these tools have limitations, notably distinguishing between varying types of masses, such as solid and cystic lesions. This diagnostic uncertainty can lead to staging and proper management problems, especially in the upper aerodigestive tract cancers, where early intervention is critical. As highlighted by current studies, the susceptibility to errors of these conventional approaches makes inquiry into more advanced imaging modalities, including ultrasound, relevant, which provides a global evaluation of soft tissue form and lymph node characteristics with greater diagnostic accuracy (Baatenburg de Jong & Rongen, 1990). Ultrasound offers an inexpensive and non-invasive approach to the assessment of neck masses, particularly as it offers real-time imaging and the ability to perform ultrasound-guided fine needle aspiration biopsy (UGFNAB). Not only does it help to obtain histological samples of suspect lymph nodes, but it also helps to differentiate between benign and metastatic lesions. Recent years have, however, witnessed some advancement in the employment of ultrasound technology in the form of high-frequency transducers that have significantly helped in visualizing surface structures and established ultrasound as a darling of clinicians. The use of thyroglobulin assays in the fine-needle aspirate washout has also been useful in circumstances where cytological sampling may yield suboptimal results. This adjunct diagnostic modality can increase confidence in the assessment of cervical lymph nodes, particularly in thyroid cancer, where precise identification of metastasis is required (Amabile et al., 2019). Utilization of ultrasound as a part of standard practice can hence transform the diagnostic work-up for neck masses and lymphadenopathy. By providing a clearer delineation of the various types of lesions present, ultrasound enhances diagnostic accuracy and minimizes unnecessary surgery. Additionally, its ability to accurately guide aspirations allows even cystic lymph nodes, which are infamous for being difficult to diagnose, to be adequately sampled for their examination. Clinicians need to become proficient in these new modalities in order to enhance patient outcomes. While research continues to confirm the effectiveness of ultrasound and its adjunctive techniques, its use in the comprehensive assessment of neck masses will likely increase, marking a milestone in clinical practice (Baatenburg de Jong & Ronge, 1990) (Figure 4.10).

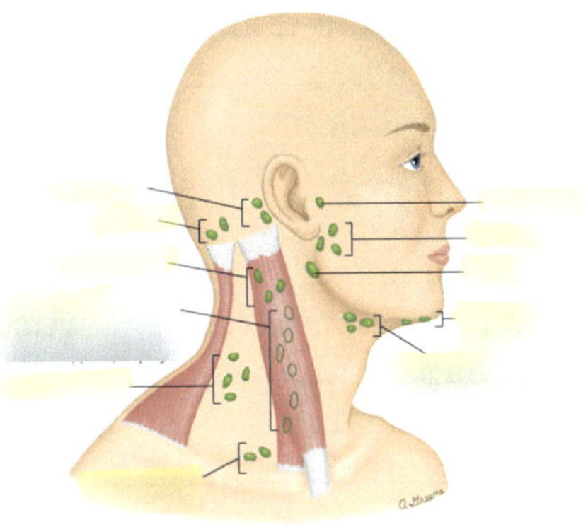

Figure 4.10. Assessment of neck masses and lymphadenopathy.

Source: https://external-content.duckduckgo.com/iu/?u=https%3A%2F%2Fo.quizlet.com%2F8JHX.2gwd3rXSAi3attKIg_b.png&f=1&nofb=1&ipt=85a67cf2e1bee2624269f1437387b263167f4a333570d148b62423778e997d6b.

4.3.3. Monitoring Thyroid Disease and Treatment Efficacy

Prognosis and surveillance of thyroid disease and treatment response have increasingly relied on advanced imaging modalities, led by ultrasound. Neck and thyroid ultrasound have become significant in thyroid disease assessment and treatment, including differentiated thyroid cancers (DTCs). DTCs' evolution has been marked by the occurrence of smaller, regional, and often asymptomatic disease that requires individualized therapeutic approaches. Applying ultrasound makes it possible for physicians to perform dynamic assessments of the thyroid and overlying tissues and hence intervene in a timely fashion. Real-time imaging not only aids in depicting disease progression accurately but also in measuring treatment response, an essential factor in an ever-changing management paradigm. The integration of ultrasound with clinical evaluation ensures that treatment planning is based on the most current evidence relative to individual patient risk profiles and disease courses. The application of neck and thyroid ultrasound is particularly fitting in post-treatment follow-up of DTC patients. With increasingly conservative clinical treatment of DTCs with less invasive procedures, routine imaging becomes a crucial component to ensure the efficacy of such interventions. Procedures like Doppler analysis of blood flow and ultrasonography of the cervix are employed presently to observe time-dependent alterations in nodules and contiguous lymphoid tissue. Such evaluation is most vital for realizing the dynamic nature of these disease threats that can change spontaneously or during treatment. The information gained through ultrasound not only guides clinical decision-making but also helps in earlier diagnosis of recurrence cases, which can lead to improved outcomes by rendering early interventions feasible in accordance with the evolving clinical situation. In some situations, for example, in the case of Hürthle cell carcinoma (HCC), follow-up after treatment with ultrasound becomes increasingly subtle due to the aggressive nature of the tumor and typical physiological characteristics. Whereas minimally invasive HCC can generally be successfully treated with lobectomy and does not always require radioactive iodine, advanced HCCs can be very problematic. Ongoing ultrasound follow-up also helps to detect any metastasis or recurrence early and assist in determining additional interventions, such as systemic therapy. Last, an understanding of the iodine-avid nature of HCC compared to other DTCs highlights the utility of individualized follow-up. The addition of robust imaging methods, including thyroid and neck ultrasound, thus has an important role to play in the overall handling of thyroid illness, allowing for effective management as well as maximizing patient outcome within a rapidly evolving clinical setting (Figure 4.11).

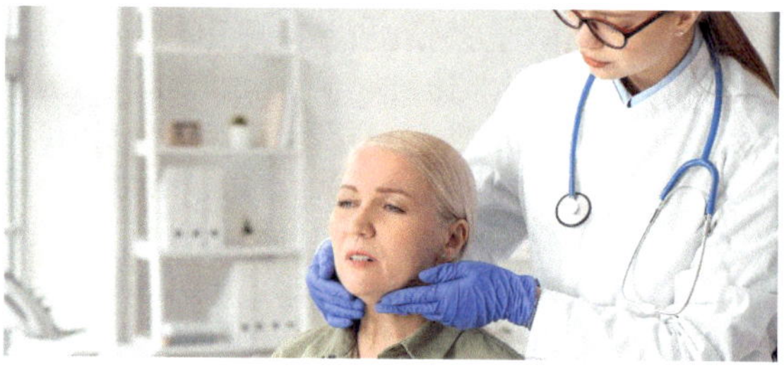

Figure 4.11. Monitoring thyroid disease and treatment efficacy.

Source: https://external-content.duckduckgo.com/iu/?u=https%3A%2F%2Fmedicalofficeofkaty.com%2Fwp-content%2Fuploads%2F2023%2F08%2FTHYROID-DISORDERS-Banner.jpg&f=1&nofb=1&ipt=f1771e2db78a1dac32e833bcd09c730bc2e3dd6cac85ca07a660437b4db02ae6.

4.4. Procedure of Neck and Thyroid Ultrasound

Neck and thyroid ultrasound is an important diagnostic test in the evaluation of thyroid and cervical masses. It is a non-invasive imaging test with high-frequency sound waves to create images of the thyroid gland and structures of the neck. The sonographer begins by putting gel on the neck of the patient to facilitate the transmission of the sound waves. A transducer, which both sends and receives such waves, is then rolled over the target area. This method is particularly helpful to recognize nodules, assess their size, structure, and vascularity, and determine if they are benign or malignant. The reliability of ultrasound in differential diagnosis continues to be confirmed by clinical data, making it a first-line imaging modality for the initial assessment of patients with thyroid symptoms or palpable neck masses. Moreover, it is at the core of the guidance of fine needle aspiration biopsies of suspicious nodules, and hence to the setting of subsequent management plans. In recent years, there has been a significant improvement in ultrasound technology to make thyroid and neck examinations more accurate and effective. Doppler ultrasound can provide information on blood flow within the nodules, which could indicate future malignancy. Such an ability makes fine-tuning the evaluation of thyroid nodules possible and eventually aids in clinical decision-making for observation versus intervention. Furthermore, high-resolution ultrasound can identify tiny lesions that would otherwise go unnoticed, validating the necessity for regular thyroid monitoring, particularly in high-risk groups. Literature indicates greater emphasis on having a multidisciplinary management approach towards thyroid nodule patients. This includes collaboration among radiologists, surgeons, and endocrinologists to ensure correlatively interpreting ultrasound findings in the broader clinical context, as supported by Mauri et al. (2021) and Planchard et al. (2018).

Apart from the role in diagnosis, the procedure of ultrasound of the neck and thyroid plays a pivotal role in monitoring patients known to have thyroid disease or following treatment. Routine follow-up with ultrasound aids the clinician in tracking the size and behavior of the nodules over time, so that intervention can be initiated early when growth or suspicious features are noted. Ultrasound also facilitates focused therapies such as ultrasound-guided radiofrequency ablation, demonstrating its value in the care of patients. Despite continued controversy as to the optimal mode of thyroid care, utilization of ultrasound remains a mainstay in the establishment of customized treatment plans. The emphasis on personalized patient care, coupled with advancements in ultrasound technology, makes it an important consideration in the full management of thyroid conditions. Thus, the neck and thyroid ultrasound process not only aids in effective diagnosis but also enhances patient outcomes in thyroid well-being (Figure 4.12).

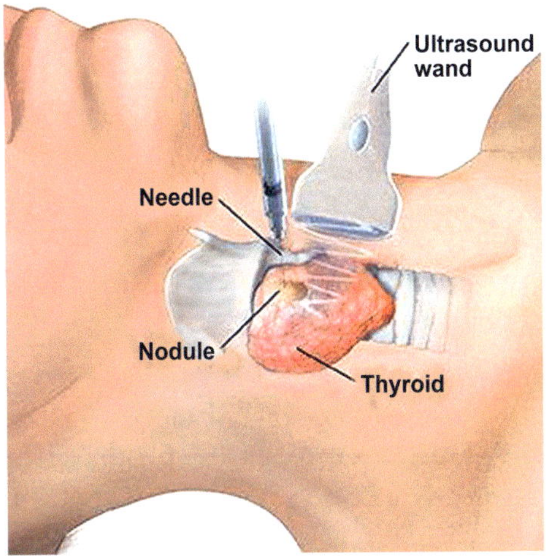

Figure 4.12. Procedure of neck and thyroid ultrasound.

Source: https://www.thyroidcancer.com/upimg/1044/side-view-of-neck-showing-thyroid-with-nodule-ultrasound-probe-is-on-skin.jpg.

4.4.1. Preparation for the Ultrasound Examination

Preparation for ultrasound scanning of the neck and thyroid is also necessary to make sure that diagnostic imaging results are accurate. Clinicians must first obtain full patient clinical histories, such as symptoms related to thyroid dysfunction or palpable neck masses. The information notifies the sonographer to specific areas of interest, which continues as a directed scan. It is also crucial that the doctor gives a clear written or electronic order for the ultrasound with clinical indications noted, as these requests enable relevant preparation of equipment and technical approach. Proper documentation, like the clinical setting, aligns with American Institute of Ultrasound in Medicine (AIUM) Practice Parameter standards that emphasize the need for systematic records to enhance the quality of care for patients undergoing neck and thyroid ultrasound tests (AIUM, 2023).

Patient positioning is another extremely critical aspect of preparation for the US exam. The AIUM recommends that the neck should be hyperextended to have optimal imaging access to the thyroid gland; this is possible by offering a towel or other supportive device for increased comfort. In those patients who cannot tolerate this position, semi-upright positioning can be useful. The sonographer must ensure the process of examination is open by making a description of the process to patients and eliminating anxiety associated with the type of ultrasound. Furthermore, preparation involves ensuring that adequate ultrasound equipment is available, such as linear transducers that allow for a high frequency range to enhance the resolution of near-surface structures. All these attributes come together to create a convenient environment for proper ultrasound scanning of the neck and thyroid (Lyon et al., 2022). Pre-examination routines also need to incorporate infection control policies to maintain the safety of patients. This includes adequate cleaning and disinfection of ultrasound machines and transducers in accordance with guidelines set. The guidelines of the AIUM favor the meticulous adherence to infection control procedures, necessary to minimize the possibility of cross-contamination when interacting with the patient. In addition, sonographers need to take note of the patient's history, especially allergy to the ultrasound gel or other substances applied for the inquiry. Through scrutinizing these pre-exam preparations, practitioners create an ideal situation that results in a productive ultrasound examination. Syncing clinical practice with planned safety measures not only guarantees well-organized flow but also maximizes patient trust and satisfaction with the diagnostic process (AIUM, 2023) (Figure 4.13).

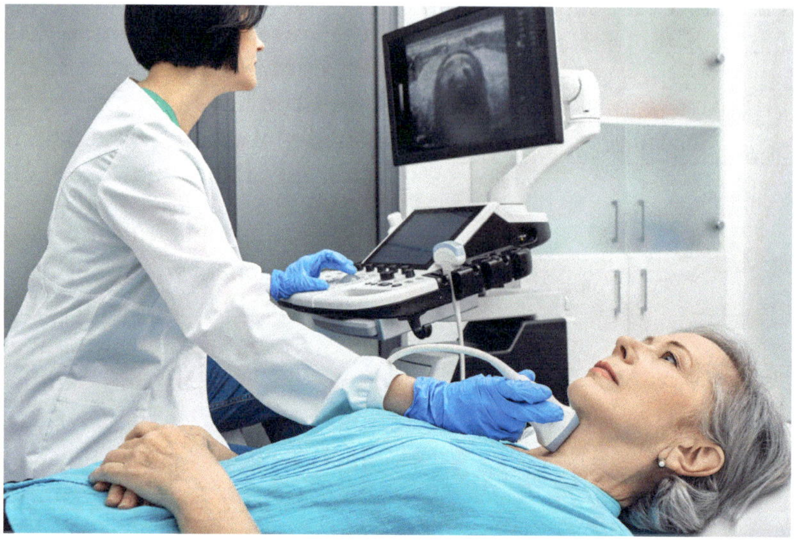

Figure 4.13. Preparation for the ultrasound examination.

Source: https://www.health.com/thmb/St3z38l7XHrRZQiTiaL60Aqj9v4=/5760x0/filters:no_upscale():max_bytes(150000):strip_icc()/Health-GettyImages-1400264257-96cad1815ad34f4794c716414fbf5efc.jpg.

4.4.2. Step-by-Step Process of Conducting the Ultrasound

The procedure of conducting a neck and thyroid ultrasound includes several systematic steps in order to be safe and accurate. The patient is first positioned in a comfortable position, typically supine, with a pillow beneath the shoulders to hyperextend the neck. This allows maximum visualization of the thyroid gland and the surrounding anatomical landmarks. A coupling gel is subsequently applied to the skin overlying the region of examination in order to provide a better transmission of sound waves and reduce artifacts. The doctor or sonographer selects a high-frequency transducer, typically in the range of 5 to 15 MHz, ideally for imaging of superficial structures. This initial step not only prepares the patient and equipment but also sets the stage for obtaining high-quality ultrasound images needed for further scrutiny and diagnosis. After preparation, the technician then sonographically scans the neck in a systematic and methodical fashion, focusing on the thyroid gland and nearby lymphatic tissue. The ultrasound is performed in set planes, the transverse and longitudinal images, to obtain comprehensive images. On scanning, the technologist evaluates the echogenicity, size, and shape of the thyroid lobes and the isthmus and checks for any irregularities in the shape in the form of nodules or cysts. The pictures so generated allow the specialist to examine not just the thyroid, but also important anatomical landmarks such as the recurrent laryngeal nerve and the lymph nodes around it. More sophisticated visualization techniques can be employed, such as Doppler ultrasound, in an attempt to assess blood flow that can provide more information about pathologies, and thereby this step becomes extremely critical for accurate assessment and proper diagnosis.

The final step after the imaging process is documentation and interpretation of the resulting ultrasound images. These are usually archived in digital format for reference in the future, and a comprehensive report is made summarizing the observations. This report should include complete measurements of the nodule, if one is present, and its characteristics and what it means for the patient's health. In some cases, recommendations for additional diagnostic testing, such as fine needle aspiration or follow-up imaging, can be included based on what is observed. This procedure not only ensures proper communication among healthcare providers but also aids in individualizing patient management according to the diagnosed pathology, thereby enhancing patient care in thyroid and neck disorders (Pfaltz et al., 2018; Mannelli, 2015) (Figure 4.14).

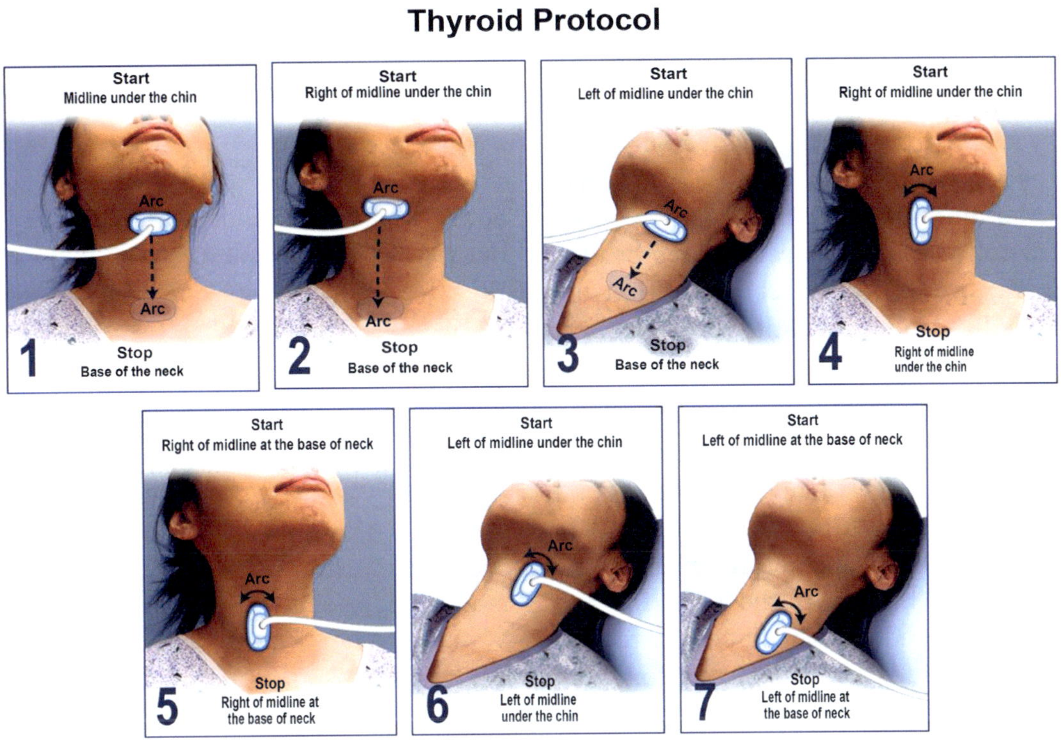

Figure 4.14. Step-by-step process of conducting the ultrasound neck and thyroid.

Source: Marini, T.J., Weiss, S.L., Gupta, A. et al. Testing telediagnostic thyroid ultrasound in Peru: a new horizon in expanding access to imaging in rural and underserved areas. J Endocrinol Invest 44, 2699–2708 (2021). https://doi.org/10.1007/s40618-021-01584-7 .

4.4.3. Post-Procedure Care and Considerations

After the neck and thyroid ultrasound, correct post-procedure care must be used to maintain patient safety and comfort. Although the procedure itself is not very invasive and usually doesn't require much time for recovery, the patient should be cautioned to watch for any immediate reaction that is adverse in nature. Unusual side effects include mild tenderness or swelling at the site of any needle punctures used for the biopsies, and such side effects can often be managed with over-the-counter pain medication. Patients are also instructed to rest and refrain from heavy lifting for a short period after the procedure. Clear instructions for care should be provided by health care professionals following the procedure, which can enhance patient compliance and satisfaction. This forward-looking practice in post-procedure care can significantly enhance the overall success of the intervention and allow for timely intervention in the event of complications.

Another crucial aspect of post-procedure issues is the follow-up protocol, particularly relevant in the follow-up of differentiated thyroid cancers (DTCs). Since the trend with DTCs is towards minimally invasive operations such as lobectomy rather than total thyroidectomy, the need for patient-specific surveillance protocols takes on a larger role. Physicians would be well advised to follow a risk-of-recurrence-based management approach with consideration of patient-specific evaluation and the dynamic nature of neoplastic growth.

This approach is informed by the evolution of imaging modalities that not only aid post-treatment staging but also aid effective short- and long-term follow-up. The melding of ultrasound with other diagnostic tests, as in current literature, highlights the need for an integrated post-procedure plan that caters to the varied needs of patients who have undergone thyroid-related procedures (Deandreis et al., 2016). With the addition of newer modalities like the Smart-touch fine needle (STFN) system, care following procedures can be elevated to new levels. The ability to pair mechanical profiling and stiffness measurements of tissue with fine needle aspiration (FNA) can even enhance diagnostic dependability and inform subsequent treatment algorithms. Education regarding the importance of these new technologies and how they help inform the treatment algorithm is necessary following the procedure. The explanation of the variations in tissue stiffness, as revealed by STFN, is histopathology-oriented and may influence post-procedure decision-making (Aguilera et al., 2019). The information regarding the availability of ongoing monitoring and follow-ups with such sophisticated techniques should be communicated to the patients so that they are also engaged in their own care. This is one factor that not only reinforces the understanding of their health status but also underscores the necessity of individualized medicine in thyroid management.

4.5. Interpretation of Ultrasound Results

Sonographic analysis of images in the context of neck and thyroid examinations plays a pivotal role in accurate diagnosis and treatment. Ultrasound is now a first-line imaging tool for the evaluation of thyroid nodules due to its lack of invasiveness and good anatomical resolution. Determination of nodule characteristics in terms of size, echogenicity, and microcalcifications is one of the most important aspects of image interpretation. Hypoechoic nodules, for example, are more often associated with increased malignancy, again underscoring the utility of using a systematic approach to defining such features. Interobserver variability, that is, different interpretations among different radiologists of otherwise similar nodules, is also a complicating factor, necessitating a strict framework in terms of maintaining consistency and accuracy of reporting (Bakshi et al., 2012).

Moreover, the value of ultrasound-guided fine needle aspiration cytology (FNAC) cannot be overemphasized in this diagnostic process. FNAC enables cytological examination of thyroid nodules, giving the clinician seminal clues as to their character. Nevertheless, it is important to note that FNAC is not perfect; non-diagnostic results can arise and can result in further clinical management conundrums. The results of repeated FNAC attempts point towards the decreasing diagnostic yield with sequential samples. Notably, while malignancy rate in the setting of non-diagnostic FNAC is low in general, careful ultrasound result interpretation is necessary to determine the best next course of action—observation, re-aspiration, or surgery (Bakshi et al., 2012).

Finally, recent advances in ultrasound technology hold promise for enhancing the predictability of the malignancy of thyroid nodules. Research indicates that quantitative measurements of echogenicity can stratify for risk of malignant change. Nodule/parenchyma median gray ratio, for instance, has been demonstrated to be a meaningful continuous measure of hypoechogenicity and predictive of malignancy rates. Incorporating such measures in the interpretive process can assist practitioners in improving diagnostic performance and therapeutic decision-making. Using an objective approach based on cautious echogenicity assessments and heterogeneity ratings may minimize interobserver variability and optimize overall clinical success in the management of suspicious thyroid nodules (Alessandrini et al., 2015) (Figure 4.15).

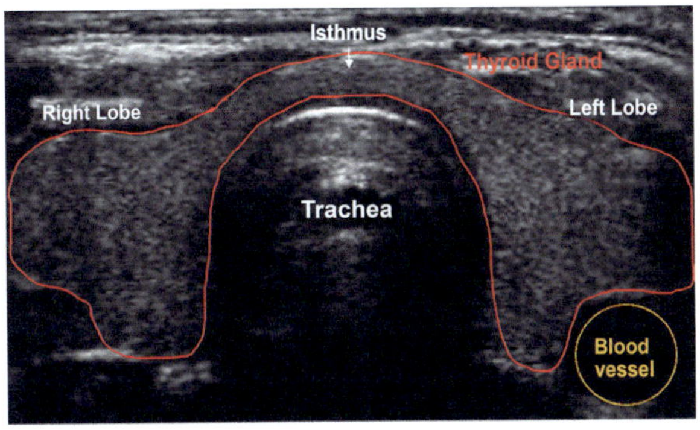

Figure 4.15. Interpretation of ultrasound results of neck and thyroid.

Source: https://rfaforlife.com/wp-content/uploads/2022/04/thyroid2.png.

4.5.1. Common Findings in Neck and Thyroid Ultrasounds

The use of ultrasound in the evaluation of thyroid and neck pathology has increased since it is not invasive and can provide real-time imaging. The most frequent findings on neck ultrasound are lymphadenopathy, cystic lesions, and thyroid masses. Lymph nodes are assessed for evidence of malignancy, such as size, shape, and vascularity. These are significant in differentiating between malignant and benign lymph nodes. Enlargements with gross irregularity or vascular abnormalities can be further examined through FNAC or biopsy so that appropriate management of potential malignancies can be achieved, particularly in head and neck cancers (Schache et al., 2021).

In the thyroid gland, ultrasound is most often able to identify nodules, either single or multiple. The prevalence of high thyroid nodules in the population underscores the necessity for accurate ultrasound evaluation. The majority of nodules are categorized based on the Thyroid Imaging Reporting and Data System (TIRADS) for malignancy risk stratification and clinical decision-making. Solid nodules, particularly larger than 1 cm with worrisome characteristics such as microcalcifications or hypervascularity, usually need FNAC to ascertain their nature. Additionally, the existence of cysts, either simple or complex, should be investigated in detail because the nature of these cysts can influence the management approach, that is, observation vs. surgery (Castroneves et al., 2018). Additionally, ultrasound also plays a vital role in the follow-up of patients after thyroid cancer treatment. Detection of new thyroid nodules, lymph node metastases, or evidence of recurrence is important in early intervention. Serial ultrasound scans complement serum thyroglobulin levels, determining the need for additional imaging or intervention. Radiologists concentrate on disease-related abnormalities, such as suspicious nodes or evidence of local recurrence, thus enhancing management protocols. With emerging advances in ultrasound technology, the ability for accurate detection and characterization of such findings will further improve care and treatment of patients with thyroid and neck diseases, and ultrasound will become a part of routine clinical practice (Schache et al., 2021) (Figure 4.16).

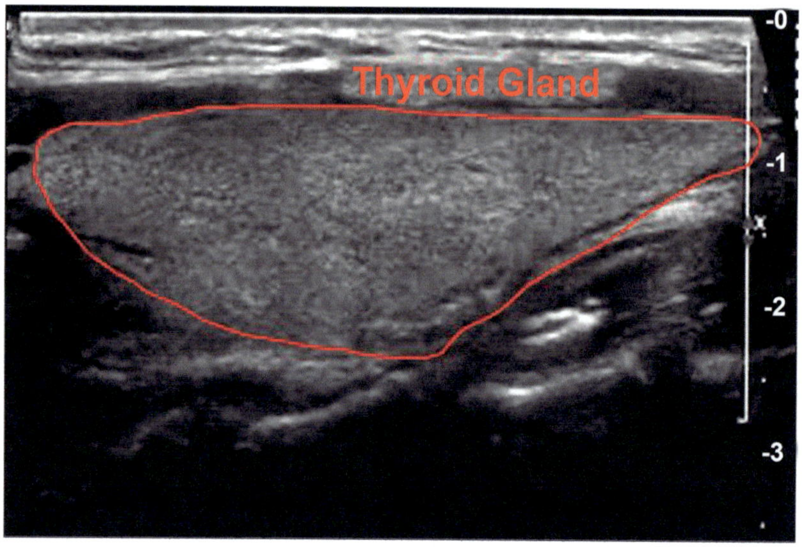

Figure 4.16. Common findings in neck and thyroid ultrasounds.

Source: https://rfaforlife.com/wp-content/uploads/2022/04/thyroid-gland.png.

4.5.2. Criteria for Benign Versus Malignant Nodules

One of the key aspects of thyroid nodule assessment is distinguishing between benign and malignant lesions, and this is considerably image-dependent, using methods like ultrasound. Ultrasound features play a significant role, and some of them indicate a higher risk for malignancy. For instance, those nodules that present with irregular borders, hypoechoicity, greater diameter, and microcalcifications have been associated with malignancy. Conversely, homogenous, cystic nodules with well-defined margins are more likely to reflect benign disease. In fact, it has been reported in the literature that a high proportion of cystic thyroid nodules can hide malignancy, with rates as high as 17–32% being reported in several reviews, such that careful ultrasound assessment is a crucial component of the diagnostic process (Hsueh et al., 2007). Besides these imaging features, history and physical examination have an important role in thyroid nodular risk assessment. Another new feature of thyroid nodule diagnosis is the application of biomarkers, for example, Galectin-3 (Gal-3), which assists further in differentiating between benign and malignant lesions. Recent systematic reviews reinforce the superior histologic validity of Gal-3 as a diagnostic marker for thyroid cancers, as testified by studies demonstrating its sensitivity and specificity levels at around 87% (Crescenzi et al., 2017). Moreover, Gal-3 positivity in FNAC samples has a pooled incidence of 94% in final cancers, as a measure of its utility as an adjunct diagnostic tool in preoperative diagnoses. Because cytological diagnoses are heterogeneous, the addition of Gal-3 testing to the diagnostic algorithm would further refine the accuracy of thyroid nodule evaluation. These more comprehensive approaches enable practitioners to make an informed decision for further treatment, including the requirement for surgical interventions or active surveillance. Ultimately, the approach to discriminating benign from malignant thyroid nodules is modified with advances in diagnostic imaging and biomarkers. Combining ultrasound findings with cytological and histological tests forms the foundation of an integrated model of diagnosis. Since techniques such as ultrasound-guided aspiration and biomarkers such as Gal-3 can be used, medical professionals have the capacity to optimize their diagnostic performance. This triad concept not only optimizes the identification of nodular characteristics but also allows for customized management plans, thereby reducing overtreatment and overdiagnosis of benign conditions. As practice evolves, the refinement of these criteria will prove crucial in optimizing patient outcomes in the assessment of thyroid nodules in the practice of thyroid and neck ultrasound (Figure 4.17).

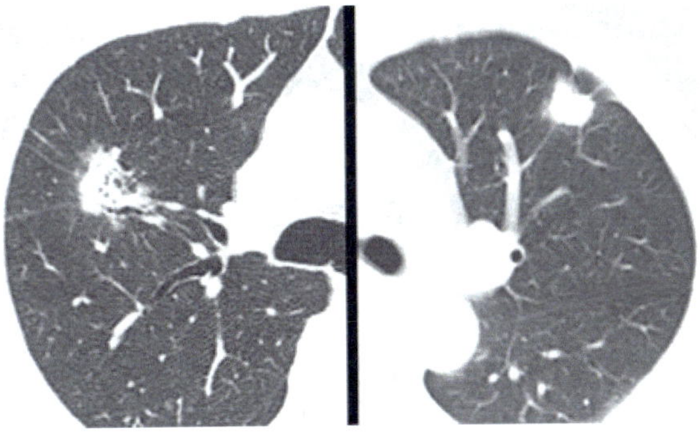

Figure 4.17. Benign versus malignant nodules.

Source: https://radiologyassistant.nl/assets/solitary-pulmonary-nodule-benign-versus-malignant/a5097977958d59_airbroncho-2.jpg.

4.5.3. Role of Radiologists in Interpreting Results

Thyroid and neck ultrasound imaging interpretation is an important responsibility placed squarely on radiologists' shoulders. Radiologists have the responsibility of interpreting ultrasound images to identify abnormalities or pathologies that may result in thyroid malignancies or other disorders. They have the practice scope of possessing such fine nuances as differentiating between benign and malignant nodules, which are important in guiding further diagnostic workup or treatment. Moreover, accurate communication of these results is essential since the interpreting radiologists must confirm that they make themselves understood to the ordering physicians so that the latter appreciate the consequences of their reports. This collaborative approach not only enhances patient care but also introduces an integrated diagnostic process that enhances the medical imaging discipline in how it can positively influence patient treatment. In such situations, where a complicated case is involved, the radiologist also plays a more significant role by correlating imaging evidence with clinical details. For example, tumors such as parotid oncocytoma, which are not uncommonly seen in the context of the thyroid network, may require being interpreted more broadly in the context of the patient's entire medical history and symptoms expressed. Use of sophisticated imaging modalities, such as 18F-Fluorodeoxyglucose Positron Emission Tomography/Computed Tomography (18F FDG PET/CT), can aid in head and neck cancer assessment. This is an indication that radiologists must remain competent not only in routine ultrasound reporting but also in integrating disparate imaging modalities to create broad-based assessments. These cross-sectional approaches avoid underestimation of the minor pathological changes, thereby safeguarding against errors in diagnosis that could affect treatment and prognostic outcome (Ahmad Saad et al., 2016). Moreover, radiologists are pivotal in developing research and innovation in ultrasound methodology. Being very well-versed in imaging equipment, they can engage in collaborations that result in better diagnostic processes and education for peers. By highlighting the role of the thyroid and surrounding structures, radiologists can help shape best practices that enhance diagnostic accuracy. Additionally, their repeated observations will help determine new criteria for the evaluation of thyroid nodules, impacting guideline directives on management. This commitment to advancing the radiology field is an important step in the management of neck pathology complications and improving the interpretative ability for future radiologists, ultimately leading to improved patient care outcomes in thyroid well-being (Focal Spot, 2007).

4.6. Limitations and Challenges

The application of the use of ultrasound in the assessment of thyroid and neck abnormalities has several significant limitations and concerns. Foremost is the operator dependency of the ultrasound technique. The validity of the results is automatically tied to the sonographer's technical capability and level of experience, which can provide susceptibility to variability in diagnostic outcomes. Inconsistent performance of skills and unequal levels of experience may result in pathologies being missed or misinterpretation of ultrasound images. This operator dependency emphasizes the need for standardized protocols and extensive training to improve diagnostic accuracy and reduce discrepancies in clinical practice, which is a must in providing maximum patient care and management. Another actual drawback in the case of neck and thyroid ultrasound is the limitation of being able to distinguish between a benign and a malignant lesion. Ultrasound sensitivity can lead to false positives, particularly when nodules possess indeterminate characteristics. The uncertainty necessitates further invasive procedures, such as biopsies, for a definitive diagnosis, which can be further harmful to the patient. Further, although ultrasound is valuable in providing initial assessment, it cannot provide in-depth information regarding the biological behavior of certain lesions. Thus, practitioners often rely on a multi-dimensional decision-making approach that intermixes ultrasound findings with clinical suspicion and other imaging modalities, as is evident from the diagnostic roles of ultrasound, CT, and MRI reported in recent literature (Dudea et al., 2013). The accuracy of ultrasound in the examination of metastatic lymph nodes of the neck also poses challenges, particularly in treatment planning and prognostic assessment. Identification of malignant lymph nodes greatly influences the decision for surgical treatment and other interventions, including chemotherapy and radiation (Dudea et al., 2013). Nonetheless, detection of such characteristics could be indefinite by ultrasound, making results interpretation cumbersome. The limitations in subclinical metastatic changes detection in ultrasound explain the need for thorough evaluation and added complexity imaging assessments to guarantee correct staging and best therapeutic outcomes. Hence, health practitioners must guard against the inherent technical constraints of ultrasound technology when integrating information from more than a single diagnostic platform in order to maximize patients' management optimally.

4.6.1. Technical Limitations of Ultrasound Imaging

Ultrasound scanning, while a wonderful asset in the evaluation of thyroid and neck abnormalities, does have its technical limitations. A significant drawback is the variability of image quality with operator dependence; the radiologist's expertise can have a tremendous influence on diagnostic outcome. For instance, in thyroid fine needle aspiration cytology (FNAC) scenarios, research indicates diagnostic yield can significantly differ based on whether the test is being performed by a head and neck radiologist or a generalist radiologist. The risk of non-diagnostic findings can reach 90% in the case of non-ultrasound guidance, highlighting the need for advanced training in the use of ultrasound skills to mitigate such risks and enhance diagnostic precision (Bakshi et al., 2012). Such reliance on operator skills thus highlights a major limitation of ultrasound imaging, particularly in complex evaluations. Further, ultrasound scanning has some anatomical limitations, particularly in the way it is supposed to evaluate deeper structures in the neck. The modality itself is limited by features such as superimposed tissues, which may prevent one from visualizing the thyroid gland and associated structures. This is especially so where there is excessive obesity or where there are large muscular neck structures that may interfere with the transmission of the sound waves. Additionally, isoechoic lesion evaluation—lesions with the same echogenicity as the surrounding tissue—is problematic and biases towards misinterpretation or overlooked abnormalities. Such anatomical factors greatly detract from the accuracy of ultrasound for final diagnoses, necessitating reinforcement diagnostic imaging such as CT or MRI when the results of ultrasound are not definitive. A second significant ultrasound limitation is the fact that it cannot provide detailed information on the biochemical composition of thyroid nodules. While ultrasound is very good at signaling nodule shape, size, and texture, it does not provide information about the cellular composition of nodules—information needed to stratify cancer risk. Studies have shown the malignancy rate of non-diagnostic FNAC findings to be negligible, where histopathological correlation is normally necessary to conclude the nature of suspected nodules (Bakshi et al., 2012). Moreover, other imaging devices, such as portable mini gamma-cameras, are more diagnostically precise compared to preoperative ultrasound, further necessitating integrative approaches in enhancing the validity of diagnosis in the management of neck and thyroid diseases. Therefore, the ultrasound limitations become a testament to the need to apply a multimodal approach in clinical practice for the sake of correct diagnosis and efficient management of patients.

4.6.2. Challenges in Differentiating Between Conditions

The subtleties regarding the discrimination between various neck and thyroid diseases pose significant problems for physicians. The difficulty primarily results from overlapping clinical presentations of thyroid diseases, including benign nodules, malignant thyroid cancer, and inflammatory thyroid disease, rendering initial diagnoses troublesome. Neck and thyroid ultrasound has been invaluable in imaging of such structures in a diagnostic role, but its usefulness is often flawed by the skill of the operators and the constraints inherent in the technology itself. For instance, the delicate line between benign and malignant nodules may not be adequately expressed through the application of ultrasound imaging, and thus may lead to misdiagnosis and undue therapeutic plans. Thus, while ultrasound seemed to be a critical component of the evaluation of neck masses, the challenges of making accurate differentiation between conditions emphasize the importance of supportive diagnostic imaging. The integration of AI and radiomics in thyroid diagnosis has promise for enhanced differentiation between conditions, albeit with some accompanying challenges. Current research highlights the diagnostic efficacy of radiomics in improving diagnostic accuracy, and there is evidence that it can identify patterns in ultrasound images that the human eye may not see. But integration is not without its challenges; explainability of AI algorithms and reliance on large datasets with good image quality remain major challenges. Moreover, operational factors such as variability in the setting of ultrasound machines and operator skill can cause AI algorithms to be biased. The convergence of findings from various studies indicates that while AI presents promising advancements in the diagnosis of diseases like thyroid cancer, the significance of standardization protocols and multicenter trials cannot be disregarded to make the process effective and reliable in clinical practice (Alizadehsani et al., 2024).

As technology relating to the application of neck and thyroid ultrasound evolves, a multi-faceted solution to the challenges in discriminating between conditions is called for. Future studies should be aimed at the collaboration of radiologists, endocrinologists, and data scientists to develop robust models that can perform better diagnostic image interpretation. Notably, the employment of explainable AI technology is able to solve some interpretability issues by allowing clinicians to interpret and have faith in algorithmic recommendations. Furthermore, personalized medicine technologies may provide customized treatment plans based on each patient's individual conditions. By enhancing a collaborative environment that gives primacy to technology-clinical convergence, the health community can advance diagnostic precision, strengthen patient outcomes, and ultimately prevent the difficulties of differentiating between varied thyroid disorders (Focal Spot, 2008).

4.6.3. Patient Factors Affecting Ultrasound Outcomes

Proper application of ultrasound in the diagnosis of neck and thyroid illness is extremely vulnerable to various patient-related ailments that influence imaging results. Age plays a critical role; older patients may have anatomical changes in the thyroid gland, such as nodules or calcifications, which complicate the interpretation of ultrasound results. In addition, physiological aging changes, such as decreased thyroid function, influence nodule vascularity and may lead to mischaracterization on assessment. Given that PHPT is commonly seen in elderly patients, such effects and systemic contributions must be carefully taken into account to prevent misdiagnosis and proper management during the ultrasound process (Armanini et al., 2015). Furthermore, patient population, such as sex and body mass index (BMI), body size and shape, has been cited to affect the outcomes of thyroid ultrasounds. Incidence of thyroid nodules has been found to be high in women by studies; hence, rates of detection are sex-differentiated. Increased BMI also brings a serious limitation, in that additional fat tissue can obscure ultrasound images and lower the quality of the results obtained, potentially risking missing diagnoses or inappropriate assessments. These are all factors in ensuring that ultrasound findings are adequately correlated to the clinical context in order to make the best patient management decisions regarding additional diagnostic testing or follow-up (Carnes et al., 2018). Additionally, ultrasound results can be interpreted by thyroid function tests, particularly in patients with indeterminate nodules. Different TSH levels, free T4, and total T3 levels in patients may present different patterns on ultrasound imaging, so it is challenging to evaluate the nodule. It has been stated that demographic characteristics and values of thyroid function are generally not sufficient to estimate malignancy risk in indeterminate nodules; hence, ultrasound characteristics still remain significant in decision-making. In managing indeterminate outcomes, it is important that clinicians consider these along with ultrasound imaging in determining whether or not surgery or observation is required, thereby enhancing the outcome of patient care for neck and thyroid ultrasound scans (Carnes et al., 2018).

SUMMARY

The incorporation of ultrasound of the neck and thyroid into clinical practice has revolutionized the treatment of thyroid ailments at its core. With progressive improvements in diagnostic imaging, the technology continues to provide greater sensitivity and specificity for identifying thyroid abnormalities. This is especially true in the changing trend in managing differentiated thyroid cancers (DTCs), which have shifted toward a more conservative management strategy. The shift is also motivated by the ability of ultrasound in providing real-time scanning of thyroid nodules and lymph nodes to enable physicians to create intervention strategies that are minimally invasive during surgery but best suited for potential malignancies. The emphasis on risk stratification in current literature highlights imaging's relevance to guiding clinical judgment to optimize patient outcomes better than previously possible with conventional means alone (Deandreis et al., 2016). Moreover, the utilization of ultrasounds within the diagnostic procedure, that is, in combination with fine needle aspiration cytology (FNAC) for evaluating thyroid nodules, reinforces its significant application in guiding therapeutic measures. Despite the challenge posed by non-diagnostic FNAC, ultrasound allows limiting the margin of error in follow-up efforts by experienced practitioners and thus enhances diagnostic yield. The evidence offers strong evidence that ultrasound guidance, especially by experienced head and neck radiologists, plays a key role in reducing rates of non-diagnostic results against generalist policy. This improvement in diagnostic certainty is tantamount to more absolute clinical decision-making and is essential in thyroid nodule malignancy risk assessment, allowing for enhanced risk stratification and management plans (Bakshi et al., 2012). Lastly, the role of neck and thyroid ultrasound in the present practice cannot be overstressed. Not only does the technology enhance diagnostic yields, but it also allows for more complex management plans for ailments like DTCs. As imaging modalities keep changing, health care systems will have to keep changing and adapting in order to be able to best treat patients. By prioritizing the use of ultrasound and ensuring that providers are adequately trained, the healthcare community will be able to improve the outcome for thyroid patients, remaining responsive to the dynamic nature of such conditions. Ultimately, continued research and improvement of ultrasound technology will continue to maximize its applications, leading to greater surveillance, earlier detection, and greater therapeutic efficacy in the area of thyroid health (Deandreis et al., 2016).

In the field of thyroid and neck ultrasound, some important observations have been made that bring out the importance of proper surgical management. Total thyroidectomy (TT) and subtotal thyroidectomy (ST) have been effective surgeries for the treatment of multinodular non-toxic goiter, with TT being a major advantage in avoiding goiter recurrence rates. Evidence has established that recurrence of goiter post-surgery is significantly less in TT, with a recurrence of only 0.2% compared to 8.4% of the ST population, demonstrating the effectiveness of TT as a method of treating this extremely common thyroid condition. The rate of re-intervention due to recurrence is also significantly less in patients with TT. These findings suggest that in the case of considering surgical options, TT can be the safer route to maintaining long-term patient health and avoiding the risk of complications due to recurrence of goiter (Arezzo et al., 2015).

Thyroid surgery unwanted effects analysis shows an interesting pattern regarding complications such as recurrent laryngeal nerve palsy and hypoparathyroidism. Though TT is associated with a higher incidence of chronic complications, such as hypoparathyroidism in 0.6% of TT patients compared to 0.1% of ST patients, recurrent laryngeal nerve injury rates are low with either approach.

This alludes to an important consideration in the risk-benefit ratio that has to be considered by clinicians when deciding between TT and ST. While decreased complication risks for ST are important, the reduced rate of recurrence observed for TT patients can ultimately lead to increased cancer surveillance and preventive interventions following surgery (Arezzo et al., 2015). Thus, the ultrasounds have become an essential part of preoperative assessment, guiding decision-making through tailored patient risk profiles. The thyroid neoplasms' challenges add further complexity to the surgical management paradigm, particularly for Hürthle cell carcinoma (HCC) instances. This cancer has a clinically aggressive behavior, and it demands meticulous evaluation and management strategies. Most significantly, minimally invasive HCC potentially can be cured by lobectomy alone for lesions that are smaller than 4 cm in diameter, reducing total patient stress. Larger lesions are best treated with total resection with follow-up radioactive iodine (RAI) therapy, as current studies suggest that RAI is effective at improving survival in those patients who have widespread metastasis. This necessitates a multidisciplinary strategy for patient management, including both ultrasound imaging for correct diagnosis and surveillance, and surgery, individually tailored to overcome the particular challenge that HCC poses. Ultimately, a complete understanding of ultrasound results directly determines surgical decisions and optimizes patient outcomes in thyroid disease.

CLOSER LOOK

DIFFERENTIATED THYROID CANCERS (DTCS)

Differentiated thyroid cancers (DTCs) are the most prevalent type of thyroid malignancies, accounting for approximately 90–95% of all thyroid cancers. They originate from the follicular epithelial cells of the thyroid gland and are termed "differentiated" because the tumor cells retain many morphological and functional characteristics of normal thyroid tissue, including the ability to absorb iodine. DTCs are broadly classified into papillary thyroid carcinoma (PTC), follicular thyroid carcinoma (FTC), and the less common Hürthle cell carcinoma (oncocytic carcinoma). PTC is the most common subtype, representing about 70–80% of DTCs. It is characterized histologically by papillary structures and distinctive nuclear features such as nuclear grooves and "Orphan Annie eye" nuclei. PTC often spreads to regional cervical lymph nodes but typically has an excellent prognosis with a 10-year survival rate exceeding 95%. FTC accounts for 10–15% of DTCs and is more likely to spread hematogenously to distant organs such as lungs and bones. Hürthle cell carcinoma, previously considered a variant of FTC, is now recognized as a distinct and more aggressive subtype, often showing reduced responsiveness to radioactive iodine therapy. The pathogenesis of DTCs involves genetic alterations such as BRAF V600E and RET/PTC rearrangements in PTC and RAS mutations in FTC. Diagnosis relies on ultrasound evaluation, fine-needle aspiration cytology (FNAC), and serum thyroglobulin measurement for follow-up. Management of DTCs typically involves total or near-total thyroidectomy followed by radioactive iodine ablation and thyroid hormone suppression therapy to reduce TSH stimulation of residual tumor cells. Targeted therapies like tyrosine kinase inhibitors are emerging options for RAI-refractory disease. Overall, DTCs are considered highly treatable malignancies with excellent long-term outcomes, although vigilant monitoring is essential to detect recurrence and manage advanced disease effectively.

References

1. Abdullah, A. M., Qaradakhy, A. J., Saeed, Y., Muhialdeen, A. S., Mohammed, R. O., Baba, H. O., Salih, A. M., et al. (2025). Kikuchi-Fujimoto disease coexistent with papillary thyroid carcinoma: A report of two cases. *Barw Medical Journal*. https://www.semanticscholar.org/paper/c94b2de8155b46719eb62f4163eb23f03a881315 (accessed on 12th July 2025).
2. Adrian, T., Alecu, L., Cristian, B., Hainarosie, R., et al. (2018). Functional radical cervical dissection for differentiated thyroid cancer: The experience of a single center. https://core.ac.uk/download/216809678.pdf (accessed on 12th July 2025).
3. Aguilera, R., Gimzewski, J. K., Rao, J. Y., Sharma, N., et al. (2019). Piezoelectric needle sensor reveals mechanical heterogeneity in human thyroid tissue lesions. https://core.ac.uk/download/323076249.pdf (accessed on 12th July 2025).
4. Ahmad Saad, F., Fikri, F., Mohtarrudin, N., Nordin, A. J., Subha, R., et al. (2016). Parotid oncocytoma in Birt-Hogg-Dube syndrome: A new pitfall in 18F-fluorodeoxyglucose positron emission tomography/computed tomography imaging study. https://core.ac.uk/download/153813493.pdf (accessed on 12th July 2025).
5. Ahmadi, S., Jiang, X. S., Sosa, J. A., Stang, M., et al. (2016). Hürthle cell carcinoma: Current perspectives. https://core.ac.uk/download/323072068.pdf (accessed on 12th July 2025).
6. AIOM-AIRTUM Working Group, AIRTUM Working Group, Alexander, A., Ali, N., Altman, A., Attia, R., et al. (2017). Comparative analysis of diagnostic performance, feasibility and cost of different test-methods for thyroid nodules with indeterminate cytology. https://core.ac.uk/download/188830446.pdf (accessed on 12th July 2025).
7. AIUM. (2023). AIUM Practice Parameter for the Performance and Interpretation of Diagnostic Ultrasound of the Thyroid and Extracranial Head and Neck. *Journal of Ultrasound in Medicine, 42*. https://doi.org/10.1002/jum.16251 (accessed on 12th July 2025).
8. Alessandrini, S., Bianchini, M., Carbottà, G., Coccaro, A., et al. (2015). Grey-scale analysis improves the ultrasonographic evaluation of thyroid nodules. Medicine. 94. e1129. 10.1097/MD.0000000000001129. https://core.ac.uk/download/54530544.pdf (accessed on 12th July 2025).
9. Alizadehsani, R., Jafari, A., Jafarizadeh, A., Maleki, M., et al. (2024). Advancements in radiomics and artificial intelligence for thyroid cancer diagnosis. http://arxiv.org/abs/2404.07239 (accessed on 12th July 2025).
10. Amabile, M. I., Arcieri, S., Ascoli, V., Baldini, E., et al. (2019). Thyroglobulin measurement in the washout of fine needle aspirates for the diagnosis of suspicious cervical lymph nodes. https://core.ac.uk/download/195776721.pdf (accessed on 12th July 2025).
11. Anari, H., Bashardoust, B., Pourissa, M. and Refahi, S. (2011). The diagnostic accuracy of high-resolution ultrasound imaging for the detection of secondary hyperparathyroidism in patients with chronic renal failure. https://core.ac.uk/download/11685402.pdf (accessed on 12th July 2025).
12. Arezzo, A., Avenia, N., Barczyñski, M., Cirocchi, R., et al. (2015). Total or near-total thyroidectomy versus subtotal thyroidectomy for multinodular non-toxic goiter in adults. https://core.ac.uk/download/54521026.pdf (accessed on 12th July 2025).

13. Armanini, D., Bordin, L., Camozzi, V., Donà, G., et al. (2015). Transient hypercortisolism and symptomatic hyperthyroidism associated to primary hyperparathyroidism in an elderly patient: Case report and literature review. https://core.ac.uk/download/53518371.pdf (accessed on 12th July 2025).

14. Assanti, A. P., Colao, A., Del Prete, M., & Faggiano, A. (2012). Thyroid nodules treated with percutaneous radiofrequency thermal ablation: A comparative study. https://core.ac.uk/download/159268412.pdf (accessed on 12th July 2025).

15. Baatenburg de Jong, R. J., & Rongen, R. J. (1990). Ultrasound examination of the head and neck. https://core.ac.uk/download/18513420.pdf (accessed on 12th July 2025).

16. Bakshi, A., Corrias, A., Mendelson, A. A., Renshaw, A. A., Fusco, A., Carmeci, C., Oertel, C. Y., et al. (2012). Malignancy risk analysis in patients with inadequate fine needle aspiration cytology (FNAC) of the thyroid. https://core.ac.uk/download/9562718.pdf (accessed on 12th July 2025).

17. Cantisani, V., Chiovato, L., Durante, C., Farina, M., et al. (2018). Thyroid ultrasonography reporting: Consensus of Italian Thyroid Association (AIT), Italian Society of Endocrinology (SIE), Italian Society of Ultrasonography in Medicine and Biology (SIUMB) and Ultrasound Chapter of Italian Society of Medical Radiology (SIRM). https://core.ac.uk/download/188833333.pdf (accessed on 12th July 2025).

18. Cappelli, C., Casella, C., Nascimbeni, R., Nessi, M., et al. (2015). Radioguided parathyroidectomy with portable mini gamma-camera for the treatment of primary hyperparathyroidism. https://core.ac.uk/download/80138964.pdf (accessed on 12th July 2025).

19. Carnes, N. (2018). Predicting risk of malignancy in patients with indeterminate thyroid nodules. https://open.bu.edu/bitstream/2144/31159/5/Carnes_bu_0017N_13608.pdf (accessed on 12th July 2025).

20. Castroneves, L. A., Coura-Filho, G. B., Freitas, R. M. C., Salles, R., Moysés, R. A., Mendoza López, R. V., Pereira, M. A. A., et al. (2018). Comparison of 68Ga PET/CT to other imaging studies in medullary thyroid cancer: Superiority in detecting bone metastases. *The Journal of Clinical Endocrinology & Metabolism, 103*, 3250–3259. https://doi.org/10.1210/jc.2018-00193 (accessed on 12th July 2025).

21. Chong, J., Sun, Y., Ning, C., Wang, H., & Yang, Z. (2017). Contrast-enhanced ultrasound characteristics of papillary thyroid carcinoma and its relationship with micro vessel density and micro vessel area. *14*, 274–279. https://www.semanticscholar.org/paper/d0ce88e50fdd6e0ab7f1fa9dda758eff64704b98 (accessed on 12th July 2025).

22. Crescenzi, A., Giovanella, L., Romanelli, F., Trimboli, P., et al. (2017). Galectin-3 performance in histologic and cytologic assessment of thyroid nodules: A systematic review and meta-analysis. https://core.ac.uk/download/158327840.pdf (accessed on 12th July 2025).

23. Daminet, S., Peremans, K., Saunders, J., Vandermeulen, E., et al. (2016). Hyperthyroidism in cats, part I: Anatomy, physiology, pathophysiology, diagnosis and imaging. https://core.ac.uk/download/74658457.pdf (accessed on 12th July 2025).

24. Deandreis, D., Durante, C., Filetti, S., Lamartina, L., et al. (2016). ENDOCRINE TUMOURS: Imaging in the follow-up of differentiated thyroid cancer: Current evidence and future perspectives for a risk-adapted approach. https://core.ac.uk/download/74318453.pdf (accessed on 12th July 2025).

25. Dudea, D., Petrovic, T., Sham, E., & Torabi, F. (2013). Application of imaging methods in the diagnostics of malignant neck lymph nodes. https://core.ac.uk/download/pdf/26978184.pdf (accessed on 12th July 2025).

26. Evidence-Based Complementary and Alternative Medicine. (2023). Retracted: Analysis of the application value of ultrasound three-dimensional speckle tracking technology combined with thyroid autoantibodies and hormones in the diagnosis and treatment of Graves' disease. *Evidence-based Complementary and Alternative Medicine: eCAM, 2023.* https://www.semanticscholar.org/paper/c073755ae7342d34d39b5256a9ca9d556d9e60f9 (accessed on 12th July 2025).

27. Focal Spot, Summer/Fall 2007, July 2007. Bernard Becker Medical Library Archives. Washington University School of Medicine. https://core.ac.uk/download/129069359.pdf (accessed on 12th July 2025).

28. Focal Spot, Spring 2008, April 2008. Bernard Becker Medical Library Archives. Washington University School of Medicine. https://core.ac.uk/download/129069364.pdf (accessed on 12th July 2025).

29. Haddad, R. I., Bischoff, L. A., Ball, D. W., Bernet, V., Blomain, E., Busaidy, N. L., Campbell, M. J., et al. (2022). Thyroid carcinoma, Version 2.2022, NCCN clinical practice guidelines in oncology. *Journal of the National Comprehensive Cancer Network, 20*, 925–951. https://doi.org/10.6004/jnccn.2022.0040 (accessed on 12th July 2025).

30. Hsueh, C., Huang, B. Y., & Lin, J. D. (2007). Application of ultrasonography in thyroid cysts. https://core.ac.uk/download/pdf/82730599.pdf (accessed on 12th July 2025).

31. Kim, J. H., Irvinn, J., & Sammut, L. (2024). P25 When fevers hide secrets: A case report of papillary thyroid carcinoma presenting as secondary hemophagocytic lymph histiocytosis. *Rheumatology Advances in Practice, 8.* https://www.semanticscholar.org/paper/84ae3eb8256d62f97b54572ff31862448f05162a (accessed on 12th July 2025).

32. Lesende, I. M., Iglesias Losada, J., González Santisteban, R., Azkarate Estevez, N., Bravo Bárcena, M., Llamosas Luengo, I., López de Heredia Gutiérrez, A., et al. (2023). Feasibility and utility of point-of-care ultrasound (POCUS) in primary care practice: EKOAP Pilot Study. *Family Medicine and Primary Care: Open Access.* https://www.semanticscholar.org/paper/10ae4f366f4c5360fcc34f15d9e2e5e1f94062f3 (accessed on 12th July 2025).

33. Lo Baido, C., Tranchina, E., & Verso, M. G. (2019). Does still exist a correlation between X-rays occupational exposure and benign nodular thyroid disease? https://core.ac.uk/download/224993285.pdf (accessed on 12th July 2025).

34. Lyon, A. R., López-Fernández, T., Couch, L. S., Asteggiano, R., Aznar, M. C., Bergler-Klein, J., Boriani, G., et al. (2022). 2022 ESC Guidelines on cardio-oncology developed in collaboration with the European Hematology Association (EHA), the European Society for Therapeutic Radiology and Oncology (ESTRO) and the International Cardio-Oncology Society (IC-OS). *European Heart Journal, 43*, 4229–4361. https://doi.org/10.1093/eurheartj/ehac244 (accessed on 12th July 2025).

35. Man, I., & Chau, K. (2018). Ultrasound diagnosis of cervical vagal schwannoma misdiagnosed as nodular goiter. *Open Journal of Radiology, 08*, 203–208. https://www.semanticscholar.org/paper/5a4105ded0d8029d29c0f3fd89f3471112204ecb (accessed on 12th July 2025).

36. Mannelli, G. (2015). Laryngeal preneoplastic lesions and cancer: Challenging diagnosis. Qualitative literature review and meta-analysis. https://core.ac.uk/download/79618239.pdf (accessed on 12th July 2025).
37. Mauri, G., Hegedűs, L., Bandula, S., Cazzato, R. L., Czarniecka, A., Dudeck, O., Fugazzola, L., et al. (2021). European Thyroid Association and Cardiovascular and Interventional Radiological Society of Europe 2021 clinical practice guideline for the use of minimally invasive treatments in malignant thyroid lesions. *European Thyroid Journal, 10*, 185–197. https://doi.org/10.1159/000516469 (accessed on 12th July 2025).
38. Pfaltz, M., Schmid, S., Steinert, H., Stoeckli, S., et al. (2018). Sentinel lymph node biopsy in thyroid tumors: A pilot study. https://core.ac.uk/download/159154743.pdf (accessed on 12th July 2025).
39. Planchard, D., Popat, S., Kerr, K. M., Novello, S., Smit, E. F., Faivre-Finn, C., Mok, T., et al. (2018). Metastatic non-small cell lung cancer: ESMO Clinical Practice Guidelines for diagnosis, treatment and follow-up. *Annals of Oncology, 29*, iv192–iv237. https://doi.org/10.1093/annonc/mdy275 (accessed on 12th July 2025).
40. Ramamoorthy, G., Thiagarajan, B., & Ulaganathan, V. (2013). Thyroglossal cyst: Our experience. https://core.ac.uk/download/pdf/9634096.pdf (accessed on 12th July 2025).
41. Schache, A., Kerawala, C., Ahmed, O. A., Brennan, P. A., Cook, F., Garrett, M., Homer, J. J., et al. (2021). British Association of Head and Neck Oncologists (BAHNO) standards 2020. *Journal of Oral Pathology and Medicine, 50*, 262–273. https://doi.org/10.1111/jop.13161 (accessed on 12th July 2025).
42. Steinberg, I., Huland, D. M., Vermesh, O., Frostig, H., Tummers, W. S., & Gambhir, S. S. (2019). Photoacoustic clinical imaging. *Photoacoustics, 14*, 77–98. https://doi.org/10.1016/j.pacs.2019.05.001 (accessed on 12th July 2025).

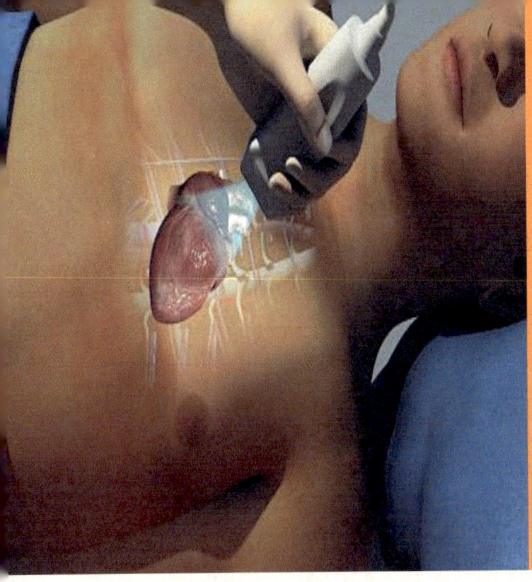

Chapter 5

CHEST AND PLEURA ULTRASOUND

Contents

Introduction

Advances in ultrasound technology have highly transformed the practice of diagnostic imaging, particularly the evaluation of chest and pleural disorders. Traditionally dominated by more invasive methods, the practice of lung diagnosis has seen a gradual shift towards non-invasive modalities with increased focus on patient safety and comfort. One such modality is pleura and chest ultrasound, which offers clinicians the possibility of viewing anatomical landmarks and identifying pathological changes in real-time. This technique has gained popularity not just due to its availability but also because it can provide significant information about various pulmonary pathologies, including pneumonia, pleural effusion, and interstitial lung disease. The application of ultrasound as a standard of clinical practice is an increasing witness to the worth of the modality in enhancing diagnostic precision and guiding management decisions, thus providing a foundation for modern thoracic practice. Further stimulus to the call for effective diagnostic processes arises from the recent outbreak of respiratory diseases, led visibly by the recent global COVID-19 pandemic. While global health systems reeled from increasing cases of respiratory conditions, the imperative for efficacious imaging techniques came to the fore. Here, deep learning in chest ultrasound presents a bright future. Researchers have set out to investigate artificial intelligence technologies to improve the diagnostic efficacy of lung ultrasonography (Roy et al., 2020). Through the utilization of large datasets and advanced algorithms, such initiatives can not only improve image interpretation but also enable the early identification of those conditions that would otherwise fall outside the reach of conventional diagnostic avenues. This transformation represents a movement toward more powerful, data-driven approaches that maximize the potential of contemporary technology to enhance outcomes for patients. In addition, with procedures such as transbronchial cryobiopsy (TBCB) available as alternatives to surgery for diffuse parenchymal lung disease, the use of chest ultrasound becomes all the more crucial (Hetzel et al., 2018). While TBCB provides a less invasive but effective alternative for sampling lung tissue, pre-procedure assessment meticulously performed using ultrasound is essential. This method allows for in-real-time assessment of lung architecture and pleural spaces, improving procedural safety and patient selection. The combination of ultrasound technology and novel diagnostic techniques brings to light the importance of ultrasound in contemporary pulmonary medicine with a focus on a future where precision and safety go hand in hand in thoracic care (Figure 5.1).

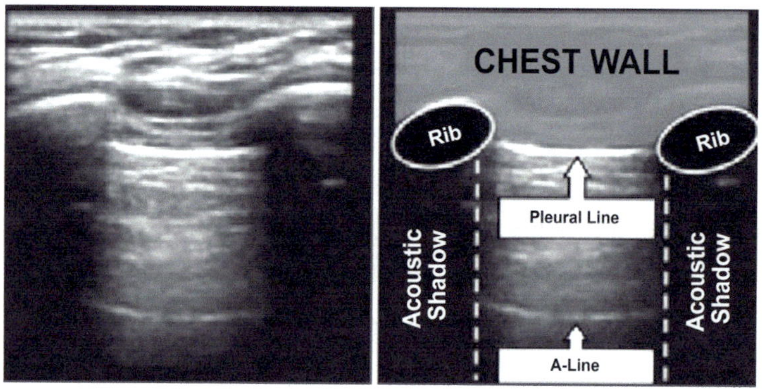

Figure 5.1. Chest and pleura ultrasound.

Source: de Souza, Tiago & Giatti, Marina & Brandão, Marcelo. (2016). Lung ultrasound for diagnosis of pneumothorax in an infant. Journal of Pediatric Critical Care. 3. xx. 10.21304/2016.0304.00149. .

Definition of Chest and Pleura Ultrasound

Chest and pleura ultrasound is an essential diagnostic imaging device that utilizes high-frequency sound waves to visualize structures in the thoracic cavity, specifically the chest and pleural membranes. It is a non-invasive technique applied to carry out real-time images, which facilitates the assessment of various pleural conditions, such as effusions, pneumothorax, and adhesions. The cost-effectiveness and accessibility approaches have made it an extremely well-liked modality compared to conventional imaging techniques, that is, chest X-ray or CT scans, especially in cases where emergent evaluation is needed. Since healthcare professionals utilize ultrasound, they are able to obtain valuable information about the fluid collection status or pleural abnormal thickening, and hence enhance their capability to make effective and timely clinical decisions. The use of chest ultrasound can be widened to the evaluation of patients with complex conditions, that is, patients on dialysis. Evidence in current literature supports that focused lung ultrasound is useful in hydration assessment through identification of B-lines associated with interstitial fluid overload (Petersen et al., 2024). This correlation highlights the use of the method in assisting in fluid balance management, which is a factor among renal patients. Furthermore, ultrasound utilization in everyday clinical practice can improve patient outcomes by detecting and treating respiratory complications early. Visualization of the interaction of lung and pleural structures adds a beneficial dimension to patient management that can deliver a more integrated form of diagnosis. In trauma and operative conditions, such as in perforation of the esophagus, the value of ultrasound is further explained. It can easily identify pleural adhesions and assess the extent of complications from esophageal trauma, particularly fistula formation (Ihnatsiuk & Karpitski, 2022). With visualization techniques that examine the barcode sign on M-mode, healthcare practitioners can distinguish among pleural dynamics, which aids in decision-making regarding intervention techniques, including drain insertion. Thus, ultrasound of the chest and pleura becomes an effective diagnostic tool as well as a useful guide for postoperative treatment, eventually resulting in better patient outcomes and reduced hospital stay. With time, standardized ultrasound protocol need to be incorporated in order to fully utilize its clinical utility.

Importance in Medical Diagnosis

The clinical significance of chest and pleura ultrasound is highlighted by its ability to provide real-time imaging and a non-invasive approach to assess several pulmonary disorders. Its application is particularly beneficial in the assessment of pleural effusions, pulmonary nodules, and consolidations. Compared with traditional imaging techniques, such as X-rays and CT scans, ultrasound offers dynamic assessment with the option for the physician to observe movement and blood flow in real time. This skill enhances the clinicians' capacity to make informed decisions regarding intervention and management of patients. Secondly, the development of newer technologies like artificial intelligence has also solidified the role of ultrasound in enhancing diagnostic accuracy through enabling automated detection of lung tissue abnormalities, consistent with current trends in the practice of medical imaging (Roy et al., 2020).

Besides, the utility of ultrasound extends beyond mere imaging. It plays a significant function in guiding interventions such as needle biopsies and thoracentesis, where proper localization is critical for success. Through the use of ultrasound, practitioners can actually minimize complications and improve patient safety when these are being done. The increasing apparent potential of ultrasound also offers pathways towards normalizing its inclusion into routine tests, particularly in emergency and critical care settings where prompt decisions must be made. With the medical environment changing, so is the demand for modalities that are effective, safe, and affordable (Adler et al., 2015). The constant exploration of the potential of ultrasound in medical diagnosis not only adds to its utility but also enhances the overall quality of care given to pulmonary patients. Also, the use of deep learning and artificial intelligence in the interpretation of lung ultrasound images has made changes in diagnostic practices by leaps and bounds. Recent advances have demonstrated that these technologies possess the potential to automate image interpretation of ultrasound with much greater velocity and precision. Development of large annotated sets enables the algorithm to learn from a broad spectrum of diseases, leading to improved detection of pulmonary pathology. These technologies are well in line with the growing emphasis on precision medicine, offering personalized treatment strategies that can be tailored to patient profiles. With the horizon of ultrasound technology continuing to widen, its utility in medical diagnosis is also set to become ever more crucial, assisting clinician proficiency and ultimately helping to result in better patient outcomes within the framework of respiratory diseases (Roy et al., 2020) (Figure 5.2).

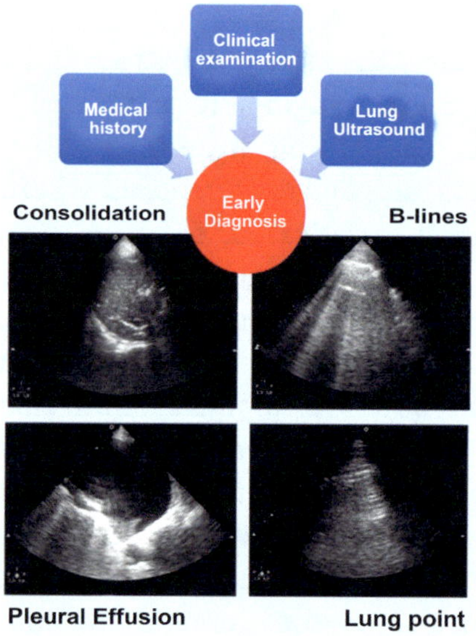

Figure 5.2. Medical diagnosis of chest and pleura ultrasound.

Source: Vetrugno, L., Biasucci, D.G., Deana, C. et al. Lung ultrasound and supine chest X-ray use in modern adult intensive care: mapping 30 years of advancement (1993–2023). Ultrasound J 16, 7 (2024). https://doi.org/10.1186/s13089-023-00351-4 .

5.1. Historical Background

The development of ultrasound technology throughout history has, to a great degree, influenced the medical specialty, particularly when it comes to assessing the chest and pleura. Early applications of ultrasound technology were for non-medical reasons, including naval sonar during World War I. It wasn't until the mid-20th century that the technology began to be applied to medical diagnostics. The introduction of the A-mode scanning technique, and subsequently that of the B-mode, revolutionized how clinicians could view internal anatomy, and this allowed them to notably excel at detecting abnormalities of the thoracic cavity. And so, the current practices for chest and pleura ultrasound arose, which not only comprised imaging but also immediate assessment of structures and fluid movement. With additional advancements, the relationship between ultrasound and other imaging modalities became self-evident in terms of comprehensive diagnostic procedures in chest disease. As technology in ultrasound progressed, so did its use in thoracic medicine. In the 1970s, technique-improved ultrasounds had appeared, like real-time echocardiography, which was vital in keeping track of cardiac conditions and cardiac anatomy. These years saw widespread exploration of using ultrasound for pleural assessment with a focus on pleural effusion and pneumothorax diagnosis. Bedside examination was also made possible by portable ultrasound machines, increasing the efficacy of emergency medicine and critical care. Clinical research began to reveal the potential role of ultrasound in making thoracentesis and other intervention procedures a paradigm shift in the management of pleural diseases. This evolution illustrates the way in which ultrasound has become a key tool for clinicians when evaluating complex thoracic disease alongside traditional imaging methods. Furthermore, the development of standardized protocols and educational enhancements has played a significant role in facilitating the use of chest and pleura ultrasound in clinical practice. Institutions worldwide have realized the necessity of training healthcare professionals in the use of ultrasound technology in thoracic assessment and have established comprehensive curricula as a result. Clinical practice guidelines supporting the use of ultrasound in the emergency department have also been forthcoming, with evidence-based validation of its use in clinical rapid diagnosis and treatment in pneumonia and pleural disease. One large study reported the success of novel techniques for de-airing during open heart surgery and cited the use of ultrasound as an intraoperative real-time guide (Smith et al., 2017). All these events represent the evolution and current state of chest and pleura ultrasound, reaffirming its significant role in modern medical practice and setting a precedent for innovation development in healthcare delivery.

5.1.1. Development of Ultrasound Technology

Ultrasound technology has significantly transformed the medical diagnostic process, particularly in respiratory medicine. Developed originally for industrial use, ultrasound began gaining traction for medical use in the mid-20th century. As a means that was versatile and not invasive, it implied safer patient evaluations without the risks of ionizing radiation. Advances in transducer technology, as well as signal processing, have made deeper tissue penetration and greater resolution images possible, which are absolutely essential to properly evaluate pleural as well as chest-related conditions. Advances have not only enhanced diagnostic precision but also augmented the list of procedures that can be conducted by pulmonologists, which has improved the overall care of pleural disease (Astoul et al., 2016). With advancements in the technology of ultrasound, so did its applications in the clinical setting. With the invention of portable and handheld ultrasound machines, the technology became more democratic, allowing point-of-care usage that could be performed in a range of clinical settings. This shift is particularly noteworthy in the treatment of pleural disease, historically reliant on interventional radiologists or thoracic surgeons to carry out interventions such as thoracentesis and closed pleural biopsy. The growing recognition of ultrasound as an integral part of the pulmonologists' toolkit has provoked research into its potential to guide these interventions. Therefore, modern ultrasound techniques have enhanced the precision of pleural procedures, minimizing complications and improving patient outcomes (Gunarathne, 2021). Furthermore, ultrasound technology has contributed to more educational programs for clinicians. Ultrasonography training has become a key part of pulmonary medicine training, embedding its use within the center of clinical decision-making for pleural disease. Continuing developments in ultrasound technology, for example, real-time imaging and enhanced software facilities, have provided access to new procedures such as medical thoracoscopy and indwelling pleural catheters. These developments signify a paradigm shift in the identification and management of pleural diseases, demonstrating the importance of staying abreast of modern advances in technology to provide optimal patient care. Studies continue to demonstrate the effect of this integration, with more recent methods holding promise in both safety and efficacy (Astoul et al., 2016) (Figure 5.3).

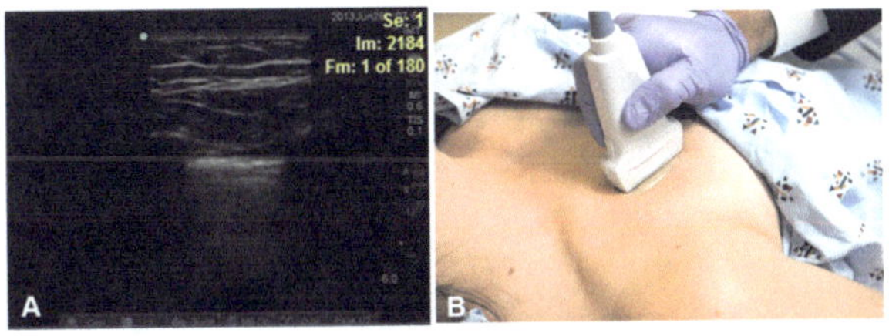

Figure 5.3. Development of ultrasound technology of chest and pleura ultrasound.

Source: Diaz-Gomez, Jose & Via, Gabriele & Ramakrishna, Harish. (2016). Focused cardiac and lung ultrasonography: Implications and applicability in the perioperative period. Romanian Journal of Anesthesia and Intensive Care. 23. 41-54. 10.21454/rjaic.7518.231.lus.

5.1.2. Evolution of Chest and Pleura Imaging

The imaging process of the chest and pleura has drastically revolutionized with the advent of thoracic-focused ultrasound technology. The classical methodology in the past used for the diagnosis of pulmonary diseases involved imaging techniques like X-rays and computed tomography (CT). But these procedures had ginormous disadvantages in the form of radiation and logistics associated with the transport of patients. Lung ultrasound (LUS) has been a game-changer in the field of modality over the last decade, particularly in critical care. Its real-time capability and non-invasive nature have enabled us to make more precise diagnoses of pleural and pulmonary pathology without the hazards entailed by conventional approaches. The continuously emerging advancements in imaging technology have required revision and enhancement of LUS guidelines by professional panels into updated recommendations to enhance education and clinical practice (Demi et al., 2022). The COVID-19 pandemic brought a significant accelerating influence on the integration of LUS into routine clinical practice, further emphasizing the utility of LUS in pleural and pulmonary complication diagnosis. Throughout the pandemic, it was observed that a significant number of patients suffered from severe pneumonia and acute respiratory distress secondary to the virus. While CT scans worked well, they posed logistical challenges due to reasons of exposure for both patient and healthcare workers. Here, LUS proved to be a gold-standard option with its capability of performing an examination at the bedside without any radiation usage. Research has pointed out LUS to detect characteristic patterns indicative of COVID-19 pneumonia, that is, thicker pleural lines and multiple B-lines, thus providing critical information for early therapeutic approaches to clinicians (Allinovi et al., 2020).

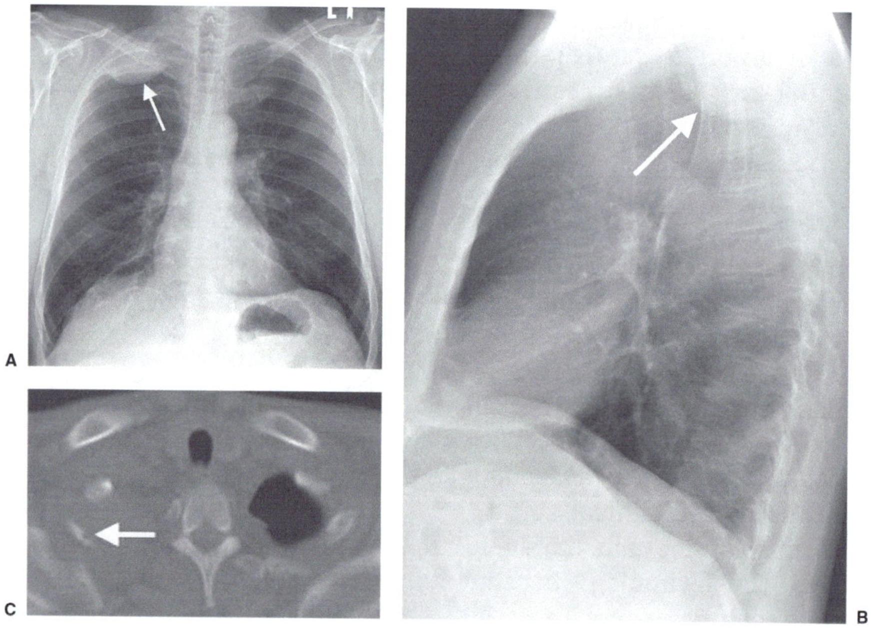

Figure 5.4. Evolution of chest and pleura imaging.

Source: https://radiologykey.com/wp-content/uploads/2016/08/image00890.jpeg.

With every developing advancement in chest imaging technology, the future of ultrasound technology promises to improve patient outcomes by further refining the diagnostic protocol and expanding its application to various healthcare settings. Experts recognized the necessity of developing explicit guidelines that define the methodological conditions of LUS while facilitating security practices necessary for effective utilization. The recent consensus statement supplemented technical and pedagogic aspects, delineating the frame of application in diverse healthcare environments (Demi et al., 2022). In addition, as technology improves, artificial intelligence can potentially be incorporated into lung ultrasound to optimize image interpretation, reducing the intellectual load on doctors and improving diagnostic accuracy. This ongoing evolution is a sign of a changing paradigm for chest imaging, with LUS in the vanguard of diagnostic innovation for pleural and pulmonary assessment (Figure 5.4).

5.1.3. Key Milestones in Ultrasound Research

The development of ultrasound imaging technology has come a long way since its inception, particularly in its application within chest and pleura diagnosis. A landmark in this field has been the utilization of lung ultrasonography as a diagnostic tool, in parallel with the development of high-frequency imaging technologies. This technique is more prized for its ability to provide instant, portable readings of pulmonary pathology and thus becomes a very valuable instrument in intensive care and emergency care facilities as well. Lung ultrasound has been proven to be as sensitive and specific as traditional imaging technologies like CT scans, thus solidifying its position as a cost-effective and safer tool. Above all, the avoidance of exposure to ionizing radiation, especially in vulnerable patient populations, is a significant benefit of ultrasound technology that promotes its practice use (Abo et al., 2019). Further more recent research also further elucidates the diagnostic utility of lung ultrasound, showing pronounced similarities between results yielded by less experienced operators and specialists. One of the early classic studies was an Indian college of medicine study that highlighted the use of bedside lung ultrasound and demonstrated 82% sensitivity in lung pathology diagnosis when it was set against a composite reference standard that included clinical evaluation and conventional imaging (Manisha, 2018). Not only does this verify the diagnostic efficacy of ultrasound, but also its applicability for its widespread use, particularly in low-resource settings. Such facts substantiate the hypothesis that investment in training for healthcare workers can directly impact patient outcomes, and lung ultrasonography is an attractive option in respiratory medicine. Continuous evolution of ultrasound science includes not only technological advances but also investigation into clinical guidelines protecting patient health. Safety is still a concern, since practitioners need to be highly trained in the techniques of ultrasound to avoid any hazards from ultrasound exposure. This tradition is aligned with the principle of as-low-as-reasonably-achievable, which promotes minimizing patient exposure while being able to get diagnostically adequate images (Abo et al., 2019). As ultrasound technology becomes increasingly integrated into routine clinical evaluation of chest and pleural illness, regulatory bodies and healthcare organizations are faced with the challenge of instituting robust training practices. Ultimately, the comprehensive understanding of both the virtues and the limitations of ultrasound imaging will lead to its expanded use and consolidate its role as a pillar in modern-day pulmonary diagnostics.

5.2. Principles of Ultrasound

The technology of ultrasound is founded on the use of high-frequency sound waves to view inner structures, and as such, it is a highly useful medical imaging modality, especially in the chest and pleura. Ultrasound operates through echolocation, whereby the transducer emits sound waves that travel through tissues and reflect once they hit interfaces of differing densities, such as fluid and air. These reflected waves are then processed into images by the ultrasound machine, giving real-time imaging of anatomical structures. The principal advantages of ultrasound include that it is non-invasive, easily available, ionizing radiation-free, and able to generate dynamic imaging of respiratory motion. In addition, these features make it particularly appropriate to evaluate conditions affecting the pleura, for example, pleural effusions, where ultrasound can help to ascertain the volume and nature of the fluid in order to guide management. In the evaluation of chest pathology, the role of ultrasound extends beyond basic imaging; it is also concerned with diagnostic and therapeutic applications. The pleural and chest ultrasound is a significant imaging tool for the assessment of various thoracic diseases, including pneumothorax and interstitial lung disease. Practitioners are able to apply procedures such as thoracentesis with the use of principles of ultrasound to aspirate excess fluid from the pleura or to obtain samples for testing. This is crucial in the clinical situation where rapid intervention is necessary. Apart from that, ultrasound provides real-time feedback, which is helpful for clinicians to adjust their approach accordingly, maintaining both accuracy and patient safety. Real-time visualization of structures facilitates quick decision -making by healthcare providers, validating the use of ultrasound as an important modality for chest assessment. Furthermore, technological advancements in ultrasound have supported its use and efficacy in thoracic assessment. Advances in imaging technology, such as Doppler ultrasound, enable evaluation of blood flow, which in certain circumstances may be essential for the diagnosis of disease related to pulmonary circulation. Increased resolution and hand-carried ultrasound devices have broadened the indication for this imaging modality to be utilized in a wide variety of settings, from emergency departments to outpatient clinics. Nevertheless, with its numerous benefits, the interpretation of ultrasound images is demanding in terms of expertise, since artifacts and operator drift can affect results. For instance, clinicians should be skilled at separating genuine pathologies from artifacts that may simulate diseases such as pleural effusions. Lastly, knowing the fundamentals of ultrasound is important for radiologists and clinicians alike in order to thoroughly understand its application in chest and pleural diseases and further propagate better patient care (Figure 5.5).

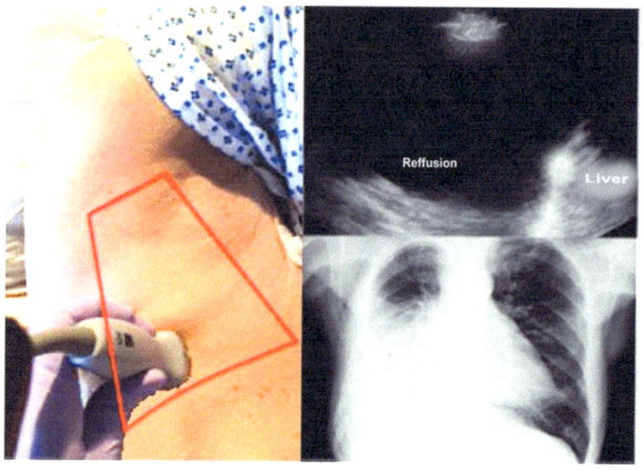

Figure 5.5. Principles of ultrasound of chest and pleura imaging.

Source: DeBiasi, Erin & Puchalski, Jonathan. (2016). Thoracentesis: State-of-the-Art in Procedural Safety, Patient Outcomes, and Physiologic Impact. PLEURA. 3. 10.1177/2373997516646554.

5.2.1. Basic Physics of Ultrasound Waves

The physical principles of ultrasound waves form an essential part of various medical imaging techniques, particularly for chest and pleura ultrasound. Ultrasound waves are highly frequent sound waves that exhibit specific properties while propagating in different biological tissues. Wavelength, frequency, and amplitude are inherent properties of ultrasound that play a very important role in image quality and diagnostic accuracy. During the passage of ultrasound through the thoracic cavity, variations in tissue density, such as air within lungs versus liquid within pleural effusions, modify the reflection and transmission of waves. This interaction yields the distinctive echogenic patterns that are assessed by technicians to differentiate between normal and pathological states. Understanding these fundamental principles is important since they dictate the application of ultrasound in clinical scenarios, for instance, the identification of pleural effusions or lung tissue consolidations. Additionally, the bioeffects of ultrasound through thermal and non-thermal interaction highlight the need for care in its clinical use. Experiments have demonstrated that ultrasound energy is capable of inducing physiological changes in tissues, and thermal and mechanical indices have thus been established for assessing safety.

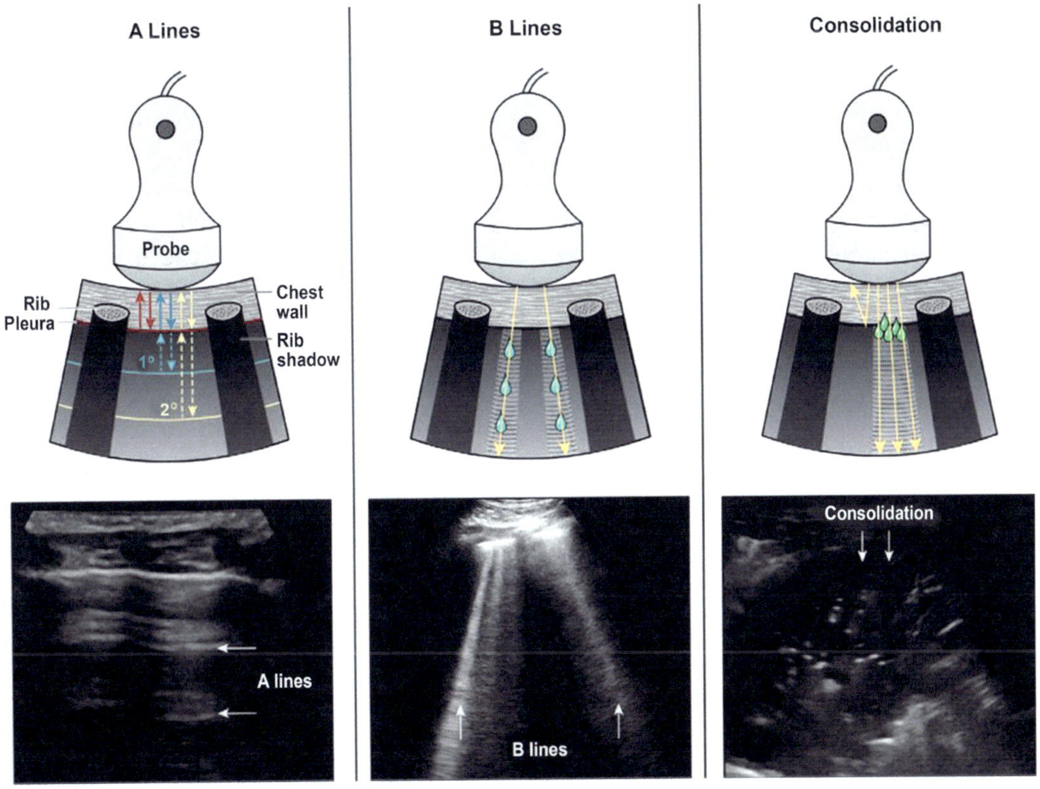

Figure 5.6. Physics of ultrasound waves of chest and pleura imaging.

Source: Marini, Thomas & Rubens, Deborah & Zhao, Yu & Weis, Justin & O'Connor, Timothy & Novak, William & Kaproth-Joslin, Katherine. (2021). Lung Ultrasound: The Essentials. Radiology: Cardiothoracic Imaging. 3. e200564. 10.1148/ryct.2021200564.

The thermal index quantifies the risk of tissue heating due to exposure, and the mechanical index quantifies possible mechanical bioeffects due to the effects of cavitation. The distinction between these two mechanisms is particularly striking in chest and pleura ultrasound, where sensitive structures such as the heart and lungs are involved. Current guidelines are likely to emphasize the ALARA (As Low As Reasonably Achievable) principle, which encourages minimizing ultrasound exposure to the barest minimum while achieving diagnostic objectives effectively. Doctors must be cognizant of the potential risks linked to the application of ultrasound, as outlined in recent literature (Quarato et al., 2023). Recent developments within lung ultrasound (LUS) have led to even more precise guidelines and consensus, leading to widespread multidisciplinary collaboration. Given the dynamic nature of ultrasound technologies, an international panel of experts critically reviewed recent practice in point-of-care LUS. This evaluation resulted in the formulation of 20 statements representing various technical, clinical, educational, and safety issues. These guidelines illustrate an emphasis on improving diagnostic accuracy coupled with enhancing patient safety, especially in relation to new ultrasound methods such as contrast-enhanced ultrasound and acoustic radiation force impulse elastography. Continuous updates of guidelines are required to ensure the management of the intersection of innovation and patient care, based on both clinical practice and technological progress (Demi et al., 2022). Joint actions provide assistance not only to the effectiveness of chest and pleura ultrasound but also to the role of strict training and education for practitioners in this rapidly evolving field (Figure 5.6).

5.2.2. Mechanism of Image Formation

The mechanism of image formation in the pleura and ultrasound of the chest is basically driven by the interaction of the ultrasound waves with body tissues. When an ultrasound probe emits sound waves, the high-frequency waves travel through the thoracic space and interact with various structures, including the pleura and lung parenchyma. The differential acoustics of the tissues according to their composition and density result in variation in reflection as well as transmission of the ultrasound waves. When the reflected waves travel back to the transducer, they are converted to electrical signals, which are then processed to generate images of the underlying anatomy. This is critical in the diagnosis of conditions such as pneumothorax and pleural effusions, where the differential between normal and pathological findings largely relies on accurate imaging techniques. Thoracic pathology diagnosis relies on certain artifacts seen in ultrasound imaging. Among these, A and B-lines are particularly valuable in the differentiation of normally aerated lung from pathological lung. A-lines appear as horizontal lines on the ultrasound screen and are indicative of well-aerated lung tissue, while B-lines are indicative of interstitial edema. The artifacts are created because of the interaction between the ultrasound waves and air-tissue interfaces and the pleural plane, which produces differential echo patterns seen on the ultrasound screen.

There is a requirement for a thorough awareness of these artifacts among clinicians via lung ultrasound, since they direct diagnostic algorithms in addition to therapy. While the clinical relevance of these artifacts has been noted, the physical principles responsible for their appearance remain an issue waiting for better clarification (Soldati et al., 2019). The recent progress in lung ultrasound has prompted an entire review of its applications and best practices. An international panel of experts from a wide range of disciplines re-visited the original guidelines for point-of-care lung ultrasound, and this led to 20 updated statements emphasizing the significance of technical, clinical, educational, and safety matters in practice (Demi et al., 2022). Such developments aim to maximize lung ultrasound as an investigative tool, particularly for the examination of parenchymal lung diseases. Elaboration of the basic mechanisms of the formation of images will further enhance the clinical use of ultrasound for the diagnosis of conditions previously challenging to assess. As the field continues to advance, ongoing education and adherence to updated guidelines will be imperative in optimizing the benefits of chest ultrasound in clinical and emergency practice (Figure 5.7).

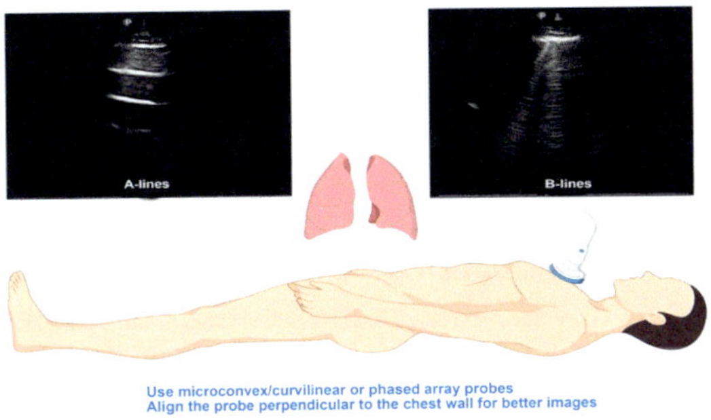

Figure 5.7. Mechanism of ultrasound image formation of chest and pleura.

Source: Lung ultrasound: A and B-lines. https://i0.wp.com/nephropocus.com/wp-content/uploads/2020/02/a-b-lines-1.png?fit=3000%2C2100&ssl=1.

5.2.3. Types of Ultrasound Equipment Used

The technology of ultrasound has considerably evolved, especially in the assessment of thoracic diseases. Various types of ultrasound units are being used in chest and pleural sonography exams to make diagnoses more accurate. Portable ultrasound machines are particularly valuable in emergency and critical care medicine. The devices have smaller sizes and user-friendly designs, making it possible to perform rapid examinations where timely intervention is required. Also, high-frequency linear transducers are employed to image superficial structures, such as the pleura and lung interfaces. Their ability to generate high-resolution images is significant in diagnosing conditions such as pleural effusion or pneumothorax, which are normally evaluated in chest ultrasounds.

Standardized frameworks and procedural guidelines maximize the use of ultrasound equipment within clinical practice. It has become essential to revise lung ultrasound (LUS) protocols in accordance with recent studies, firmly endorsing the implementation of evidence-based practice for enhanced diagnostic performance. Recent international consensus statements have shown in recent times that recent accuracy in the classification of ultrasound applications has informed the development of technical, clinical, and educational guidelines for professionals. This categorization ensures the employment of relevant results in various kinds of ultrasound in a variety of clinical contexts, hence improving patient care. Modern ultrasound equipment with advanced imaging resources enables physicians to assess varied thoracic abnormalities rapidly and effectively, making sure that timely diagnosis and therapy are within reach. Technological advancements also contribute to the armory at the clinician's disposal by incorporating features such as Doppler imaging and 3D ultrasound. Doppler ultrasound gives essential information regarding blood flow dynamics, helping to diagnose vascular disorders involving the thoracic area. Similarly, 3D ultrasound enables one to get a better perception of anatomical structure, making it easier to examine complicated pleural diseases in detail. These developments represent a move in the direction of an integrated application of ultrasound, with more recent suggestions calling for utilizing sophisticated technology to enhance patient safety and care. Lastly, the integration of different ultrasound modalities appropriately aligns with the added emphasis on evidence-based practice in current medical environments, so that clinicians are adequately trained to meet patient needs (Bodenham et al., 2016; Demi et al., 2022) (Figure 5.8).

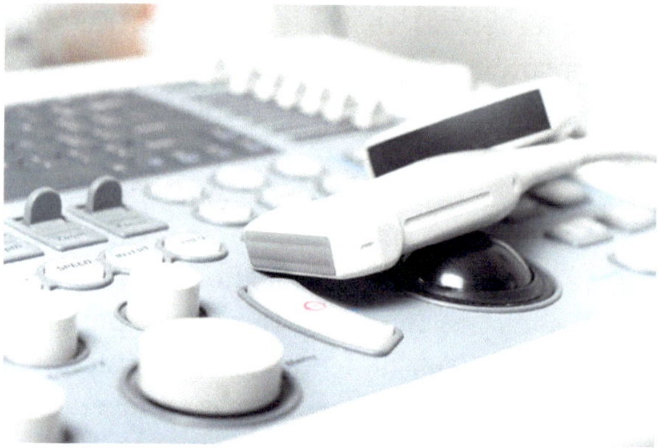

Figure 5.8. Types of ultrasound equipment used of chest and pleura.

Source: https://www.emra.org/contentassets/441f24af0d864f3e8c23c048e6ab6d67/ultrasound.png?w=600.

5.3. Indications for Chest and Pleura Ultrasound

Chest and pleura ultrasound is an important diagnostic aid in many clinical scenarios, particularly the assessment of pathology affecting the lungs. Pleural effusion assessment is one of the primary indications for the use of this imaging modality and can be caused by a vast array of etiologies, including congestive heart failure, infection, or malignancy. Proper diagnosis is important as treatment and prognosis depend on accurate identification of the cause. With ultrasound, providers can probe the pleural space, gauge the level of fluid collection, and even assist in therapeutic interventions such as thoracentesis. Further advances in deep learning techniques also acknowledge the potential of increased automation of ultrasound interpretation, increasing diagnostic efficiency, especially in emergency situations, making patient care easier (Roy et al., 2020). In combination with pleural effusions, chest and pleura ultrasound is increasingly applied to evaluate patients with pneumonia or empyema suspected of occurring. The visualization of lung pleural surfaces provides information on complications that may develop from infectious disease. Ultrasound findings are able to show the presence of fluid or loculations that characterize empyema and require early treatment to prevent further morbidity. In addition, the non-invasive nature of ultrasound promotes serial assessment in the critically ill patient, providing critical information without the risks associated with more invasive imaging procedures. Therefore, incorporating ultrasound as a component of routine pneumonia and complication assessment can significantly influence patient outcomes, since early detection and treatment of the aforementioned conditions are critical to recovery (Jany & Welte, 2019). Furthermore, ultrasound plays a crucial role in the direction of various interventional procedures for pleural and chest uses, including biopsies, catheter placement, and drainage of fluid accumulations. The precision of high-resolution ultrasound provides accurate localization of the lesion or the fluid to be addressed, minimizing the chance of complications with blind techniques. With continued growth in clinical practice, the addition of technologies such as image-guided deep learning has the potential to enhance the evaluation of ultrasound images, thereby enhancing diagnostic confidence and procedural efficiency. Thus, training healthcare professionals in cutting-edge ultrasound techniques and their applications in the clinic becomes essential to maximize patient care in all specialties, ultimately paving the way for broader application of this useful imaging modality for the evaluation of chest and pleura pathology (Roy et al., 2020) (Figure 5.9).

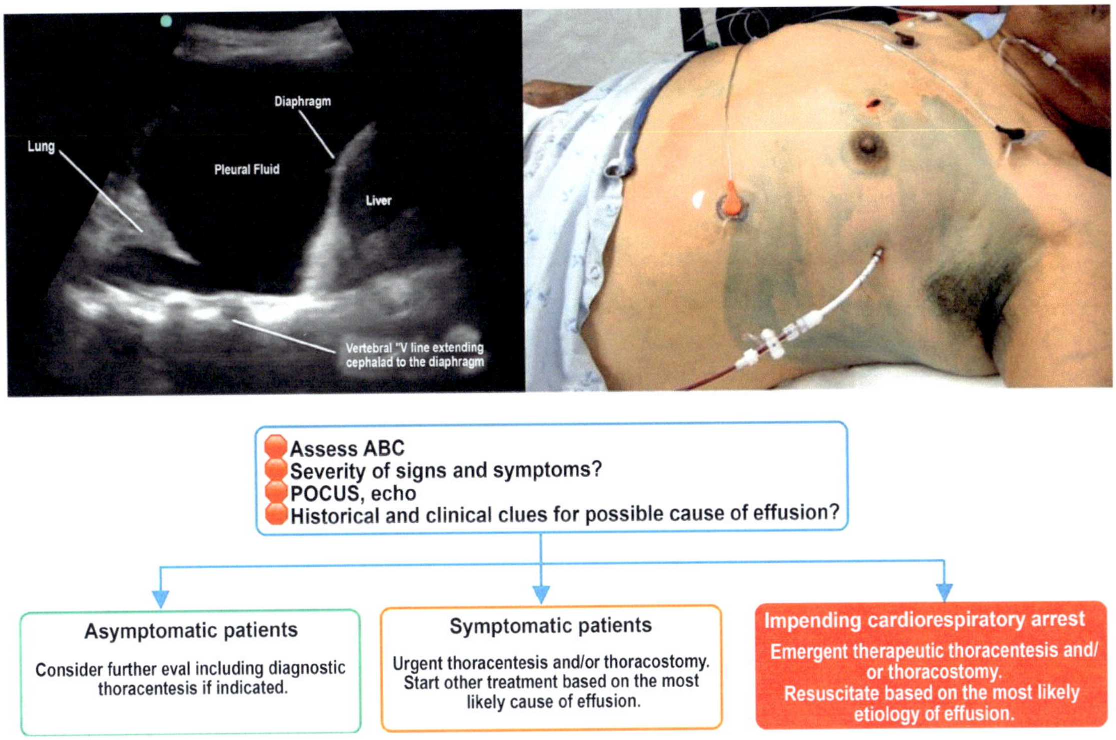

Figure 5.9. Indications for chest and pleura ultrasound.

Source: Shahriar Lahouti (2023). Pleural Effusion in Critically ill Patients. https://recapem.com/wp-content/uploads/2023/06/pleural-effusion.png.

5.3.1. Diagnosis of Pleural Effusion

Accurate diagnosis of pleural effusion is critical in clinical practice since the pathologies with prognostic potential for obscuring existing diseases like congestive heart failure, pneumonia, and malignancy. Clinicians traditionally utilize chest X-rays (CXR) as a first modality for initial evaluation. However, studies indicate that point-of-care ultrasound (POCUS) is of greater diagnostic utility and hence serves as a valuable instrument in pleural effusion assessment. Specifically, POCUS demonstrated 97.88% sensitivity and 94.54% specificity when compared to CXR's low values, signifying a conclusive advantage in bedside diagnosis (Zaki et al., 2024). This shift toward the implementation of POCUS in standard practice requires redesigning current diagnosis procedures, particularly in emergency and intensive care departments where rapid decision-making is crucial. Aside from its high diagnostic accuracy, POCUS is particularly recognized for its real-time imaging that enables quick assessment that can shape resultant treatment plans. The modality has good sensitivity in identifying not only the absence or presence of pleural effusion but also whether it is of a specific type and what the potential reasons for it are, which can make clinical decision-making optimal. Furthermore, there is high specificity in varied positions of the patient during examination of ultrasound with supine and erect procedures, providing particularly good results (Zaki et al., 2024). With the older techniques such as CXR still holding relevance, the incorporation of ultrasound in diagnostic processes can help physicians make more accurate diagnoses without losing time in handling patient care. Even though POCUS has several advantages, there is a need to value other imaging techniques like computed tomography (CT) in the full diagnosis of pleural effusion. Though POCUS has an advantage in the emergency room, CT offers more anatomical detail hat can be essential in complex cases, for instance, when malignancy or gross complication is suspected. Additionally, standard imaging techniques like CXR are still valid, particularly when used in combination with ultrasound. Lastly, an integrated approach wherein the particular strengths of each of the diagnostic tools are utilized will most likely have the best outcomes in the management of pleural effusions and hence result in correct diagnosis and appropriate therapeutic interventions (Figure 5.10).

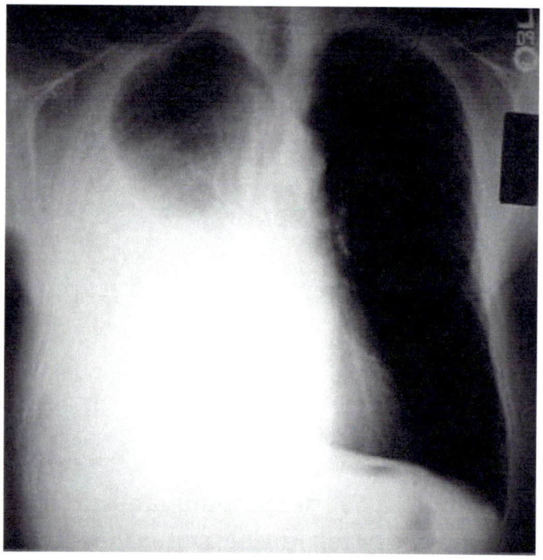

Figure 5.10. Diagnosis of pleural effusion.

Source: https://img.medscapestatic.com/pi/meds/ckb/65/38665tn.jpg.

5.3.2. Evaluation of Lung Pathologies

Lung pathologies assessment has been significantly enhanced by the application of chest and pleura ultrasound (LUS). The technique offers an imaging method that is non-invasive and devoid of radiation, which is a suitable alternative for the assessment of varied lung and pleural disorders. The characterization of normal and pathological lung patterns is essential in the diagnosis of conditions such as pneumonia, pleural effusion, and pneumothorax. Notably, ultrasound is able to detect the occurrence of B lines, an indication of interstitial fluid and impending pulmonary edema, whereas the absent lung sliding shows pneumothorax. Advances in point-of-care ultrasound (POCUS) have further improved, making rapid diagnoses possible, allowing clinicians to institute timely interventions that improve patient outcomes significantly (Kalagara et al., 2021). Besides, the use of artificial intelligence (AI) and deep learning techniques represents a groundbreaking development in the evaluation of lung pathologies. The literature has begun to explore deep learning techniques applied directly to lung ultrasonography (LUS), promising the potential for automated diagnosis with enhanced diagnostic efficacy. With the creation of highly annotated datasets from various clinical settings, the application of deep neural networks is now capable of localizing and detecting pathological artifacts cost-effectively. The process not only aids in the diagnosis of traditional lung diseases but also has excellent scope for identification of emerging diseases, significantly boosting clinicians' ability to manage intricate cases effectively in real-time (Roy et al., 2020). Besides improving the accuracy of diagnosis, ultrasound evaluation of lung conditions is possible with ongoing patient follow-up and monitoring. Traditional imaging modalities like chest X-ray or CT scanning might not be feasible in acute situations, either due to logistics or time required for deployment. Nonetheless, LUS is convenient and can be performed at the bedside, where examinations can be done quickly within emergency conditions. It allows constant observation of lung function, which allows immediate clinical decision-making regarding patient treatment. The advantages of bedside ultrasonography in combination with the emergence of AI technologies illustrate the future line of development for improving patient care by means of enhanced diagnostic models for pulmonary diseases (Kalagara et al., 2021) (Figure 5.11).

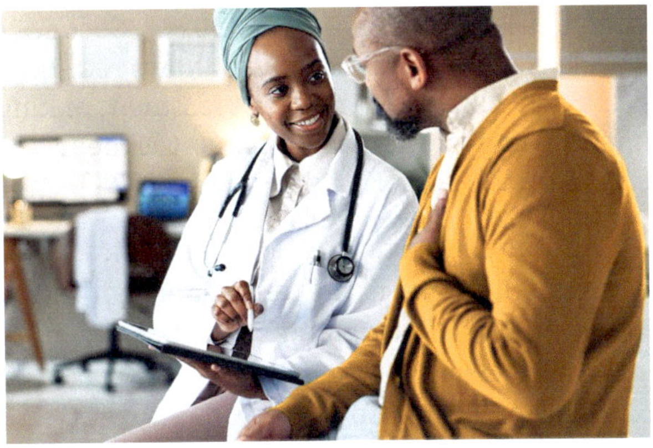

Figure 5.11. Evaluation of lung pathologies.

Source: spirometry.com. The Role of Spirometry in the Evaluation of Interstitial Lung Disease. https://spirometry.com/media/images/the-role-of-spirometry-in-the-evaluation-of-in.width-770.jpg.

5.3.3. Guidance for Thoracentesis Procedures

With thoracentesis procedures in mind, ultrasound guidance has revolutionized the practice of managing pleural effusions through greater accuracy and fewer complications. Making use of ultrasound in the procedures allows the pleural space to be seen in real-time, thus potential identification of the optimal sites of puncture and preservation of vital structures such as vessels and lung tissue. The ultrasound can detect dynamic pleural changes and effusion patterns and enable clinicians to establish the amount and nature of the fluid—transudative or exudative—by providing valuable pre-intervention diagnostic data. This evidence-based practice not only increases thoracentesis safety but also directly equates to patient comfort enhancement and reduced post-procedure complications as a result of incorrect needle placement, further supporting the importance of methodical training in ultrasound-guided procedures in contemporary medical education (Biggins et al., 2021).

Lastly, the success of the procedures in the majority of instances depends on many variables, including the appropriate positioning of the patient and the experience of the operator. Proper positioning, typically with the patient sitting, optimizes fluid drainage and minimizes the risk of lung puncture. Ultrasound guidance is particularly valuable in complicated or loculated effusions where the standard landmarks are unreliable or poor. Furthermore, ultrasound-guided thoracentesis allows the puncture to be performed in the correct intercostal space and visually verifies entry into the pleural space. This evidence-based methodology aligns with the overall principles found in clinical guidelines that advocate for the standardization of thoracentesis procedures for the maintenance of patient safety and procedure success (Biggins et al., 2021). In conclusion, the incorporation of ultrasound guidance into thoracentesis is a significant new innovation in pulmonary medicine and part of a broader trend toward the use of point-of-care ultrasound (POCUS). Subsequent recommendations should focus on training and experience of ultrasound skills by healthcare providers who conduct thoracentesis to optimize the management of pleural effusion across various clinical settings. Such evidence is attainable via systematic reviews and expert consensus, as illustrated by recent attempts at establishing formal guidelines solely for pediatric and neonatal populations who have undergone similar procedures. With the progressing research, the role of ultrasound must be further defined and demarcated in the field of thoracentesis and its significance expressed in terms of ensuring improved patient outcomes in respiratory care (Singh et al., 2020) (Figure 5.12).

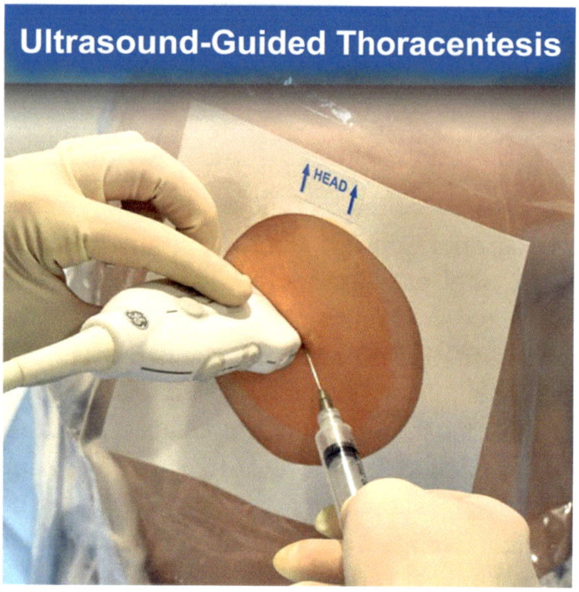

Figure 5.12. Guidance for thoracentesis procedures.

Source: https://cdn2.sonosim.com/wp-content/uploads/2020/02/thoracentesis_product_image_blue_ribbon.jpg.

5.4. Advantages of Ultrasound in Chest Imaging

Ultrasound use in chest imaging has several advantages that are extremely valuable in optimizing diagnostic capability and patient care. One of the most striking is the modality's relative portability and ease of use. Point-of-Care Ultrasound (POCUS) machines are easily available and can be utilized directly at the bedside, allowing rapid assessment in emergent situations. Such emergent use is extremely beneficial in the emergency department, where rapid diagnosis may literally be a lifesaver. POCUS can evaluate various conditions of the lungs, including pleural effusions, pneumothorax, and lung parenchymal diseases, typically with increased sensitivity compared to conventional imaging methods like the chest X-ray or CT scan, which may be time-consuming or lead to patient delay (Kalagara et al., 2021). Secondly, the release of ultrasound sound allows real-time imaging, facilitating dynamic assessment of lung function and pathology without the need for ionizing radiation (Kalagara et al., 2021).

Another important advantage of ultrasound in chest imaging is its affordability, which remains making it an indispensable asset in acute as well as in chronic care. Ultrasound examinations are also cheaper than computed tomography (CT) and can be acquired without the associated costs that accompany patient transport for imaging or with contrast agent hazards linked to certain diagnoses. These cost savings translate to increased access to reliable diagnostic imaging, particularly in resource-poor environments. The capacity for bedside evaluation also reduces the time to wait for diagnosis, which is critical in cases where expeditious treatment intervention can drastically alter outcome. Additionally, the non-invasive nature of ultrasounds ensures comfort for patients throughout the procedure, resulting in a paradigm change in clinicians' handling of respiratory exams (Kalagara et al., 2021). Moreover, the ability of ultrasound to provide real-time visual information regarding extravascular lung water (EVLW) accumulation further supports its application in the management of diseases such as heart failure. Through detection of B-lines, which signify interstitial pulmonary edema, ultrasound enables clinicians to dynamically evaluate fluid status and formulate evidence-based decisions for diuretic treatments. This capability supports enhanced patient management by allowing intervention earlier in the progression of clinical deterioration, a critical consideration in the acute environment. In addition, as clinicians grow more familiar with ultrasound technology, its integration into routine practice not only empowers professionals but also speeds a culture of evidence-based, real-time decision-making diagnosis. Lastly, the advantages of using ultrasound in chest imaging underscore its central role in modern medicine, remodeling the provision of chest pathology and care for patients by healthcare providers (Figure 5.13).

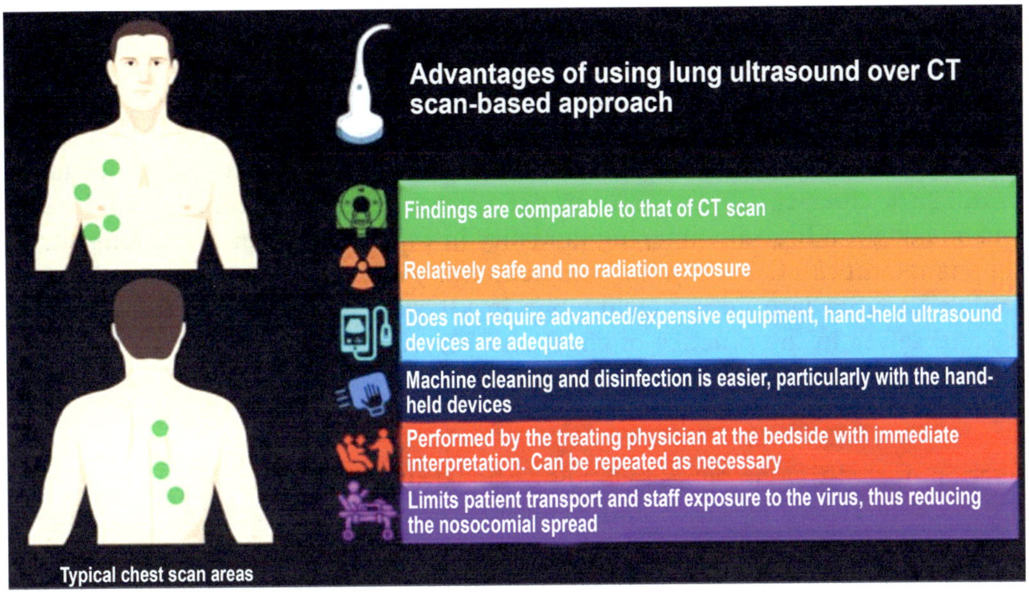

Figure 5.13. Advantages of ultrasound in chest imaging.

Source: Reisinger, N., Koratala, A. Lung ultrasound: a valuable tool for the assessment of dialysis patients with COVID-19. Clin Exp Nephrol 24, 850–852 (2020). https://doi.org/10.1007/s10157-020-01903-x

5.4.1. Non-Invasiveness and Safety

The non-invasive nature of chest and pleura ultrasound (CPU) is an important advantage of its growing use in clinical practice. In contrast to traditional imaging techniques, for example, computed tomography (CT) or magnetic resonance imaging (MRI), the application of ultrasound does not subject patients to ionizing radiation or pose a risk of complications secondary to invasive procedures. This capability is particularly helpful when monitoring conditions like spontaneous pneumothorax, where serial imaging may be needed to assess lung re-expansion and pleural integrity. Additionally, bedside ultrasound capacity can accelerate diagnosis and treatment, which will once more enhance patient safety and comfort (Roberts et al., 2023). Thus, the non-invasive nature of ultrasound not only accords with the patient-centered care philosophy but also addresses the extremely relevant questions about long-term health risks from other diagnostic modalities. Safety in medical procedures is of critical concern, particularly in sensitive areas such as the chest and pleura. Ultrasound techniques have been well established through scientific studies, hence making them safe for patients with an extensive range of clinical diseases. Recent developments within the field are that the integration of lung ultrasound will be able to assist clinicians in the early detection of those conditions needing urgent management, reducing the need for more invasive diagnostic techniques

(Demi et al., 2022). Ultrasound's use in accurately measuring pleural effusion and pneumothorax and its real-time imaging feature encourages timely decision-making, critical in emergency cases. This extra safety profile, combined with focus on non-invasive methods, emphasizes the role of ultrasound in modern diagnostic practice and results in an overall reduction in procedural risk and patient anxiety related to testing. The technological advances for ultrasound have supported its utility in thoracic disease diagnosis without affecting patient safety. The current agreement among international experts has introduced improved methods of employing lung ultrasound, focusing on technical developments ensuring high-quality images while maintaining non-invasive priorities (Demi et al., 2022). Clinicians become more proficient in the use of ultrasound techniques and are able to diagnose pathology more efficiently with minimal or no interference with the patient, facilitating a more reassuring examination procedure. Furthermore, this safety-focused approach helps to establish a clear-cut distinction between ultrasound and more invasive techniques of imaging, thus making it a first-line imaging modality in the diagnosis of conditions such as pleural effusion and pneumothorax. Generally, the complementary effect between the non-invasive methods and continuous research into newer technology in ultrasound helps enhance the overall rise in patient care and safety in the practice of chest and pleura ultrasound.

5.4.2. Real-Time Imaging Capabilities

The introduction of real-time imaging technology has dramatically altered the diagnostic imaging landscape, especially regarding chest and pleural ultrasound. Conventional imaging techniques frequently necessitate long procedures and can require patient sedation, particularly in children. Real-time magnetic resonance imaging (rtMRI) appears as a worthwhile substitute, allowing for immediate, sedation-free evaluation of thoracic anatomy. With the ability to capture up to 50 images every second, rtMRI significantly lowers motion artifacts associated with respiration or patient movement. This new capability is critical in order to accurately see diseases such as pneumonia or chest wall malignancies, allowing clinicians to make prompt, informed decisions regarding patient treatment. Furthermore, the efficiency and speed of rtMRI enable quick triage, thereby ensuring timely intervention in emergency situations, thus underscoring its status as a future-looking instrument in the imaging of pediatric thorax (Hirsch et al., 2025). Aside from rtMRI, the development in ultrasound technology has made it possible to achieve significant leaps in real-time imaging for lung evaluations. With techniques such as directed intercostal scanning, lung ultrasound allows doctors to scan over the intercostal spaces with precision, thereby eliminating the interference caused by rib shadowing. This technique plays a vital role in obtaining optimal image quality with the least diagnostic error in the context of lung pathology. Also, automation of scanning procedures through robotic ultrasound systems has been promising in enhancing diagnostic accuracy. With the use of high-level path planning algorithms and adjustable probe placement, these systems provide high-quality images with optimal positioning against the pleural line. Implementation of such robot-based solutions in clinical environments is a step forward in guaranteeing consistent and efficient lung disease evaluations, emphasizing the critical role that real-time imaging technology plays in contemporary medicine (Lei et al., 2025). As the health care industry continues to embrace technological advancements, the implications of real-time imaging capacity extend beyond individual modalities. Intermodality interactions provide a scenario for enhanced diagnostic certainty and patient safety. With the combined strength of rtMRI and lung ultrasound capacities, health care professionals can better assess a range of thoracic afflictions, from pleural effusion to congenital malformations, with a greater overall patient experience. The creation of these imaging modalities is a sign of a paradigm shift toward greater patient-centered care and the necessity to decrease distress in relation to diagnostic procedures. While development and research keep extending, a bright future is also in sight for real-time imaging as a standard practice in chest and pleura ultrasound, in which diagnoses are readily made and reliable with utmost precision and timeliness (Hirsch et al., 2025; Lei et al., 2025) (Figure 5.14).

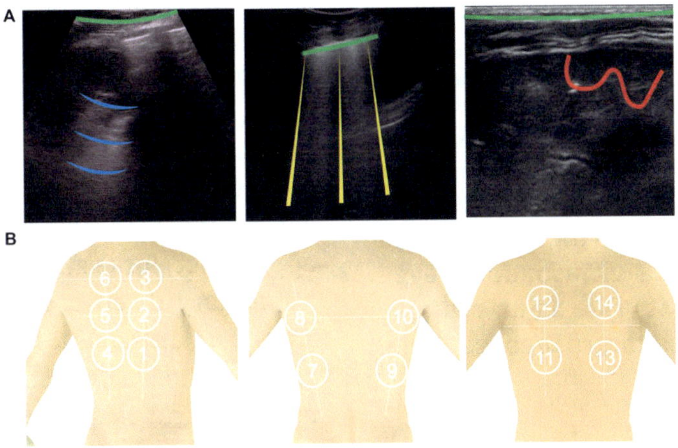

Figure 5.14. Real-time imaging capabilities of ultrasound in chest imaging.

Source: McDermott C, Łącki M, Sainsbury B, Henry J, Filippov M and Rossa C (2021) Sonographic Diagnosis of COVID-19: A Review of Image Processing for Lung Ultrasound. Front. Big Data 4:612561. doi: 10.3389/fdata.2021.612561 -

5.4.3. Cost-Effectiveness Compared to Other Modalities

CPU has been revealed as a cost-effective modality, particularly when compared to other traditional imaging modalities such as computed tomography (CT) and chest X-rays. CPU offers a less invasive approach with fewer accompanying costs, such as lower radiation exposure costs and contrast media costs. In addition, the portability of ultrasound machines permits bedside use, which can simplify patient management and waiting times dramatically. Such immediacy is particularly important in emergency situations where timely diagnosis can actually affect the outcome for the patient. The financial benefits of CPU include not only the prevention of more expensive imaging techniques but also the reduction of hospital stays and other follow-up treatments, hence representing a budget-friendly choice within limited healthcare budgets. In addition, the increased use of thoracic ultrasound in clinical practice is facilitated by evidence demonstrating its effective use in various medical conditions. Clinical experience has demonstrated that CPU can diagnose pneumothorax, pleural effusions, and consolidations of the lung with good efficacy, leading to higher diagnostic yield. With this, ultrasound application may permit timely, appropriate intervention, enhancing real-time clinical decision-making. The European Respiratory Society's evidence supports the increasing recognition of thoracic ultrasound as an important tool for pulmonologists. These developments not only signify an improvement in the quality of patient care but also have economic benefits by reducing unnecessary investigations and treatments. Lastly, with the accumulation of more evidence backing the efficacy of ultrasounds, it reaffirms its position as an economical alternative for more invasive forms of diagnostic procedures (Laursen et al., 2020). Also, continuous updating of consensus statements for lung ultrasound itself indicates evolving appreciation of its potential and applications.

Expert panels today have written guidelines favoring technical and clinical innovation that are harmonizable with the standardization of ultrasound use in varied medical environments. CPU is not only cost-effective but also reusable as equipment durability outlives single-use or low-use alternatives. Accordingly, the overall cost of care can be reduced without compromising the quality of diagnosis. These technologies, when adopted in clinical practice, not only improve patient management but also improve better utilization of healthcare resources. Keeping these advancements in mind, the argument in favor of chest and pleura ultrasound is even stronger, substantiating its role as an example of economically sound healthcare practice (Demi et al., 2022).

5.5. Limitations of Chest and Pleura Ultrasound

Even with the development of chest and pleura ultrasound technology, there are some drawbacks that limit its use as an independent diagnostic tool. One of the main disadvantages is the technician dependency of ultrasound, which may result in variations in readings depending on the skill and experience of the technician. Variable outcomes may be encountered when various practitioners utilize their skills in different clinical scenarios, risking misdiagnosis. Additionally, factors such as patient anatomy, for example, obesity or the amount of excess thoracic gas, can hide ultrasound visualization, reducing the diagnostic capability. In addition, certain pathologies have similar ultrasound appearances, which are challenging to make proper diagnoses from and require more reliance on ancillary imaging modalities, for instance, chest X-ray or CT scans, to confirm diagnoses. These observations emphasize the requirement for adherence to standardized protocols when accepting possible interpretive variations in routine clinical practice (Mojoli et al., 2018). Another significant limitation of chest and pleura ultrasound relates to its inability to replace exhaustive diagnostic workup in certain acute medical conditions. While ultrasound may identify pleural effusions, consolidations, and pneumothorax, it may not be sensitive enough to identify early or subtle pathology. The diagnostic specificity of the ultrasound can be greatly compromised when evaluating conditions that have no unique sonographic appearance, for example, malignancies or diffuse pulmonary disease. Additionally, the temporal aspect of ultrasound imaging can be limiting, as it provides a snapshot at an instant moment of lung status instead of real-time examination, possibly resulting in lags in clinical thinking. For example, the absence of specific ultrasound findings is not conclusive to exclude pulmonary embolism conditions. Clinicians should therefore exercise caution in using ultrasound in acute settings and add it to a holistic diagnostic strategy as part of incorporating other imaging techniques and clinical assessment (Diaz-Gomez et al., 2018).

Lastly, there are practical obstacles encountered in practice while using chest and pleura ultrasound in different clinical contexts that must be overcome. Restrictions of mass application can be brought about by the availability of advanced ultrasound equipment and the need for expert training. Health facilities, in some cases, may have to resort to conventional imaging methods, occasioning a delay in diagnosis and treatment. Also, while the ultrasound enjoys the portability benefit of having immediate results, its effectiveness is thwarted where it is challenging to achieve optimal imaging conditions, such as in surgical procedures. Surgical drapes or confined windows of access restrict extensive probing, leading to incomplete assessment. With increasing use of ultrasound in clinical practice, these limitations should be kept in mind to prevent misinterpretation of data in different patient populations (Mojoli et al., 2018).

5.5.1. Operator Dependency and Skill Levels

The effectiveness of lung ultrasound (LUS) as a diagnostic tool is significantly influenced by operator dependency and skill levels. The proficiency of the operator plays a critical role in the accurate interpretation of ultrasound images, as novice practitioners may struggle to recognize essential artifacts or patterns indicative of pathological conditions. This reliance on human expertise underscores the necessity for standardized training modules that can develop consistent competencies across practitioners. Moreover, variations in skill levels may lead to discrepancies in diagnostic accuracy, potentially impacting treatment decisions. Enhanced operator training can mitigate these challenges, ensuring that healthcare providers are equipped with the requisite knowledge to utilize LUS effectively, particularly in complex cases such as neonatal respiratory distress syndrome (RDS) (Costa et al., 2024). The integration of simulation technology in medical education has emerged as a promising solution to address operator dependency in LUS. Utilizing advanced medical simulations, healthcare professionals can develop and refine their ultrasound skills in a risk-free environment. During situations like the COVID-19 pandemic, such simulations have provided invaluable training opportunities without endangering patient or practitioner safety. Simulators not only allow for repetitive practice but also create scenarios that exhibit key diagnostic artifacts, aiding in the recognition of lung conditions. As operators gain confidence and competency through simulated experiences, the variability linked to individual skill levels may be reduced, fostering a higher standard of care in ultrasound diagnostics (Szostek et al., 2023). Despite the benefits of improved training and simulation, the successful implementation of LUS in clinical practice faces specific challenges unique to diverse healthcare settings. Access to high-quality training resources can be limited, particularly in resource-limited environments. Hence, addressing these disparities in training availability is crucial for broadening the accessibility of lung ultrasound. Initiatives aimed at standardizing training protocols and developing comprehensive guidelines for LUS can further enhance its utility across varying skill levels. As ultrasound technology continues to evolve, fostering collaboration among healthcare educators, practitioners, and technology developers will be essential in promoting operator competency and maximizing the diagnostic potential of LUS in managing conditions like neonatal RDS (Costa et al., 2024; Szostek et al., 2023) (Figure 5.15).

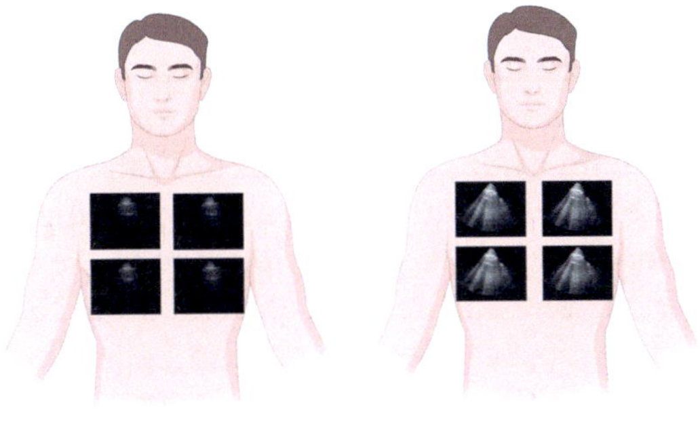

Figure 5.15. Operator dependency and skill levels of chest and pleura ultrasound.

Source: Vetrugno, L., Biasucci, D.G., Deana, C. et al (2024). Lung ultrasound and supine chest X-ray use in modern adult intensive care: mapping 30 years of advancement (1993–2023). Ultrasound J 16, 7. https://doi.org/10.1186/s13089-023-00351-4.

5.5.2. Limited Visualization of Deep Structures

The application of chest and pleura ultrasound (US) has evolved significantly over the past few years, providing useful information regarding several pulmonary diseases. Despite one of the major limitations, however, one of the main issues remains: the limited visibility of deep structures within the thorax. This is usually due to the intrinsic behavior of ultrasound waves, with these waves not being able to penetrate through multiple layers of tissue or air spaces, resulting in poor imaging of deeper anatomical structures. For effective diagnosis and assessment, practitioners depend heavily on the image quality obtained during examination. As such, the majority of pathologies located in deeper regions could remain undetected, pointing to a need for sophisticated imaging techniques. This shortcoming underscores the importance of ongoing research aimed at developing better ultrasound technologies and applications in the clinical environment, especially the diagnosis of conditions such as pneumonia or pleural effusions, which may not be visualized well using conventional ultrasound techniques. In the past 10 years, there have been considerable developments in lung ultrasound (LUS) that can potentially remedy some of the limitations of limited visualization. A global group of multidisciplinary LUS experts has revisited and revised previous guidelines, and this represented an organized effort to maximize the effectiveness of ultrasounds in practice (Demi et al., 2022). The new statements are intended to maximize technical imaging parameters along with clinical and educational guidelines that illuminate practitioners about best practices. Nevertheless, even with such advancements, challenges persist in visualizing deep structures. One fascinating avenue of investigation is applying deep learning (DL) techniques to image interpretation of LUS. The new techniques are intended to better interpret images and can lead to improved diagnostic performance, although early on, they were reported to be plagued with some of the same drawbacks as conventional ultrasound imaging. Integration of deep learning approaches into interpreting LUS images offers a radical solution to the challenge of inadequate visualization of deep structures. Recent studies have established the efficacy of DL-based systems to identify and quantify various lung diseases even from images that cannot be adequately acquired by conventional ultrasound (Roy et al., 2020). Based on large annotated databases, the algorithms can identify patterns not apparent to humans, thus providing a greater insight into underlying pathologies. Furthermore, the new algorithms can also localize pathological artifacts and give frames severity scores, which will allow for extensive analysis of conditions that are not easily visualized. Ongoing research, combining enhanced ultrasound techniques with advanced computational techniques, can provide an even more powerful diagnostic tool, allowing for the chest and pleura ultrasound to become an even more versatile tool in pulmonary medicine.

5.5.3. Challenges in Obese Patients

The challenges that one faces in the case of obese patients when it comes to chest and pleura ultrasound are many and significant. A key impediment is the increased difficulty of obtaining adequate ultrasound images. Obesity generally results in a thicker covering of adipose tissue that may impair the transmission of sound waves, resulting in poor imaging quality. Displacement of anatomical structures by redundant body tissue complicates the identification of important landmarks for further effective evaluation. As a result, healthcare providers can be hindered in their capacity to make effective evaluations, and diagnosis may be delayed with resultant effect on patient care. Also, the inherent challenges with ultrasound technology necessitate closer examination of techniques and protocols to ensure efficient application in this patient population, making ongoing education and training of clinicians within this evolving field of medical imaging increasingly important. In addition to imaging issues, the management of obese patients also has particular clinical considerations in the application of chest and pleural ultrasound.

Positioning these patients during the procedure may prove difficult, with the standard methods maybe being unsuitable or unsafe in those with higher body mass index (BMI). This can lead to longer examination times, reduced overall patient comfort, and increased rates of procedural complications. Moreover, interpretation of the sonograms for obese patients can be inclusive of adjusting normal reference ranges or special sonographer training so that misreading of the data being collected is minimized. All these issues highlight the necessity for special guidelines and adaptation of current protocols to suit this category efficiently without compromising the quality of care that addresses the specific needs of obese patients. The evolving scenario of lung ultrasound (LUS) has been under the limelight, particularly in light of the ongoing challenges in managing obesity patients.

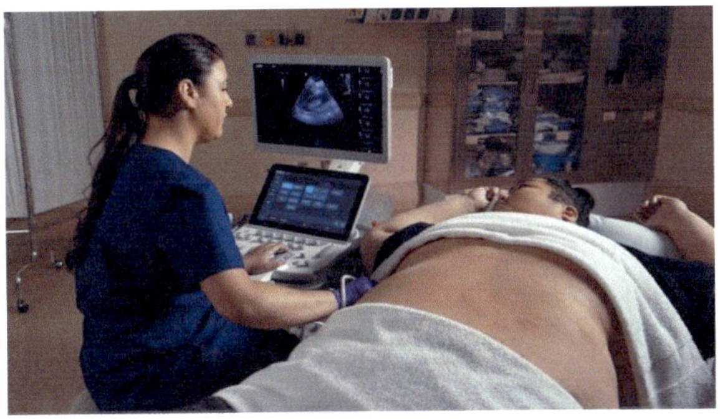

Figure 5.16. Challenges in imaging obese patients.

Source: Biswas S. (2023). Challenges in imaging the obese patients. Series Clin Med Case Rep Rev; 1(1):6-12. DOI: 10.54178/2993-3579.v1i1a1994

The developments showcased and the development of international consensus statements by a multidisciplinary panel are indicative of the desire to optimize procedures for point-of-care LUS in diverse clinical environments. The statements, having both technical and clinical recommendations, give high priority to the need for individualized processes during ultrasound examinations among obese patients. As per the recent reports, understanding where and how to utilize LUS for optimal results can make a big difference in the outcomes, especially when dealing with conditions that disproportionately affect this population. This focus on maximizing LUS effectiveness not only serves to increase the quality of patient care but also promotes interdisciplinarity among healthcare professionals looking to overcome obesity-related challenges in clinical practice (Demi et al., 2022; Gargani et al., 2020) (Figure 5.16).

5.6. Future Directions in Ultrasound Technology

The future of ultrasonic technology, especially chest and pleura ultrasound, is full of promise for developments that will increase diagnostic yields and improve patient outcomes. Most important to development may be the marriage of artificial intelligence (AI) and machine learning algorithms. These tools can accelerate image interpretation, enabling real-time analysis and automated detection of such conditions as pneumonia and pleural effusions. As described in recent research, the reliability of ultrasound technology integrated with AI capabilities has the potential to enable early detection of community-acquired pneumonia because of its high mortality rate in high-risk groups such as infants and elderly patients (Kanwal et al., 2024). This convergence of AI and ultrasound has the potential to transform point-of-care diagnosis into rapid, non-invasive solutions that have the potential to significantly improve clinical workflows and patient care. Advances in small-footprint ultrasound equipment also hold the promise of a new frontier for ultrasound technology in thoracic exams. With the advent of handheld, battery-powered ultrasound systems, clinicians can perform examinations across multiple sites, ranging from remote and emergency care settings. The increased availability of the equipment makes it possible to conduct timely examination of the pleura and the lungs by medical practitioners, making them more effective at making rapid and accurate diagnoses. For instance, the mobility of ultrasound equipment can make it possible to conduct instantaneous tests of patients with respiratory distress, thereby identifying critical issues such as pneumothorax or pleural effusions. Thanks to these new technologies, physicians are able to provide immediate interventions, which is particularly important in emergency conditions where immediate decision-making can be the key to saving lives. Therefore, a rise in ingenuity in portable ultrasound machines is a breakthrough of traditional barriers to easy diagnostics.

Another path that is promising much in chest and pleura ultrasound technology is the combination of ultrasound with robotic platforms. As more minimally invasive surgeries become commonplace, the marriage of ultrasound and robotically assisted surgery might hold its full share of benefits in terms of accuracy and safety to patients. For example, the use of ultrasound guidance for robotic thoracic procedures can help localize tumors or pleural diseases with greater accuracy, thereby enhancing surgical outcomes. The provided evidence suggests the incorporation of loco-regional anesthesia techniques into robotic interventions to optimize pain management during the recovery process, which is paramount for post-operative recovery (La Via et al., 2024). Streamlining these robotic devices through enhancing their ability to integrate ultrasound imaging should be the area of future development. This hybrid strategy not only emphasizes heightened procedural efficiency but also places ultrasound technology at the forefront of advancing surgical practices in thoracic medicine (Figure 5.17).

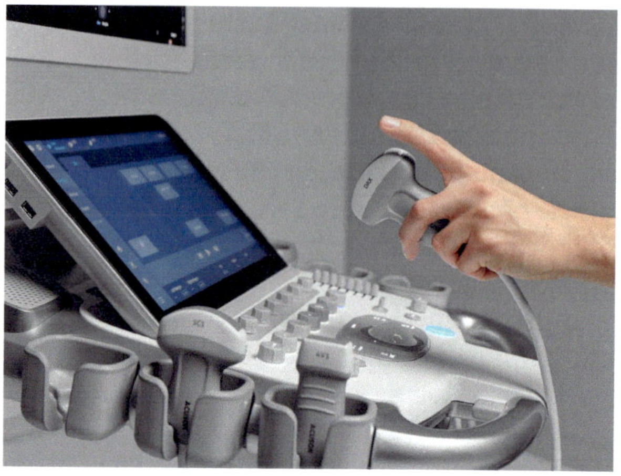

Figure 5.17. Future directions in ultrasound technology of the chest and pleura.

Source: https://avatars.mds.yandex.net/get-altay/4042551/2a0000017aea006093b624fb17b437066f1b/XXXL

5.6.1. Advancements in Imaging Techniques

The introduction of advanced imaging modalities has changed the face of diagnostic medicine and, more specifically, in the case of chest and pleural ultrasound. Advanced technology, apart from enhancing the resolution of images, has made these modalities simpler and easier to use. For example, ultrasound machines are now portable, and this enables doctors to perform point-of-care studies as easily as never before. This shift to real-time imaging capabilities allows clinicians to make prompt and informed decisions, particularly under urgent circumstances. In addition, advances in ultrasonic technology, exemplified by the progression in transducers and sophisticated signal processing, have greatly improved chest imaging quality and dependability. The expansion of these modalities underscores their significance in managing pleural disorders, an aspect increasingly being identified as at the heart of respiratory medicine (Astoul et al., 2016).

In addition to this, advances in ultrasound technology have made a broader range of interventional procedures available for pulmonologists. Technological innovations such as medical thoracoscopy and image-guided closed pleural biopsies have revolutionized the management of pleural diseases to allow for minimally invasive yet highly effective treatments. Practice with indwelling pleural catheters is merely one illustration of how advances in imaging not only facilitate diagnosis but also improve the therapeutic possibilities for patients with advanced pleural disease. Ultrasonography lies at the heart of real-time visual guidance during procedures, minimizing complications and maximizing patient outcomes. As clinical understanding of pleural disease increases, use of these new imaging modalities has become imperative, a reflection of ongoing progress within the specialty (Astoul et al., 2016).

Furthermore, ongoing developments in ultrasonic imaging fuel increased developments and applications in pleural diagnostics. Scientists are continually looking for new ways and technologies, particularly towards the goal of increasing diagnostic accuracy and extending the scope of ultrasound in the clinic. Advances in electronics, computers, and algorithms are all enabling ultrasound to be a front-line diagnostic tool in its own right. Techniques such as chemical pleurodesis and thoracentesis are also developing in tandem with these technologies, supported by increasingly more robust clinical evidence of effectiveness. The convergence of technological progress and heightened awareness of pleural disease highlights a profound transformation in the geography of respiratory medicine. As pleural medicine continues to develop, the future holds tremendous potential for further integrating innovation in imaging to maximize patient management and outcomes.

5.6.2. Integration with Artificial Intelligence

The integration of Artificial Intelligence (AI) in chest and pleura ultrasound represents a significant advancement in the diagnostic capabilities of medical practitioners. With the advent of point-of-care ultrasound (PoCUS), emergency medicine has embraced AI as an auxiliary tool, enhancing the precision of ultrasound applications in critical care settings. AI algorithms can streamline image acquisition and interpretation, effectively assisting clinicians during time-sensitive emergencies. By employing machine learning techniques, these systems can analyze ultrasound images in real time, identifying relevant anatomical structures and pathologies with greater accuracy than traditional methods. As AI continues to evolve, its capacity to support clinical decision-making processes ensures that physicians can deliver timely diagnoses, consequently improving patient outcomes in an ever-complex medical landscape (Österwalder &Hoffmann, 2023). Furthermore, AI's role extends into the realm of lung cancer screening, where early detection is crucial for successful intervention. Advanced AI systems facilitate risk stratification by analyzing extensive imaging data, enabling healthcare professionals to identify high-risk patients who require further investigation. In chest ultrasound, AI can aid in the early detection of abnormalities associated with lung cancer, thus improving the chances of initiating effective treatment strategies at earlier disease stages. Through intelligent algorithms, ultrasound images can be assessed for potential malignancies, acting as a second reader that enhances diagnostic accuracy and reduces interpretation time. By incorporating these AI-driven methodologies, healthcare providers can standardize screening programs, ultimately leading to better management of patients at risk for lung cancer and ensuring timely access to care (Cellina et al., 2023). Moreover, the future trajectory of AI in chest and pleura ultrasound is characterized by ongoing innovation. The integration of AI technologies into ultrasound practices aligns with the necessity for continuous adaptation in medical care, particularly amidst rapidly changing technological environments. Innovations such as cloud-based solutions, augmented reality applications, and interoperable systems promise to expand the operational capabilities of ultrasound in both acute and outpatient settings. As clinicians learn to navigate these advanced tools, they can enhance their diagnostic practice by merging traditional clinical skills with cutting-edge technology. The synergy between AI and ultrasound not only augments the clinician's ability to deliver accurate diagnoses but also fosters an environment where patient care becomes more efficient and personalized. As this integration progresses, it holds the potential to redefine standard practices in lung assessment and management (Österwalder & Hoffmann, 2023) (Figure 5.18).

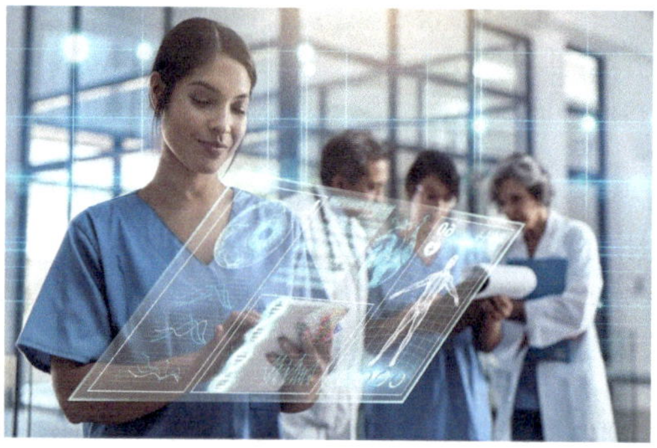

Figure 5.18. The integration of artificial intelligence (AI) in chest and pleura ultrasound.

Source: https://graphlogic.ai/wp-content/uploads/2025/06/737.jpg

5.6.3. Potential for Enhanced Diagnostic Accuracy

The integration of chest and pleura ultrasound into practice has shown an unprecedented potential for enhanced diagnostic accuracy, with a major impact on respiratory care. Compared to the traditional imaging technologies, ultrasound is a dynamic, real-time assessment modality that enables immediate decision-making. It has been shown in studies that point-of-care ultrasound enables clinicians to detect pleural abnormalities and lung pathologies with high sensitivity and specificity, which is particularly important in cases such as acute respiratory failure or dyspnea. The key diagnostic characteristic not only facilitates the detection of the occurrence of conditions such as pleural effusions but also allows for the assessment of associated complications. Therefore, the real-time nature of ultrasound enhances the diagnostic precision, leading to faster treatments and better patient outcomes, demonstrating how imaging technological advancements can benefit clinical practice and patient management maximally (Hew et al., 2016).

Besides, enhanced diagnostic accuracy also has a significant impact on decision-making efficacy within the clinical setting, making ultrasound a valuable tool in the provision of therapeutic intervention guidance. For instance, there is evidence to show that ultrasound can precisely direct pleural interventions such as thoracentesis or chest tube placement by locating fluid accumulation in the exact position and assessing its nature. This application minimizes procedural complications and maximizes therapeutic gain for patients. Further, while ultrasound facilitates quick diagnosis and decision-making, the clinician's role remains the most critical; clinicians must integrate ultrasound imaging into clinical wisdom to manage challenging cases successfully. The combination of enhanced diagnostic accuracy with informed decision-making increases the position of ultrasound to not just complement clinical practice but also maximize respiratory medicine outcomes (Adler et al., 2015). With further research on the entire potential of ultrasound capabilities, there is a possibility of validating its merit in quantifying beyond simple diagnostic accuracy measures. This innovation requires careful studies to find out the health outcomes of point-of-care ultrasound, particularly among diverse patient populations. Through capturing improvements in results due to timely and effective diagnoses made by ultrasound, the medical community can make an effective case for its application in respiratory care on a regular basis. Lastly, this validation will not only enhance clinical practice but also direct larger maternal and public health interventions. The demand for exploring the complicated dynamic between diagnosis and actual health outcomes can pave the way to the development of ultrasound as a cornerstone in respiratory diagnostics (Hew et al., 2016).

SUMMARY

In summarizing findings on chest and pleura ultrasound, it can be seen that the diagnostic modality is of high advantage in various clinical contexts, particularly in respiratory emergencies such as COVID-19. The rapid growth in ultrasound technology has made it possible to get better imaging capability that compares to traditional methods like computed tomography (CT). Experiments have demonstrated that lung ultrasound (LUS) may detect certain sonographic patterns typical of lung injury typical of SARS-CoV-2 pneumonia, such as multifocal confluent B-lines and irregular pleural markings. The findings indicate that LUS is not onlyas sensitive and specific as CT but also provides timely examination of patients' conditions in an out-of-hospital setting, which practically enhances patient treatment during acute respiratory attacks (Lakhin et al., 2021). Moreover, the utilization of lung ultrasound extends beyond diagnostic purposes. Given the established drawbacks related to imaging methods that are capital-intensive and potentially incorporating cross-contamination risks, LUS provides a safer alternative for patients as well as healthcare workers. In recent research, the adoption of portable ultrasound devices has been found to be of significant value in limiting the time spent in isolation rooms and thereby decreasing viral transmission risk. This access is a significant factor in facilitating greater utilization of ultrasound as a first-line diagnostic modality for the evaluation of pulmonary conditions. As testified, the high sensitivity and specificity of LUS for SARS-CoV-2 pneumonia diagnosis confirm its role as a principal component of contemporary clinical practice (Jalil et al., 2020). In conclusion, the integration of chest and pleura ultrasound into routine clinical evaluation is a paradigm shift in respiratory disease management practice. The integration of ultrasound findings with traditional imaging modalities, along with the advantages of logistics, positions LUS as a valuable tool in critical care settings. With studies continually progressing and confirming the effectiveness of ultrasound in detecting and monitoring pulmonary pathologies, healthcare workers now have no choice but to embrace this technology. On a long-term basis, the commitment to using advanced ultrasound techniques will not only expand the accuracy of diagnoses but also improve the overall outcome of patient care in respiratory health management in general, especially in the event of continued existing challenges such as the COVID-19 pandemic (Lakhin et al., 2021).

In pleura and chest ultrasound, understanding the significance of this imaging technique is key to providing proper clinical assessment and management. The fact that the technique is non-invasive offers real-time imagery of thoracic organs, with early detection of many pulmonary pathologies, including pneumothorax and pleural effusion. One of the highlights is that ultrasound can be an excellent first line of imaging diagnosis since it is portable and accessible and can provide immediate results at the bedside. As noted in the literature, spontaneous pneumothorax can be effectively managed with ultrasound-guided interventions, which are very accurate for the detection of air leaks and for guiding drainage (Roberts et al., 2023). Thus, inclusion of ultrasound in routine examinations enhances clinical practice and results in expedited therapeutic decisions. The role of ultrasound in thoracic examination extends its usefulness beyond diagnosis to the guidance of treatment procedures. It is a valuable adjunct, for instance, in chest tube placement, which is of direct importance in treating complications like pleural effusion and hemothorax. As clinicians progress towards improving their proficiency in this area, it is crucial to appreciate that the validity of ultrasound findings largely depends on the operator's familiarity and experience with thoracic anatomy. Additionally, teaching initiatives to enhance proficiency in ultrasound procedures can have a dramatic influence on patient care. This would bring dividends in the form of faster response times and fewer complications due to invasive processes, going with current advice for the management of spontaneous pneumothorax and other respiratory illnesses (Roberts et al., 2023). Developing the practice of radiology through improved technology in the form of artificial intelligence is another developing topic in the context of chest and pleura ultrasound. Current studies have shown that technology like ChatGPT has the capacity to enhance the delivery of complicated medical outcomes by translating elaborate radiology reports into more palatable formats for patients and clinicians alike. Such a change does not just make radiology results less enigmatic, but it also promotes informed patient participation in their own medical care. Furthermore, such technology can aid clinicians by providing them with brief prompts derived from ultrasound reports, thereby streamlining clinical decision-making protocols. In all, the integration of ultrasound and artificial intelligence promises greatly to improve the quality of care delivered in the evaluation of chest and pleura, once again highlighting the importance of continued research and education in this evolving field.

CLOSER LOOK

TRANSBRONCHIAL CRYOBIOPSY (TBCB)

Transbronchial cryobiopsy (TBCB) is an advanced bronchoscopic technique that collects larger and better-preserved lung tissue samples from peripheral airways and lung parenchyma, primarily for the diagnosis of interstitial lung diseases (ILDs) and diffuse parenchymal lung disease. TBCB is a less invasive method than surgical lung biopsy (SLB) with optimal diagnostic yield and procedural risk. The procedure involves the use of a cryoprobe that is flexible and is placed through a bronchoscope within the location to be treated in the lung, guided either by fluoroscopy or by radial endobronchial ultrasound (r-EBUS). The cryoprobe is subsequently activated (most commonly with liquid carbon dioxide or nitrous oxide), which, in seconds, cools at the tip to approximately −80°C. This results in freezing of the adjacent lung tissue, which adheres to the probe and is excised en bloc on removal, leaving a relatively large and intact tissue specimen with little crush artifact—a definite improvement over forceps biopsies.

The primary clinical application of TBCB lies in the diagnosis of ILDs, especially when high-resolution computed tomography (HRCT) findings are indeterminate. Histological patterns such as usual interstitial pneumonia (UIP), nonspecific interstitial pneumonia (NSIP), and organizing pneumonia (OP) can be more accurately identified with cryobiopsies than with standard transbronchial forceps biopsies, which often produce small and fragmented samples. Compared to SLB, TBCB is a less invasive method of obtaining diagnostically sufficient tissue, therefore reducing the need for general anesthesia, in-patient admission, and associated morbidity. While not completely risk-free, the rate of complications with TBCB is generally acceptable in skilled centers. The most common side effects are pneumothorax (10–20% incidence) and moderate bleeding. For avoidance of these risks, balloon occlusion catheters (such as Fogarty balloons) are usually used to control hemorrhage during the procedure of biopsy removal, and fluoroscopic guidance is utilized to insert the probe carefully away from the pleura and great vessels.

TBCB should be done cautiously in carefully chosen patients and withheld in patients with severe hypoxemia, bleeding diathesis, pulmonary hypertension, or impaired lung function. The optimal results are achieved when performed within a multidisciplinary diagnostic algorithm by pulmonologists, pathologists, and radiologists correlating imaging, histology, and clinical presentation. Recent data suggest that if it is properly performed, TBCB can have diagnostic yields as high as SLB, 70% to 85%, and minimal complications. The technique is currently included in numerous international guidelines as an indicated diagnostic test for assessment of ILD when HRCT and clinical findings are indeterminate.

For all that it has to offer, standardization of technique remains problematic with variations in biopsy size, freezing time, sample number, and location between centers. Attempts go on to characterize procedural protocols, assess long-term outcomes, and determine the utility of cryobiopsy for the diagnosis of lung cancers, rejection in transplant patients, and granulomatous disease. As procedural wisdom spreads and technology advances, TBCB will be a staple of pulmonary diagnosis, offering clinicians a high-yield, relatively safe, and cost-effective way in which to find their way through diffuse lung disease's subtleties.

References

1. Abo, A., Abramowicz, J., Bigelow, T., Bigelow, E., et al. (2019). Diagnostic ultrasound safety review for point-of-care ultrasound practitioners. https://core.ac.uk/download/286268919.pdf (accessed on 12th July 2025).
2. Adler, Y., Charron, P., Imazio, M., Badano, L. P., Barón-Esquivias, G., Bogaert, J., Brucato, A., et al. (2015). 2015 ESC Guidelines for the diagnosis and management of pericardial diseases. *European Heart Journal, 36*, 2921–2964. https://doi.org/10.1093/eurheartj/ehv318 (accessed on 12th July 2025).
3. Allinovi, M., Parise, A., Giacalone, M., Amerio, A., Delsante, M., Odone, A., Franci, A., et al. (2020). Lung ultrasound may support the diagnosis and monitoring of COVID-19 pneumonia. *Ultrasound in Medicine & Biology, 46*, 2908–2917. https://doi.org/10.1016/j.ultrasmedbio.2020.07.018 (accessed on 12th July 2025).
4. Astoul, P., Bhatnagar, R., Corcoran, J. P., Feller-Kopman, D., et al. (2016). Advanced medical interventions in pleural disease. https://core.ac.uk/download/73983410.pdf (accessed on 12th July 2025).
5. Biggins, S. W., Angeli, P., García-Tsao, G., Ginès, P., Ling, S. C., Nadim, M. K., Wong, F., et al. (2021). Diagnosis, evaluation, and management of ascites, spontaneous bacterial peritonitis, and hepatorenal syndrome: 2021 Practice guidance by the American Association for the Study of Liver Diseases. *Hepatology, 74*, 1014–1048. https://doi.org/10.1002/hep.31884 (accessed on 12th July 2025).
6. Bodenham, A., Babu, S., Bennett, J., Binks, R., Fee, P. A., Fox, B., Johnston, A. J., et al. (2016). Association of Anesthetists of Great Britain and Ireland: Safe vascular access 2016. *Anesthesia, 71*, 573–585. https://doi.org/10.1111/anae.13360 (accessed on 12th July 2025).
7. Cellina, M., Cacioppa, L. M., Cè, M., Chiarpenello, V., Costa, M., Vincenzo, Z., Pais, D., et al. (2023). Artificial intelligence in lung cancer screening: The future is now. *Cancers, 15*, 4344–4344. https://doi.org/10.3390/cancers15174344 (accessed on 12th July 2025).
8. Costa, F., Titolo, A., Ferrocino, M., Biagi, E., Dell'Orto, V., Perrone, S., & Esposito, S. (2024). Lung ultrasound in neonatal respiratory distress syndrome: A narrative review of the last 10 years. *Diagnostics, 14*, 2793–2793. https://doi.org/10.3390/diagnostics14242793 (accessed on 12th July 2025).
9. Demi, L., Wolfram, F., Klersy, C., De Silvestri, A., Ferretti, V. V., Müller, M., Miller, D. L., et al. (2022). New international guidelines and consensus on the use of lung ultrasound. *Journal of Ultrasound in Medicine, 42*, 309–344. https://doi.org/10.1002/jum.16088 (accessed on 12th July 2025).
10. Díaz-Gómez, J. L., Renew, J. R., Ratzlaff, R. A., Ramakrishna, H., Via, G., & Torp, K. D. (2017). Can lung ultrasound be the first-line tool for evaluation of intraoperative hypoxemia? *Anesthesia & Analgesia, 126*, 1769–1773. https://doi.org/10.1213/ane.0000000000002578 (accessed on 12th July 2025).
11. Ganti, A. K., Loo, B. W., Bassetti, M., Blakely, C. M., Chiang, A. C., D'Amico, T. A., D'Avella, C., et al. (2021). Small cell lung cancer, Version 2.2022, NCCN clinical practice guidelines in oncology. *Journal of the National Comprehensive Cancer Network, 19*, 1441–1464. https://doi.org/10.6004/jnccn.2021.0058 (accessed on 12th July 2025).

12. Gargani, L., Soliman-Aboumarie, H., Volpicelli, G., Corradi, F., Pastore, M. C., & Cameli, M. (2020). Why, when, and how to use lung ultrasound during the COVID-19 pandemic: Enthusiasm and caution. *European Heart Journal – Cardiovascular Imaging, 21*, 941–948. https://doi.org/10.1093/ehjci/jeaa163 (accessed on 12th July 2025).
13. Haddad, R. I., Bischoff, L. A., Ball, D. W., Bernet, V., Blomain, E., Busaidy, N. L., Campbell, M. J., et al. (2022). Thyroid carcinoma, Version 2.2022, NCCN clinical practice guidelines in oncology. *Journal of the National Comprehensive Cancer Network, 20*, 925–951. https://doi.org/10.6004/jnccn.2022.0040 (accessed on 12th July 2025).
14. Hetzel, J., Maldonado, F., Ravaglia, C., Wells, A. U., Colby, T. V., Tomassetti, S., Ryu, J. H., et al. (2018). Transbronchial cryobiopsies for the diagnosis of diffuse parenchymal lung diseases: Expert statement from the Cryobiopsy Working Group on safety and utility and a call for standardization of the procedure. *Respiration, 95*, 188–200. https://doi.org/10.1159/000484055 (accessed on 12th July 2025).
15. Hew, M., & Tay, T. R. (2016). The efficacy of bedside chest ultrasound: From accuracy to outcomes. *European Respiratory Review, 25*, 230–246. https://doi.org/10.1183/16000617.0047-2016 (accessed on 12th July 2025).
16. Hirsch, F. W., Sorge, I., Roth, C., Anders, R., Frahm, J., Voit, D., Prenzel, F., et al. (2025). Real-time MRI of the chest wall, diaphragm, and lungs in children. *Pediatric Pulmonology, 60*(6), e71133. https://www.semanticscholar.org/paper/e30a6db21ddacde4f7ed9062ccedda6f9889e269 (accessed on 12th July 2025).
17. Ihnatsiuk, A., & Karpitski, A. (2022). Ultrasound diagnosis in the formation of esophagopleurocutaneous fistulas. *Journal of the Grodno State Medical University*. https://www.semanticscholar.org/paper/64c83cbdea6f4df3a59320ebd56a1ea43743cbc5 (accessed on 12th July 2025).
18. Jalil, B., Khan, A., Kugasia, I. R., & Ijaz, M. (2020). Lung ultrasound in early SARS-CoV-2 pneumonia and the LUS-CoV criteria. *Baylor University Medical Center Proceedings, 34*, 1–4. https://doi.org/10.1080/08998280.2020.1834658 (accessed on 12th July 2025).
19. Jany, B., & Welte, T. (2019). Pleural effusion in adults—Etiology, diagnosis, and treatment. *Deutsches Ärzteblatt International*. https://doi.org/10.3238/arztebl.2019.0377 (accessed on 12th July 2025).
20. Kalagara, H., Coker, B. J., Gerstein, N. S., Kukreja, P., Deriy, L., Pierce, A., & Townsley, M. M. (2021). Point-of-care ultrasound (POCUS) for the cardiothoracic anesthesiologist. *Journal of Cardiothoracic and Vascular Anesthesia, 36*, 1132–1147. https://doi.org/10.1053/j.jvca.2021.01.018 (accessed on 12th July 2025).
21. Kanwal, K., Asif, M., Khalid, S. G., Liu, H., Qurashi, A. G., & Abdullah, S. (2024). Current diagnostic techniques for pneumonia: A scoping review. *Sensors, 24*, 4291–4291. https://doi.org/10.3390/s24134291 (accessed on 12th July 2025).
22. La Via, L., Cavaleri, M., Terminella, A., Sorbello, M., & Cusumano, G. (2024). Loco-regional anesthesia for pain management in robotic thoracic surgery. *Journal of Clinical Medicine, 13*, 3141–3141. https://doi.org/10.3390/jcm13113141 (accessed on 12th July 2025).
23. Laursen, C. B., Clive, A., Hallifax, R., Pietersen, P. I., Asciak, R., Davidsen, J. R., Bhatnagar, R., et al. (2020). European Respiratory Society statement on thoracic ultrasound. *European*

Respiratory Journal, 57, 2001519–2001519. https://doi.org/10.1183/13993003.01519-2020 (accessed on 12th July 2025).

24. Lei, L., Hu, Y., Jiang, Z., Miao, J., Luo, X., Zhang, Y., Wang, Q., et al. (2025). Toward lung ultrasound automation: Fully autonomous robotic longitudinal and transverse scans along intercostal spaces. *IEEE Transactions on Medical Robotics and Bionics, 7*, 768–781. https://www.semanticscholar.org/paper/c667c75b66e0c922fcb1b1b462d9a5f734455580 (accessed on 12th July 2025).
25. Lyu, Q., Tan, J., Zapadka, M. E., Ponnatapura, J., Niu, C., Myers, K. J., Wang, G., et al. (2023). Translating radiology reports into plain language using ChatGPT and GPT-4 with prompt learning: Results, limitations, and potential. *Visual Computing for Industry Biomedicine and Art, 6*. https://doi.org/10.1186/s42492-023-00136-5 (accessed on 12th July 2025).
26. Manisha, A. (2018). Bedside lung ultrasonography in a general medical ward: Comparison with chest radiography (BLUR). https://core.ac.uk/download/235668996.pdf (accessed on 12th July 2025).
27. Mojoli, F., Bouhemad, B., Mongodi, S., & Lichtenstein, D. A. (2018). Lung ultrasound for critically ill patients. *American Journal of Respiratory and Critical Care Medicine, 199*, 701–714. https://doi.org/10.1164/rccm.201802-0236ci (accessed on 12th July 2025).
28. Focal Spot, Fall/Winter 2002/2003, October 2003. Bernard Becker Medical Library Archives. Washington University School of Medicine. https://core.ac.uk/download/129069325.pdf (accessed on 12th July 2025).
29. Gunti Gunarathne (2021). *Advancements and Breakthroughs in Ultrasound Imaging*. https://core.ac.uk/download/478140644.pdf (accessed on 12th July 2025).
30. Österwalder, J., Polyzogopoulou, E., & Hoffmann, B. (2023). Point-of-care ultrasound—History, current and evolving clinical concepts in emergency medicine. *Medicina, 59*, 2179–2179. https://doi.org/10.3390/medicina59122179 (accessed on 12th July 2025).
31. Petersen, N. A., Falster, C., Schultz, A. Ø., & Kampmann, J. (2024). #1906 Lung ultrasound as a valid tool for fluid assessment in dialysis patients: A systematic review. *Nephrology Dialysis Transplantation*. https://www.semanticscholar.org/paper/34dab6c7259645229cd930d731c073b0fef075d4 (accessed on 12th July 2025).
32. Picaño, E., & Pellikka, P. A. (2016). Ultrasound of extravascular lung water: A new standard for pulmonary congestion. *European Heart Journal, 37*, 2097–2104. https://doi.org/10.1093/eurheartj/ehw164 (accessed on 12th July 2025).
33. Quarato, C. M. I., Lacedonia, D., Salvemini, M., Tuccari, G., Mastrodonato, G., Villani, R., Fiore, L. A., et al. (2023). A review on biological effects of ultrasounds: Key messages for clinicians. *Diagnostics, 13*, 855–855. https://doi.org/10.3390/diagnostics13050855 (accessed on 12th July 2025).
34. Roberts, M., Rahman, N. M., Maskell, N., Bibby, A., Blyth, K. G., Corcoran, J., Edey, A., et al. (2023). British Thoracic Society guideline for pleural disease. *Thorax, 78*, s1–s42. https://doi.org/10.1136/thorax-2022-219784 (accessed on 12th July 2025).
35. Roslan, N. L., Lim, N., & Wahab, M. A. (2023). Massive pleural effusion post-emergency cesarean in an undiagnosed congenital diaphragmatic hernia. *International Journal of Case Reports and Images*. https://www.semanticscholar.org/paper/bdf990227abbb8f299c2389deac9fec9868f8360 (accessed on 12th July 2025).

36. Roy, S., Menapace, W., Oei, S., Luijten, B., Fini, E., Saltori, C., Huijben, I. A. M., et al. (2020). Deep learning for classification and localization of COVID-19 markers in point-of-care lung ultrasound. *IEEE Transactions on Medical Imaging, 39*, 2676–2687. https://doi.org/10.1109/tmi.2020.2994459 (accessed on 12th July 2025).

37. Singh, Y., Tissot, C., Fraga, M. V., Yousef, N., González, R., López, J., Sánchez-de-Toledo, J., et al. (2020). International evidence-based guidelines on point of care ultrasound (POCUS) for critically ill neonates and children issued by the POCUS Working Group of the European Society of Pediatric and Neonatal Intensive Care (ESPNIC). *Critical Care, 24*. https://doi.org/10.1186/s13054-020-2787-9 (accessed on 12th July 2025).

38. Smith, M. L. (2017). Lund concept for de-airing of the left heart. Clinical evaluation. https://core.ac.uk/download/83722437.pdf (accessed on 12th July 2025).

39. Soldati, G., Demi, M., Smargiassi, A., Inchingolo, R., & Demi, L. (2019). The role of ultrasound lung artifacts in the diagnosis of respiratory diseases. *Expert Review of Respiratory Medicine, 13*, 163–172. https://doi.org/10.1080/17476348.2019.1565997 (accessed on 12th July 2025).

40. Szostek, K., Lasek, J., & Piórkowski, A. (2023). Real-time simulation of wave phenomena in lung ultrasound imaging. *Applied Sciences, 13*, 9805–9805. https://doi.org/10.3390/app13179805 (accessed on 12th July 2025).

41. Zaki, H. A., Albaroudi, B., Shaban, E. E., Shaban, A., Elgassim, M., Almarri, N. D., Basharat, K., et al. (2024). Advancement in pleural effusion diagnosis: A systematic review and meta-analysis of point-of-care ultrasound versus radiographic thoracic imaging. *The Ultrasound Journal, 16*. https://www.semanticscholar.org/paper/417494a1ca87600b8fe20bc8a5984354a69f35c8 (accessed on 12th July 2025).

42. Lakhin, P. E., Zhirnova, E. A., Shchegolev, A. V., Jovanikić, O., Zheleznyak, I. S., Menkov, I. A., Salukhov, V.V., et al. (2021). Lung ultrasound in COVID-19 pneumonia: Comparison with computed tomography. An observational prospective clinical trial. *Annals of Critical Care*. https://doi.org/10.21320/1818-474x-2021-2-82-93 (accessed on 12th July 2025).

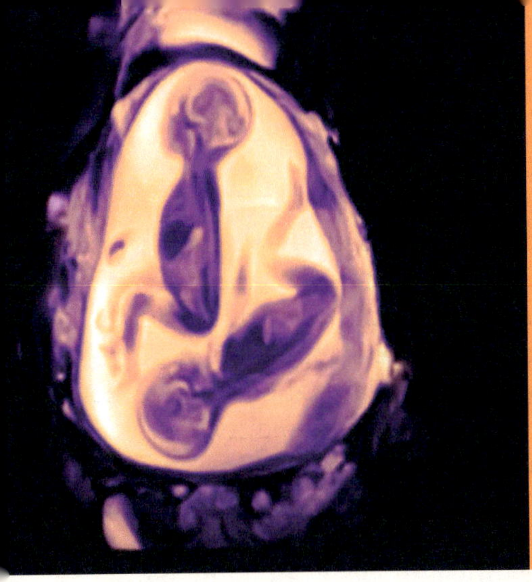

Chapter 6

BASIC CARDIAC ANATOMY VIA ULTRASOUND

Contents

Introduction

An understanding of cardiac anatomy is essential to effective clinical practice and instruction, particularly within cardiovascular medicine. The intricate anatomy of the heart, four chambers, valves, and associated vasculature, is basic to sustaining life through its critical mechanism of circulatory blood flow. As technology advances, ultrasound has evolved into a significant non-surgical method of imaging cardiac structure, and real-time imaging enhances diagnosis and therapeutic management. This essay will explore the fundamentals of cardiac anatomy from the heart of ultrasound technology, noting its central role in modern cardiology and increasing applicability to practice in acute and chronic disease. Use of ultrasound not only aids the detection of structural abnormalities but also allows clinicians to visualize dynamic cardiac function, thereby improving patient management and gaining a better understanding of cardiovascular health. Over the past few years, there has been a significant emphasis on enhancing techniques in real-time cardiac imaging. Application of ultrasound technology makes it possible for cardiac structures to be imaged as they function and to have parameters such as chamber size, wall motion, valve function, and blood flow patterns measured. The diagnostic utility of dynamic imaging to recognize processes such as congenital heart disease, valvular heart disease, and cardiomyopathies is invaluable. Secondly, technological advances in ultrasound imaging, like the application of three-dimensional imaging, enhance the resolution that can be achieved and provide clinicians with a complete view of the heart's anatomy. With the application of these advanced techniques, practitioners are able to make informed decisions regarding patient treatment and care. Therefore, a precise understanding of cardiac anatomy, combined with quality imaging modalities, is crucial in the expectation of improving diagnostic accuracy and optimizing therapeutic intervention. The contribution of ultrasound to the understanding of cardiac anatomy nuances cannot be understated. With advances in deep learning and advanced image segmentation software, the identification of cardiac structures and defects has been significantly enhanced, enabling better diagnoses and treatment planning (Hesamian et al., 2019). Besides, the importance of collaborative work in this field is also evident from the contribution of organizations such as the Heart Rhythm Society and the European Heart Rhythm Association to bring focus on the synthesis of new evidence and techniques to improve patient care (Calkins et al., 2017). This essay aims to bring to light the convergence of cardiac anatomy and ultrasonographic technology in describing how these elements converge to contribute to the field of cardiology. Ultimately, a detailed review of these concepts will reiterate the important role that ultrasound serves in allowing for a sophisticated understanding of cardiac wellness and the accurate treatment of cardiovascular disease (Figure 6.1).

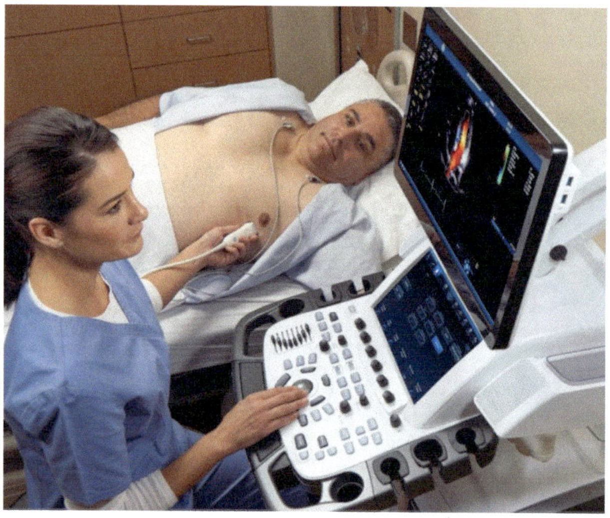

Figure 6.1. Focused cardiac ultrasound.

Source: https://external-content.duckduckgo.com/iu/?u=https%3A%2F%2Fsghanaesthesiaeducation.files.wordpress.com%2F2022%2F07%2F50163.jpg%3Fw%3D816&f=1&nofb=1&ipt=a1b57f4d63c463c44101a21cd0a9c3774815583c064d95dd0a93efb817a0f4de.

Importance of Cardiac Anatomy in Medical Practice

An understanding of cardiac anatomy is critical for medical professionals, particularly with complex imaging modalities such as ultrasound. A thorough comprehension of the anatomy of the heart, chambers, valves, and significant vessels allows clinicians to accurately diagnose various cardiovascular diseases through ultrasound findings. This knowledge enhances the clinician's skills to accurately diagnose various cardiovascular conditions. For instance, determination of left ventricle and right atrial position and other critical structures aids in the identification of pathologies such as valvular disease or cardiomyopathy. Moreover, as point-of-care ultrasound (POCUS) becomes more embedded in medical school curricula, education in cardiac anatomy reinforces fundamental principles that serve as the foundation for application in practice and, in the end, bridging the gap between theory and practice (Knopfholz et al., 2023). The role of cardiac anatomy is not only diagnostic but also assessment and patient management, planning of treatment. The right knowledge of anatomy enables physicians to assess the function of the heart and decide on time-bound interventions. Physicians can gauge parameters such as left ventricular function and pericardial effusion at bedside with POCUS (Peters & Patil, 2018). Such direct applicability not only aids in improved decision-making but also maximizes patient outcomes through the ability to rapidly identify important conditions. Secondly, inclusion of ultrasound in practice also serves to reinforce the importance of anatomy by making it directly relevant to clinical cases, maximizing the abilities of students and practitioners alike to grasp its usefulness in managing cardiovascular health. Educating medical professionals in cardiac anatomy through ultrasound enhances their diagnosis and, eventually, the quality of patient care. Additionally, education in cardiac anatomy through ultrasound is a very effective teaching strategy in medical education. Compared to traditional methods, ultrasound offers a dynamic, real-time image of anatomical structures, making learning more participatory and less theoretical. As noted, the use of ultrasound as a learning medium not only emphasizes anatomy but also includes basic principles of physiology and semiology, making the learning process more efficient for students (Knopfholz et al., 2023). For the future generation of health professionals, the process develops a greater understanding of the cardiac system and its intricacies, allowing them to manage various clinical cases more efficiently. With med school curricula now adapting to include POCUS training, emphasis will be on cardiac anatomy, and students will acquire priceless skills in making this transition into professional practice as they continue to utilize ultrasound in their daily work.

Role of Ultrasound in Visualizing Cardiac Structures

Ultrasound has played a crucial role in imaging of cardiac structures with fetal anatomy assessment. This imaging method relies on sound waves to generate real-time images and allows clinicians to measure the size, structure, and function of fetal hearts with great accuracy. High-resolution transducers significantly enhance image quality, and detailed features like chamber size, wall thickness, and valvular morphology can be identified. Routine scans typically include detection of the four-chamber view, which is important for determining the heart's position within the thorax and the presence of structural defects. Additionally, advanced imaging techniques,such as color Doppler, identify patterns of blood flow, providing essential information regarding hemodynamics that can indicate potential congenital heart disease (Bilardo et al., 2023). Such preclinical identification can impact later clinical management and counseling of the parents for possible interventions. In prenatal ultrasonography, evaluation of cardiac anatomy is not only routine but is also very important in prenatal screening protocols. The International Society of Ultrasound in Obstetrics and Gynecology (ISUOG) has developed guidelines that describe the systematic approach to fetal cardiac surveys. The guidelines strongly highlight the need for combining grayscale and color Doppler imaging to assess the anatomy of the heart in detail. The combination of these imaging modalities enables clinicians to visualize important associations between the cardiac chambers and evaluate any pathologies in great vessel associations. Also, the scanning of some of these indicators, such as aortic and pulmonary outflow tracts, further improves the diagnosis of abnormalities such as tetralogy of Fallot or transposition of the great arteries, hence facilitating better patient outcomes through the early interventions (Salomon et al., 2022).

Aside from that, the operator experience and expertise cannot be overstated in ultrasound assessment of cardiac structures. Successful imaging relies on a combination of anatomical knowledge and technical proficiency in ultrasound technique. As sonographers become more adept at utilizing systematic scanning regimens, detection rates for cardiac abnormalities improve markedly. Advances in ultrasound technology certainly have improved the capacity to detect even small abnormalities, which can be crucial to the early detection of conditions affecting neonatal health. It is most important to establish an ongoing training setting in order to keep practitioners up to date on state-of-the-art practice and advances within ultrasound technology. Such devotion, subsequently, increases the standard of care in fetal cardiac evaluation, which optimizes benefit to pregnant parents (Bilardo et al., 2023; Salomon et al., 2022) (Figure 6.2).

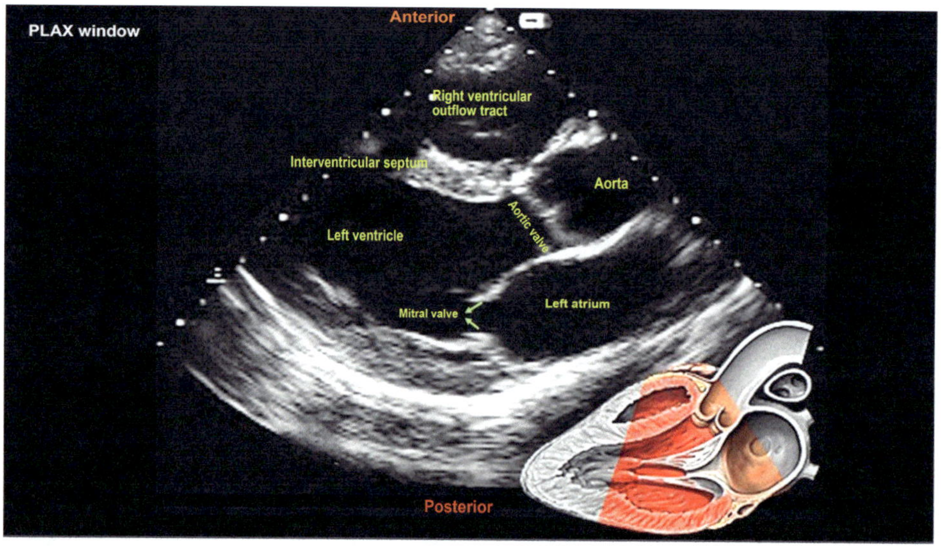

Figure 6.2. Role of ultrasound in visualizing cardiac structures.

Source: https://external-content.duckduckgo.com/iu/?u=https%3A%2F%2Fwww.renalfellow.org%2Fwp-content%2Fuploads%2F2019%2F06%2FFigure-5-1024x576.jpg&f=1&nofb=1&ipt=dc81557ef48c64ee2b240783bcaa0baf7fc5a0d6b7649e6c32566c0c06273b4a.

6.1. Fundamentals of Cardiac Anatomy

The intricacies of cardiac anatomy are imperative to understand the physiological mechanisms and clinical presentations of the heart in normality and disease. Pioneering the cardiac anatomy research are the four chambers of the heart: the right atrium, right ventricle, left atrium, and left ventricle. These four chambers act in concert to enable the flow of blood through the body. Each of the two chambers possesses distinct structural features that enable it to function in this manner; for instance, the left ventricle is muscular and thick-walled to eject oxygenated blood with great force from the aorta into the systemic circulation, while the right ventricle is thin-walled and pumps the blood into the lungs via the pulmonary artery to be oxygenated. These structural differences must be noted when analyzing ultrasound scans depicting cardiac function and morphology in order to enhance diagnostic precision for many cardiovascular diseases. The cardiac anatomy is complemented by a valvular system that is made to regulate the flow of blood and to prevent backflow between the chambers. The atrioventricular valves, tricuspid and mitral, are between the atria and ventricles and ensure one-way blood flow during heart contraction and relaxation phases. The semilunar valves, like the pulmonary and aortic valves, carry out a similar function at the ventricular outflow tracts. The functioning of these valves is imperative as any structural or functional defect will have severe hemodynamic implications, for example, stenosis or regurgitation. Ultrasound imaging, in the form of echocardiography, is also a central instrument for evaluating valvular function, enabling clinicians to examine functional in addition to structural parameters of the heart in real time and thus contribute to life-saving decision-making in cardiac care. Emerging imaging technologies, such as ultrasound, have revolutionized cardiac anatomy knowledge by providing non-invasive, high-resolution pictures of the structural elements of the heart. Advances in deep learning have also advanced cardiac imaging segmentation performance, allowing for greater accuracy in anatomical structure delineation, such as the ventricles, atria, and major vessels (Bai et al., 2025). Through application of sophisticated algorithms, physicians are now in a position to review complicated cardiac images more quickly, with higher diagnostic precision and to direct therapy. Challenges remain, though, especially in model generalizability between different imaging modalities and patient cohorts. As research continues, there should be a continued optimization of such technologies and breaking through barriers to achieve optimum utilization of ultrasound for cardiac anatomy research and pave the way for improved patient care in cardiovascular medicine (Figure 6.3).

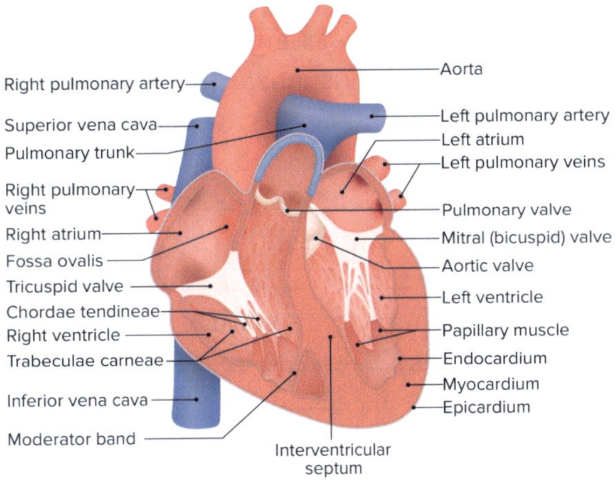

Figure 6.3. Cardiac anatomy.

Source: Heart: Anatomy-Lecturio. https://cdn.lecturio.com/assets/Anterior-view-of-the-internal-cardiac-structures-1200x933.jpg

6.1.1. Overview of the Heart's Structure

The human heart is a highly developed organ with a multilayered structure built to accommodate its essential role in circulation. It has four major chambers: the right and left atria, and the right and left ventricles. The atria are the receiving chambers that receive blood before the entry of the blood into the ventricles, the pumping chambers that eject blood to the rest of the body. Inside each chamber lies a thin wall of tissue known as the endocardium, creating a smooth inner surface that lessens friction when blood moves through. The myocardium, a thick muscular tissue layer, surrounds the heart, allowing it to contract forcefully for the circulation of blood. The pericardium wraps around the heart in the final position, providing protection and supporting it in the thoracic cavity. In addition to its chambers, the heart contains a set of valves that are important to prevent bidirectional blood flow. Included among them are tricuspid and mitral valves, which separate the atria from the ventricles, and pulmonary and aortic valves, which occur at the exits of the ventricles. Careful functioning of these valves is extremely crucial since they prevent the blood from flowing backwards, thus ensuring the maximum efficiency of the heart's pumping action. Failure of these valves results in severe health issues like valvular heart disease, which can be evaluated employing imaging techniques, such as ultrasound. The dynamic nature of the heart's structure allows it to adapt to various physiological demands, illustrating just how important it is to the process of homeostasis maintenance within the body (Bao, 2024).

Cardiac anatomy is significantly enhanced through the use of ultrasound technology, which provides real-time visualizations of the structural characteristics of the heart. Ultrasonography allows health professionals to visualize the heart's chambers and valves, allowing for complete measurements of their size, shape, and function. It is very effective at diagnosing congenital cardiac malformations as well as acquired illnesses like valvular heart disease. Also, methods such as Doppler ultrasound can quantify blood flow and pressure differences through valves and within chambers, allowing for complete comprehension of cardiac function. In general, the use of ultrasound technology in cardiac assessment not only enables accurate diagnostic testing but also contributes significantly to ongoing research regarding cardiovascular disease and cardiovascular health (Wang et al., 2025).

6.1.2. Most Important Components of the Cardiovascular System

The cardiovascular system is a highly developed network that is the body's lifeline, enabling blood, nutrients, and hormones to move into and out of cells. The major components of this system are the heart, blood vessels, and blood. The central pump is the heart itself, which is made up of four chambers: the right atrium, right ventricle, left atrium, and left ventricle. Each of the chambers has a distinct role in the transmission of blood; for example, the left ventricle distributes oxygenated blood to the body, and the right ventricle carries deoxygenated blood to the lungs for refilling. Understanding these chambers and their roles is crucial for interpreting cardiac ultrasound images, which provide distinct images of cardiac motion and structure, thereby enhancing diagnostic value in cardiovascular health evaluation. The heart is surrounded by the blood vessels, including arteries, veins, and capillaries, each with specific functions in the circulatory system. Arteries, for example, are strong vessels that contain high-pressure oxygen-rich blood from the heart to tissues with high efficiency. Veins, however, carry oxygen-poor blood back to the heart, made possible by valves that prevent backflow. Capillaries, on the other hand, are tiny vessels where the exchange of gases, nutrients, and waste occurs between tissues and blood. The addition of these vessels to ultrasound evaluations provides essential information about hemodynamics, enabling medical professionals to detect abnormalities in blood flow that can be indicative of underlying pathologies, such as atherosclerosis or valve insufficiency, thus highlighting the importance of extensive cardiac imaging. Besides, blood is an essential component of the cardiovascular system, consisting of red blood cells, white blood cells, platelets, and plasma. Red blood cells are responsible for the transport of oxygen, essential for metabolism in the cells, and white blood cells are responsible for the immune defense. Platelets are responsible for clotting, that prevents excessive bleeding when the body is injured, while plasma acts as the carrier medium for chemicals in the body. The dynamic equilibrium between these factors is critical to cardiovascular well-being, and any disruption from the norm can have significant repercussions for worldwide health. Through the ultrasound procedure, techniques such as Doppler imaging enable one to quantify blood flow and vascular function, providing a complete profile of cardiovascular dynamics. Such findings turn out to be invaluable in the diagnosis of diseases like coronary artery disease and heart failure, thereby establishing the intense interdependence between cardiac anatomy and ultrasound diagnostics in modern medicine (Arango et al., 2022; Riley et al., 2020).

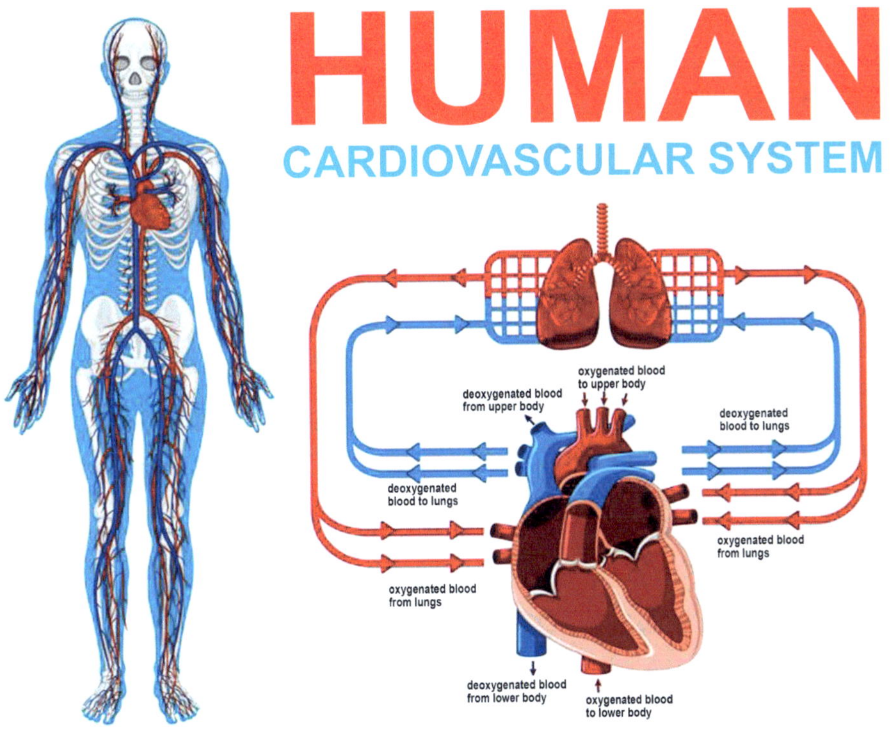

Figure 6.4. Major components of the cardiovascular system.

Source: https://external-content.duckduckgo.com/iu/?u=https%3A%2F%2Fcdn3.vectorstock.com%2Fi%2F1000x1000%2F74%2F22%2Fdiagram-showing-human-cardiovascular-system-vector-42357422.jpg&f=1&nofb=1&ipt=af1d291d84ed4c7ca2960dbc7addbf5594e577da9dd1535dd2a008bed0a2f707.

6.1.3. Importance of Understanding Cardiac Anatomy for Diagnosis

A thorough knowledge of cardiac anatomy is essential for medical personnel since it directly affects diagnostic precision and patient outcomes. Echocardiography, the indispensable non-invasive imaging technique, is highly dependent on accurate anatomical knowledge to recognize possible pathologies and congenital abnormalities. The structure of the heart, including its chambers, valves, and vascular connections, needs to be well appreciated in order to efficiently interpret ultrasound images. Misinterpretations may result in wrong diagnoses, potentially worsening patient conditions. As can be demonstrated through regions of other medical imaging modalities, for example, orofacial cleft detection, the ability to observe and properly assess anatomical structures early in the diagnostic pathway can have a significant impact on management outcome and overall patient care (Deliverska et al., 2025). Comprehending cardiac anatomy is not then an ivory tower exercise but an indispensable tool for efficient, practical application within clinical settings. Application of simulation technology to the teaching of cardiac anatomy once again emphasizes its esteemed position in enhancing echocardiographic skills in medical students. Evidence has determined that ultrasound simulation of sectional human anatomy provides several distinct advantages, such as an enhanced and interactive form of learning, potentially lost in traditional education methodologies. For example, students exposed to high-fidelity simulations demonstrate increased retention of cardiac anatomical structures and enhanced active learning. The results of the latest educational interventions revealed to have a pronounced increase in the post-test scores of students after undergoing simulated practices compared to conventional teaching practices (Ding et al., 2024). This is a reflection of ongoing progress in medical education that enhances the importance of proper pedagogical practice, especially when it comes to intricate subjects like cardiac anatomy that have a direct impact on diagnostic skills. Briefly speaking, the intersection of cardiac anatomy and diagnostic practices reveals vast significance to clinical practice. A good grounding in the topic enhances the diagnostic ability of health workers to identify various cardiac conditions, varying from simple to complex. With the advancement of the medical field towards more sophisticated imaging techniques, the importance of knowing cardiac structures will become even greater. The convergence of knowledge development and technological innovation, such as ultrasound, demonstrates a bimodal approach to learning and application. Implementing such approaches will allow practitioners to deliver efficient and timely diagnosis, thereby improving patient management and outcomes in cardiovascular practice (Ding et al., 2024). The establishment of this knowledge base is critical to producing an efficient healthcare workforce that can manage the complexity of cardiac disease (Figure 6.5).

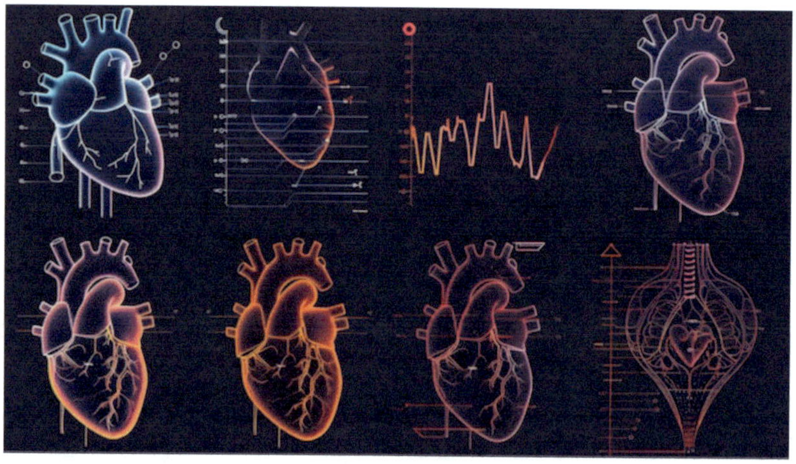

Figure 6.5. Cardiac anatomy and diagnostic.

Source: https://external-content.duckduckgo.com/iu/?u=https%3A%2F%2Fimg.freepik.com%2Fpremium-photo%2Fdetailed-cardiac-anatomy-diagnostic-infographics_38013-43419.jpg&f=1&nofb=1&ipt=422d026e640d23db2dbdfc38596924eebcd2174949d750e68e83d9940023ddd6.a

6.2. Principles of Ultrasound Technology

The quality of ultrasound technology is what makes cardiac imaging so effective, especially when assessing cardiac anatomy and function. Essentially, ultrasound utilizes high-frequency sound waves generated by a transducer. When these sound waves travel through the body and strike different tissues, they reflect off the tissues and back toward the transducer in the form of echoes. This is achieved through a scanning technique with real-time imaging that generates two-dimensional (2D) or even three-dimensional (3D) images of the heart's structures. The interpretation of the images relies on anatomic information and comprehension of how differing tissues will reflect sound waves, such that clinicians are able to visualize cardiac chambers, valves, and adjacent structures effectively. This accurate imaging is central to the diagnosis of a broad range of cardiac conditions and gives insight into both structural abnormalities and functional impairment. At the heart of ultrasound in cardiology is the Doppler effect, which makes it possible to investigate hemodynamics in the heart. By capitalizing on the change in frequency of the sound wave that is reflected, Doppler ultrasound can measure blood flow velocity, direction, and turbulence. This method is essential in valvular heart disease diagnosis, where altered blood flow patterns may indicate stenosis or regurgitation. Furthermore, the integration of Doppler with conventional echocardiography offers a complete cardiac assessment for both structure and function in a single setting. Therefore, the integration of Doppler and traditional echocardiographic modes enhances diagnostic accuracy, making ultrasound a cornerstone in contemporary cardiology practice, particularly in describing complex cardiovascular dynamics (Wiegers et al., 2019).

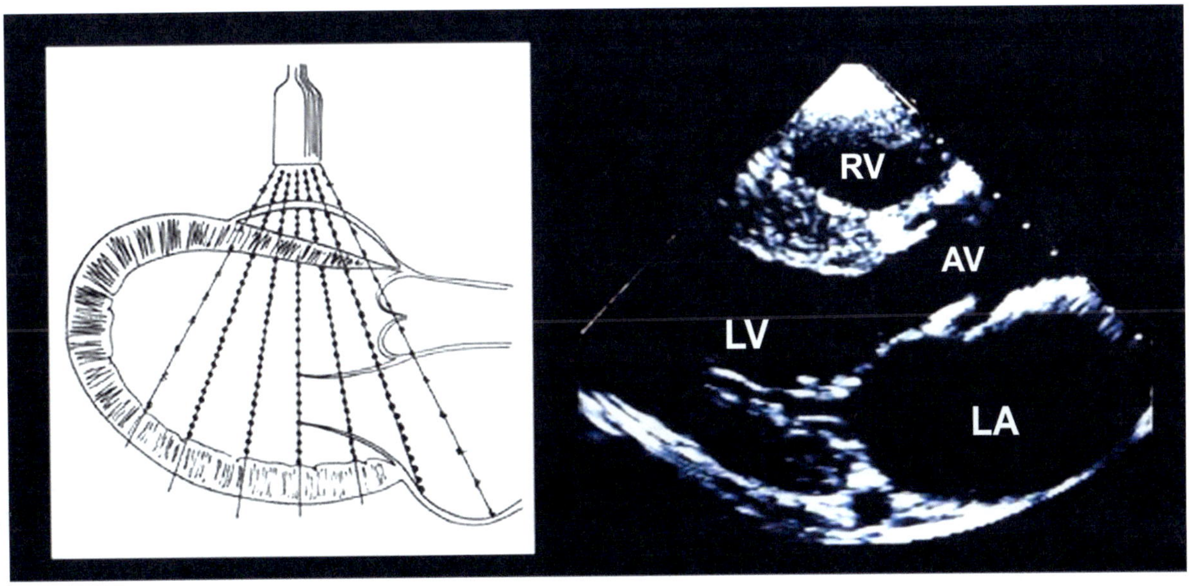

Figure 6.6. Principles of cardiovascular ultrasound.

Source: thoracickey.com, Principles of Cardiovascular Ultrasound. https://thoracickey.com/wp-content/uploads/2016/06/image00877.jpeg.

Although it has many advantages, the application of ultrasound technology requires a deep understanding of the supporting physics and potential pitfalls. The images formed are regulated by several variables, including patient anatomy, body habitus, and operator technique, which can influence the accuracy and quality of echocardiographic measurement. Furthermore, the artifact phenomenon—unwanted echoes that can obscure or simulate disease—creates yet another layer of challenge to accurate interpretation. As discussed in advanced applications, image registration and fusion algorithms significantly enhance echocardiographic diagnostic accuracy by eliminating certain vagaries of the conventional imaging (Brock et al., 2017). Ultimately, proficiency in ultrasound technology not only demands technical skill but also a robust knowledge base that engages both the physiological and anatomical intricacies of heart structures. This comprehensive comprehension ensures that practitioners can make the fullest use of ultrasounds in clinical practice and thereby maximize patient outcomes (Figure 6.6).

6.2.1. Basics of Ultrasound Imaging

The concepts of ultrasound imaging lie in its ability to employ high-frequency sound waves to generate real-time two-dimensional visual representations of interior anatomy. The process is one that is not invasive and makes use of the properties of sound waves, which are emitted by a transducer and reflected back by body tissue to produce images. The varying intensities of reflection, or echogenicity, are dependent on tissue composition and density. In cardiac anatomy, ultrasound scanning has numerous benefits, such as cost-effectiveness, accessibility, and absence of ionizing radiation, thereby itis widely used in diagnosing various cardiovascular diseases. With modalities such as two-dimensional (2D) and three-dimensional (3D) echocardiography, physicians can visualize anatomical features such as chamber dimensions, wall motion, and valvular function, essential to comprehend cardiac health and disease onset. Particularly, echocardiography is a must in defining cardiac anatomy and demonstrating the physiological basis of cardiac function. The incorporation of Doppler techniques enhances the diagnostic potential of ultrasound by measuring blood flow velocities and thereby gaining insight into hemodynamics. This is enabled with a comprehensive evaluation of structural heart disease, like congenital defects and acquired valvular heart diseases. Moreover, technological improvements, such as the development of contrast agents and strain imaging, have significantly contributed to the visual evaluation of myocardial function. Echocardiography is not only a critical tool for initial diagnosis but also for disease monitoring and therapeutic intervention guidance (Wiegers et al., 2019). As ultrasound imaging technology improves, the application of cardiac anatomy expands to redefine cardiovascular disease treatment by clinicians. With the application of three-dimensional imaging in a novel manner, the limitations of traditional two-dimensional assessment are reduced, giving a more accurate impression of cardiac morphology. This can be particularly beneficial in the case of complex cases of congenital cardiac defects or post-operative assessment. The need for more training and skills in specialized echocardiography procedures is mandatory for practitioners. As stated in the current guidelines, specialized training in ultrasound imaging is essential for cardiologists to offer correct interpretation and implement adequate management plans. The growing advancement and integration of ultrasound imaging into clinical practice point to its pivotal role in the support of cardiac diagnostics and therapeutic decision-making procedures (Rychik et al., 2019).

6.2.2. Types of Ultrasound Used in Cardiology

In cardiology, ultrasound offers different pioneering modalities that enable doctors to visualize cardiac anatomy and function in complete detail. Transthoracic echocardiography

(TTE) is the most common type, where the chest wall transducer emits sound waves that produce images of the heart. This technique is non-invasive, allowing real-time assessment of cardiac chambers, valves, and the pericardium, and providing critical information regarding heart failure and valve disease. Ease of use and widespread availability of TTE make it a first-line investigation in all but the most unusual clinical situations. Moreover, technological advances in TTE, such as minimally invasive Doppler imaging, enhance its diagnostic potential by quantifying flow and detecting abnormalities like stenosis or regurgitation, further solidifying it in the full cardiac evaluation, as per updated guidelines (Virani et al., 2023).

Transesophageal echocardiography (TEE) is a more sophisticated variety offering better resolution when scanning posterior to lungs or bones. In TEE, the transducer is inserted into the esophagus, allowing for nearness to the heart. The invasive method is particularly utilized in assessing atrial structures and thrombi and providing guidance for interventional cases such as catheter ablation for atrial fibrillation. Clear images render TEE very useful for pre-operative assessments and in patients with suspected endocarditis, where valves need to be imaged in detail. With ongoing development in TEE techniques and applications, its integration into clinical practice reflects the growing awareness of its value in advanced cardiology (Calkins et al., 2017). Another comparatively new technique in cardiac ultrasound is three-dimensional echocardiography, which offers volumetric data and enhances spatial understanding of cardiac anatomy. By reconstructing three-dimensional heart images, this modality provides a more precise evaluation of heart morphology and function. It permits precise measurement of chamber volume and size, which are critical to effective cardiomyopathy and congenital heart disease diagnosis and management. Though still not as well accepted as TTE or TEE, advances in imaging software and technology increasingly integrate 3D echocardiography as part of routine cardiac assessment. Finally, these different ultrasound methods together augment the cardiologists' diagnostic repertoire, enabling a sophisticated appreciation of cardiac disease and advancing patient benefit through individualized treatments (Virani et al., 2023) (Figure 6.7).

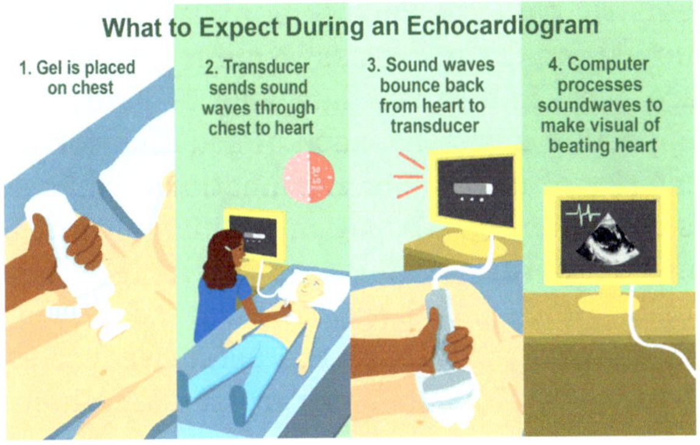

Figure 6.7. Types of ultrasound used in cardiology.

Source: Richard N. Fogoros (2023. What to Expect during an Echocardiogram, www.verywellhealth.com. *https://www.verywellhealth.com/the-echocardiogram-1745246*

6.2.3. Advantages of Ultrasound in Cardiac Assessment

Ultrasound has emerged as an integral modality in cardiac anatomy evaluation with its non-invasive character and absence of ionizing radiation. It employs high-frequency sound waves to create images of heart structures in real time, allowing for extensive study of cardiac chambers, valves, and surrounding tissues. One of the greatest advantages is its ability to present dynamic images that illustrate the function of the heart during various phases of the cardiac cycle. In doing so, clinicians are not only able to visualize static anatomical data but also the working mechanics of the heart, an aspect that is key in diagnosing heart valve failure or cardiomyopathies. The real-time imaging by ultrasound enhances immediate evaluation capacity, leading to early therapeutic interventions that can significantly influence patient outcomes. Ultrasound further enables precise examination of intricate cardiac anatomy and is therefore essential for specific patient groups. As an example, it is especially valuable in pediatric cardiology, whereby the absence of invasiveness minimizes stress and risk to pediatric patients. Furthermore, its portability allows for bedside assessment in critical care, with immediate data able to guide life-supporting decisions. Lack of sedation for the majority of ultrasound examinations enhances its convenience, with patients remaining awake and cooperative, hence optimizing image quality and diagnostic performance. These advantages underscore the extensive variety of uses of ultrasound in cardiac assessment, and it is therefore a method of preference for initial assessment and ongoing monitoring of various cardiac disease processes. In addition to its functions as a diagnostic tool, ultrasound offers some notable advantages in the steering of therapeutic interventions, which enhance its worth in clinical use. For instance, during interventions such as pericardiocentesis or catheter insertions, real-time ultrasound imaging may lower complications, thus ensuring patient safety. Precise accuracy of ultrasound guarantees interventions are performed with accuracy, less likely to result in damage to adjacent tissues. Its capacity for instant feedback to interventions is also facilitating the need for quick decision-making in emergencies. As outlined in recent reports on laboratory-based innovation in imaging medicine, the fusion of ultrasound with other techniques has the possibility of further improving its effectiveness in cardiac assessment, recording a sustained decrease in the discipline (Das & Yip, 2017) and depicting the infinite potential for patient care advancement (Focal Spot, 2007).

6.3. Standard Views in Cardiac Ultrasound

Standard views in cardiac ultrasound play a vital role in the assessment of the anatomy and function of the heart as building blocks. These views, which are predominantly two-dimensional (2D) assessments, include the four-chamber view, the left ventricular outflow tract (LVOT) view, and the short-axis view. Of these, the four-chamber view is highly important as it provides visual inspection of both the right and left atria, ventricles, and septal structures of the heart. It also provides information not just regarding chamber size and morphology but also regarding the timing and mechanism of cardiac contractions. The standardized technique in ultrasound facilitates clinicians to identify congenital heart abnormalities accurately, assess ventricular function, and monitor myocardial performance, thus making the views pivotal under prenatal and postnatal care (Bilardo et al., 2023). Left ventricular outflow tract view, another standard ultrasound view, is significant in the evaluation of the aortic arch and the evaluation of left ventricular outflow dynamics. This view is achieved by tilting the ultrasound probe from the four-chamber view. It provides a close-up visualization of the aortic valve and how close it is to the pulmonary artery. Abnormalities at the LVOT can suggest significant cardiac malformations, including outflow tract obstruction or aortic coarctation. Furthermore, detection of the arterial connections using color Doppler imaging enhances understanding of blood flow within cardiac structures and provides valuable data regarding hemodynamics and potential congenital heart disease (Salomon et al., 2022).

Furthermore, the short-axis view is included in a comprehensive assessment of cardiac anatomy with ultrasound. This view is obtained by rotating the transducer 90° from the position of the LVOT, giving a cross-sectional image of the left ventricle at varying levels, like the papillary muscles and apex of the ventricle. It is utilized to evaluate the contractility of the walls of the ventricle and can be used to demonstrate regional wall motion defects indicative of ischemia or remote myocardial infarcts. The comprehensive echo information obtained from the short-axis views helps in the complete assessment of cardiac function and clinical decisions in both the acute and chronic contexts. Thus, the systematic incorporation of these standard views not only improves diagnostic efficiency but also reflects the role of high-quality ultrasound protocols in the assessment of cardiac anatomy (Bilardoet al., 2023) (Figure 6.8).

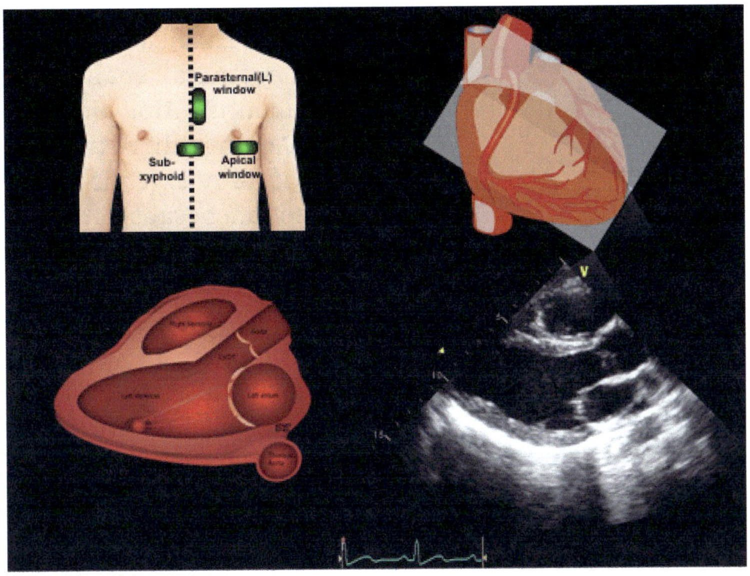

Figure 6.8. Standard views in cardiac ultrasound.

Source: https://www.albertasono.ca/wp-content/uploads/2021/06/PLAX_21.gif.

6.3.1. Parasternal Long-Axis View

Parasternal long-axis view (PLAX) is a crucial image of the heart in cardiac ultrasound that provides invaluable information about the anatomy and function of the heart. By placing the transducer on the left sternal border in either the third or fourth intercostal space, sonographers can visualize key anatomical structures, including the left ventricle, right ventricle, left atrium, aortic outflow tract, and mitral and tricuspid valves. It is particularly convenient for the assessment of chamber sizes, morphology of the valves, and overall cardiac function, thus forming a basis in echocardiographic examinations. Properly obtained PLAX view, along with complete awareness of the echocardiographic windows, optimizes the uniformity of the diagnostic information provided by the ultrasound, again illustrating its potential for implementation in clinical use and cardiac disease treatment. Other than anatomy, the parasternal long-axis view is applied in evaluating cardiac function in a number of clinical scenarios. Registration of the left ventricles ejection fraction using this view is required during the diagnosis of heart failure or cardiomyopathy. Point-of-care ultrasound (POCUS) technology has made it possible to integrate echocardiographic techniques in routine clinical practice, allowing for real-time cardiac function evaluation during patient examination. These skills underscore the need for inclusion of ultrasound training in medical schools, as indicated by research showing improvement in POCUS competencies in subsequent clinical students versus prior clinical peers

(Bingisser et al., 2019). Effective use of the PLAX view also supports rapid decision-making and enhances patient care in acute settings, again underscoring its utility in modern cardiology. Further still, ongoing research also continues to indicate the uses of the parasternal long-axis view beyond basic measurements. For instance, studies on the mechanistic therapeutic uses of mesenchymal stromal cells (MSCs) following myocardial infarction (MI) have utilized ultrasound to monitor changes in cardiac performance over extended time frames (Borgarelli et al., 2013). With the use of the PLAX view, researchers are able to quantify ejection fraction and other function parameters over time, providing a more accurate indication of treatment effect. Such visualization of structural adaptation correlating with functional recovery reflects the range of application of parasternal long-axis imaging beyond immediate in-the-moment clinical diagnosis to extended research use. As the field of cardiac ultrasound evolves, the integration of these advanced imaging techniques becomes imperative for enhancing patient care and advancing cardiology practices (Figure 6.9).

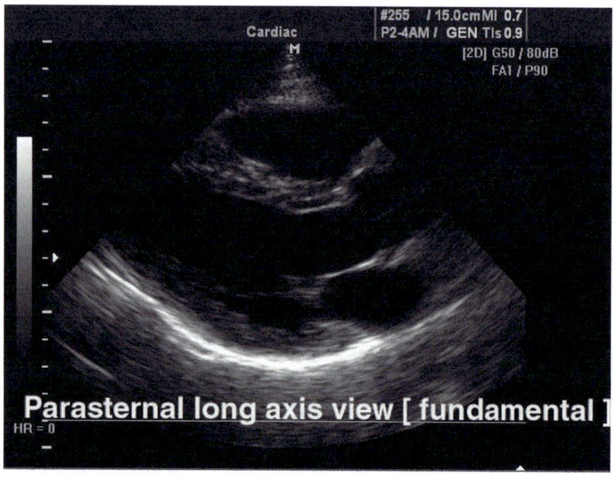

Figure 6.9. Parasternal long-axis view in cardiac ultrasound.

Source: https://www.medison.ru/uzi/img/p110.jpg

6.3.2. Apical Four-Chamber View

The apical four-chamber view (A4CV) is an important component of cardiac anatomy assessment with ultrasound to render a one-view, holistic image of the heart's structure. It allows clinicians to measure the left and right atria, left and right ventricles, and interatrial and interventricular septa all in one plane. This type of visualization is critical both in prenatal and postnatal evaluation because it aids in the identification of congenital heart defects (CHDs) and other structural abnormalities. The use of A4CV extends beyond simple anatomical depiction because it facilitates assessment of the dynamics of the blood stream through the atrioventricular valves, communicating to specialists the element of hemodynamic stability and whether there are problems associated with regurgitation. In summary, the A4CV remains an important tool in cardiac ultrasound, providing sharp details on the morphometry and function of hearts. Utilization of color Doppler technology in combination with the A4CV can play an important role in the detection of hemodynamic abnormalities, especially atrioventricular valve regurgitation (AVVR). It is possible to measure blood flow across the atrioventricular valves accurately using this application, which is essential in the diagnosis of such diseases as atrioventricular septal defects (AVSDs). Studies have identified that AVVR detection by the 4CV is better than traditional two-dimensional ultrasound procedures and has strong correlations with increased nuchal translucency thickness, further contributing to fetal cardiac complexity early in pregnancy. For instance, recent studies highlighted that AVVR identified during the first trimester had a stronger correlation with AVSD compared to other markers, thereby highlighting the significance of the A4CV in prenatal screening. Its efficiency as a screening tool highlights the necessity of extensive evaluation of intracardiac and extracardiac status on initial ultrasounds. Besides, the A4CV forms an essential part of high-standard cardiac assessment protocols, particularly in those centers that specialize in early cardiac screening. Professionals are likely to include this view as part of extensive evaluations aimed at identifying suspected congenital heart diseases (CHDs) in fetuses in a methodical approach. In a multicenter retrospective study, experienced operators performing first-trimester scans followed prolonged follow-up protocols with priority to A4CV and other views. Subsequent fetal echocardiography following initial suspicious findings in the study had a high percentage of cases that confirmed or ruled out CHD. This is an important process that highlights the role of A4CV in preventing misdiagnosis on the positive side and determining correct judgments, restating its importance in prenatal cardiac echocardiography. In the end, the union of sound assessment processes around the A4CV can lead to improved outcomes and improved fetal cardiac anomaly management (Figure 6.10).

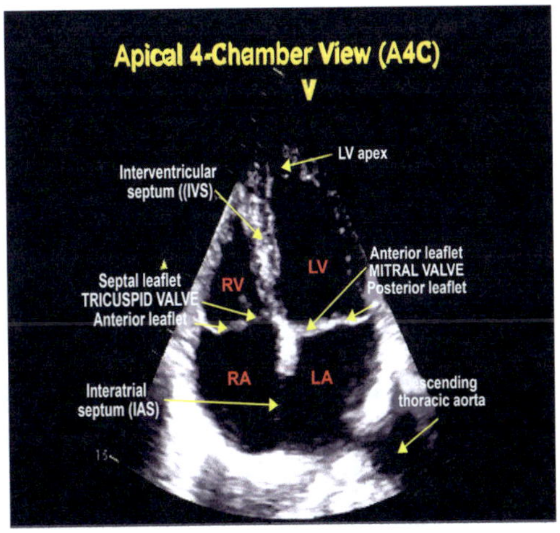

Figure 6.10. Apical four-chamber view.

Source: Michal Pazderník (2021). Apical views. www.pragueicu.com. https://cdn.prod.website-files.com/5ff99f5f7aec6fe4770f6b92/616f144e8b372e2724a33eb0_Apical%204-Chamber%20View%20(A4C).png.

6.3.3. Subcostal View

The subcostal view is one of the important angles employed in ultrasound imaging, particularly cardiac anatomy examination. It is obtained through positioning the ultrasound transducer below the xiphoid process and angled to the left shoulder in an upward direction. All this is done to bring structures like the inferior vena cava, right atrium, and ventricular septum into view, thereby allowing complete assessment of cardiac function. The subcostal view is valuable in cases with poor acoustic windows in alternative views and is a crucial tool for sonographers and clinicians. It is also a portal for hemodynamic assessment, predominantly for measuring the collapsibility and diameter of the inferior vena cava, a critical parameter to decide fluid status in patients with heart failure or volume overload states. Apart from its advantages anatomically, the subcostal view has significant roles in Doppler ultrasound studies, enhancing the understanding of heart blood flow patterns. The subcostal position offers unhindered observation of the inferior vena cava and the right atrial inflow, providing invaluable information regarding right heart performance. Through the application of Doppler imaging, doctors can quantify the blood flow velocities across the pulmonary and tricuspid valves and aid in the diagnosis of illnesses such as tricuspid regurgitation or pulmonary hypertension. This sometimes difficult analysis by Doppler in other planes illustrates the value of subcostal views in total cardiac evaluation. By enabling the visualization of structural and functional parameters equally, the subcostal view is an essential component of cardiac ultrasound, further solidifying its value in clinical practice. Aside from its clinical applications, the subcostal view also plays an educational function in ultrasonography training programs. It offers trainees an opportunity to become familiar with three-dimensional cardiac anatomy as they practice their technical skills in ultrasound imaging. The simplicity of obtaining the subcostal view, in contrast to the apical or parasternal views, promotes self-assurance among students and healthcare professionals. Furthermore, the proven accuracy of the subcostal view in adults and children increases its didactic significance, as new sonographers can learn to master the procedure and its diagnostic importance with ease. With use both in clinical and teaching environments, the subcostal view not only supports the diagnosis of cardiac pathologies but also promotes a new era of effective practitioners in conducting advanced echocardiography to produce proper patient care, reaffirming its place in cardiac imaging (Höglund, 2007; Paterson, 1990) (Figure 6.11).

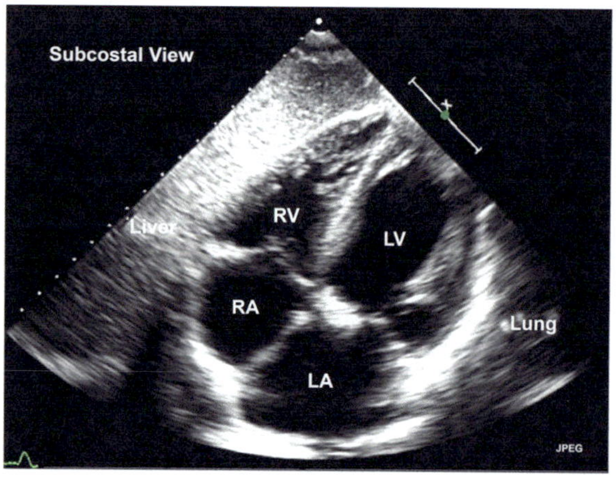

Figure 6.11. Subcostal view in cardiac ultrasound.

Source: https://img1.wsimg.com/isteam/ip/3d8964c4-d4ee-44be-980a-64900a374e01/SubCostal.png.

6.4. Visualization of Cardiac Chambers

The ultrasound imaging of cardiac chambers remains a mainstay of cardiac anatomy assessment. With the development of two-dimensional (2D) echocardiography, clinicians have the ability to create real-time images of heart structure, allowing for careful evaluation of cardiac chamber anatomy and function. This imaging modality not only enhances the identification of normal cardiac structures but also aids in the diagnosis of a number of conditions, such as valvular heart disease and cardiomyopathies. By the application of Doppler techniques, echocardiography offers dynamic insight into hemodynamics, further influencing diagnostic decisions. Despite improvements achieved in imaging quality, there are still constraints with respect to good visualization in patients suffering from a large body habitus or respiratory disease, leading to worse outcomes in some patients (Sorrell & Kumar, 2011). Thus, the further improvement of imaging methods is of key importance to increase echocardiographic examination diagnostic potential and overall accuracy. Moreover, new methods are also being used to improve the cardiac anatomy visualizations, like the use of contrast agents. The American Society of Echocardiography has stressed the usefulness of the agents in improving endocardial visualization, particularly with the advent of suboptimal ultrasound images. Contrast-enhanced echocardiography is useful in augmenting the detection of pathologies in challenging areas of anatomy, such as the left ventricular apex, facilitating delineation of conditions such as apical variant hypertrophic cardiomyopathy and left ventricular thrombus. By means of signal enhancement, contrast agents augment the validity of echocardiographic evaluations, which eventually translate into better clinical outcomes. Additionally, these agents enhance spectral Doppler signals, thus providing valuable information about diastolic function and general cardiovascular hemodynamics, which are critical in overall patient assessment in the clinic setting (Sorrell & Kumar, 2011).

Also, extensive education and training on how to use advanced ultrasound techniques-including contrast echocardiography, are required by medical personnel interested in optimizing cardiac chamber visualization. As ultrasound technology becomes increasingly advanced, so too does the technical expertise and knowledge required to analyze such complex images. This may be supplemented through mutual co-operation among cardiologists and medical physicists in order to enhance training programs to promote sufficient proficiency in technical and clinical aspects of echocardiography. Such interdisciplinarity leads towards standardization in imaging protocols and reading and, as a result, enhanced patient care. Educational resources, such as higher-level textbooks that focus on imaging physics and cardiac anatomy, may be critical tools in bridging this knowledge gap and helping facilitate an upgrade in the medical profession of cardiac ultrasound (Figure 6.12).

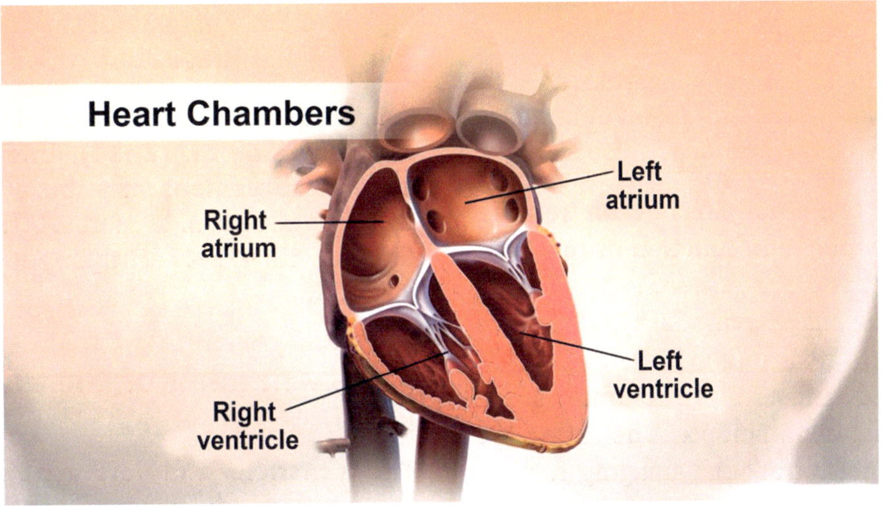

Figure 6.12. Visualization of cardiac chambers.

Source: https://external-content.duckduckgo.com/iu/?u=https%3A%2F%2Fmedmovie.com%2F_uploads%2Fcvml_0014a_HeartChambers_1280x720-1.jpg&f=1&nofb=1&ipt=e8404c544ba550d545c8c18cc026b44e2a3a00ea6eff54d2aab19dbece548fb1.

6.4.1. Anatomy of the Right Atrium and Ventricle

The right atrium is a central component of the circulatory system since it is the large chamber into which the body's deoxygenated blood is routed prior to being pumped into the right ventricle. It takes in blood through two large veins, the superior and inferior vena cavae, which receive blood from the upper and lower parts of the body, respectively. Anatomically, the right atrium is divided by the interatrial septum containing the fossa ovalis, an embryonic remnant. In the application of ultrasound techniques, their identification comes first, since it makes it possible to evaluate the size of the right atrium, movement of its wall, and also any disease, such as atrial septal defects or thrombi. An adequate evaluation of the right atrium should be done, as its function is crucial in maintaining efficient forward flow and preventing heart failure or arrhythmia among patients. Proceeding to the right ventricle, this chamber's function is crucial in pumping deoxygenated blood to the lungs to be oxygenated via the pulmonary arteries. The right ventricle is uniquely structured with a crescent shape, facilitating contraction and the movement of blood through systole. Knowledge of the chamber's anatomical complexities, consisting of three distinct segments—infundibulum, trabecular portion, and outflow tract—is crucial as well as for accurate echocardiographic evaluation. Emerging imaging modalities, particularly ultrasound-based methods, enable right ventricular size, wall thickness, and function to be assessed. In the clinical setting, pathology such as right ventricular dilatation or pressure overload is crucial to account for in the management of the patient, and therefore, the anatomical data derived using ultrasound is very critical in diagnosis and follow-up of cardiovascular disease, particularly in patients with pulmonary hypertension or congenital heart disease.

Ultrasound technology has revolutionized the way the anatomy and function of the right atrium and ventricle are researched. With the addition of this imaging modality, clinicians are able to attain real-time visualizations that can aid in the diagnosis of structural disease and functional impairment. The dynamic three-dimensional ultrasound imaging further enhances the understanding of cardiac dynamics as well as provides rich insight into the intraventricular patterns of flow. For instance, deep learning has seen extensive use in cardiac image segmentation so that a person can have more accurate analyses of both the atria and ventricles, as cited in recent research (Bai et al., 2025). Techniques based on computational fluid dynamics also emphasize the requirement to understand dynamic flow patterns inside the right ventricle and, therefore, emphasize the importance of real-time imaging in routine practice, as pointed out in echocardiography research (Bavo et al., 2016). Overall, an interdisciplinary solution through the application of ultrasound is required to further clarify right atrial and ventricular anatomy and its clinical significance (Figure 6.13).

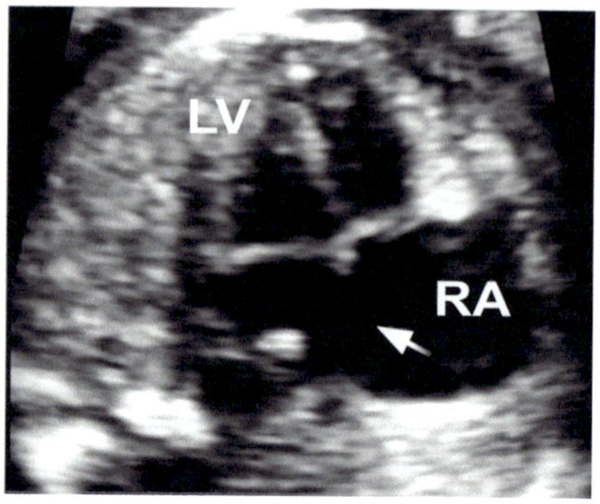

Figure 6.13. Anatomy of the right atrium and ventricle in ultrasound.

Source: Paladini, D., Tiesi, M., Buffi, D., Tuo, G. and Marasini, M. (2014), Unexplained right atrial enlargement may be a sign of Holt–Oram syndrome in the fetus. Ultrasound Obstet Gynecol, 43: 475-476. https://doi.org/10.1002/uog.13238

6.4.2. Anatomy of the Left Atrium and Ventricle

The ventricle and left atrium are critical components of cardiac anatomy and are responsible for the flow of blood within the human system. The left atrium is occupied by oxygenated blood through pulmonary veins, which is directed to the left ventricle during systole when the ventricle squeezes. The left atrium, morphologically, possesses a clear-cut morphology with its large appendage and smooth walls. This appendage, or left atrial appendage, is of clinical relevance in that it has the potential to develop thrombi, particularly in the case of patients with atrial fibrillation. Understanding such anatomical information is significant since it influences not only the efficacy of diagnostic procedures such as ultrasound but also subsequent therapeutic interventions (Arango et al., 2022). Atrium to the left ventricle, we observe that it is the primary pumping chamber of the heart with the responsibility of generating the pressure necessary to circulate oxygenated blood into systemic circulation.

Walls of the left ventricle are thicker in relation to the atrium, which shows its critical function throughout the cardiac cycle. The anatomy of the ventricles consists of important structures such as the mitral valve, which allows for one-way blood flow from the atrium during diastole, and papillary muscles, which hold the chordae tendineae in place in order to prevent prolapse of the valves. Surprisingly, advances in imaging modalities, especially through the application of ultrasound, have provided unparalleled information on the dynamic movements of these structures through the cardiac cycle (Chen et al., 2020). Understanding this anatomy is essential to medical professionals for the diagnosis and management of cardiac disease.

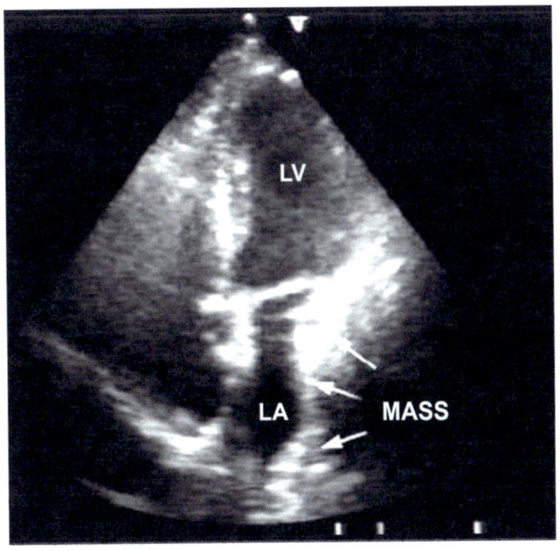

Figure 6.14. Anatomy of the left atrium and ventricle in ultrasound.

Source: Siu, David & Jim, Man & Ho, Hee & Chu, F & Chan, H-W & Lau, C-P & Tse, Hanh. (2005). Recurrent acute heart failure caused by sliding hiatus hernia. Postgraduate medical journal. 81. 268-9. 10.1136/pgmj.2004.023416.

Further, the interaction between the left atrium and ventricles is complicated, both in function and pathology. For instance, increased pressure in the left atrium can lead to pulmonary congestion, and hypertrophy of the left ventricle is typically a result of conditions like hypertension or aortic stenosis. Understanding of these interdependent processes is especially important in clinical assessment of cardiac function. New modalities with the application of ultrasound have enhanced visualization of the chambers and their associated structures, along with increased diagnostic precision and patient outcomes. Echocardiography, therefore, has become a vital part of perioperative management, and this reveals that practitioners need to develop competency in recognizing and interpreting left atrial and ventricular anatomy (Arango et al., 2022). This information is critical for the best possible care of patients and for avoiding complications of cardiac interventions (Figure 6.14).

6.4.3. Importance of Chamber Size and Function Assessment

Assessment of the size and function of the chambers is critical to cardiac anatomy and physiology through the application of ultrasound technology. Chamber measurement of the hearts, that is, the left ventricle and right ventricle and atria, enables the most critical data about the overall health of the cardiovascular system. Ultrafast imaging technology, such as echocardiography, makes it possible to detect diseases such as hypertrophy or dilation, which may signify underlying disease. With the use of more than one imaging modality, clinicians are able to measure cardiac volumes and ejection fractions, which are vital to the diagnosis of valvular heart disease or heart failure. Apart from informing clinical decision-making, assessment is vital in longitudinal follow-up of a patient's heart status over time, thus the enhancement of patient outcomes by interventions made in a timely manner. Moreover, technical advancements in imaging have revolutionized the assessment of chamber performance. Deep learning methods and convolutional neural networks have greatly improved the measurement accuracy of chamber size. The latest techniques can segment cardiac morphology from echocardiography images automatically and approximate functional parameters with high precision, surpassing traditional manual estimations. For instance, the EchoNet model was able to accurately identify enlarged left atria and left ventricular hypertrophy, according to (Ghorbani et al., 2020). These innovations not only optimize the workflow in clinical practice but also enhance the interpretability of cardiac images. These innovations emphasize bridging innovative technology with routine ultrasound exams to improve diagnostic accuracy and patient management. Measurement of chamber function and size also carries significant implications for risk stratification and cardiovascular disease management. This assessment provides the ability to recognize at-risk patients for adverse outcomes due to specific chamber abnormalities. An example would be dilatation of the left ventricle as an indication of a high cardiac workload and thereby the possible need for heightened monitoring or intervention123. As has been shown, echocardiographic markers of chamber size and function are able to predict systemic phenotypes for cardiovascular risk variables such as age and body weight, demonstrating an intimate connection between structural cardiac assessment and general well-being consequences (Ghorbani et al., 2020). Hence, knowing the chamber size and function by ultrasound not only benefits individual patient care but also public health by influencing risk assessment and preventive measures in the general population.

6.5. Valvular Anatomy and Function

The anatomy of the valvular heart includes large structures that are in charge of the control of blood flow inside cardiac chambers, which causes effective circulation and hemodynamic stability. The four large heart valves include the aortic, mitral, pulmonary, and tricuspid valves. They all play a role in the unidirectional flow of blood. The tricuspid and mitral valves, located between the atria and ventricles, open to allow blood flow during diastole and close during systole to prevent regurgitation. The aortic and pulmonary valves, placed on the ventricular exits, open during contraction of the ventricles to allow ejection of blood into the systemic and pulmonary circulations, respectively. Dedicated ultrasound techniques enable visualization and assessment of such valves, and diagnostic evaluation of valvular diseases such as stenosis and regurgitation, and the creation of successful management plans on that basis. The functional capability of heart valves is essential, as even minimal abnormalities can cause a significant clinical impact. Valve stenosis, or narrowing of the valve opening, can impede blood flow and increase cardiac workload, resulting in heart failure if left untreated. Regurgitation, or failure of the valves to close, allowing blood to go backward, can, in time, result in volume overload in the heart. Evaluation of these dynamics by cardiac ultrasound is extremely useful, as it provides instant data on valve function, morphology, and hemodynamic impact. Moreover, technical advancements in ultrasound technology have made it possible to acquire high-resolution images and Doppler data with greater ease, which not only enables clinicians to make a diagnosis of valvular disease but also allows them to assess the efficacy of therapeutic interventions. Understanding of the combined interaction of valvular anatomy and function is most important for clinicians with patients of cardiovascular disease. For instance, congenital cardiovascular disease patients may present with unique valvular configurations that make traditional anatomical and functional concepts unworkable. Ultrasonographic evaluation may also exhibit not only structural defects but also the functional repercussions on overall cardiac function. Active studies in this field also highlight the need for ongoing education on the nuances of valvular physiology as interventions, such as surgical interventions and percutaneous interventions, continue to change. With more patients suffering from acquired or congenital valvular heart disease, the use of ultrasound imaging in clinical practice to ensure early intervention and improved patient outcomes is imperative to clearly define the practice of cardiology in today's healthcare (Riley et al., 2020; Rychik et al., 2019) (Figure 6.15).

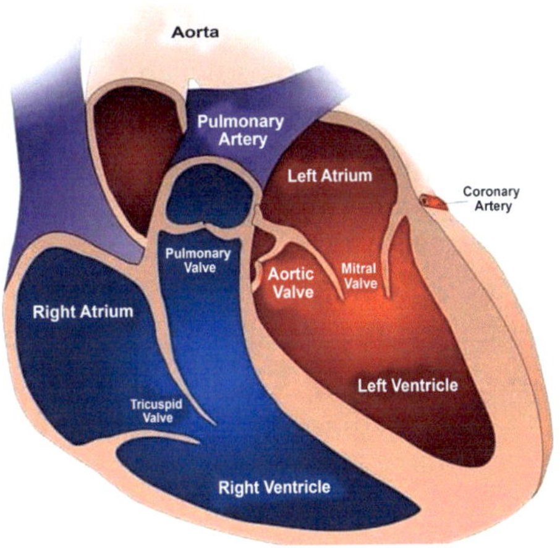

Figure 6.15. Valvular anatomy and function.

Source: https://www.sportzyogi.com/wp-content/uploads/2021/04/valves-of-heart-2.jpg.

6.5.1. Structure of the Heart Valves

The valves of the heart are needed to control the efficient flow of blood within the heart as well as into the major arteries. They are four in number: the mitral valve, tricuspid valve, aortic valve, and pulmonary valve. The mitral valve, between the left atrium and left ventricle, consists of two leaflets opening to allow blood to flow from the atrium into the ventricle and closing to prevent backflow with contraction of the ventricle. The tricuspid valve, situated between the right atrium and right ventricle, consists of three leaflets and operates similarly, providing unidirectional flow of blood. The positioning of such valves, together with their corresponding chordae tendineae and papillary muscles, contributes significantly to normal function, and any form of anomaly can lead to severe cardiovascular issues. Aortic and pulmonary valves are semilunar valves that are found at the junctions where ventricles are attached to the aorta and pulmonary arteries, respectively. The valves in both have three cusps, half-moon in shape that open to expel blood with ventricular systole. During ventricular relaxation, the cusps close to prevent regurgitation into the ventricles. Remarkably, the aortic valve is specifically designed to withstand higher pressures than the pulmonary valve because it delivers oxygenated blood to the systemic circulation. Understanding the specific structural adaptations of these valves is essential to evaluating potential pathological states, as imaging modalities such as ultrasound can precisely represent valve morphology and function in both the healthy and diseased heart. Ultrasound, and particularly Doppler techniques, have revolutionized the assessment of heart valve structure and function.

Through the application of echocardiography, practitioners can obtain complete images of heart valves in real-time, enabling them to assess such factors as valve size, mobility, and blood flow pattern. Advanced imaging devices like three-dimensional echocardiography even enhance the structural visualization of valves. This is particularly relevant in disorders like valvular stenosis or regurgitation, where structural lesions can affect valve performance. Visualization of heart valves with ultrasound not only aids in diagnosis but also improves preoperative planning and postoperative management of patients undergoing surgery for repair or replacement of valves, addressing some critical problems in cardiac health management as posed by Bilardo et al. (2023); Arango et al. (2022) (Figure 6.16).

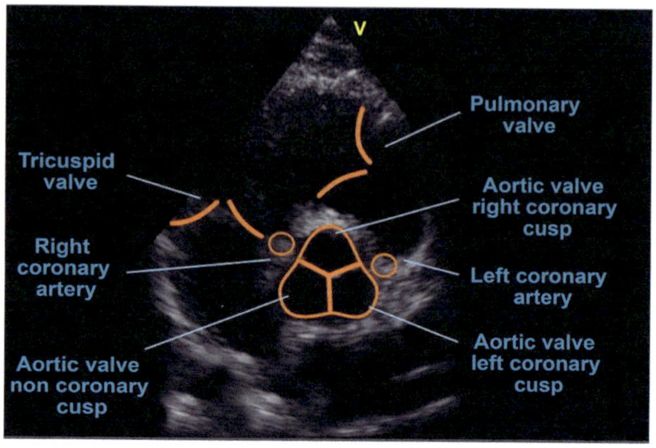

Figure 6.16. Structure of the heart valves.

Source: Parasternal Short Axis; icuecho.com. https://icuecho.com/images/psax_basal_3.jpg

6.5.2. Role of Valves in Cardiac Function

The heart valves are crucial to ensure efficient cardiac function by regulating blood flow through the chambers of the heart. Comprising the atrioventricular (AV) valves—that is, mitral and tricuspid valves—and the semilunar valves—that is, the aortic and pulmonary valves—these valves ensure backflow prevention as well as one-way blood flow. During the cardiac cycle, the valves open and close during pressure fluctuations due to ventricular contraction and relaxation. This precise timing is essential; for instance, the mitral valve opens to allow left ventricular filling during diastole, while the aortic valve opens for ejection of blood into the aorta during systole. Understanding valvular function by ultrasound imaging can provide insights about the efficient operation of these structures and determine abnormalities that may jeopardize overall cardiac functioning. Dysfunction of valves can severely compromise cardiac efficiency in the form of stenosis or regurgitation. Stenosis occurs when a valve fails to open normally, causing increased pressure in the cardiac chambers and ultimately heart failure. Alternatively, regurgitation or a leaky valve causes backward blood flow and decreases cardiac output. These conditions can be identified via ultrasound, which allows real-time assessment of valve function and structure. This allows clinicians to evaluate hemodynamic impact and decide on therapy. Because of the intricacy of valvular disease and its potential to negatively alter conditions such as coronary artery disease or congestive heart failure, a detailed understanding of valve function within cardiac performance is critical. The valvular examination thus forms an integral component of cardiac ultrasound investigations, enabling enhanced prognostication and management of affected patients. Contemporary cardiac practice emphasizes the incorporation of valvular integrity into the total assessment of cardiac anatomy and function. The intricate relationship between valvular and ventricular performance necessitates a multidisciplinary approach to patient management. For instance, patients with concomitant coronary artery disease and valve pathology are at risk for adverse outcomes, including mortality. The value of a multidisciplinary heart team is critical in the management of such complexity, as it ensures that each patient's individual needs are met with tailored treatment strategies. Collaboration of this sort is particularly valuable when it comes to planning interventions for valvular repair or replacement, where procedural risk must be weighed against possible benefit. With technology advance on ultrasound, its application to guide and monitor valvular interventions will likely be increasingly important in enhancing patient outcomes, as well as how valves remain the axis of cardiac function and well-being (Riley et al., 2020; Rychik et al., 2019).

6.5.3. Common Valvular Diseases Assessed by Ultrasound

Assessment of the prevalent valvular illness is a critical application of ultrasound technology in the understanding of basic cardiac anatomy. Valvular heart disease, such as aortic stenosis, mitral insufficiency, and tricuspid insufficiency, can significantly impact cardiac function and overall health. Ultrasound, particularly echocardiography, provides real-time visualization of structures within the heart, allowing clinicians to assess valve anatomy and function with unforeseen accuracy. Aortic stenosis, characterized by aortic valve narrowing, can be reliably evaluated using Doppler ultrasonography for the measurement of blood velocity across the valve. Quantification allows calculation of the stenosis degree, facilitating early intervention and treatment planning. Lastly, ultrasound allows for early diagnosis and planning of treatment, preventing long-term consequences of untreated valvular disease and optimizing patient outcomes in cardiovascular disease treatment. Mitral regurgitation is another prevalent valvular illness usually evaluated via ultrasound. Abnormal closure of the mitral valve produces the condition, leading to regurgitation back into the left atrium with ventricular systole. Echocardiography plays a pivotal role in diagnosing and determining the severity of mitral regurgitation using several techniques, including color Doppler imaging, which provides a visual evaluation of regurgitant flow. Second, ultrasound makes possible the assessment of ventricular performance and left atrial enlargement as complications of chronic mitral regurgitation. The inclusion of a complete echocardiographic assessment, therefore, assists in providing correct decisions on operative intervention or treatment. By enabling accurate visualization of the condition, ultrasound not only enhances the diagnostic effectiveness but also helps provide customized treatment strategies for patients suffering from mitral regurgitation. Tricuspid regurgitation is yet another serious valvular heart disease problem that can be ideally followed up using the support of ultrasound imaging. More often secondary to left heart failure or pulmonary hypertension, tricuspid regurgitation poses unique diagnostic and therapeutic challenges. Doppler quantification of regurgitant flow across the tricuspid valve provides valuable data regarding the hemodynamic severity of the disease. Moreover, echocardiography may even specify possible contributing factors, for example, dilatation or right ventricular dysfunction, thereby enabling clinicians to evaluate the overall impact of tricuspid regurgitation on patients' well-being. The updated guidelines, according to competence, recognize the preeminence of ultrasound in the assessment of valvular disease, specifically that of tricuspid regurgitation, in confirming its primacy in guiding therapy and optimizing results for the corresponding patients (Halvorsen et al., 2022; Levitov et al., 2016) (Figure 6.17).

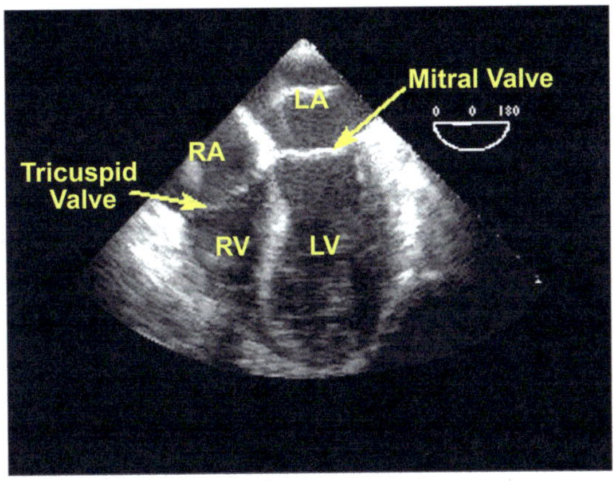

Figure 6.17. Structure of the heart valves in ultrasound.

Source: Echocardiogram; www.daviddarling.info. https://www.daviddarling.info/images/echocardiogram.gif.

6.6. Assessment of Cardiac Motion and Function

Cardiac motion and function measurement is at the core of heart mechanics comprehension and the diagnosis of numerous cardiovascular conditions. One such novel technique that has gained prominence is two-dimensional (2D) speckle tracking imaging. In this case, myocardial deformation is assessed by tracking the speckle pattern motion within the ultrasound images. This allows for a quantitative assessment of wall motion abnormality based on strain value measurements. Recent studies have shown the significance of quantifying left ventricular strain, specifically "global longitudinal strains," with speckle tracking echocardiography. Not only does such an analysis enhance prognostic estimates for cardiac events in heart failure patients, but it also identifies subclinical myocardial damage in various myocardial illnesses, illustrating the methods' scope in cardiology diagnosis (Takigiku, 2016). Based on standard methods, three-dimensional echocardiography is a keynote technology of cardiac motion and function measurement. It provides a clearer view of endocardial structures and allows accurate sonographic angle determination than its two-dimensional counterpart. The regular visualisation of cardiac anatomy of living organisms, including animals, has been facilitated through the use of hi-tech ultrasound machines, for instance, the SONOS 7500. The machine has proven efficient in the pursuit of obtaining accurate representations of cardiac anatomy, and this has helped us understand the heart working in a living state better. Advantages of three-dimensional imaging also comprise its ability to fuse multiple views in a single image, valuable for close anatomical assessment, particularly in small animals like dogs and cats (Nautrup, 2005). Further, the clinical utility of these new imaging techniques cannot be overemphasized. It is a welcome advantage that heart structures are visible in real-time, making it easier for clinicians to comprehend cardiac function and likely pathologies. Recent work has moved toward the description of new concepts and methods for measuring cardiac performance that were not previously possible with two-dimensional echocardiography. The ability to incorporate real-time data in a continuous manner provides the potential for increased accuracy in localizing pathologic motion of the heart and in evaluating the function of heart valves and muscular walls. With ongoing research, these imaging modalities will definitely find an integral place in pediatric cardiology as well, with early diagnosis of congenital heart defects and other related conditions, thus transforming cardiovascular medicine (Takigiku, 2016; Nautrup, 2005).

6.6.1. Evaluation of Wall Motion Abnormalities

Ultrasound evaluation of wall motion abnormalities (WMAs) is extremely crucial in the evaluation of cardiac health, particularly in the diagnosis of myocardial infarction and coronary artery disease. The evaluation is largely based on cardiac motion dynamics, where the contraction and relaxation of the heart muscle are shown. Characterization of normal versus abnormal wall motion relies on a clear understanding of rudimentary cardiac anatomy, since even a small deviation of motion is indicative of underlying disease. Echocardiographic examination allows physicians to visualize regional wall motion and its implications for global cardiac function, providing vital information required in treatment planning and prognostic evaluation. Assessments of this kind are paramount in modern-day cardiology because the prevalence of heart disease in the aged continues to rise, further supporting the need for enhanced training in echocardiography among clinicians, like PAs seeking to specialize in this field (Moon, 2017). One of the main advantages of utilizing ultrasound for the assessment of WMAs is that it is a non-invasive test, coupled with the capacity to image in real time. The ability to simultaneously visualize both structure and function of the heart enables physicians to identify specific regions of myocardium that do not contract adequately and therefore may indicate ischemic heart disease or other cardiac abnormalities. In addition to maximizing diagnostic sensitivity, these assessments also guide therapeutic intervention. For instance, awareness of the specific WMAs' patterns immediately influences therapeutic management, ranging from medical treatment to consideration of revascularization therapy. Furthermore, with the development of therapeutic methods, continuing innovation in echocardiographic technologies and methodologies has the possibility to improve further the validity and sophistication of the evaluation of wall motion abnormality, toward better understanding of the mechanics of the heart in various clinical situations (Kitsiou et al., 2013).

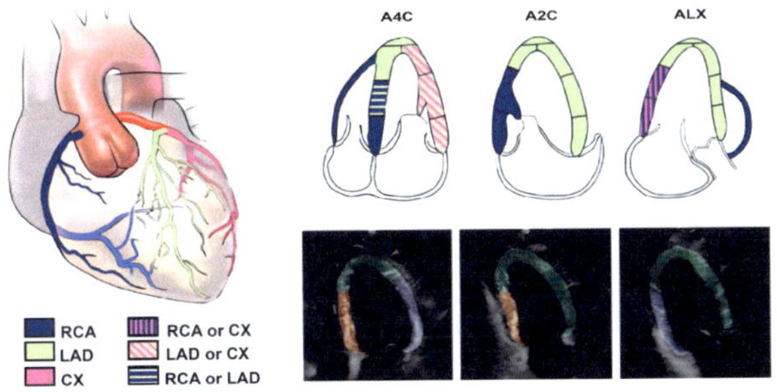

Figure 6.18. Evaluation of wall motion abnormalities.

Source: Lin X, Yang F, Chen Y, et.al (2022). Echocardiography-based AI detection of regional wall motion abnormalities and quantification of cardiac function in myocardial infarction. Front. Cardiovasc. Med. 9:903660. doi: 10.3389/fcvm.2022.903660

The growing recognition of the necessity for WMAs has generated interest in formal training programs that will improve echocardiography skills among healthcare providers, particularly physician assistants (PAs). Such a standardized curriculum that trains PAs in this area can address the current workforce shortage in cardiology and enhance patient care. This type of curriculum would cover not only the technical competence necessary to conduct echocardiograms but also result interpretation within the context of wall motion analysis. Leveraging models such as Entrustable Professional Activities (EPA), which can provide scaffolded learning objectives, future versions of this training might lead to practitioners who are able to both conduct and interpret ultrasound studies independently. In the long term, empowering healthcare workers with specialty skills in the evaluation of wall motion abnormalities can significantly improve the quality and access to cardiovascular care (Moon, 2017) (Figure 6.18).

6.6.2. Measurement of Ejection Fraction

Ejection fraction (EF) measurement is a critical component of assessing cardiac function and one of the key components in diagnosing and treating heart illnesses. Ejection fraction is the proportion of blood expelled from the ventricles with each beat, hence serving as an indicator of myocardial contractility. In practice, ultrasound technologies like echocardiography are preferred methods in the measurement of this value as they are non-invasive and real-time imaging is possible. Clinicians can further correctly calculate EF using the measurements of left ventricular dimensions during diastole and systole. This measurement not only serves a role of utmost importance in diagnosing diseases such as heart failure but also in determining the effectiveness of treatments in the long term, further emphasizing its significance in present-day cardiology. Moreover, the implications of ejection fraction extend beyond simple numeric values because they enable clinicians to evaluate the intrinsic pathophysiology of heart disorders. A low EF typically signifies compromised myocardial function, which may be triggered by multifarious pathological conditions, such as ischemic heart disease or dilated cardiomyopathy. For example, during an experiment performed to investigate the impact of mesenchymal stromal cells (MSCs) on cardiac function in the context of myocardial infarction

(MI), treated animals showed significantly better EF values. This once again justifies the use of EF measurements in research contexts, where they are critical endpoints for assessing therapeutic interventions and recovery processes within the heart (Borgarelli et al., 2013). Lastly, ejection fraction is valuable information in the diagnostic and prognostic indications of heart disease. Beyond its clinical application, ejection fraction measurement can also contribute to cardiac anatomy and ventricular mechanics. Ventricular structure and EF are mutually related to each other in a complex fashion and are generally described using models such as the helical ventricular myocardial band (HVMB) model.

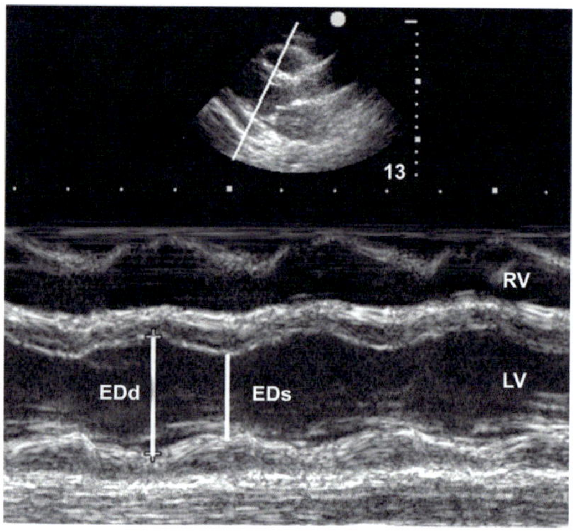

Figure 6.19. Measurement of the ejection fraction using M-mode.

*Source: Gaspar, Heloisa & Morhy, Samira & Lianza, et.al. (2014). Focused cardiac ultrasound: A training course for pediatric intensivists and emergency physicians. BMC medical education. 14. 25. 10.1186/1472-6920-14-25. *

This model attempts to connect the turning motion of the heart, which is attributable to myocardial fiber structure, to effective function (Hoffman, 2017). Understanding these complexities enriches our appreciation of ejection fraction data, enabling us to distinguish between diseased and normal states. The integration of ejection fraction, cardiac anatomy, and advanced imaging modes by employing ultrasound offers the multi-modal technique required to truly understand and evaluate cardiac function, offering a foundation for improved clinical outcomes (Figure 6.19).

6.6.3. Importance of Diastolic Function Assessment

Diastolic function assessment is highly crucial in the assessment of the overall well-being of the heart in patients, particularly in heart failure and other cardiovascular diseases. Diastolic function refers to the efficiency of the heart chambers in filling with blood during relaxation, which is critical in maintaining a healthy cardiac output. An extensive evaluation of diastolic function is typically conducted with echocardiography, which allows clinicians to directly observe myocardial properties and blood flow dynamics. Advances in the technical aspects of ultrasound allow for the identification of subtle impairments in diastolic function which can significantly affect patient management in patients with potential for heart failure. This makes diastolic function assessment an integral part of cardiac evaluation, providing data that can guide therapeutic intervention and improve patient outcome, and highlighting the intricacy of cardiac anatomy, essential to the understanding of underlying pathology and adjustment of treatment (Halvorsen et al., 2022).

Moreover, diastolic function assessment contributes to the diagnosis of hypertension, diabetes, and coronary artery disease, all of which can impede myocardial relaxation. They generate ventricular stiffness and changes in compliance, thus resulting in diastolic dysfunction. Healthcare practitioners utilize some echocardiographic metrics, such as E/A ratios, deceleration times, and tissue Doppler imaging, to quantify diastolic function. Omission or misinterpretation of these metrics would lead to underdiagnosis and inappropriate management of heart failure with preserved ejection fraction (HFpEF), an ailment that is ever-increasing in the geriatric population. Thus, an in-depth understanding of diastolic function is required, with a multidisciplinary approach involving patient-related factors and comorbidities, ultimately facilitating better disease control in more complex cases (Riley et al., 2020). Integration of diastolic function assessment into daily practice also emphasizes the necessity for early intervention among susceptible patients. By identifying diastolic dysfunction based on routine echocardiographic assessment, clinicians can target lifestyle modification, pharmacologic management, and other preventive measures to avert disease progression. Such early interventions have been associated with reduced rates of morbidity and mortality. Evidence increasingly also favors that effective treatment of diastolic dysfunction can dramatically enhance the quality of life of heart failure patients. Overall, evaluation of diastolic function yields a wealth of information that is essential to cardiac health understanding, making it a standard component of ultrasound studies designed to clarify basic cardiac anatomy and function (Halvorsen et al., 2022).

SUMMARY

In integrating data gathered with the examination of fundamental cardiac anatomy with ultrasound, it is evident that the imaging process forms a cornerstone in clinical practice. Ultrasound gives the potential for real-time and non-invasive observation of cardiac structures, with early detection of anomalies that would otherwise not be identified. Its dynamic imaging enhances clinicians' power of evaluation of cardiac morphology and function, emphasizing the value of ultrasound in everyday and critical care settings. In addition, technological advancements are accelerating the potential of ultrasound, broadening its applications and enhancing diagnostic precision, thus consolidating its central position in modern cardiovascular practice. The integration of deep learning methods in ultrasound imaging is a revolutionary leap forward in cardiac diagnosis. By using the power of machine learning, healthcare providers are now able to handle complex image data more easily, which translates into more precise segmentation of cardiac lesions and structures. Notably, automation's application can greatly relieve clinicians of their computational burden and reduce the likelihood of errors caused by humans, thus leading to improved patient outcomes. Additionally, with the continued improvement of the methods, they eliminate issues such as variability in interpretations and standardization in measurements, thus enhancing the reliability of ultrasound diagnostics in cardiology (Hesamian et al., 2019). In the future, the fate of cardiac ultrasound will undoubtedly be shaped by persistent technological advancements and the increasing incorporation of artificial intelligence into medical imaging. This development can potentially further refine ultrasound techniques such that cardiac anatomy evaluations become more precise and accessible. As deep learning penetrates this domain further, it not only empowers clinicians with greater diagnostic tools but also opens doors to new avenues of research that could potentially reshape therapeutic methods. The collective knowledge realized with the integration of cardiac anatomy via ultrasound and new technologies suggests a solid foundation for cardiovascular management in the future, promising developments that will deeply affect patient care and treatment plans (Shen et al., 2017).

While assessing simple cardiac structure using ultrasound, it is essential to highlight the significance of the process of learning structures being investigated in echocardiography. This non-invasive imaging technique provides an in-depth view of morphology and cardiac function. Such details like the chambers of the heart—the right and left atria and ventricles—and related structures like the valves are thoroughly investigated. The successful imaging of these structures enables clinicians to identify abnormalities such as valvular stenosis or regurgitation, which are decisive in diagnosing heart disease. Moreover, ultrasound makes it possible the measurement of ejection fraction so that practitioners can quantify the heart's pumping capacity. By emphasizing such structural and functional particulars, a more comprehensive understanding of cardiac anatomy is possible, ultimately leading to clinical decision-making and improved patient care. The application of ultrasound in the evaluation of cardiac anatomy extends beyond mere visualization and also includes dynamic observation of blood flow patterns. Echo Doppler technology enables doctors to measure the velocity and direction of blood flow across heart valves and chambers and thus derive valuable information regarding hemodynamic status. Such an evaluation is crucial for diagnosing conditions such as congenital heart defects and heart failure. Specifically, altered patterns of flow may represent turbulence that may be a sign of underlying cardiac disease. Integration of these hemodynamic tests with structural tests renders cardiac function and diagnosis more comprehensible and accurate. The complementarity between static images and dynamic flow analysis reminds us of the multiplanar nature of cardiac evaluations and reasserts the supremacy of ultrasound in contemporary cardiology. Lastly, the employment of ultrasound in teaching cardiac anatomy cannot be overemphasized. With its real-time imaging ability , ultrasound is a useful teaching tool for residents and students. By virtue of seeing live demonstrations and interactive simulations, the process of learning is enhanced so that students can bridge theoretical principles to practice. That ultrasound scanning is a hands-on process also supports the development of skills and retention of cardiac anatomy that may otherwise be hard to communicate through other methods. Therefore, ultrasound proficiency not only enhances the anatomical expertise of students but also equips students with skills that can be universally applied in various clinical environments. Drawing attention to this learning component reaffirms the place of ultrasound as a cornerstone in understanding fundamental cardiac anatomy, which in turn leads to improved patient care and advancement of medical practice.

CLOSER LOOK

POINT-OF-CARE ULTRASOUND (POCUS)

Point-of-care ultrasound (POCUS) refers to the use by the responsible clinician at the bedside of ultrasonography to answer targeted diagnostic questions or guide immediate medical interventions. In contrast with the traditional ultrasound performed in radiology facilities by sonographers or radiologists, POCUS becomes part of the clinical workflow and allows for instant evaluation and real-time decision-making. It has become an essential tool in a broad range of specialties, including emergency medicine, critical care, internal medicine, anesthesiology, pediatrics, and primary care. The inherent advantage of POCUS lies in its immediacy and ability to provide dynamic, non-invasive anatomical structure and physiological function visualization without the time lag and logistics of formal imaging. POCUS can be utilized by clinicians to evaluate cardiac function, detect pneumothorax or pleural effusions, evaluate abdominal free fluid, detect hydronephrosis, guide vascular access, and scan fetal well-being, among many other applications. In emergency settings, for example, POCUS can be utilized in an effort to perform the Focused Assessment with Sonography in Trauma (FAST) evaluation to effectively detect internal bleeding. It helps in critical care by providing assessment of volume status, cardiac output, and causes of shock through measurement of ventricular contractility, IVC variation, and pericardial effusion.

Technological advances have been the reason behind the revolution of POCUS. There are now wireless, handheld ultrasound machines that are compact, very portable, and simple to use, so clinicians can simply put them in their pockets and utilize them as a routine aspect of everyday practice. The machines give excellent-resolution imaging, Doppler, and cloud connectivity, and some of them even contain artificial intelligence to assist with image acquisition and interpretation. The expansion of POCUS is also driven by its value in procedural guidance. Clinicians can use ultrasound to make central line placement more successful and safe, as well as thoracentesis, paracentesis, nerve blocks, and joint injections, decreasing complications and enhancing patient comfort. Furthermore, POCUS is of significant educational value, making it easier for medical students and learners to better learn anatomy, physiology, and pathophysiology through direct visualization.

Even with growing utility, POCUS is not without limitations. Operator-dependent, it depends on proper training, experience, and interpretive ability to be effective. Erroneous results can lead to errors of diagnosis or missed diagnosis unless used in the context of appropriate clinical correlation. Thus, formal training programs, standardized protocols, and mechanisms for quality control are needed to allow for safe and effective utilization. Professional accrediting organizations and medical societies currently emphasize the requirement for competency-based education and certification in POCUS. The future of POCUS is being transformed with integration into electronic medical records, AI-enhanced imaging, and increased application in remote or resource-constrained settings where access to high-end imaging is restricted. In global health, POCUS is revolutionary because it enables frontline providers to diagnose and track conditions such as tuberculosis, heart failure, and obstetric emergencies when other modalities are unavailable. Finally, point-of-care ultrasound is transforming clinical diagnosis practice by bringing imaging to the patient, enhancing physical examination, streamlining diagnosis time, guiding therapy, and enhancing outcomes in a broad variety of healthcare environments.

References

1. Andrietti, S., D'Agostino, S., Panarelli, M., Sarno, L., Pisaturo, M. L., & Fantasia, I. (2024). False-positive diagnosis of congenital heart defects at first-trimester ultrasound: An Italian multicentric study. *Diagnostics, 14*. https://www.semanticscholar.org/paper/e59e2acff83c33611c4f880b53915baec5e3360e (accessed on 12th July 2025).
2. Arango, S., Gorbaty, B., Buyck, D., Johnson, J. E., Porter, S., Iaizzo, P. A., & Perry, T. E. (2022). A free-access online interactive simulator to enhance perioperative transesophageal echocardiography training using a high-fidelity human heart 3D model. *Journal of Cardiothoracic and Vascular Anesthesia, 37*, 308–313. https://doi.org/10.1053/j.jvca.2022.10.012 (accessed on 12th July 2025).
3. Arango, S., Gorbaty, B., Tomhave, N., Shervheim, D., Buyck, D., Porter, S., Iaizzo, P. A., et al. (2022). A high-resolution virtual reality-based simulator to enhance perioperative echocardiography training. *Journal of Cardiothoracic and Vascular Anesthesia, 37*, 299–305. https://doi.org/10.1053/j.jvca.2022.09.004 (accessed on 12th July 2025).
4. Bai, W., Chen, C., Duan, J., et al. (2025). Deep learning for cardiac image segmentation: A review.https://core.ac.uk/download/266989979.pdf (accessed on 12th July 2025).
5. Bao, Z. (2024). Application of ultrasound diagnosis in cardiac and liver diseases. *Applied and Computational Engineering*. https://www.semanticscholar.org/paper/8407d5d3f54376 9f5eeb0cc30d7c107cdb30399a (accessed on 12th July 2025).
6. Bavo, A.M., Pouch, A.M., Degroote, J., Vierendeels, J., Gorman, J.H., Gorman, R.C. & Segers, P. Patient-specific CFD simulation of intraventricular haemodynamics based on 3D ultrasound imaging. BioMed Eng OnLine 15, 107 (2016). https://doi.org/10.1186/s12938-016-0231-9 (accessed on 12th July 2025).
7. Bilardo, C. M., Chaoui, R., Hyett, J., Kagan, K. O., Karim, J., Papageorghiou, A. T., Poon, L. C., et al. (2023). ISUOG Practice Guidelines (updated): Performance of 11–14-week ultrasound scan. *Ultrasound in Obstetrics and Gynecology, 61*, 127–143. https://doi.org/10.1002/uog.26106 (accessed on 12th July 2025).
8. Bingisser, R., Byrne, C., Fox, J. C., et al. (2019). A prospective evaluation of point-of-care ultrasound teaching in Switzerland. https://core.ac.uk/download/231897443.pdf (accessed on 12th July 2025).
9. Borgarelli, M., Hageman, K. S., Lutjemeier, B., et al. (2013). Wharton's jelly or bone marrow mesenchymal stromal cells improve cardiac function following myocardial infarction for more than 32 weeks in a rat model: A preliminary report. https://core.ac.uk/download/10653310.pdf (accessed on 12th July 2025).
10. Brock, K. K., Mutic, S., McNutt, T., Li, H., & Kessler, M. L. (2017). Use of image registration and fusion algorithms and techniques in radiotherapy: Report of the AAPM Radiation Therapy Committee Task Group No. 132. *Medical Physics, 44*, e43–e76. https://doi.org/10.1002/mp.12256 (accessed on 12th July 2025).
11. Calkins, H., Hindricks, G., Cappato, R., Kim, Y. H., Saad, E., Aguinaga, L., Akar, J. G., et al. (2017). 2017 HRS/EHRA/ECAS/APHRS/SOLAECE expert consensus statement on catheter and surgical ablation of atrial fibrillation: Executive summary. *Journal of Arrhythmia, 33*, 369–409. https://doi.org/10.1016/j.joa.2017.08.001 (accessed on 12th July 2025).

12. Chen, C., Qin, C., Qiu, H., Tarroni, G., Duan, J., Bai, W., & Rueckert, D. (2020). Deep learning for cardiac image segmentation: A review. *Frontiers in Cardiovascular Medicine, 7*. https://doi.org/10.3389/fcvm.2020.00025 (accessed on 12th July 2025).

13. Claassen, J. A. H. R., Thijssen, D. H. J., Panerai, R. B., & Faraci, F. M. (2021). Regulation of cerebral blood flow in humans: Physiology and clinical implications of autoregulation. *Physiological Reviews, 101*, 1487–1559. https://doi.org/10.1152/physrev.00022.2020 (accessed on 12th July 2025).

14. Das, N., & Yip, M. (2017). Robot autonomy for surgery. http://arxiv.org/abs/1707.03080 (accessed on 12th July 2025).

15. Deliverska, E., Aleksandrova, M., & Chaveeva, P. (2025). Importance of prenatal diagnosis and multidisciplinary care in orofacial cleft: Report of three cases. Embryology understanding and risk factors. *Pharmacia*. https://www.semanticscholar.org/paper/9ecf6f6a31012261020e928e87615806e28e6bb7 (accessed on 12th July 2025).

16. Ding, K., Chen, M., Li, P., Xie, Z., Zhang, H., Kou, R., Xu, J., et al. (2024). The effect of simulation of sectional human anatomy using ultrasound on students' learning outcomes and satisfaction in echocardiography education: A pilot randomized controlled trial. *BMC Medical Education, 24*. https://www.semanticscholar.org/paper/f17a4db870733e5a8583ac3c6316131c82b09711 (accessed on 12th July 2025).

17. Ghorbani, A., Ouyang, D., Abid, A., He, B., Chen, J. H., Harrington, R. A., Liang, D., et al. (2020). Deep learning interpretation of echocardiograms. *npj Digital Medicine, 3*. https://doi.org/10.1038/s41746-019-0216-8 (accessed on 12th July 2025).

18. Guo, Z., Yan, Y., Zhili, Y., Juhua, X., Xiao, X., Jia, C., Luo, H., et al. (2024). Evaluation of atrioventricular valve regurgitation in detection of atrioventricular septal defects at first trimester ultrasound. *International Journal of Clinical Practice*. https://www.semanticscholar.org/paper/a3c26c2e151540e2ff396e5df536893def840062 (accessed on 12th July 2025).

19. Halvorsen, S., Mehilli, J., Cassese, S., Hall, T. S., Abdelhamid, M., Barbato, E., De Hert, S., et al. (2022). 2022 ESC Guidelines on cardiovascular assessment and management of patients undergoing non-cardiac surgery. *European Heart Journal, 43*, 3826–3924. https://doi.org/10.1093/eurheartj/ehac270 (accessed on 12th July 2025).

20. Hesamian, M. H., Jia, W., He, X., & Kennedy, P. (2019). Deep learning techniques for medical image segmentation: Achievements and challenges. *Journal of Digital Imaging, 32*, 582–596. https://doi.org/10.1007/s10278-019-00227-x (accessed on 12th July 2025).

21. Hoffman, J. I. E. (2017). Will the real ventricular architecture please stand up? Physiol Rep. 5(18):e13404. doi: 10.14814/phy2.13404. https://core.ac.uk/download/323072376.pdf (accessed on 12th July 2025).

22. Höglund, K. (2007). Systolic ejection murmurs and the left ventricular outflow tract in boxer dogs. https://core.ac.uk/download/11695170.pdf (accessed on 12th July 2025).

23. Kitsiou, A., Caforio, A. L. P., Porta-Sanchez, A., Vahanian, A., Iung, B., Carrera, C., Szymanski, C., et al. (2013). ESC core curriculum for the general cardiologist (2013). https://core.ac.uk/download/55756305.pdf (accessed on 12th July 2025).

24. Knopfholz, J., Margraf, L. B., Nadalin Júnior, O., & Machado, A. B. (2023). Importance of incorporating ultrasonography into undergraduate medicine practices. *Concilium*. https://

www.semanticscholar.org/paper/2f84c6b0c04948daba759c0ce57ef92abd0cfc99 (accessed on 12th July 2025).

25. Levitov, A., Frankel, H. L., Blaivas, M., Kirkpatrick, A. W., Su, E., Evans, D. P., Summerfield, D. T., et al. (2016). Guidelines for the appropriate use of bedside general and cardiac ultrasonography in the evaluation of critically ill patients—Part II: Cardiac ultrasonography. *Critical Care Medicine, 44*, 1206–1227. https://doi.org/10.1097/ccm.0000000000001847 (accessed on 12th July 2025).

26. Moon, S. (2017). Echocardiography curriculum development for physician assistants using entrustable professional activities. https://core.ac.uk/download/215924737.pdf (accessed on 12th July 2025).

27. Focal Spot, Summer/Fall 2007 (2007). Bernard Becker Medical Library Archives. Washington University School of Medicine https://core.ac.uk/download/129069359.pdf (accessed on 12th July 2025).

28. Focal Spot, Fall/Winter 2010/2011. Bernard Becker Medical Library Archives. Washington University School of Medicine. https://core.ac.uk/download/129069384.pdf (accessed on 12th July 2025).

29. Nautrup, C. P. (2005). Real-time three-dimensional echocardiography, a new approach to cardiac anatomy in live dogs and cats. *Anatomia Histologia Embryologia, 34*, 40–40. https://www.semanticscholar.org/paper/505116799c016af7d1d4bf4ddb80181b167eea4c (accessed on 12th July 2025).

30. Paterson, C. (1990). The normal canine heart: Anatomical criteria for the study of real-time ultrasonography and Doppler echocardiography. https://core.ac.uk/download/286711348.pdf (accessed on 12th July 2025).

31. Peters, A., & Patil, P. V. (2018). Tele-echocardiography: Enhancing quality at the point-of-care. *Heart, 105*, 264–265. https://www.semanticscholar.org/paper/02ea308b23b31a48474d1d55038c338f12641db7 (accessed on 12th July 2025).

32. Riley, R. F., Henry, T. D., Mahmud, E., Kirtane, A. J., Brilakis, E. S., Goyal, A., Grines, C. L., et al. (2020). *SCAI* position statement on optimal percutaneous coronary interventional therapy for complex coronary artery disease. *Catheterization and Cardiovascular Interventions, 96*, 346–362. https://doi.org/10.1002/ccd.28994 (accessed on 12th July 2025).

33. Rychik, J., Atz, A. M., Celermajer, D. S., Deal, B. J., Gatzoulis, M. A., Gewillig, M., Hsia, T. Y., et al. (2019). Evaluation and management of the child and adult with Fontan circulation: A scientific statement from the American Heart Association. *Circulation, 140.* https://doi.org/10.1161/cir.0000000000000696 (accessed on 12th July 2025).

34. Salomon, L., Alfirević, Ž., Berghella, V., Bilardo, C. M., Chalouhi, G. E., da Silva Costa, F., Hernández-Andrade, E., et al. (2022). *ISUOG* Practice Guidelines (updated): Performance of the routine mid-trimester fetal ultrasound scan. *Ultrasound in Obstetrics and Gynecology, 59*, 840–856. https://doi.org/10.1002/uog.24888 (accessed on 12th July 2025).

35. Shen, D., Wu, G., & Suk, H. I. (2017). Deep learning in medical image analysis. *Annual Review of Biomedical Engineering, 19*, 221–248. https://doi.org/10.1146/annurev-bioeng-071516-044442 (accessed on 12th July 2025).

36. Sorrell, V., & Kumar, S. (2011). Doppler contrast echocardiography. https://www.semanticscholar.org/paper/8ee9e1ade2e5698d2148f031dddaf82e717166f6 (accessed on 12th July 2025).

37. Tabakov, S. (2010). Handbook of Physics in Medicine and Biology. *Physics in Medicine and Biology, 55*, 6571–6572. https://www.semanticscholar.org/paper/d057838895196dd133c61f27afc3490065392315 (accessed on 12th July 2025).

38. Takigiku, K. (2016). Two-dimensional speckle tracking echocardiography and its application to children. *Pediatric Cardiology and Cardiac Surgery, 32*, 473–484. https://www.semanticscholar.org/paper/87811483748b2d230d451693b12a27b41ee963bc (accessed on 12th July 2025).

39. Virani, S. S., Newby, L. K., Arnold, S. V., Bittner, V., Brewer, L. C., Demeter, S. H., Dixon, D. L., et al. (2023). 2023 AHA/ACC/ACCP/ASPC/NLA/PCNA guideline for the management of patients with chronic coronary disease: A report of the American Heart Association/American College of Cardiology Joint Committee on Clinical Practice Guidelines. *Circulation, 148*. https://doi.org/10.1161/cir.0000000000001168 (accessed on 12th July 2025).

40. Wang, Q., Wang, F., Jiang, C., & Guo, J. (2025). The role of cardiac ultrasound virtual simulation technology in the construction of clinical diagnostic reasoning of structural heart diseases. *BMC Medical Education, 25*. https://www.semanticscholar.org/paper/161dca8f70d62a3317ab8f01ea460c250ed208ab (accessed on 12th July 2025).

41. Wiegers, S. E., Ryan, T., Arrighi, J. A., Brown, S. M., Canaday, B., Damp, J. B., Díaz-Gómez, J. L., et al. (2019). 2019 ACC/AHA/ASE advanced training statement on echocardiography (revision of the 2003 ACC/AHA clinical competence statement on echocardiography). *Catheterization and Cardiovascular Interventions, 94*, 481–505. https://doi.org/10.1002/ccd.28313 (accessed on 12th July 2025).

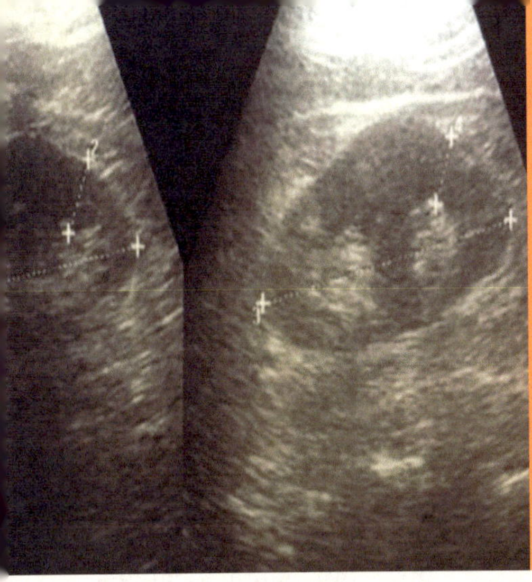

Chapter 7

ABDOMINAL WALL AND PERITONEUM ULTRASOUND

Contents

Introduction

The use of ultrasound to evaluate the abdominal wall and peritoneum is an important milestone in the history of diagnostic imaging modalities. It is a non-invasive tool that has emerged as an important asset for clinicians aiming to comprehend many of the abdominal disorders, thus rendering itself invaluable in the practice of gastroenterology and surgery. Ultrasound offers real-time imaging, which not only enhances visualization of the organs but also facilitates enhanced decision-making on diagnosis and treatment. That it can evaluate both superficial abdominal wall structures, such as muscles and fat, as well as deeper anatomical layers, such as the peritoneum, highlights its effectiveness and versatility in practice. In addition, as abdominal ultrasound technology advances, it is essential to examine its clinical applications in depth, particularly in identifying pathologies that would have otherwise gone undetected. To realize the role of abdominal wall and peritoneum ultrasound, it is essential to look at its application in varying clinical settings. This imaging technique helps in hernia, abscess, and tumor diagnosis and also in therapeutic procedures that enhance the outcome for patients. Observational studies emphasize the superiority of ultrasound over other imaging techniques, especially where local expertise exists, which supports its inclusion in the practice routine. For instance, ESGE recommends specific ultrasound-guided interventions in the case of obstructed biliary drainage, emphasizing the need for skill and experience in carrying out such interventions effectively. Accordingly, the addition of ultrasound not only enhances diagnostic effectiveness but also procedural safety and efficacy in the management of complex conditions within the abdominal cavity. Besides being specific to diagnosis, the role of ultrasound is evolving in therapeutic purposes. The importance of ultrasound in solving problems in abdominal disorders cannot be overstated. Techniques such as high-intensity focused ultrasound (HIFU) are explored for their promise in non-surgical oncological therapies, demonstrating the potential of the technology beyond imaging. This has led to a growing body of research looking into improving localized treatment for peritoneal and abdominal wall malignancies, hence increasing the use of ultrasound in cancer treatment protocols. In agreement with current literature, utilization of techniques like thermal ablation can enhance outcomes in the treatment of patients when integrated with proper imaging guidance, and thus further narrow the divide between therapeutic and diagnostic practices. As abdominal ultrasound evolves as a field, ongoing research into its applications will definitely impact the future of abdominal management and care (Figure 7.1).

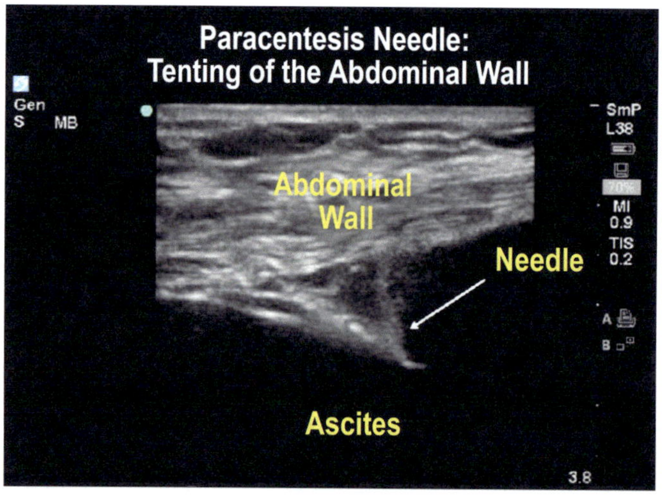

Figure 7.1. Abdominal wall and peritoneum ultrasound.

Source: Ennis, Josh & Schultz, Geoffrey & Perera, et.al. (2014). Ultrasound for Detection of Ascites and for Guidance of the Paracentesis Procedure: Technique and Review of the Literature. International Journal of Clinical Medicine. 05. 1277-1293. 10.4236/ijcm.2014.520163.

Definition of Abdominal Wall and Peritoneum Ultrasound

The abdominal wall and peritoneum ultrasound is a fundamental non-invasive imaging technique utilized to assess various medical conditions affecting the abdominal structures and organs. The abdominal wall ultrasound, through the application of high-frequency sound waves, creates images of the abdominal wall, which encompasses fascial layers, muscle, and skin, as well as the peritoneum, the lining of the abdominal cavity. With the ability to provide real-time images, ultrasound facilitates the evaluation of such conditions as hernias, tumors, and infection. Its use in identifying fluid collections or changes in abdominal wall shape also indicates its usefulness in medical applications as a diagnostic aid. Its advantages are the lack of ionizing radiation and the ability to perform studies at the bedside, increasing access to required diagnostic capability for patients, particularly in emergency and outpatient settings. The value of ultrasound as a tool in diagnosis is also augmented by its application in monitoring postoperative states. For instance, in rectus diastasis surgical repair patients, abdominal wall ultrasounds are at the core of monitoring healing status, as outlined in current research. The modality allows practitioners to assess linea alba contraction—a primary predictor of successful surgical outcome—while guiding follow-up rehabilitation protocol. A trial of postpartum patients with rectus diastasis revealed through ultrasound studies that 82.2% achieved complete repair of the linea alba after four months of surgery, confirming the utility of this process to quantify postoperative recovery (Olsson et al., 2022). Such findings support the employment of ultrasound in standardized follow-up care for improved long-term results in such patient populations. In addition, ultrasound is an essential instrument in evaluating not just the abdominal wall but also peritoneal structures and bordering organs. Visualization of the peritoneum is very important, especially for diseases like abdominal aortic aneurysms (AAA), whose undiagnosed existence could cause severe health consequences. Research indicates that variability in diagnostic criteria and methods can lead to variations in AAA prevalence detection, backing the necessity of standardized ultrasound protocols in clinical practice (Wanhainen et al., 2001). The inclusion of abdominal wall and peritoneum ultrasound findings in an overall diagnostic scheme can enhance abdominal conditions comprehension, thereby encouraging timely interventions. Finally, the definition and usage of this imaging modality attest to its integral contribution to contemporary diagnostic medicine and surgical planning.

Importance of Ultrasound in Abdominal Assessments

Ultrasound scanning has become an essential imaging tool in abdominal exams due to its non-invasive nature and real-time scanning. The use of high-frequency sound waves enables abdominal wall and peritoneum visualization, which aids in the detection of several conditions. It is particularly valuable for the detection of fluid accumulations, gallstones, and organ abnormalities without subjecting patients to ionizing radiation. Additionally, the ability of ultrasound to visualize blood flow by Doppler methods increases its value in the assessment of vascular structures and also in the detection of complications like thrombosis. The ease and speed of ultrasound investigations make it a very valuable tool in emergency situations, where speed can impact clinical decision-making considerably. In gynecologic pathology, the role of ultrasound is especially valuable in the diagnosis of endometriosis, one of women's most serious health problems, which influences women's lives in a significant way. The threat of abdominal pain and infertility at risk makes it crucial to make an early and accurate diagnosis. Ultrasound allows visualization of endometriotic lesions in the abdominal cavity, enhancing the knowledge of the scope of the disease and therapeutic modalities. As highlighted in recent literature, endometriosis etiological factors, such as several factors, can improve patient outcomes by intervening (Targeted interventions). Ultrasound application within the diagnosis protocol of such intricate pathologies is an obligation, emphasizing its relevance in ensuring reproductive health care (Smolarz et al., 2021). Furthermore, the ERAS guidelines emphasize the importance of using advanced imaging modalities, including ultrasound, in optimizing postoperative results after colorectal surgery. By guaranteeing precise assessments of the peritoneum and the abdominal wall, ultrasound optimizes surgical planning as well as postoperative care. The ERAS protocol requires multimodal care pathways where imaging contributes a revolutionary step towards patient management. For instance, preoperative ultrasound can identify possible complications such as intra-abdominal abscesses, thus allowing early interventions. The use of ultrasound in clinical practice is important, with significant evidence brought forth in the comprehensive guidelines formulated by the ERAS Society, based on quality evidence to support its recommendations (Gustafsson et al., 2018). This procedural focus on ultrasound within surgical contexts echoes its increasing appreciation as a foundation in today's abdominal evaluations (Figure 7.2).

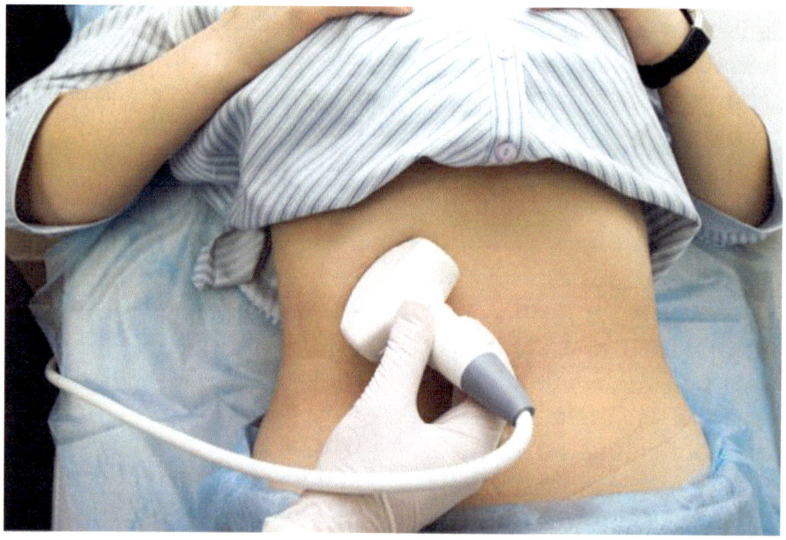

Figure 7.2. Ultrasound in abdominal assessments.

Source: https://cdn-apbgn.nitrocdn.com/TJhToCeBdthTVvVQvsfvpvDNSNjYOavZ/assets/images/optimized/rev-2df6489/ultrasound.ie/wp-content/uploads/2015/05/Abdominal-Ultrasound-Scans-Dublin-2.jpg.

7.1. Anatomy of the Abdominal Wall

Abdominal wall anatomy is a significant part of the total abdominal structure and function. Abdominal wall anatomy consists of several layers, including skin, subcutaneous tissue, muscular layers, and peritoneum. Muscular layers are particularly vital as they consist of external oblique, internal oblique, transversus abdominis, and rectus abdominis muscles, each playing distinct roles regarding intra-abdominal pressure maintenance and movement. These muscles create a critical protective covering for the organs inside and assist in respiration and posture functions. Understanding these layers through ultrasound scans forms the core of the diagnosis of many conditions, including hernias and other complications arising from surgical procedures (Santos et al., 2025). This stratified approach not only enhances their functional significance but also indicates the necessity of using ultrasound technology in the clinical setting to evaluate these structures as a whole. Ultrasound technology has revolutionized the approach to imaging the abdominal wall and its components. With real-time imaging, clinicians are able to evaluate the anatomy of the abdominal wall with excellent accuracy. This painless procedure allows dynamic evaluation of muscle contraction, blood flow, and potential pathology. The utility of ultrasound is more than imaging; ultrasound can be employed to guide therapeutic interventions, such as the placement of local anesthetics for postoperative pain management. Ultrasound-guided interventions have the potential to enhance treatment accuracy, thereby diminishing complications and improving patient outcomes (Vereen et al., 2025). These advances underscore the necessity of making imaging modalities available in clinical practice in order to enable better understanding of the anatomy of the abdominal wall and its utility in various clinical contexts. Moreover, the complexity of the abdominal wall underscores the necessity for comprehensive anatomical training among health care providers, particularly among surgeons. Complications such as ventral incisional hernias indicate the fine balance between the anatomy of abdominal walls and surgical outcomes. Anatomy layers can be compromised with surgical interventions to lead to complications after surgery, which need to be addressed with great deal of caution. Examples are procedures such as the administration of botulinum toxin A under ultrasound guidance, which has been devised to decrease tension and promote healing after operations (Santos et al., 2025). In addition, the use of regional analgesic procedures, such as ultrasound-guided abdominal wall blocks, has become increasingly popular, providing effective pain management options and facilitating recovery paths for patients (Vereen et al., 2025). Overall, an in-depth understanding of the abdominal wall is crucial for the advancement of surgical methods and better patient care in abdominal surgery (Figure 7.3).

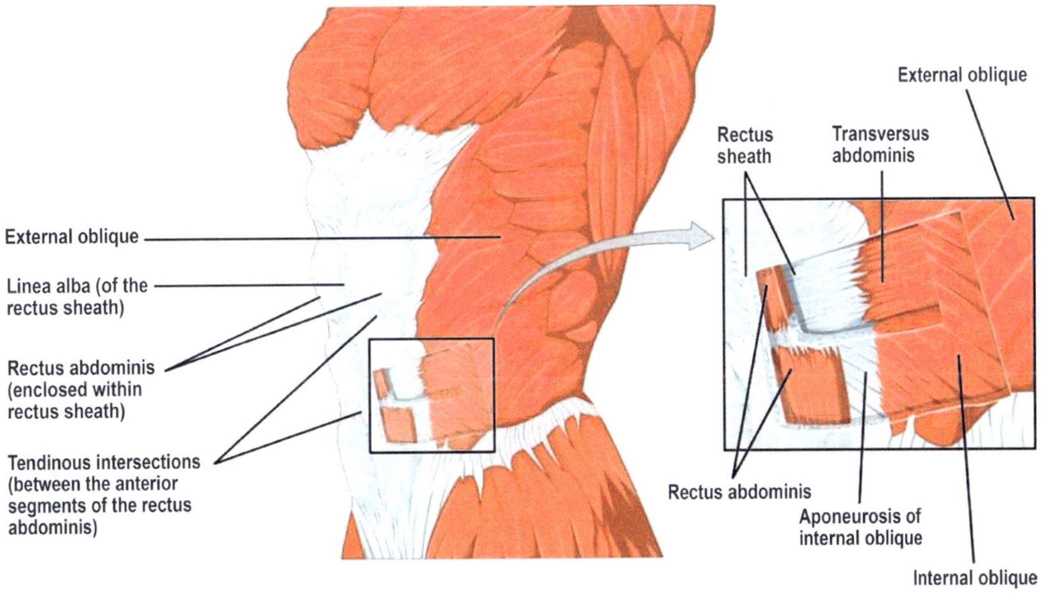

Figure 7.3. Anatomy of the abdominal wall.

Source: Oliver Jones (2024). The Anterolateral Abdominal Wall. teachmeanatomy.info https://teachmeanatomy.info/wp-content/uploads/Muscles-of-the-Anterolateral-Abdominal-Wall-1024x604.jpg.

7.1.1. Layers of the Abdominal Wall

The wall of the abdomen consists of a number of layers responsible for its structure, function, and covering function over internal organs. Understanding these layers is significant in diagnosis as well as surgery, particularly in ultrasound scans. The most external of these layers is the skin, which acts as an environmental covering. Under the superficial fascia is a fatty suprapubic layer and a membranous layer, which are also subdivisions of the superficial fascia. This subdivision allows for movement and flexibility, and a storage place for fat. Under the superficial fascia are muscles such as the rectus abdominis, external oblique, and internal oblique, which strengthen the wall as well as assist with some of the body's movements, including respiration and rotation of the trunk. Such multi-level intricacy is a must in assessing pathologies using ultrasound technology. Below the muscular layer, the transversalis fascia is located, a crucial yet very thin layer that cushions the abdominal muscles against the peritoneum. The fascia plays a role in intra-abdominal pressure maintenance and abdominal wall support. Furthermore, its architectural properties are needed for ultrasound imaging as it helps demarcate the abdominal wall from the internal organs. Within the clinical setting, recognition of the layers of the abdominal wall becomes paramount, especially in assessing conditions such as endometriosis or hernia, where pathology can occur within these layers. The ability of ultrasound to generate images of these discrete layers allows clinicians to assess potential pathologies in real time, making it an important tool within preoperative diagnosis and planning. More understanding of these layers is important, particularly with respect to surgical operations and outcomes. The peritoneum lining the abdominal cavity must also be considered in terms of the abdominal wall's layers. Two layers are formed: the parietal peritoneum that lines the abdominal wall and the visceral peritoneum that envelops the internal organs. The interface between the two layers is crucial for the diagnosis of a number of clinical conditions, and ultrasound is a suitable modality to visualize this delicate structure. Alteration in the peritoneum may be a reflection of pathological processes like ascites, infection, or malignancy. Further, research has come into perspective the importance of universal classification systems like the #Enzian classification that not only includes endometriosis but also its relationship with the peritoneum and surrounding structures (Smolarz et al., 2021; Keckstein et al., 2021). Understanding both the anatomy of the defective abdominal wall in layers as well as its relationship with the peritoneum enhances the efficiency of diagnostics, thus improving patient management outcomes (Figure 7.4).

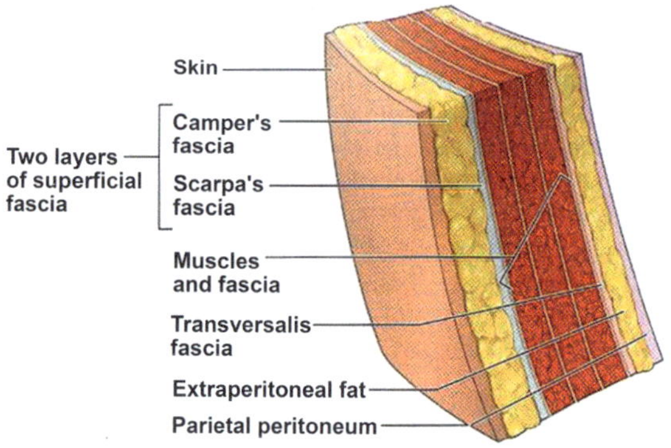

Figure 7.4. Abdominal wall layers.

Source: https://i.pinimg.com/564x/4e/c1/2c/4ec12c69ed371294566fe1bb93446de2.jpg.

7.1.2. Key Muscles Involved

The intricate anatomy of the abdominal wall consists of some significant groups of muscles that assist in core stability, protecting the internal organs, and facilitating different movements. The chief muscles involved are the rectus abdominis, internal obliques, and external obliques, along with the transverse abdominis. The rectus abdominis, or the six-pack muscle, is a vertically-oriented muscle within the abdominal cavity that assists with flexion of the trunk and helps maintain posture. The external and internal obliques, positioned laterally, function synergistically to assist with rotation and lateral flexion of the trunk. The innermost of the three abdominal muscle layers, the transverse abdominis, acts as a natural corset and is involved in the control of intra-abdominal pressure and, hence, not just in movement, but also in the structural integrity of the abdominal wall. Ultrasound imaging is a primary modality for the assessment of the anatomy and the function of these abdominal muscles, both in healthy and symptomatic subjects. It has been established through research that ultrasonic muscle thickness measurement can reveal significant differences in muscle structure, particularly in conditions such as bruxism. As is illustrated by a study into abdominal muscle thickness among patients with and without bruxism, ultrasound yielded useful information in relation to oral health and the activation of abdominal muscles. More specifically, statistically significant increases in muscle thickness with voluntary grinding were found in the bruxism group compared to their non-bruxism counterparts, demonstrating how neurological and muscular interactions may influence the dynamics of the abdominal wall (Yela-Lorenzo et al., 2025). This demonstrates the possible applications of ultrasound in the clinic to enhance knowledge of muscle function and behavior. Furthermore, the role of ultrasound is more than just its anatomical assessment; it gives vital information regarding the functional efficacy of various interventions attempting to enhance abdominal wall integrity. For instance, therapeutic interventions such as high-intensity focused ultrasound (HIFU) have been employed in treating conditions such as abdominal wall endometriosis (AWE). Studies have shown HIFU treatment as an effective way for lesion size reduction and pain relief, with lesion diameter and sonication power being key factors in determining treatment outcomes (Cheng et al., 2024). As ultrasound technology continues to evolve, its use in clinics should also improve our present understanding of the abdominal musculature and contribute to the development of more accurate therapeutic approaches against some abdominal wall diseases (Figure 7.5).

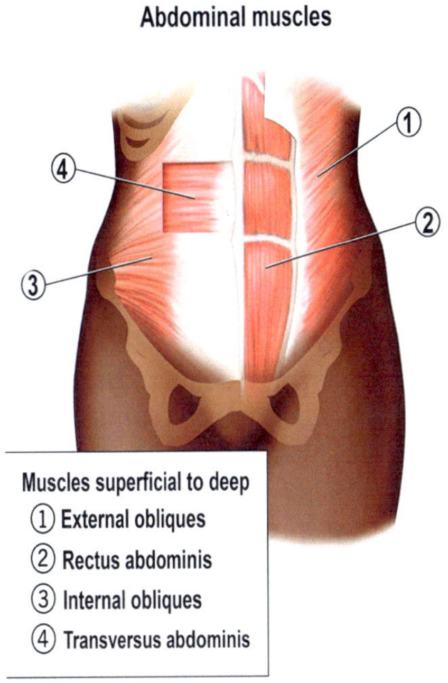

Figure 7.5. Key muscles involved in the abdominal wall.

Source: Abdominal Muscles. my.clevelandclinic. org. https://my.clevelandclinic.org/-/scassets/images/org/health/articles/abdominal-muscles.jpg.

7.1.3. Role of Fascia and Connective Tissue

Understanding the role of fascia and connective tissue is valuable in abdominal wall and peritoneum ultrasound, as these tissues provide essential support and integrity to the abdominal cavity. Fascia is a thick connective tissue that envelops muscles, organs, and other structures and is central in supporting their placement and function. Fascia serves as a conduit for vessels and nerves, providing continuity between various parts of the body. Above all, the fascia in the abdominal wall is crucial to providing the structural support for the abdominal organs and preventing excessive mobility and potential injury. Identification of fascia features during the performance of ultrasound imaging can aid in detecting pathologies, that is, hernias or tumors that could disrupt normal fascial architecture, warranting further investigation and management strategies (Alvarez-Hornia et al., 2022). That between fascia and the surrounding connective tissue is also essential in operative conditions, especially abdominal. Laparotomy exposes the interactions of the two tissues and accentuates the roles played by them during recovery and healing. Repair modalities for vault prolapse are a good example, in which a proper understanding of fascial mechanics and their coordination with connective tissues is necessary. Research suggests that the use of autologous fascia, such as fascia lata, offers comparable results with synthetic meshes in surgical reconstruction due to its inherent strength and ability to conform to host tissues. All of these factors are important in avoiding complications, improving patient outcomes, and preserving the long-term structural characteristics of the abdominal wall following surgery (Seethalakshmi, 2018). Moreover, the function of fascia extends beyond mere structural support, such as its involvement in the physiological processes of the abdominal cavity. Fascia's elasticity and durability facilitate dynamic organ movement with respiration and digestion. Pathological changes within the fascial sleeves, such as from trauma, inflammation, or surgery, can lead to functional disorders such as diminished motion or pain syndromes. High-resolution ultrasound imaging can provide valuable information regarding such changes, allowing for early detection and targeted interventions. With greater knowledge of fascia and connective tissue in the abdominal cavity, medical professionals can develop more robust diagnostic and therapy strategies, ultimately leading to improved patient outcomes in abdominal wall and peritoneal conditions (Alvarez-Hornia et al., 2022).

7.2. Anatomy of the Peritoneum

Peritoneal anatomy plays an important role in the utilization of ultrasound imaging, particularly in evaluating patients with pain in the abdomen. The peritoneum, a serous membrane, is the lining of the abdominal cavity and envelops the visceral organs. The two principal layers are the parietal peritoneum, which lines the abdominal wall, and the visceral peritoneum, which envelops the organs. One of the peritoneum's fundamental functions is facilitating movement between the organs during the process of digestion and preventing friction through the secretion of serous fluid. Its intricate anatomy forms a necessary part of clinicians' knowledge who employ ultrasound technology because it assists in making accurate diagnoses of diverse abdominal diseases and pathologies, and as a consequence, facilitates the administration of specific treatment regimens that can improve patient outcomes. During ultrasound examination, peritoneum can be evaluated for diseases such as ascites, peritoneal inflammation, or masses compressing the abdominal wall. The sonographic characteristics will be based on the condition, hence making the physicians knowledgeable on normal and abnormal anatomical structures. Abdominal wall thickness and fluctuations in the level of peritoneal fluid can also be identified. It has been studied that in some cases, such as the site of laparotomy, the thickness of the abdominal wall may represent physiological change, particularly in pregnancy (Amrozi et al., 2014). This serves to draw attention to the fact that both normal anatomical variation and disease can be sonographically imaged, enhancing diagnostic accuracy and informing surgical intervention. Additionally, the interrelation between the peritoneum and adjacent structures cannot be overstated. Specifically, studies have indicated that diseases like adenomyosis have been demonstrated to produce ectatic lymphatics, indicating a dynamic relationship between peritoneum and other abdominal cavity organs. This is notably relevant in the assessment of the risk of recurrence of endometriosis following surgery, and emphasizes the need for detailed imaging not just of the peritoneum itself but also adjacent structures (Bonaccorsi et al., 2019).

A broad understanding of such anatomical relationships is necessary for medical professionals performing ultrasound scans as it can tell us a great deal about the causation of gastrointestinal and reproductive pathologies. Thus, having knowledge of the peritoneum's anatomy contributes to clinicians' potential in providing the optimal level of care for the patient (Figure 7.6).

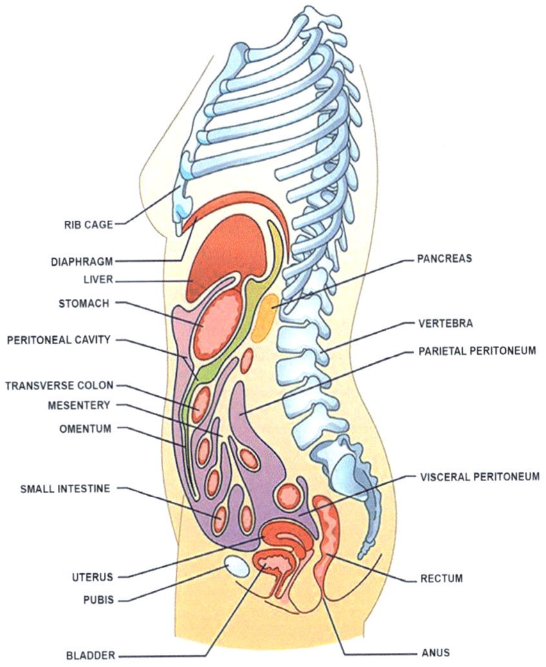

Figure 7.6. Anatomy of the peritoneum.

Source: https://assets.lybrate.com/imgs/tic/enadp/image-of-the-peritoneum.jpg.

7.2.1. Structure and Function of the Peritoneum

The peritoneum is a serous membrane that lines the abdominal cavity and covers the abdominal organs, playing a key role in structure and function. The double layer of the peritoneum membrane is made up of the parietal peritoneum, which is fixed on the wall of the abdomen, and the visceral peritoneum, which covers the organs. The space between these layers, or peritoneal cavity, contains a small amount of lubricating fluid that enables easy movement of organs during digestion and other physiological processes. Ultrasound imaging has now become central in imaging peritoneal architecture, which aids in assessing conditions such as ascites, adhesions, and infections. The accuracy with which ultrasonography defines the structural features of the peritoneum optimizes its value as a noninvasive diagnostic tool in abdominal wall and peritoneal disease applications in clinical practice. The functional role of the peritoneum transcends basic structural support; it is a key element of the body's immune defense and fluid balance. Its mesothelial cells exhibit features that enable the passage of leukocytes and proteins, facilitating the protection of the body against peritoneal infections. Ultrasound may also be applied in operating rooms to evaluate postoperative states, such as adhesion formation and fluid accumulation. Studies indicate that the imaging characteristics of abdominal tissues are determined by pathologic and physiological changes, thus emphasizing the importance of the realization of these variations. For instance, research outlined in Amrozi et al. (2014) indicate that layer thickness changes of the abdominal muscles during pregnancy unfold information concerning functional peritoneal adaptations, illustrating its significance in relation to the abdominal walls' structures dynamics. Moreover, the peritoneum's role in fibrosis and adhesion development influences patient recovery following surgery as well as long-term patient recovery. Elevated expression of fibrogenic factors may lead to postoperative adhesions, and this may lead to significant morbidity. Studies employing ultrasound-microbubble-mediated gene transfection, as discussed in Chan et al. (2009), have achieved promising results in the prevention of such side effects by targeting essential pathways in fibrogenesis. To have the ability to intervene and alter the biochemical environment of the peritoneal cavity would have the potential to revolutionize postoperative care practice, reducing the frequency and severity of adhesions. Hence, understanding the full scope of the peritoneums structural and functional characteristics is not only critical in diagnosis of abdominal disease but also in maximizing surgical technique and patient recovery (Figure 7.7).

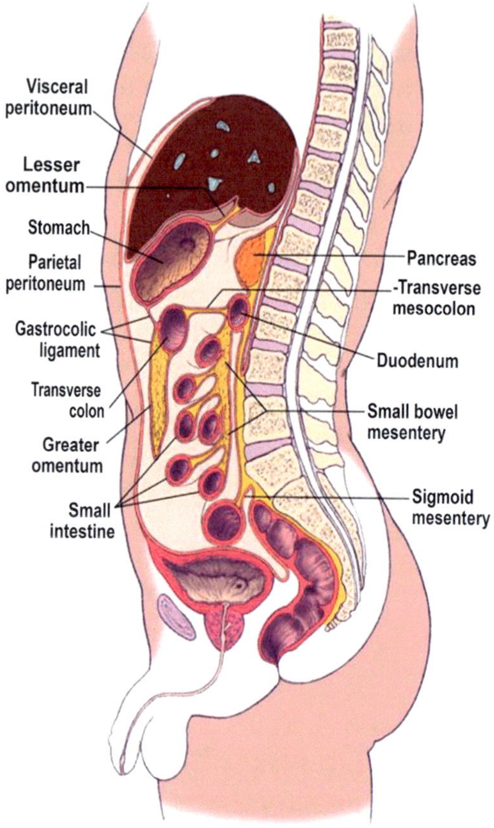

Figure 7.7. Structure and function of the peritoneum.

Source: Hull, Nathan & Granberg, Candace & Gargollo, Patricio & Thacker, Paul. (2022). Imaging of pre- and post-cytoreductive surgery and hyperthermic intraperitoneal chemotherapy for pediatric intraperitoneal malignancy. Pediatric Radiology. 52. 1-13. 10.1007/s00247-022-05424-5.

7.2.2. Types of Peritoneal Membranes

The peritoneum, which is a serous membrane, forms a vital barrier within the abdominal cavity by investing the viscera and lining the abdominal wall. It can be broadly categorized into two parts: the parietal peritoneum and the visceral peritoneum. The parietal peritoneum is a protective covering which is interposed with the abdominal wall, consisting of a dense network of connective tissues and blood vessels. Its sensory nerve fibers are pain, temperature, and pressure sensitive; thus, parietal layer inflammation tends to cause severe abdominal pain, a diagnostic symptom in most clinical presentations. Contrary to this, the visceral peritoneum lines the inner organs, which gives them a smooth surface that facilitates them to glide during physiological movement. It is essential to comprehend such differences, especially for ultrasound imaging which provides information regarding the pathology and structure of such membranes. The peritoneum's intricate structure also allows for various physiological processes, including the secretion of serous fluid, which lubricates the peritoneal cavity. Such fluid reduces friction among the abdominal organs and allows them to move easily, and it is evident that the peritoneal membranes are crucial in organ function preservation. Intra-abdominal alterations in the peritoneal cavity, such as inflammation or fluid accumulation, could have a significant impact on ultrasound examinations and clinical assessment. For instance, ascites or peritonitis can lead to pathologic alteration that is identifiable with ultrasound, which in turn could necessitate certain treatment. Moreover, the peritoneum's response to conditions such as endometriosis demonstrates the complex dynamics at play between the peritoneal membranes and reproductive health, in that endometrial cells can implant within the peritoneal cavity after reflux, defying traditional presumptions of female reproductive diseases (Smolarz et al., 2021).

Peritoneal membranes are also essential in therapeutic interventions, notably in the process of mitigating cancer therapies. Here, not only do they serve a protective role but also act as carriers for therapeutic agents during hyperthermia and thermal ablation therapies, which are increasingly being employed for the treatment of solid tumors. With the ability to selectively target and heat specific areas within the peritoneal cavity, chemotherapeutic activity can be enhanced with less systemic exposure and resultant side effects (Kok et al., 2020). As the technology of ultrasound advances, its application extends beyond simple visualization to enable real-time monitoring of therapeutic effect. The dynamic capability of ultrasound may be employed to observe thermal effects or to guide the administration of local therapies, and thus exhibit the peritoneal membranes' key role within modern protocols for cancer therapy. Understanding the varying types of peritoneal membranes enhances diagnostic and therapeutic functionality within abdominal medicine.

7.2.3. Clinical Significance of Peritoneal Anatomy

Understanding the clinical significance of peritoneal anatomy is essential for achieving maximum ultrasound use in abdominal condition assessment. Peritoneum, composed of parietal and visceral layers, is an essential interface between various abdominal organs and the abdominal wall. Its complexity allows such physiological processes as fluid movement and insulation of organs to occur. When using ultrasound technology, the operator needs to understand the anatomical relationships between structures within the peritoneal cavity to recognize pathological alterations in the form of free fluid collection, inflammatory processes, or neoplastic growth. Effective interpretation of ultrasonography images relies on recognizing the peritoneum and its normal anatomy related structures, which in turn is fundamental to accurate diagnosis and management of abdominal pathology, thereby amplifying the need for comprehensive education of peritoneal anatomy among ultrasound practitioners. Visualization in ultrasound scanning may have a significant role to play in diagnostic findings, particularly in acute abdomen or chronic pain conditions within the abdomen. Diaphragmatic ultrasonography is one such method that has been found to be an important development, offering to assess both peritoneal conditions and diaphragmatic function. Of note, identification of normal peritoneal anatomy assists cliniciansin differentiating among various pathologies, including differentiation of ascites from other fluid collections. Recent consensus statements have attempted to establish methodological standards in diaphragm ultrasonography, emphasizing the importance of correct measurement methodology and recognition of anatomical landmarks. Coupled with a greater understanding of peritoneal anatomy and newer ultrasound technologies, thus, it can be followed by enhanced clinical evaluation and enhanced management of patients, particularly in intensive care setups where evaluation within the shortest duration and maximum precision is of utmost importance (Haaksma et al., 2022). The relevance of peritoneal anatomy extends to therapeutic interventions as well, particularly when it comes to endoscopic ultrasound (EUS). EUS becomes the lead in the management of various procedures, such as biliary drainage and gastroenterostomy which are pivotal in disease management like malignant obstructions. Anatomical precision facilitated by ultrasound enables clinicians to assess biliary tree anatomy and choose the best approach for interventions. Besides, guidelines and recommendations emphasize the need for specialists to have profound knowledge of peritoneal anatomy to minimize complications and enhance patient safety throughout procedures (Van der Merwe et al., 2021). Consequently, a solid foundation in peritoneal anatomy benefits not only diagnostic intervention with ultrasound but also supports a robust base for effective therapeutic interventions and sophisticated surgery procedures in diversified clinical practices (Figure 7.8).

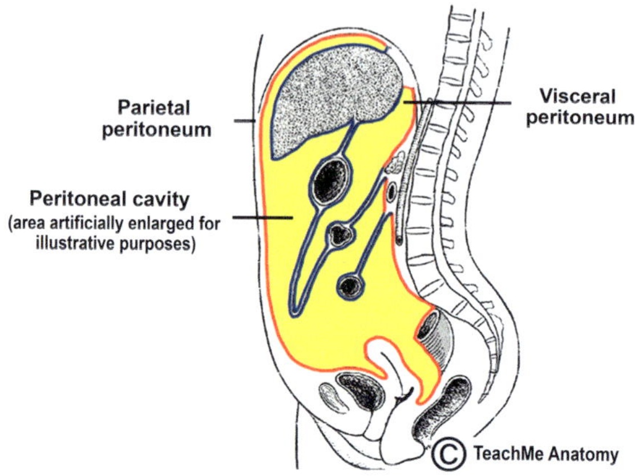

Figure 7.8. Clinical significance of peritoneal anatomy.

Source: https://teachmeanatomy.info/wp-content/uploads/Overview-of-the-Peritoneal-Abdominal-Cavity.png.

7.3. Ultrasound Technology Overview

Ultrasound technology is the cornerstone of medical imaging, offering real-time, non-invasive imaging of internal organs and structures. The technology is based on the principle of sound waves, which are transmitted through tissues to reflect and create images on the screen. This capability is particularly useful in assessing abdominal wall and peritoneal conditions, as the technology provides critical information on the morphology and function of these areas. The rapid evolution of ultrasound equipment and methods has significantly advanced diagnosis accuracy, allowing for better differentiation of various pathologies. Moreover, the portability of ultrasound equipment allows for bedside assessment, thus broadening the scope of this imaging modality in clinical settings. Specific to ultrasounds of the abdominal wall and peritoneum, technical effectiveness is illustrated through the ability to identify a variety of pathologies, such as hernias, abscesses, and fluid collections. The addition of Doppler ultrasound increases the diagnostic capabilities by providing insight into blood flow and vascular integrity. These advanced technologies can be combined, enabling medical professionals to assess cases that will be subject to surgery or nonsurgical intervention. Notably, as the medical community inches towards more embracing standardised terminologies and classifications of disease, such as endometriosis, the role of ultrasound technology remains paramount. For instance, the achievement of consensual terminology in the characterization of endometriosis underscores the importance of possessing proper imaging techniques for the identification of disease presentations, which may best be provided by an ultrasound (Tomassetti et al., 2021). In addition, the effects of ultrasound technology reach into patient management and intervention monitoring on an ongoing basis. As clinicians become more aware of developing conditions from the use of ultrasound testing, they are better able to make informed decisions regarding surgical timing and intervention. This is part of an overall trend toward personalized medicine, whereby treatment routes are determined by patient-specific considerations. The constant evolution of the use of ultrasound is borne out in efforts to develop commonly accepted description systems for numerous medical conditions so that there can be enhanced physician-to-physician communication. Lastly, the role of ultrasound technology in abdominal wall and peritoneum assessment is an expression of commitment to providing quality, patient-centered care while advancing the boundaries of medical knowledge (Tomassetti et al., 2021) (Figure 7.9).

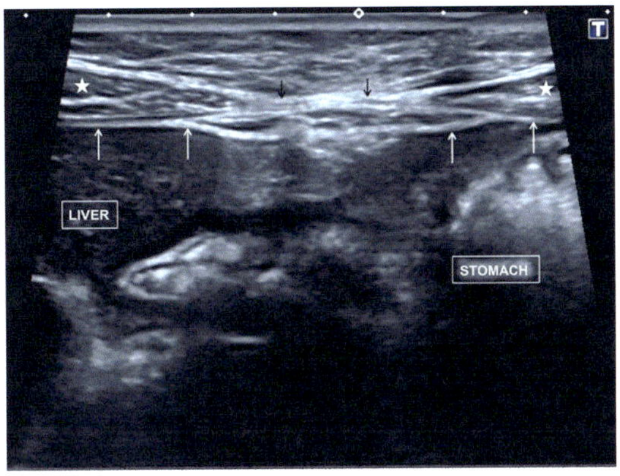

Figure 7.9. Ultrasound technology overview of peritoneal anatomy.

Source: https://encrypted-tbn0.gstatic.com/images?q=tbn:ANd9GcTXUpFrdbH2mfhUTDsMlObv17nOXyOzhg3ibg&s.

7.3.1. Principles of Ultrasound Imaging

The physiology of ultrasound imaging rests on the fundamental principles of the propagation and reflection of sound waves, which are essential in the production of images of the internal organs. Abdominal wall and peritoneum ultrasound in the form of high-frequency sound waves originates from a transducer, passing through the skin and other tissues. When such waves strike boundaries between tissues of different types, say fluid, fat, or solid organs, they are reflected back to the transducer. The duration that these echoes take to return and their strength allow the computation of the distance and formation of a two-dimensional image that outlines the anatomical structure. This imaging modality is applied as a non-invasive method for visualizing the peritoneum and abdominal wall to aid in the detection of abnormalities or conditions of these regions. Additionally, the successful utilization of ultrasound to assess the abdominal wall and peritoneum is through familiarity with the various imaging methods and their applications. Selection of appropriate frequency settings is necessary to achieve the highest image resolution since higher frequency offers more detail but with limited penetration depth. Low frequency, however, has greater penetration but gives lower resolution images. Doppler ultrasound is also used to assess arterial and venous flow into and out of abdominal organs, aiding in the diagnosis of vascular disease. The real-time evaluation made possible through the dynamic qualities of ultrasound imaging allows for the evaluation of moving structures, such as the diaphragm with breathing or peristaltic intestinal movement.

This enhances diagnostic accuracy and results in optimal patient care. In some conditions, application of the principles of ultrasound imaging can be extremely informative in the assessment of various abdominal wall and peritoneal abnormalities. For instance, ultrasound plays an important role in the diagnosis of soft tissue sarcomas, which could present as masses within the abdominal cavity, based on the NCCN Clinical Practice Guidelines for Soft Tissue Sarcoma (von Mehren et al., 2022). Also, endometriosis diagnosis requires careful imaging to distinguish between several forms of lesions, such as peritoneal endometriosis and deep endometriosis, implying the relevance of employing a comprehensive classification system together with ultrasound imaging (Keckstein et al., 2021). These examples illustrate the way in which the principles of ultrasound imaging not only contribute to the diagnosis of peritoneal and abdominal illnesses but also create opportunities for tailor-made treatment protocols, showcasing ultrasound's flexibility and medical importance (Figure 7.10).

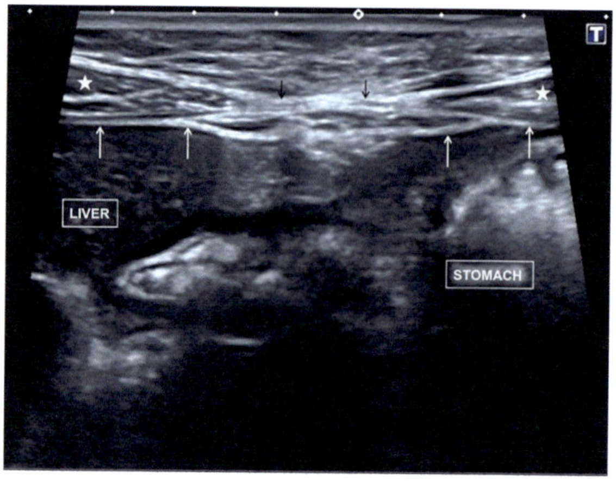

Figure 7.10. Principles of ultrasound imaging of peritoneal anatomy.

Source: Pilcher, J. M., & Patel, P. (2022). Abdominal Ultrasound—Bowel and peritoneum. In Springer eBooks (pp. 209–229). https://doi.org/10.1007/978-3-030-71742-1_13

7.3.2. Types of Ultrasound Equipment Used

In ultrasound of the abdominal wall and peritoneum, a number of machines are in the limelight when it comes to diagnosis and treatment. The fundamental machine employed is the standard ultrasound machine that employs high-frequency sound waves to create scans of internal organs. The machines are typically equipped with an array of transducers in the shape of linear and curvilinear probes. Linear transducers work well for imaging superficial structures such as the abdominal wall and are invaluable in detecting pathology such as hernias. Curvilinear probes have increased penetration and are more useful for imaging deeper organs and anatomic structures within the peritoneal cavity. This relative versatility makes it important to select the appropriate ultrasound equipment depending on the clinical scenario and depth of imaging required. Endoscopic ultrasound (EUS) is an advanced imaging tool employed in the evaluation of abdominal disease that provides high-resolution images of the lesions within and around the gastrointestinal tract. It is a modality that incorporates endoscopic vision with ultrasound imaging and allows practitioners to precisely evaluate lesions of the abdominal wall and peritoneum. EUS is particularly valuable when conventional imaging does not provide clear results, that is, in cases of suspected abdominal cavity fluid collections or malignancies. Equipment used during EUS presents high-resolution images that make it possible to identify minimal pathologies and enable procedures such as EUS-guided drainage of abscesses or cysts. According to evidence supporting the use of EUS in biliary obstruction and other complex cases, its addition enhances clinical decision-making and patient outcomes for patients with challenging-to-treat abdominal conditions (Van der Merwe et al., 2021). Apart from conventional and endoscopic ultrasound, portable ultrasound equipment has significantly influenced abdominal imaging practice, particularly in emergency and point-of-care settings. These tiny machines yield superb images with the added facility of mobility and same-time evaluation in several clinical environments. In acute assessment, for instance, assessment of trauma or acute abdominal pain, portable ultrasound can quickly detect free fluid and other complications involved and direct immediate clinical intervention. Moreover, the simultaneous application of sophisticated software and digital technology with mobile equipment facilitates telemedicine and remote diagnosis, thus extending the reach of quality care even more. Such convenience is not only very valuable in emergencies but also ensures continuous monitoring of patients whose abdominal pathologies are already established, ultimately resulting in more effective management plans in abdominal wall and peritoneum ultrasound (Henriksen et al., 2020) (Figure 7.11).

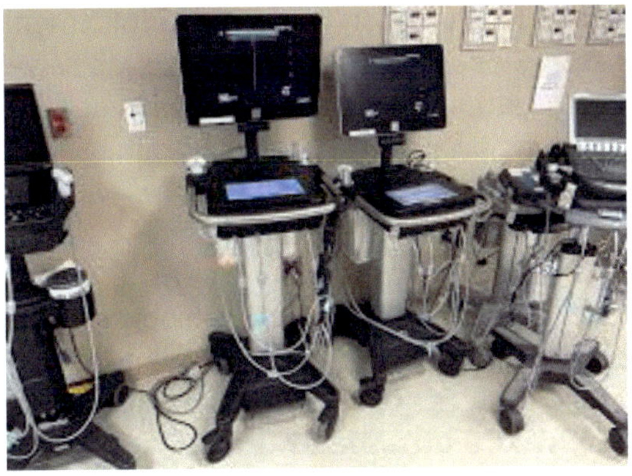

Figure 7.11. Types of ultrasound equipment used for peritoneum ultrasound.

Source: https://www.saem.org/images/default-source/academy-images/cdem/picture232dc49f4-ae13-4706-8480-6023e928ebf7.png?sfvrsn=6f1bbdbe_1.

7.3.3. Advantages of Ultrasound in Abdominal Imaging

Abdominal imaging with the aid of ultrasound has numerous advantages that increase its applicability as an option imaging modality for most clinical scenarios. A major advantage is that it is not invasive, and this ensures maximal patient comfort and safety through avoidance of ionizing radiation employed with other imaging modalities such as computed tomography (CT) and X-rays. This is particularly relevant in high-risk groups, such as pregnant women and children, where exposure to radiation must be avoided. Ultrasound is also readily accessible and can often be performed bedside, with immediate results beneficial for acute decision-making. Such pragmatic advantages position ultrasound as a useful component in the diagnosis and management of abdominal disease, facilitating rapid assessment and intervention where indicated. Another significant characteristic of ultrasound imaging of the abdomen is its real-time imaging, by which physicians are able to visualize dynamic processes in the gastrointestinal tract. It is very helpful while investigating abnormalities like bowel obstruction or peristalsis because it is able to provide real-time information regarding the functioning and mobility of the organs under investigation. Furthermore, ultrasound has proven useful in guiding certain therapeutic procedures, such as drainage of fluid collections or biopsy of abdominal masses. Real-time visualization by ultrasound ensures the accuracy and safety of these interventions with a decrease in complications. Following changes over time further add to its application, especially with chronic conditions requiring follow-up studies to observe the evolution or resolution of abnormalities. In certain clinical situations, ultrasound may have an advantage over other imaging modalities since it excels in showing soft tissue and fluid dynamics. An example is the case of gastrointestinal stromal tumors (GIST) or bladder hernias, as seen in (Babicky et al., 2014) and (Autieri et al., 2015), where ultrasound provides critical information about tumor size and vascularity that may be crucial to treatment planning and follow-up. The modality's sensitivity to fluid accumulations and solid masses and its ability to differentiate complex structures such as the peritoneum and abdominal wall are essential for accurate diagnoses. Overall, the advantages afforded by ultrasound in abdominal imaging, including safety, availability, real-time imaging capacity, and specificity for pathology visibility, highlight the value of ultrasound in contemporary practice (Figure 7.12).

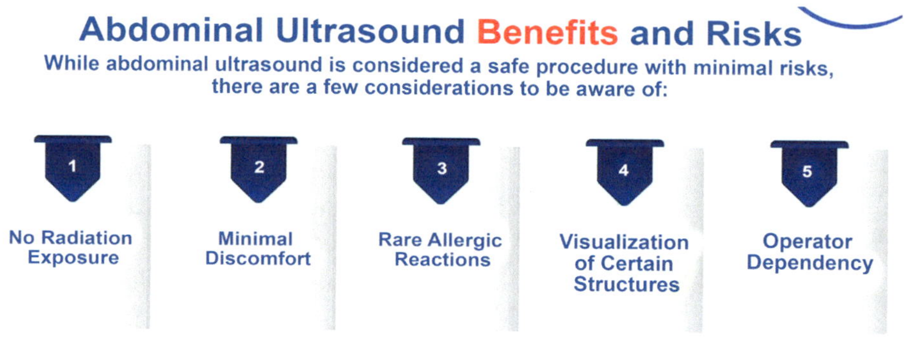

Figure 7.12. Advantages of ultrasound in abdominal imaging.

Source: Abdominal Ultrasound: Purpose, symptoms, risk, and procedure, 2024. www.theaccesshealthcare.com. https://www.theaccesshealthcare.com/images/blog/abdominal-ultrasound-purpose-symptoms-risk-and-procedure/01.webp.

7.4. Indications for Abdominal Wall Ultrasound

The use of abdominal wall ultrasound (AWUS) indications has increased due to its minimally invasive method and ability to produce real-time images of structures in the abdominal wall. One of the key indications is abdominal wall hernia assessment, in which the ultrasound can adequately detect the presence and character of protrusions, that is, size and composition. This imaging method is useful in the evaluation of inguinal and femoral hernias, enabling early surgery if necessary. Furthermore, AWUS may also be useful in identifying any associated complications, such as incarceration or strangulation that have a significant impact on clinical management. In a recent clinical guideline, it has been recommended that the differentiation of these conditions with proper imaging is crucial in deciding the right treatment modalities (Hashiguchi et al., 2019). Another key indication of abdominal wall ultrasound is the evaluation of abdominal wall masses, which may have a variety of etiologies, including tumors, abscesses, or hematomas. Ultrasound is a first-line imaging test that can determine the etiology of such masses and distinguish between benign and malignant lesions on the basis of their vascularity and echogenicity. In addition, its use applies to steering biopsies in case of suspicious lesions detected, thus increasing diagnostic precision while reducing patient discomfort. The non-invasive nature of AWUS enables repetitive examination, which can prove pivotal in the assessment of changes over time in malignant as well as benign diseases. Clinical practice guidelines underscore the application of ultrasound alongside patient history and physical examination to facilitate a detailed assessment of abdominal masses (ten Broek et al., 2018).

Lastly, ultrasound of the abdominal wall is key in the evaluation of postoperative complications, such as seroma or abscess development. Following surgical interventions, ultrasound is able to rapidly evaluate any pathology in the operative site, providing valuable information regarding fluid accumulation or infection features. This applies particularly to patients undergoing surgical interventions on the abdominal wall, as the detection of complications at an early stage is likely to have a significant impact on patient outcomes. The ability to do bedside ultrasound scans results in more rapid decision-making and intervention, with a reduced dependence on more invasive imaging modalities like CT scans. The application of AWUS as part of postoperative care protocols is increasingly gaining acceptance as a routine procedure, which is in line with prevailing practice for enhancing patient recovery and reducing the length of hospital stay (Hashiguchi et al., 2019) (Figure 7.13).

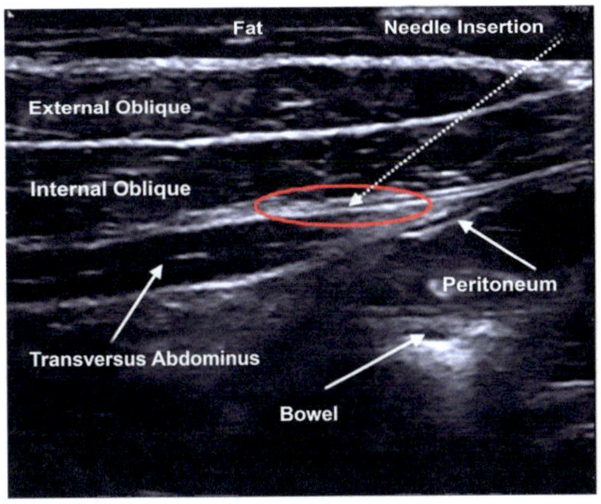

Figure 7.13. The indications for abdominal wall ultrasound (AWUS).

Source: Azawi, Nessn & Mosholt, Karina & Fode, Mikkel. (2016). Unilateral Ultrasound-Guided Transversus Abdominis Plane Block after Nephrectomy; Postoperative Pain and Use of Opioids. Nephro-Urology Monthly. In Press. 10.5812/numonthly.35356.

7.4.1. Evaluation of Abdominal Wall Hernias

Evaluation of the hernias of the abdominal wall is crucial in clinical diagnosis as well as in planning treatment. Abdominal wall hernias are a situation where the tissues, typically portions of the intestine, bulge through a weak portion of the abdominal wall. Ultrasonography is a valuable non-surgical diagnostic tool due to its ability to generate real-time images as well as assess the morphology and dynamics of the hernial sac. High-frequency ultrasound can nicely visualize hernias, differentiate the contents of hernial sacs, and identify concomitant complications, and it has a useful role in preoperative planning and postoperative outcome. Ultrasound has been proven to be not only very specific and sensitive for the diagnosis of hernias but also to enable clinicians to probe concomitant conditions such as hydroceles or varicoceles, which might coexist with hernias and complicate their clinical presentation. Thus, ultrasound is an essential part of the entire evaluation of abdominal wall hernias. Besides, the application of emerging ultrasound techniques extends to regions of surgery, filling in accuracy of surgical procedures. Techniques like laparoscopic ones need total preoperative imaging for optimal outcomes, as can be proven in laparoscopic orchiopexy for cryptorchidism research (You et al., 2020). In these cases, ultrasound helps establish anatomical relationships and identify potential complications such as a patent processus vaginalis, which is usually present with inguinal hernias. Through the use of information from ultrasound images, surgeons can more effectively plan interventions, fashioning procedures to optimize effectiveness and reduce patient recovery time. In addition, the ability for detection and subsequent treatment of any resultant issues intraoperatively illustrates the broader application of ultrasound beyond the diagnostic setting, with a definitive preemptive approach towards the treatment of abdominal wall hernias. In the long term, the evaluation of abdominal wall hernias by ultrasound not only assists in enhanced diagnosis and management but also assists in the delivery of an enhanced recovery model within surgical care. This model emphasizes multimodal perioperative care that includes optimized diagnostics and early surgical treatment, according to the ERAS guidelines (Gustafsson et al., 2018). Evidence-based practices derived from these guidelines have established a standard of care aimed at minimizing postoperative complications and promoting rapid recovery with early mobilization and nutrition. By utilizing ultrasound as a first-line imaging modality, clinicians can provide correct diagnoses, therefore optimizing the outcome of surgery and reducing reliance on more invasive diagnostic studies. Thus, the application of ultrasound in the evaluation of abdominal wall hernias is an anchor advance in patient care, which unites efficacy with enhanced clinical outcomes (Figure 7.14).

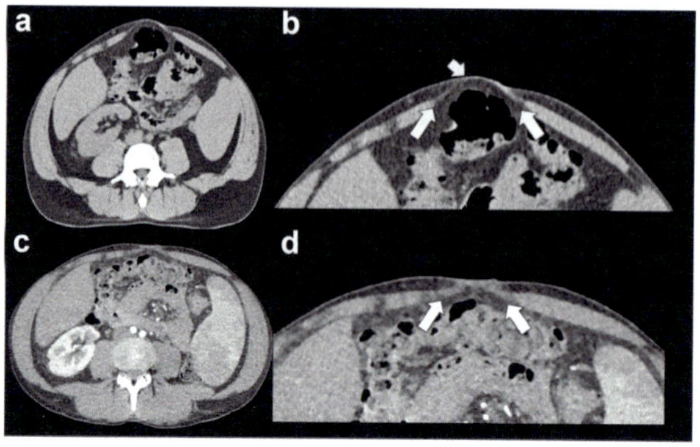

Figure 7.14. Evaluation of abdominal wall hernias.

Source: Ghafoor, S., Hoppe, A. T., Lange, M., et.al. (2024). Computed tomography for evaluation of abdominal wall hernias—what is the value of the Valsalva maneuver? Hernia. https://doi.org/10.1007/s10029-024-03036-6

7.4.2. Assessment of Fluid Collections

Assessment of fluid accumulations within the peritoneum and abdominal wall ultrasound evaluation, is important in the diagnosis of various clinical conditions. The imaging technique is non-invasive and offers real-time evaluation of peritoneal fluid, hematomas, and other accumulations, which is useful in the care of post-surgical patients and patients with abdominal trauma. Using high-frequency ultrasound imaging, health care professionals can identify characteristics such as location, size, and echogenicity of fluid accumulations. These features also play a crucial role in distinguishing among different fluid types, such as serous, hemorrhagic, or infected fluids, and their subsequent influence on management. Early detection through ultrasound can help facilitate early intervention and mitigate complications, further underscoring its function as an initiating diagnostic imaging in abdominal medicine. Furthermore, the influence of surgical techniques on fluid accumulations renders ultrasound a valuable tool in post-surgical assessments. Studies have also indicated that intra-operative visceral peritoneum handling during cesarean delivery can significantly impact fluid accumulation in the vesico-uterine space (VUS) (Farine et al., 2025). Specifically, studies have identified that visceral peritoneum closure is linked with increased fluid collection rates, which are further linked with increased post-operative complications such as febrile morbidity and increased length of stay. Therefore, understanding the interaction of surgery with fluid dynamics is critical in directing clinical practice with patient outcome as the top priority. Ultrasound is a valuable follow-up procedure to visualize these collections and to guide subsequent interventions based on patients' altered clinical status. Apart from cesarean delivery, ultrasound assessment has an important role to play in other conditions, such as complication assessment after a pancreas transplant. Graft issues detected early through imaging can significantly enhance graft survival and patient benefit (Alves et al., 2010). Ultrasound provides hints of the expected appearances and variations in grafts that are suggestive of complications, such as fluid collection at or close to the graft bed, which can also result in further morbidity if not addressed. As the number of pancreas transplants for the management of type 1 diabetes mellitus has been increasing, the role of ultrasound in post-operative complication assessment and management becomes increasingly valuable. It justifies the inclusion of ultrasound assessment in the multi-modal care plan of patients undergoing major abdominal procedures.

7.4.3. Diagnosis of Abdominal Wall Mass

Diagnosis of abdominal wall masses mandates a multidisciplinary strategy, often beginning with careful patient history and physical examination. The clinician must systematically assess any palpable mass, delineating size, shape, consistency, and, if present, concomitant symptoms like tenderness or changes in bowel function. Ultrasound is an important diagnostic imaging tool in the procedure, yielding real-time images to facilitate differentiation between solid and cystic masses and to facilitate correct diagnosis and treatment. The incorporation of ultrasound not only allows for the visual observation of the masses but also potential intervention guidance, such as aspiration or biopsy, which can be critical in determining the nature of the mass—benign or malignant. This dual utility highlights the central role of ultrasound in the algorithm of diagnosis for abdominal wall masses. When masses are considered to be malignant, complete characterization is extremely significant. Ultrasound can record vascularity or irregular borders, both of which are suggestive of malignancy. Besides, the modality permits evaluation of contiguous structures and spread to lymph nodes, aiding in staging and treatment planning. For instance, imaging characteristics of gastrointestinal stromal tumors (GISTs) are such that they can be well evaluated with ultrasound. Understanding these features is important in the effective planning of the surgery and treatment of the tumors because early detection significantly impacts prognosis and outcomes. Use of ultrasound, therefore, empowers physicians to manage complex cases of abdominal wall masses more accurately and with confidence. The diagnostic evaluation doesn't end with imaging, but one must also factor in laboratory studies, especially with suspected malignancy. Ascitic fluid analysis, performed by paracentesis, is a helpful adjunct that can provide data regarding abdominal mass pathology. Ascites may complicate the presentation and can be secondary to cirrhosis or advanced malignancies. For instance, ascites may be an indicator of hepatic decompensation and necessitate immediate treatment to prevent serious complications like spontaneous bacterial peritonitis (Harvey et al., 2022). Moreover, knowledge of immunohistochemical profiles will help differentiate among various tumors whenever pathology is involved. The combination of imaging and laboratory data offers a comprehensive diagnosis format, central in guiding treatment regimens for abdominal wall masses and patient outcomes (Casali et al., 2018) (Figure 7.15).

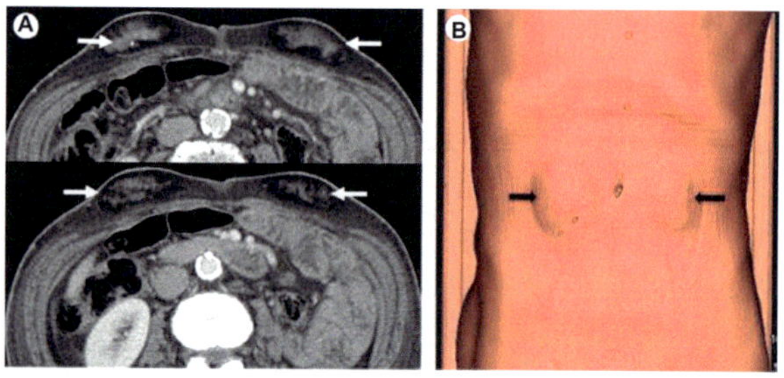

Figure 7.15. Diagnosis of abdominal wall masses.

Source: https://ars.els-cdn.com/content/image/1-s2.0-S0887217118300039-gr28.jpg.

7.5. Indications for Peritoneal Ultrasound

Peritoneal ultrasound is an important imaging modality to evaluate many conditions of the abdominal cavity. Fluid accumulation, whether due to infection, malignancy, or inflammation, is one of the primary reasons to use this imaging tool to evaluate it. Fluid accumulation may manifest as ascites, the proper evaluation of which is critical for therapeutic intervention decisions. Peritoneal ultrasound is particularly valuable in that it is a non-invasive technique, allowing clinicians to visualize intra-abdominal structures without exposing patients to toxic radiation. Its capacity to distinguish between free fluid and loculated collections not only facilitates diagnosis but also informs subsequent management plans, such as drainage or further investigation of the potential underlying pathology, thereby maximizing patient outcomes in clinical practice (Bilican et al., 2025). Another important indication of peritoneal ultrasound involves the evaluation of adhesive disease, which is a common complication of intra-abdominal surgery. Adhesions may lead to chronic pain, bowel obstruction, and other gastrointestinal symptoms, making the patient harder to treat. Traditional imaging devices are not sufficient in detecting these intra-abdominal adhesions due to their variability. Peritoneal ultrasound provides a dynamic, real-time assessment of the abdominal cavity and assists in determining changes associated with adhesive disease. Through the demarcation of the degree and severity of adhesions, ultrasound facilitates decisions regarding conservative treatments or intervention using surgery. This combined evaluation of adhesive disease demonstrates the importance of peritoneal ultrasound in advancing diagnostic accuracy and treatment efficacy for patients with adhesive disease (Andreev et al., 2017). Furthermore, peritoneal ultrasound plays a part in the follow-up of disease activity in diseases like inflammatory bowel disease (IBD). As IBD has a tendency to lead to complications like fistulas or abscesses, it is important to image early in order to manage adequately. Peritoneal ultrasound provides a valuable tool in the detection of the thickness and vascularity of the bowel wall, which are good predictors of active disease. Its ability to make repeat, non-invasive measurements allows for the potential of tracking treatment outcomes longitudinally, and peritoneal ultrasound thus becomes integral to the chronic management of IBD. This not only delivers personalized care but also enhances patient quality of care for patients with chronic gastrointestinal disease in general, eventually culminating in better health outcomes and quality of life (Bilican et al., 2025).

7.5.1. Detection of Peritoneal Fluid

Peritoneal fluid detection is a critical part of abdominal wall and peritoneum ultrasound and is a central diagnostic tool in the repertoire of clinicians. Ultrasound is a minimally invasive imaging method that allows for real-time imaging, thereby allowing clinicians to identify the presence of fluid accumulation in the peritoneal cavity. This is of specific use in a wide variety of clinical contexts, including trauma, ascites, or infection, where prompt detection can meaningfully alter management. High-resolution ultrasound may disclose the location, volume, and even nature of the fluid and help differentiate between the transudative and exudative processes. By using concise imaging modalities, clinicians can make wise decisions about possible therapeutic interventions, such as drainage or more intricate surgical procedures, improving patient care standards in acute and elective scenarios. Because of the complexity involved in peritoneal fluid detection, experts' expertise shouldered special examination techniques being designed to enhance accuracy. The European Federation of Societies for Ultrasound in Medicine and Biology (EFSUMB) facilitated this by establishing a Gastrointestinal Ultrasound (GIUS) task force whose mandate was to harmonize procedures in ultrasound imaging. This combined endeavor has provided us with current guidelines emphasizing the importance of systematic scanning protocols, such as imaging dependent areas of the peritoneal cavity where fluid is most likely. The effective application of these methods allows sonographers to maximize their diagnostic potential while ensuring that the examination conforms to established clinical guidelines, ultimately benefiting abdominal conditions (Calabrese et al., 2016). In addition, improved ultrasound technology enhances the sensitivity of peritoneal fluid detection, improving diagnostic precision. The use of high-frequency transducers has increased the resolution of images, which allows for differentiation between small volumes of fluid and other structures in the abdomen, which can frequently interfere with the interpretation of results. The new use of Doppler ultrasound also has the potential to assess vascular tissues around the fluid, providing additional information that is valuable to understand the etiology of the fluid accumulation. Through a combination of data from various imaging modalities, medical professionals are able to gain an integrated comprehension of the status of patients and, therefore, make tailored plans of management aimed at the aetiology of the accumulation of peritoneal fluid (Calabrese et al., 2016). Lastly, the ongoing advancement in ultrasound modalities and application of evidence-based guidelines enhances clinical confidence, thus enhancing detection as well as peritoneal fluid management (Figure 7.16).

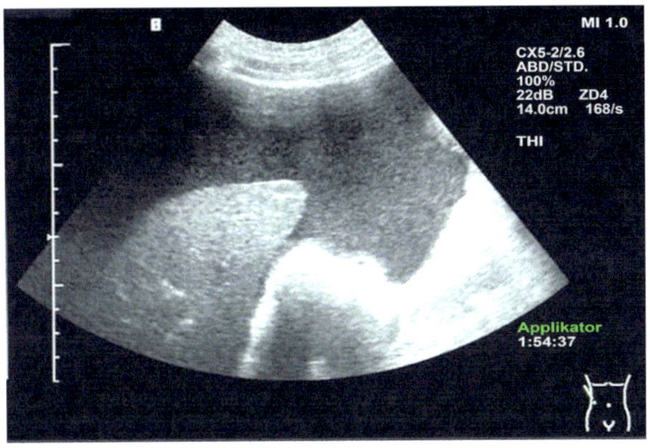

Figure 7.16. Detection of peritoneal fluid in ultrasound.

Source: https://radiologykey.com/wp-content/uploads/2016/01/9783131708212_013_003.tif_epub1.jpg.

7.5.2. Identification of Peritoneal Disease

Peritoneal disease identification through ultrasound is a significant advance in imaging diagnosis, particularly in the evaluation of abdominal pathology. Through the employment of high-frequency sound, ultrasound provides real-time imaging of the peritoneal cavity in order to allow physicians to assess for fluid, masses, or lesions. It is a non-invasive method that is particularly beneficial in emergency applications where there need to be speed of diagnosis. Of particular interest is the ability of ultrasound to differentiate between various types of fluid collections, for example, hemorrhage and ascites, which occur as a result of traumatic injury or other disease states. The utility of this imaging technique is further heightened by its capability for guiding procedural intervention, such as paracentesis, that can further assist in the diagnosis and treatment of peritoneal pathology. Lastly, ultrasound's value here enhances clinical decision-making and may maximize patient outcomes (Spahnet al., 2019). In addition to fluid dynamics evaluation, ultrasound is valuable in diagnosing peritoneal neoplastic processes. Carcinomatosis of the abdomen, or the spreading of malignant cells inside the peritoneal cavity, may be observed on ultrasound, which can contribute to tumor burden and distribution measurement. It is crucial to identify peritoneal metastases since they affect the treatment mode and prognosis directly. Ultrasound, being capable of giving a dynamic assessment, can also detect peritoneal surface nodules and delineate tumor borders, both of which will contribute to treatment planning. The modality can also involve evaluation for associated lymphadenopathy, which may provide information on the spread of the disease. This information substantiates the position of targeted imaging in the treatment of cancer patients, preventing delays in interventions (Prakash &Chakrabarti, 2019). Detection of infectious processes, e.g., abscesses or peritonitis, constitutes another essential component of peritoneal disease detection via ultrasound. Visualization of inflammatory changes within the peritoneum is useful in the establishment of a proper diagnosis, particularly in acute abdominal pain patients. Ultrasound can define peritoneal fluid pattern changes and allow identification of complex collections indicative of abscesses. These are significant as they determine further therapeutic interventions, including the need for surgery or antibiotics. Furthermore, the utility of ultrasound enables ongoing evaluation of treatment response, enabling clinicians to assess the resolution of infectious processes effectively. The addition of ultrasound to the diagnostic workup of peritoneal disease not only enhances the clinical outcome but also assists in the overall management of pathology in the abdomen (Spahn et al., 2019).

7.5.3. Assessment of Intra-Abdominal Organs

In abdominal ultrasound, intra-abdominal organ evaluation is of utmost significance in condition diagnosis, particularly trauma cases. The rapid evaluation provided by ultrasound, particularly with the Focused Assessment with Sonography for Trauma (FAST), enables clinicians to detect free intra-peritoneal fluid along with solid organ trauma. A study that continued over several months highlighted the validity of FAST when compared with contrast-enhanced computed tomography (CECT) and established CECT as the gold standard for determining the severity of visceral injury and vascular compromise. While FAST offers rapid information, its limitations need careful interpretation and often necessitate further investigation by the use of advanced imaging techniques. This heightened sense of rapid diagnostic processes can significantly alter management in acute abdominal trauma, ultimately improving patient outcomes (Manzoor et al., 2025). Also essential is the awareness of how various afflictions of the abdominal wall and peritoneum can influence intra-abdominal organ assessment. For instance, the presence of inguinal hernias, lateral inguinal hernias specifically, can render visual assessment of intra-abdominal structures during ultrasound more difficult. Since these hernias are caused by deficiencies in the abdominal wall, they also occur with increased intra-abdominal pressure, which can distort normal anatomical landmarks. Altered anatomy can cause interference with the accurate evaluation of adjacent organs. Not only is the incorrect assessment of these organs risky in terms of misdiagnosis, but it alsoemphasizes the need for practitioners to be competent to diagnose and manage hernias as a component of comprehensive abdominal ultrasound (Fitriani et al., 2025). The nature of such conditions necessitates extensive training and comfort in abdominal wall anatomy in an effort to make ultrasound imaging more useful. Finally, the continuous progress in ultrasound technology has transformed intra-abdominal organ evaluation to offer increased diagnostic accuracy. Such developments have seen the introduction of high-resolution imaging and portable ultrasound devices, which enable real-time assessment in various settings, particularly in urgent care. Such technologies can allow earlier detection of abdominal pathologies, allowing timely intervention that can avert disease complications like hemorrhagic shock or acute peritoneal disease. Its complementarity with clinical evaluations based on pre-defined protocols enhances its value in acute conditions. Lastly, the application of ultrasound in intra-abdominal organ assessment not only facilitates acute diagnostic processes but also provides health care providers with a multifunctional tool for repeated assessment and management throughout a patient's care pathway (Manzoor et al., 2025).

7.6. Interpretation of Ultrasound Findings

Sonographic interpretation of ultrasound findings on abdominal wall and peritoneal assessment is an essential component of the diagnosis of various conditions and is made possible by high-resolution imaging of anatomical structures. By means of real-time imaging techniques, ultrasound delineates anatomic deficits like hernias, abscesses, and fluid collections. Lack of identification or misinterpretation of subtle sonographic findings can have serious clinical implications, including delayed therapy or unnecessary surgery. Furthermore, the operator's experience and skill contribute greatly to diagnostic precision, which emphasizes the significance of specialized training in abdominal ultrasound. With advancing technology, the use of Doppler imaging enhances the capacity to assess vascular structures and identify blood flow pathologies, thereby increasing the diagnostic scope of ultrasound in the evaluation of abdominal illness. In gastrointestinal tumors, ultrasound is a poor-sensitive modality that helps in the choice of the best surgical management and monitoring for response to therapy. For instance, the evaluation of gastrointestinal stromal tumors (GISTs) with ultrasound has elucidated their growth patterns, as demonstrated by a study presenting how ultrasound can be used in following up tumor growth in patient-derived xenografts. The ability to make repeated measurements of tumor size and appearance with the use of ultrasound is correlated directly with actual tumor volume and offers useful insight into the biologic behavior of GISTs. It highlights the importance of ultrasound not only as a diagnostic tool but as part of an active continuum of care of abdominal tumor patients that allows immediate feedback on therapeutic efficacy and aids in clinical decision-making. Secondly, the sonographic assessment of diagnoses in abdominal tuberculosis underscores the modality's crucial function in diagnosing a condition with varied presentations. In regions where abdominal tuberculosis is common, ultrasound significantly aids in the detection of pregnant pathologies, that is, strictures and fluid collections that need to be operated upon. The characteristic signs of abdominal tuberculosis, including thick bowel wall and lymphadenopathy, can be detected by examining ultrasound pictures. An investigation into the surgical results of abdominal tuberculosis shows that an early diagnosis assists in offering timely intervention, which improves patient survival. Clinicians, hence, need to acquire high suspicion and skill in interpreting the ultrasound, particularly in environments where there is poor resource availability and abdominal tuberculosis constitutes a public health issue, necessitating early and effective interventions for management (Singhal et al., 2013) (Figure 7.17).

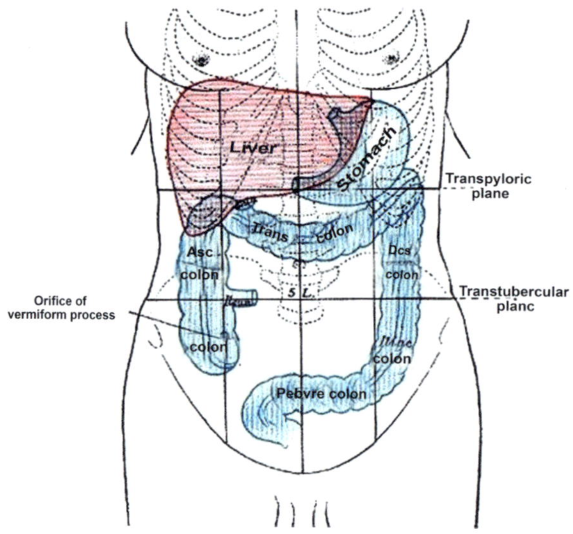

Figure 7.17. Intra-abdominal organs.

Source: Gray1223.png Wikimedia Commons. https://prod-images-static.radiopaedia.org/images/23537/ccc929df91a5bab900db886805b835_gallery.jpeg.

7.6.1. Normal Ultrasound Appearances

Ultrasound examination is an important diagnostic technique utilized to assess the peritoneum and abdominal wall so that health practitioners can see normal anatomical structures and identify potential abnormalities. In abdominal ultrasonography, normal views of the structures like organs, muscles, and connective tissues are significant in providing a baseline for comparison if pathologies are suspected. Characteristic ultrasound features usually depict echogenic (bright) appearances for tissues such as fat and connective tissue, and degrees of echogenicity for solid organs like the liver and kidneys based on their composition. Elucidation of these characteristic appearances not only aids in the evaluation of the abdominal wall, but also provides a groundwork for identifying abnormalities of morphology that may represent disease processes. In normal conditions, there are multiple layers of the abdominal wall with distinct ultrasound characteristics. Both skin and subcutaneous fat form the outermost layer, with both of them being echogenic. There are superficial and deep fascia layers underneath this with varying echogenic contents; the deep fascia layer is particularly important due to its structural support of the muscles underneath. Muscle layers, such as rectus abdominis and external oblique, are typically of intermediate echogenicity. Familiarity with these normal appearances will help differentiate from normal tissue the various forms of pathology, which can exist within the abdominal wall, that is, hernias or abscesses, by observing alterations in texture, contour, and echogenicity.

Also, evaluation of the peritoneum via ultrasound is helpful with respect to the integrity and function of the abdominal cavity. The peritoneal lining is a thin echogenic membrane that is optimally visualized in the context of fluid or pathology. In healthy individuals, the peritoneum should be free of excess fluid, and any focal collections could be pathological, for example, infection or malignancy. Ultrasound also evaluates peritoneal pathologies, such as endometriosis, and thus demonstrates its role as a test of diagnosis. It is vital to comprehend the normal ultrasound characteristics because it allows accurate interpretation of the results, thereby providing timely and effective clinical interventions in case abnormalities are observed (Pascoal et al., 2022; Tomassetti et al., 2021).

7.6.2. Common Pathological Findings

In peritoneum and abdominal wall ultrasound, there are many pathological features that can have a significant impact on management and diagnosis. Pathological features consist of tumors, abscesses, and hernias, each with its distinctive ultrasound appearance. Hernias, for instance, are typically recognized as defects in the abdominal wall and displaced or bulging overlying structures. Ultrasound offers a convenient way of viewing these defects noninvasively, determining size and contents. In addition, abscesses may also appear as multiplanar fluid collections that range from anechoic to echogenic, typically having variable amounts of debris within the fluid, indicating infection. Their identification through ultrasound guarantees early treatment, which is crucial to prevent complications such as perforation or sepsis.

Peritoneal and abdominal wall tumors constitute another vast category of pathologic findings that appear under ultrasound. Benign and malignant neoplasms can both be evaluated successfully with the aid of this imaging method, which provides accurate details regarding the size, location, and extent of lesions. GISTs, for instance, can be identified on the basis of their characteristic appearance as typically well-circumscribed, solid, hypoechoic masses. Growth and response to therapy followed by ultrasound have become increasingly popular, showing its utility in a clinical setting. As described in current literature, PDXs have provided hints on the tumor's biology, further elucidating the way ultrasound can facilitate research and clinical application in the detection and management of such illnesses (Babicky et al., 2014).

Furthermore, ultrasound application is involved in the evaluation of pregnancy complications in the provided populations, such as mares during late gestation. Diseases like uterine torsion can potentially result in severe distress and require immediate veterinary attention, and ultrasound is a very valuable diagnostic tool in these cases. Through the provision of real-time pictures of the uterus and related structures, clinicians can make a diagnosis of abnormal presentations, such as uterine body torsion or fetal positioning defects. Identification of such complications at an early stage by ultrasound can be life-saving for both mare and foal, making the greater significance of using ultrasound in the assessment of some of several pathological abnormalities in the abdominal cavity (Chiers et al., 2008).

7.6.3. Limitations of Ultrasound in Abdominal Assessments

Ultrasound scanning is also widely employed for imaging abdominal organs and pathology, albeit with certain intrinsic limitations that can undermine diagnostic accuracy. Operator dependency is one of the principal limitations, whereby the technical skill and experience level of the individual performing the examination can significantly affect the quality and image definition of the ultrasound. Variation in scanning technique will generate patchy images, potentially leading to misleading clinical management. Furthermore, the amount of excess adipose tissue that obese subjects accumulate can obscure relevant anatomical information and interfere with the visualization of underlying structures, rendering the assessment of the abdominal wall and peritoneum difficult. Because ultrasound is fundamentally an imaging method that involves using sound waves to travel through soft tissues, the process is hindered by the excess amount of body fat, which makes it necessary to employ other imaging methods in such situations. In addition, the use of ultrasound is also limited by its capacity for evaluating some pathological conditions. The modality uses a principle of reflecting sound waves, and this may lead to a problem in discriminating among complex abdominal masses or between benign and malignant lesions. Soft tissue sarcomas, for instance, present a unique challenge to ultrasound examination; their heterogeneous nature and growth patterns may not lead to conclusive characterization by ultrasound alone.

This nonspecificity is illustrated in the case of abdominal examinations, where cysts, abscesses, or tumors can be virtually indistinguishable from one another in ultrasound appearances, and thus become difficult to diagnose. As the NCCN Guidelines for Soft Tissue Sarcoma discloses, a thorough understanding of the clinical setting, augmented by other imaging procedures such as CT or MRI, is crucial to accurate diagnosis and the best treatment plan in complicated abdominal mass situations (von Mehren et al., 2022).

Even more, the limitations of ultrasound are follow-up studies and the inability to assess disease progression. While the ultrasound can be useful for initial evaluation, effectiveness is lost when it is applied to track the course of certain conditions over time. The suggestions provided in the Enhanced Recovery After Surgery (ERAS) guideline note the application of a multimodal regimen for the management of patients, particularly in a surgical setting. Follow-up imaging will typically demand more precise modalities with higher resolution and detail, such as computed tomography or magnetic resonance imaging, which will quantify changes in tumor size and shape more accurately than ultrasound. Therefore, while ultrasound is an excellent first-line imaging modality in abdominal condition assessment, its shortcomings underscore the importance of a multimodal imaging approach that combines various modes to ensure an accurate diagnosis, management, and follow-up of peritoneum- and abdominal wall-related pathologies (Gustafsson et al., 2018).

SUMMARY

The peritoneum and abdominal wall ultrasound scanning has been a goldmine of information in the medical diagnostics and surgical planning arenas. It is a non-surgical technique that provides important information regarding the structural and functional integrity of the abdominal cavity, facilitating early detection and follow-up of various pathologies like hernias, adhesions, and neoplastic lesions. As discussed in a study using ultrasound to investigate postoperative complications, such as inhibition of fibrogenesis associated with Smad7 transgene administration in adhesions of the abdomen, clinical practitioners can access the significance of these results for the purpose of improving patient outcomes (Chan et al., 2009). Ultimately, the capacity of ultrasound technology to guide clinical intervention justifies its ongoing utility and efficacy in surgical settings. Further, while the application of ultrasound in the assessment of the peritoneum and abdominal wall is largely driven by traditional imaging modalities, ongoing investigations continue to reveal its potential to revolutionize therapeutic intervention. For instance, research into adenomyosis and its relation to endometriosis recurrence reveals the significance of identifying lymphatic drainage patterns in designing appropriate treatment regimens (Bonaccorsi et al., 2019). The integration of ultrasound with other imaging techniques maximizes the diagnostic accuracy and treatment planning, marking a milestone in patient care. Such observations also encourage the incorporation of ultrasound as a routine process in preoperative assessment and postoperative follow-ups. In conclusion, the multimodality of abdominal wall and peritoneum ultrasound transcends diagnosis; it includes a holistic approach to patient management that allows practitioners to adequately manage complicated clinical situations. As the field evolves, combining new methods and research developments will likely enhance the utilization of ultrasound to deliver anticipatory intervention protocols for the advancement of patient care. Embracing continuous learning and adaptation of ultrasound techniques will be critical to address future challenges in abdominal pathology and towards a bolder paradigm for diagnosis and therapy. This vision towards the future is supportive of the necessity for evolving ultrasound practice so that patients can benefit from the fruits of advanced medical science meant to serve their unique health needs.

The application of ultrasound in assessing the abdominal wall and peritoneum is relevant to modern medical practice, primarily due to its non-invasive aspect and real-time imaging provided. Clinicians can use this modality to study the myriad intra-abdominal pathologies, such as hernias, fluid collections, and tumors, for data regarding the structural integrity of the abdominal wall. With an enhanced consensus statement set of ultrasonography skills, as identified by experts in intensive care, the abdominal ultrasound position has been upgraded. Not only do these guidelines standardize practices, but they also identify essential competencies necessary for effective abdominal examination, thus ensuring proper abdominal diagnosis and treatment (Robba et al., 2021). Moreover, the application of ultrasound extends beyond fundamental anatomical imaging; it also serves to guide therapeutic procedures. To illustrate, ultrasound may assist with focused aspirations of fluid collections or assist with mass localization for the sake of biopsy. This function reflects the importance of skill in ultrasound techniques, as they may really optimize patient outcomes through prompt and accurate interventions. The growing body of agreement studies highlights the practical benefits of integrating ultrasound in routine abdominal assessment, encouraging doctors to adopt such a practice in the numerous clinical settings (Robba et al., 2021). Endometriosis becomes a timely concern here because it can be greatly enhanced by ultrasound diagnosis. The condition, which is characteristically found by endometrial-like tissue in a location outside the uterus, diagnostic challenges in ways that traditional imaging methods may not be able to fully address. With the use of focused ultrasound methods, healthcare providers can better assess endometriosis-related lesions and cysts. Improved diagnosis of such conditions is important not only for optimal treatment of symptoms but also for alleviation of attendant complications such as infertility. Appreciation for the multifaceted nature of endometriosis, as well as its numerous etiological causes and effects on women's health, only underscores the importance of competent ultrasound practitioners within clinical settings.

CLOSER LOOK

HIGH-INTENSITY FOCUSED ULTRASOUND (HIFU)

High-Intensity Focused Ultrasound (HIFU) is a new, non-surgical therapeutic process using focused ultrasonic energy to heat or mechanically destroy targeted tissue deep within the body without damaging the surrounding structures. HIFU works by converging several beams of high-frequency ultrasound onto a focal point in a tissue mass where the temperature rapidly increases (typically to 60–100°C) and produces coagulative necrosis and cell death. The peripheral tissues are not damaged because the ultrasound beams deposit a large amount of energy only at the convergence point, similar to a burning glass focusing sunbeam energy. In addition to thermal effects, HIFU may also produce mechanical effects such as cavitation and radiation force, which can be employed to induce cell disruption. The two mechanisms in tandem render HIFU particularly appealing in curing tumors and focal diseases with high accuracy and little collateral damage.

Originally developed for prostate cancer, HIFU today is applied in numerous clinical conditions like uterine fibroids, liver cancer, kidney tumors, breast cancer, pancreatic cancer, and even neurological disorders like essential tremor and Parkinson's disease. In the treatment of cancer, HIFU is most often employed in patients who are not suitable candidates for surgery or who prefer to avoid surgery. It has come to be accepted for its ability to reduce tumor burden, relieve symptoms, and in some cases, offer local control of the tumor. Its most widely accepted application is in uterine fibroids, in which HIFU offers an outpatient, uterus-sparing alternative to hysterectomy or myomectomy, with low recovery. In neurology, MR-guided HIFU has received clearance in treating essential tremor, where focused ultrasound is delivered to certain brain nuclei, such as the thalamus, for tremor relief without the need for brain surgery.

One of the major developments in HIFU is the integration of imaging guidance, most notably Magnetic Resonance Imaging (MRI) or real-time ultrasound, which enables accurate targeting and concurrent temperature and treatment effect monitoring during the procedure. This enhances efficacy and safety and allows clinicians to adjust parameters in real time. One of the best advantages of HIFU is that it is not surgical—patients will have fewer complications, faster recovery, and shorter hospitalization compared to standard surgery. Moreover, it obviates the hazards of radiation and systemic chemotherapy and is therefore an optimal option for certain patients, including elderly patients or those with comorbidities.

However, HIFU also has limitations. Its effectiveness can be lost in the treatment of deeply seated or highly vascular tumors due to issues regarding energy delivery and heat dissipation. It is also less suitable for disseminated or metastatic disease. Proper patient selection, adequacy of anatomy, and availability of appropriate imaging modalities are crucial for success. Existing studies are exploring combinations of HIFU with chemotherapy or immunotherapy to enhance systemic anti-tumor efficacy, and new advances in microbubble technology to achieve maximum delivery of energy and targeting to the tumor.

References

1. Alvarez-Hornia Pérez, E., Brancatelli, G., Cannella, R., Porrello, G., & Vernuccio, F. (2022). The benign side of the abdominal wall: A pictorial review of non-neoplastic diseases. https://core.ac.uk/download/576922546.pdf (accessed on 12th July 2025).
2. Alves, F., Castro-Henriques, A., Certo, M., França, M., et al. (2010). Imaging of pancreas transplantation and its complications. https://core.ac.uk/download/71742276.pdf (accessed on 12th July 2025).
3. Amrozi, A., Noordin, M., Panjaitan, B., Setiadi, B., et al. (2014). Sonographic appearance of the abdominal wall at the left flank of laparotomy incision site in Ettawah grade does. https://media.neliti.com/media/publications/157374-EN-sonographic-appearance-of-abdominal-wall.pdf (accessed on 12th July 2025).
4. Andreev, A., Alexander A. A., Ostroushko, A., Ostroushko A. P, Sotnikova, E. S., Sotnikova E. C., Kiryanova, D. V., et al. (2017). Adhesive disease of the abdominal cavity. *Vestnik of Experimental and Clinical Surgery, 10*, 320–326. https://www.semanticscholar.org/paper/7a1d15e1ba4c3d2b05c8df511d547869c6792656 (accessed on 12th July 2025).
5. Autieri, D., Axer, S., Basilico, G., Bertoglio, G., et al. (2015).: Rare and special cases, the real "Strange cases." https://core.ac.uk/download/54524712.pdf (accessed on 12th July 2025).
6. Babicky, M. L., French, R. P., Hoh, C. K., Jaquish, W., et al. (2014). Generation of orthotopic patient-derived xenografts from gastrointestinal stromal tumor. https://core.ac.uk/download/323066735.pdf (accessed on 12th July 2025).
7. Bilican, G., Karakan, T., Eğritaş Gürkan, Ö., Sabhan, H., Hedin, C., Forss, A., Petrousis, G., et al. (2025). P0376 Advancing intestinal ultrasound for IBD in Turkey: Results of a national survey. *Journal of Crohn's and Colitis*. https://www.semanticscholar.org/paper/30611e47cd0b36def50c23f1da2c6676be6ab456 (accessed on 12th July 2025).
8. Bonaccorsi, G., Greco, P., Noventa, M., Pesci, F., et al. (2019). Dye diffusion during laparoscopic tubal patency tests may suggest a lymphatic contribution to dissemination in endometriosis: A prospective, observational study. https://core.ac.uk/download/286075797.pdf (accessed on 12th July 2025).
9. Calabrese, E., Dietrich, C. F., Dirks, K., Gilja, B., et al. (2016). EFSUMB recommendations and guidelines for gastrointestinal ultrasound–Part 1: Examination techniques and normal findings (Long version). https://core.ac.uk/download/74321241.pdf (accessed on 12th July 2025).
10. Calabrese, E., Dietrich, C. F., Dirks, K., Gilja, B., et al. (2016). EFSUMB recommendations and guidelines for gastrointestinal ultrasound–Part 1: Examination techniques and normal findings (Short version). https://core.ac.uk/download/74321243.pdf (accessed on 12th July 2025).
11. Casali, P. G., Abecassis, N., Bauer, S., Biagini, R., Bielack, S., Bonvalot, S., Boukovinas, I., et al. (2018). Gastrointestinal stromal tumors: ESMO–EURACAN Clinical Practice Guidelines for diagnosis, treatment and follow-up. *Annals of Oncology, 29*, iv68–iv78. https://doi.org/10.1093/annonc/mdy095 (accessed on 12th July 2025).
12. Chan, L. Y. Y., Cheung, J. S., Guo, H., Lai, W., et al. (2009). Non-viral Smad7 gene delivery and attenuation of postoperative peritoneal adhesion in an experimental model. https://core.ac.uk/download/37953559.pdf (accessed on 12th July 2025).

13. Cheng, H., Zhu, X., He, Y., Liu, M., Xue, M., & Sun, X. (2024). Efficacy and influencing factor analysis of high-intensity focused ultrasound therapy for abdominal wall endometriosis: A case series. *International Journal of Hyperthermia, 41*. https://www.semanticscholar.org/paper/703423cacaf4b1c0506ba56c281c36139236abbd (accessed on 12th July 2025).

14. Chiers, K., de Kruif, A., Govaere, J., Hoogewijs, M., et al. (2008). Uterine torsion in the mare: A review and three case reports. https://core.ac.uk/download/55757870.pdf (accessed on 12th July 2025).

15. Farine, D., Guido, M., Malvasi, A., Stark, M., et al. (2025). Should the visceral peritoneum at the bladder flap be closed at caesarean sections? A postpartum sonographic and clinical assessment. https://core.ac.uk/download/pdf/37831103.pdf (accessed on 12th July 2025).

16. Fitriani, A., Istiqamah, S. Y., & Lismayanti, L. (2025). Implementation of wound care with simple island dressing technique in inguinal hernia lateralis postoperative patients. *JURNAL KESEHATAN STIKes Muhammadiyah Ciamis*. https://www.semanticscholar.org/paper/cfe6b35310987e139cb95414a894c6b7daaf287a (accessed on 12th July 2025).

17. Gustafsson, U., Scott, M. J., Hübner, M., Nygren, J., Demartines, N., Francis, N., Rockall, T., et al. (2018). Guidelines for perioperative care in elective colorectal surgery: Enhanced Recovery After Surgery (ERAS®) Society recommendations: 2018. *World Journal of Surgery, 43*, 659–695. https://doi.org/10.1007/s00268-018-4844-y (accessed on 12th July 2025).

18. Haaksma, M. E., Smit, J. M., Boussuges, A., Demoule, A., Dres, M., Ferrari, G., Formenti, P., et al. (2022). EXpert consensus On Diaphragm UltraSonography in the critically ill (EXODUS): A Delphi consensus statement on the measurement of diaphragm ultrasound-derived parameters in a critical care setting. *Critical Care, 26*. https://doi.org/10.1186/s13054-022-03975-5 (accessed on 12th July 2025).

19. Harvey, J. J., Prentice, R., & George, J. (2022). Diagnostic and therapeutic abdominal paracentesis. *The Medical Journal of Australia, 218*, 18–21. https://doi.org/10.5694/mja2.51795 (accessed on 12th July 2025).

20. Hashiguchi, Y., Muro, K., Saitô, Y., Ito, Y., Ajioka, Y., Hamaguchi, T., Hasegawa, K., et al. (2019). Japanese Society for Cancer of the Colon and Rectum (JSCCR) guidelines 2019 for the treatment of colorectal cancer. *International Journal of Clinical Oncology, 25*, 1–42. https://doi.org/10.1007/s10147-019-01485-z (accessed on 12th July 2025).

21. Henriksen, N. A., Montgomery, A., Kaufmann, R., Berrevoet, F., East, B., Fischer, J. P., Hope, W. W., et al. (2020). Guidelines for treatment of umbilical and epigastric hernias from the European Hernia Society and Americas Hernia Society. *British Journal of Surgery, 107*, 171–190. https://doi.org/10.1002/bjs.11489 (accessed on 12th July 2025).

22. Keckstein, J., Sarıdoğan, E., Ulrich, U., Sillem, M., Oppelt, P., Schweppe, K. W., Krentel, H., et al. (2021). The #Enzian classification: A comprehensive non-invasive and surgical description system for endometriosis. *Acta Obstetrician Et Gynecological Scandinavica, 100*, 1165–1175. https://doi.org/10.1111/aogs.14099 (accessed on 12th July 2025).

23. Kok, H. P., Cressman, E. N. K., Ceelen, W., Brace, C. L., Ivkov, R., Grüll, H., ter Haar, G., et al. (2020). Heating technology for malignant tumors: A review. *International Journal of Hyperthermia, 37*, 711–741. https://doi.org/10.1080/02656736.2020.1779357 (accessed on 12th July 2025).

24. Manzoor, H., Ara, I., Maqsood, S., Khan, M. T., Maqsood, M., & Lone, T. (2025). Diagnostic accuracy of FAST scan in patient with blunt abdominal trauma keeping CECT abdomen as gold standard. *Journal of Medical & Health Sciences Review*. https://www.semanticscholar.org/paper/1ecd46225d406ddf12fdc5cdcd76285c1d0e8d33 (accessed on 12th July 2025).

25. Olsson, A., & Woxnerud, K. (2022). P-096 Assessment of the fascia healing process after suture plication of rectus diastasis–Measured with ultrasound at one, two, three- and four-months following surgery. *British Journal of Surgery*. https://www.semanticscholar.org/paper/f84ab9c52a8ef8a914f7529a1e0a08dbe154a795 (accessed on 12th July 2025).

26. Pascoal, E., Wessels, J. M., Aas-Eng, M. K., Simões Abrão, M., Condous, G., Jurkovic, D., Espada, M., et al. (2022). Strengths and limitations of diagnostic tools for endometriosis and relevance in diagnostic test accuracy research. *Ultrasound in Obstetrics and Gynecology, 60*, 309–327. https://doi.org/10.1002/uog.24892 (accessed on 12th July 2025).

27. Prakash, H., & Chakrabarti, A. (2019). Global epidemiology of mucormycosis. *Journal of Fungi, 5*, 26. https://doi.org/10.3390/jof5010026 (accessed on 12th July 2025).

28. Robba, C., Wong, A., Poole, D., Al Tayar, A., Arntfield, R., Chew, M. S., Corradi, F., et al. (2021). Basic ultrasound head-to-toe skills for intensivists in the general and neuro intensive care unit population: Consensus and expert recommendations of the European Society of Intensive Care Medicine. *Intensive Care Medicine, 47*, 1347–1367. https://doi.org/10.1007/s00134-021-06486-z (accessed on 12th July 2025).

29. Santos, A. P., Matos, S., & Reis, L. (2025). Anesthesiology and ultrasound-guided injection of botulinum toxin in the abdominal wall: A state-of-the-art and technical adaptation. *Cureus, 17*. https://www.semanticscholar.org/paper/f5c7a7d37dc8be889166b0298fb417f81913851f (accessed on 12th July 2025).

30. Seethalakshmi, K. (2018). Randomized controlled clinical trial comparing the clinical outcome of autologous fascia lata to synthetic mesh for abdominal sacrocolpopexy among successfully repaired vault prolapse patients. https://core.ac.uk/download/270241659.pdf (accessed on 12th July 2025).

31. Singhal, A., Soylu, A., Zafar, A., Arif, A. U., Anuradha, B., Mawalla, B. M., Bolukbas, C., et al. (2013). Clinicopathological profile and surgical treatment of abdominal tuberculosis: A single center experience in northwestern Tanzania. https://core.ac.uk/download/pdf/16666714.pdf (accessed on 12th July 2025).

32. Smolarz, B., Szyłło, K., & Romanowicz, H. (2021). Endometriosis: Epidemiology, classification, pathogenesis, treatment and genetics (Review of literature). *International Journal of Molecular Sciences, 22*, 10554. https://doi.org/10.3390/ijms221910554 (accessed on 12th July 2025).

33. Spahn, D. R., Bouillon, B., Černý, V., Duranteau, J., Filipescu, D., Hunt, B. J., Komadina, R., et al. (2019). The European guideline on management of major bleeding and coagulopathy following trauma: Fifth edition. *Critical Care, 23*. https://doi.org/10.1186/s13054-019-2347-3 (accessed on 12th July 2025).

34. ten Broek, R. P. G., Krielen, P., Di Saverio, S., Coccolini, F., Biffl, W. L., Ansaloni, L., Velmahos, G. C., et al. (2018). Bologna guidelines for diagnosis and management of adhesive small bowel obstruction (ASBO): 2017 update of the evidence-based guidelines from the World Society of Emergency Surgery ASBO working group. *World Journal of Emergency Surgery, 13*. https://doi.org/10.1186/s13017-018-0185-2 (accessed on 12th July 2025).

35. Tomassetti, C., Johnson, N., Petrozza, J. C., Simões Abrão, M., Einarsson, J. I., Horne, A. W., Lee, T. T. M., et al. (2021). An international terminology for endometriosis, 2021. *Journal of Minimally Invasive Gynecology, 28*, 1849–1859. https://doi.org/10.1016/j.jmig.2021.08.032 (accessed on 12th July 2025).

36. Tomassetti, C., Johnson, N., Petrozza, J. C., Simões Abrão, M., Einarsson, J. I., Horne, A. W., Lee, T. T. M., et al. (2021). An international terminology for endometriosis, 2021. *Facts Views and Vision in ObGyn, 13*, 295–304. https://doi.org/10.52054/fvvo.13.4.036 (accessed on 12th July 2025).

37. Van der Merwe, R. L. J., van Wanrooij, M., Bronswijk, M., Everett, S., Lakhtakia, S., Rimbaş, M., Hucl, T., et al. (2021). Therapeutic endoscopic ultrasound: European Society of Gastrointestinal Endoscopy (ESGE) guideline. *Endoscopy, 54*, 185–205. https://doi.org/10.1055/a-1717-1391 (accessed on 12th July 2025).

38. Vereen, M. S., Bidault, V. J., Krabbendam, E., Hoeks, S. E., Stolker, R., & Dirckx, M. (2025). The effectiveness of liposomal bupivacaine in ultrasound-guided abdominal wall blocks after open abdominal surgery: A systematic review. *Pain Practice, 25*. https://www.semanticscholar.org/paper/46ba47381a555a0499ceacc7d8565c57bc20f48d (accessed on 12th July 2025).

39. von Mehren, M., Kane, J. M., Agulnik, M., Bui, M. M., Carr, J. R., Choy, E., Connelly, M., et al. (2022). Soft tissue sarcoma, Version 2.2022, NCCN Clinical Practice Guidelines in Oncology. *Journal of the National Comprehensive Cancer Network, 20*, 815–833. https://doi.org/10.6004/jnccn.2022.0035 (accessed on 12th July 2025).

40. Wanhainen, A., Björck, M., Boman, K., Rutegård, J., & Bergqvist, D. (2001). Influence of diagnostic criteria on the prevalence of abdominal aortic aneurysm. *Journal of Vascular Surgery, 34*(2), 229–235. https://www.semanticscholar.org/paper/eed574e30d36fe2620f3622a55c8033b59ead5a0 (accessed on 12th July 2025).

41. Yela-Lorenzo, P., Montes-Arenas, P., Abuín-Porras, V., Gónzalez-de-la-Flor, Á., González-Fernández, L., Villafañe, J., & Mínguez-Esteban, I. (2025). Bruxism repercussions in muscular activation: Ultrasound differences in abdominal wall between women with and without bruxism. A cross-sectional study. *PLOS ONE, 20*. https://www.semanticscholar.org/paper/45524b37e39256606d88eab2d0f30c012987098f (accessed on 12th July 2025).

42. You, J., Li, G., Chen, H., Wang, J., & Li, S. (2020). Laparoscopic orchiopexy of palpable undescended testes: Experience of a single tertiary institution with over 773 cases. *BMC Pediatrics, 20*. https://doi.org/10.1186/s12887-020-2021-6 (accessed on 12th July 2025).

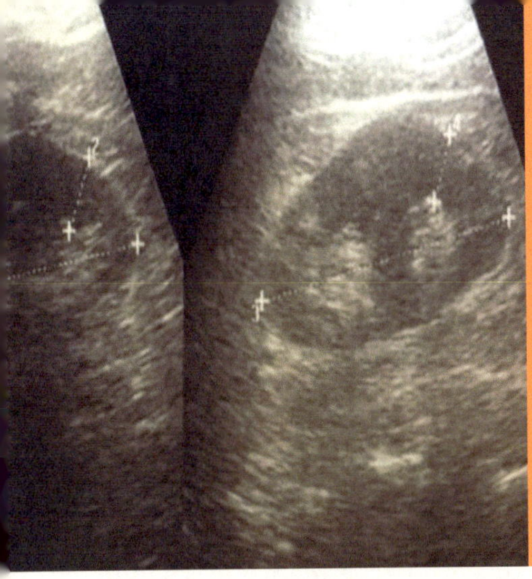

Chapter 8

LIVER AND BILIARY SYSTEM ULTRASOUND

Contents

Introduction

The biliary tree and liver play crucial roles in providing metabolic homeostasis and detoxification of a broad range of compounds and are therefore central to human health. With advancements in imaging technologies, ultrasound has emerged as a dominant diagnostic modality, providing us with useful insights into the anatomy and disease of these systems. Convenient, non-invasive, and sensitive, liver and biliary ultrasound is invaluable in diagnosing from mild inflammation to severe diseases like cirrhosis and hepatocellular carcinoma. By utilizing sound waves to generate real-time images of the liver and surrounding structures, ultrasound enables clinicians to make precise clinical decisions. This fundamental knowledge forms the background for the clinical and technical appropriateness of liver and biliary ultrasound, ultimately guiding effective management of the patients. In addition to being diagnostic, liver and biliary ultrasound play a crucial role in screening potential complications of a given disease. For instance, the diagnosis of gallstones, bile duct obstruction, and pathologic liver lesions is important in the initial management of acute conditions that can lead to severe morbidity. Conditions such as viral hepatitis and liver fluke infection are known to significantly impair liver function. In the impoverished regions, the incidence of liver fluke infection, for instance, illustrates the need for effective diagnostic practices, particularly given the implication of such infections' complications, which can encompass significant carcinogenic threats (Harrington et al., 2017). Accordingly, the application of ultrasound technology not only enhances understanding of pathology in the liver but also facilitates the reduction of likely healthcare costs through early identification and treatment. Finally, the integration of ultrasound with other diagnostic modalities can further stratify liver and biliary tract pathology knowledge. While the intrinsic sensitivity of ultrasound in detecting fluid collections and vascular disease is unique, integration with techniques like CT or MRI can provide comprehensive studies necessary for difficult cases. As has been seen with drug-induced liver injury, including that which occurs with long-term linezolid treatment, ultrasound may reveal significant morphologic changes that need further evaluation (Benoit et al., 2010). The ultrasound is thus an important gateway to more invasive diagnostic tests if and when needed, enabling clinicians to effectively navigate the complexities of liver pathologies. In brief, the merits of liver and biliary ultrasound encompass diagnostic precision, therapeutic intervention potential at an early stage, and facilitating comprehensive patient management, hence the cornerstone of modern hepatology (Figure 8.1).

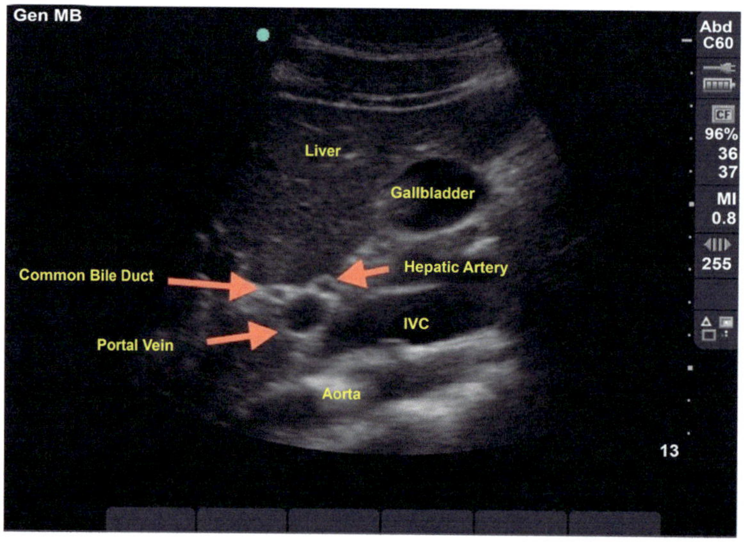

Figure 8.1. Liver and biliary system ultrasound.

Source: https://coreem.net/content/uploads/2019/05/GB2.png.

Definition of Ultrasound in Medical Imaging

Ultrasound is a non-invasive imaging technique based on the use of high-frequency sound waves to create real-time images of the interior structures of the body. It follows the principle of acoustic echo, whereby sound waves emitted by a transducer travel through tissues and are reflected back when they encounter different media densities. This back-reflection creates images of organs and soft tissues in minute detail, making ultrasound a valuable instrument in medical diagnostics. In liver and biliary system ultrasonography, the modality is very helpful as it can visualize liver pathology, obstructive biliary ducts, and other pathologies. The safety profile is excellent; ultrasound does not involve ionizing radiation, which is a bonus compared to other imaging studies. It is not invasive, so it can be repeated as often as needed for monitoring over time. In imaging of the liver and biliary tract, ultrasound is a primary modality for the detection and characterization of tumors, cysts, and gallstones. It not only allows practitioners to examine the morphology of these organs and structures but also allows them to assess blood perfusion via Doppler ultrasound, an enhanced modality that investigates hepatic and biliary vessel hemodynamics. In addition, diagnostic productivity is also facilitated by advances in ultrasound technology, such as the coming of 3D imaging and elastography, which measures the stiffness of tissues—a determinant factor in liver fibrosis assessment. Ultrasound is therefore an eminent tool in hepatology, enabling doctors to come to sensible decisions on management and treatment based on sonographic findings. On top of that, ultrasonographic use within a multidisciplinary process yields the highest diagnostic accuracy for liver disease. Multidisciplinary collaboration with specialists in other disciplines—that is, radiology, gastroenterology, and oncology—ensures that ultrasonographic diagnoses are consistent with the overall clinical context. Pancreatic neuroendocrine neoplasms are an example of the multidisciplinary process of diagnosis and treatment since their management is typically supplemented by elaborate imaging and biochemical testing. The intricate interplay between clinical expertise and more recent imaging technologies emphasizes the place of ultrasound in current medical practice, particularly in the liver and biliary apparatus (Focal Spot, 2003; Almar et al., 2019). Lastly, ultrasound is not merely a diagnostic tool but also a method to enhance patient care through its ability to provide timely and proper information.

Importance of Liver and Biliary System Assessment

Liver and biliary tree evaluation is crucial in modern medicine due to the complexity of the organs' functions in metabolism, storage, and detoxification. The introduction of novel imaging techniques, particularly ultrasonography, allows for non-invasive liver disease and biliary tract disease assessment. Imaging of organs such as gallbladders, hepatic arteries and veins, and hepatic parenchyma is crucial in the diagnosis of conditions such as cirrhosis, fatty liver, and obstruction of the bile ducts. Also, ultrasound is a prime investigation method, with immediate feedback to enable clinicians to determine whether more advanced imaging or therapeutic intervention is needed. Early diagnosis dramatically enhances outcomes for patients, justifying the importance of routine liver and biliary system evaluation in high-risk populations. Lastly, the benefit of liver and biliary system evaluation goes beyond diagnostic capability to encompass preventive health. With increasing rates of liver disease incidence globally, especially in economically developing nations, detection at an early stage is essential in managing and stopping further development. It has been documented that infections like liver fluke infection, prevalent in specific geographical regions, have high morbidity rates and are a significant risk factor for liver cancer. Identification of the epidemiology of such infections can inform public health policy to minimize exposure and increase screening activity. The integration of liver and biliary ultrasound into routine examinations can be an indispensable step toward identifying high-risk individuals, motivating early intervention, and reducing the load of liver ailments. Moreover, the implementation of technologies such as Contrast-Enhanced Ultrasound (CEUS) has revolutionized the landscape of liver examinations by making diagnosis more efficient while minimizing the risks associated with radiation exposure. CEUS provides a noninvasive alternative that is especially useful in pediatric patients, where conventional imaging modalities may risk damage from ionizing radiation. As has been emphasized by recent evidence, CEUS is increasingly being used for the evaluation of focal liver lesions in children, demonstrating its potential utility in several different clinical situations. As medicine evolves through the use of technology like CEUS, not only will precision in diagnosis increase, but clinical practice will become progressively more patient-focused, further highlighting the necessity for comprehensive liver and biliary assessment in modern healthcare practice (Cantisani et al., 2016; Harrington et al., 2017) (Figure 8.2).

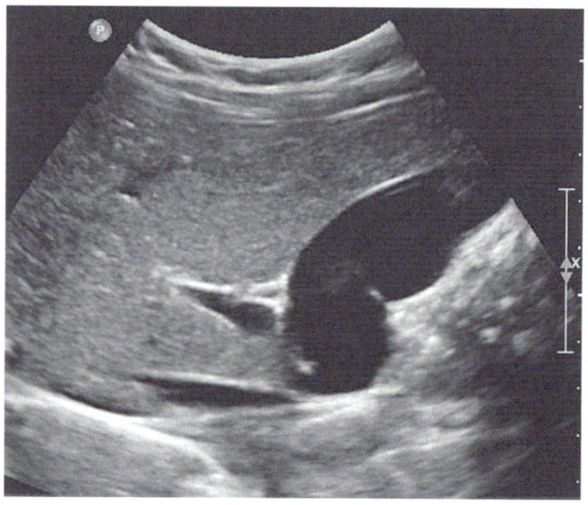

Figure 8.2. Liver and biliary system assessment.

Source: https://radiologykey.com/wp-content/uploads/2020/06/10-1055-b-003-122515_009_001.jpg.

8.1. Anatomy of the Liver

The liver is a highly organized organ that plays a critical role in many physiological processes like metabolism, detoxification, and digestion. The liver is anatomically divided into two major lobes called the right lobe and the left lobe, and each of these lobes is further divided into smaller units called lobules. These lobules consist of hepatocytes, the liver's functional cells, which are arranged around central veins. The characteristic spatial organisation of the liver's vascular pathways, including the hepatic artery and portal vein, facilitates effective oxygen and nutrient delivery. It is a rudimentary understanding of such anatomy that underlies the understanding of ultrasound scans, as differences or deviations can represent underlying pathologies. A well-developed comprehension of the anatomy of the liver is important in medical practice, especially for the usage of imaging modalities in the assessment of the health and function of the liver. In liver and biliary tract ultrasonography, liver visualization entails attention to both the parenchyma and related structures of the liver. The normal liver parenchyma is uniform on ultrasonography, demonstrating an echogenicity that separates it from adjacent tissues. However, pathologies such as cirrhosis, fatty liver, and neoplasms can potentially alter this echogenic pattern, and difficulties in diagnosis can arise, requiring specialist interpretation of ultrasound images. Furthermore, the biliary tree of bile ducts and gallbladder is intimately related to liver anatomy. Disease or obstruction of the biliary tract potentially alters liver function and ultrasound appearances, such as cholangitis or choledocholithiasis. The ability to visualize these relationships on imaging is essential to making appropriate clinical impressions. Ultrasound and other imaging modalities are employed not only to visualize anatomical structures but also to assess potential complications of liver transplantation. Transplantation introduces new anatomical arrangements, particularly with respect to the surgical anastomoses that connect new supplies of blood with the liver. Radiologists must be well-versed with these settings to appropriately evaluate normal vs. pathological results after transplantation. For instance, imaging modalities can identify vascular and biliary complications rapidly, which are critical in the prevention of such devastating events as hepatic artery thrombosis or portal vein stenosis, and directly affect graft survival. Selective arterial portography and other angiographic examinations play an important role in post-transplant diagnostics, particularly in those with indeterminate ultrasound findings. Appreciation of these all-crucial connections highlights the anatomical complexity of the liver and stresses the importance of imaging to management and outcome in the patient, as illustrated in the pertinent research of liver transplantation (Anzidei et al., 2016) and post-angiographic outcome (Bron et al., 1985) (Figure 8.3).

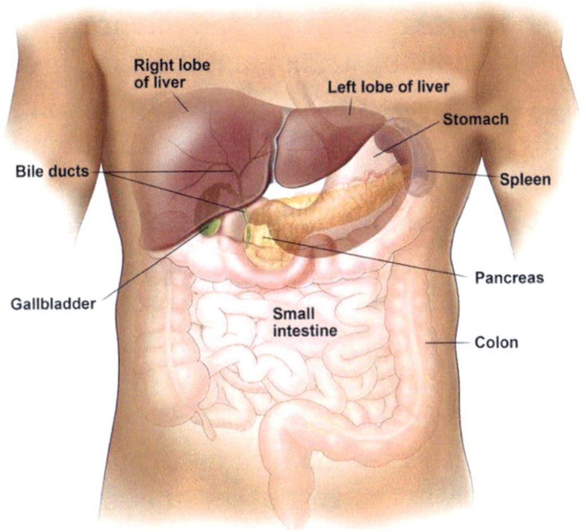

Figure 8.3. Anatomy of the liver.

Source: https://visualsonline.cancer.gov/retrieve.cfm?imageid=9077&dpi=72&fileformat=jpg.

8.1.1. Lobes and Segments of the Liver

The liver is anatomically divided into lobes and segments, a terminology that is of paramount importance for surgery and diagnosis, above all in the ultrasound of the liver and biliary system. The liver has two large lobes: the right and left lobes. The right lobe is considerably larger and divided into segments according to the vascular supply of the liver. This division is primarily based on the portal vein and hepatic artery supply nourishing the liver and allowing it its innumerable functions. These divisions anatomically are well-known to the ultrasound technicians, and they can properly evaluate and visualize liver pathology, which increases the efficacy of diagnostic imaging and interventional maneuvers. Furthermore, segmentation provides a foundation for liver procedures, that is, resections, for which an extremely precise understanding of the liver's configuration is essential to patient safety and greatest surgical success. Exploring liver segmentation further, Couinaud's classification system remains a cornerstone of liver anatomy, segmenting the liver into eight functionally independent segments. All of these segments also possess their own vascular inflow, outflow, and biliary drainage, which are particularly relevant when one is thinking about liver lesions or surgical access planning. As an example, understanding segmental anatomy is useful in distinguishing between benign and malignant lesions on ultrasound examination because certain pathologies can appear differently based on their location within the liver. With advancing technology, three-dimensional imaging, particularly with the use of real-time ultrasound, optimizes visualization of these segments. Clinicians and radiologists are thus given equipment that allows better evaluation, thereby making decision-making in patient management and surgical planning feasible, thus bringing to focus the role of basic liver anatomy in clinical practice (Hirai et al., 2015).For the purpose of ultrasound imaging, adequate patient preparation and knowledge of transducer choice are important in successful imaging of the liver segments and lobes. Fasting is commonly advised to minimize gas within the gastrointestinal tract to prevent the obscuration of liver imaging. The selection of a transducer is also essential, as different patients might need different frequencies depending on their body habitus. For instance, the use of lower-frequency transducers in obese patients is possible since they penetrate deeper. The scanning technique has to be meticulous and cautious to check the liver comprehensively so that all segments and lobes are scanned appropriately. Use of extensive patient history also aids ultrasound technicians in determining specific areas of anatomy that would require more detailed evaluation. This concentration increases accurate diagnoses and positive patient outcomes in the case of liver and biliary system ultrasound tests (Fatchett, 1997) (Figure 8.4).

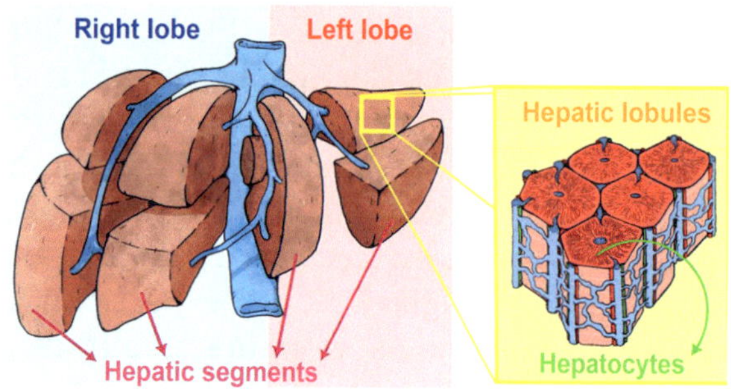

Figure 8.4. Lobes and segments of the liver.

Source: Luque, Luciana & Carlevaro, Manuel & Llamoza Torres, Camilo & Lomba, Enrique. (2023). Physics-based tissue simulator to model multicellular systems: A study of liver regeneration and hepatocellular carcinoma recurrence. PLOS Computational Biology. 19. e1010920. 10.1371/journal.pcbi.1010920.

8.1.2. Blood Supply and Drainage

Understanding the blood supply and drainage of the liver is important in comprehending its function and pathophysiology, especially in the context of liver and biliary system ultrasound. The liver has a double blood supply: approximately 75% from the portal vein and 25% from the hepatic artery. The portal vein supplies the gut-derived high-nutrient blood that helps metabolite processing, and the hepatic artery supplies oxygenated blood required for hepatocyte function. The single dual supply makes many biochemical activities, including detoxification and the production of essential proteins, possible. Anomalies in this intricate system may result in fatal clinical complications that may manifest as a disturbance in blood supply or even hepatic transplant failure, thus providing huge importance to ultrasound evaluation of blood vessels in diagnostic imaging. Complications of hepatic artery thrombosis (HAT) and portal vein thrombosis (PVT) are of grave concern in liver transplantation. As realized in recent publications, HAT has been termed the Achilles heel of orthotopic liver transplantation due to its cataclysmic effects, including fulminant hepatic necrosis and bacteremia. It is crucial to diagnose HAT early at a prevalence of 6.8% in grafts following transplantation, to prevent septic complications and mortality in the patient. Moreover, PVT is rare but could be highly injurious to graft viability, necessitating vigilant surveillance with imaging techniques such as ultrasound. Continuous assessment can guide early interventions to mitigate risk from such vascular complications, improving patient outcomes and graft survival rates (Gordon et al., 1987). The evolution of ultrasound modalities, in particular contrast-enhanced ultrasound (CEUS), promises great potential in the evaluation of liver blood flow and drainage. Previously, CEUS had been extensively applied in adults; however, its application in pediatric patients has only recently begun to gain momentum, considering the critical imaging benefit with minimal dose of exposure to ionizing radiation. This is especially relevant as the vascular organs of the liver and any pathological changes must be watched closely in children, who may have their own individualized conditions. Greater sensitivity in imaging can render a more distinct picture of hepatic perfusion and drainage issues, which can assist in diagnosing vascular disease, tumors, as well as potential liver disease and transplantation complications. The promising results of CEUS use demonstrate a greater acceptability and need for integration into routine ultrasound practice, thereby making it vital for liver evaluation in various patient populations (Cantisani et al., 2016).

8.1.3. Association with Surrounding Organs

Understanding the proximity of the liver to surrounding organs is critical when analyzing the ultrasound results in relation to the biliary system. The liver is in close proximity to the gallbladder, pancreas, and right kidney, and disease in each of the above organs can directly affect liver function and morphology. For instance, diseases such as cholecystitis have been implicated in causing gallbladder inflammation, which may appear as liver or altered echogenicity on ultrasound. Furthermore, the pancreas, particularly the head, is anatomically close to the liver, and thus a multimodal imaging approach is needed to identify any lesion with accuracy. This is possible because with knowledge of the anatomical surround, radiologists will be able to differentiate between those pathologies that may either be from the liver itself or the surrounding organs, and with that, all conditions in the abdomen will be assessed thoroughly. The biliary system, which is a part of the liver's architecture, makes the relationship even tougher. Structures such as the common bile duct and hepatic arteries are vital components of the biliary apparatus that exist in intimate anatomical relationship with both the pancreas and the liver. Disorders such as biliary obstruction can manifest as sonographic abnormalities in the liver parenchyma, for example, intrahepatic biliary dilatation. In pancreatitis, typically presented as peritoneal inflammation, the resulting effects have a chance to precipitate biliary complications affecting liver ultrasound findings. Imaging techniques like ultrasound are therefore not only critical in assessing liver pathology but also in observing how the surrounding organs interact or influence liver well-being. Precise measurement of these relationships enhances diagnostic accuracy, guiding subsequent management and treatment in patients presenting with abdominal pain or other gastrointestinal symptomatology. The usefulness of ultrasound for assessment of the liver and visceral organs extends beyond mere anatomical representation. Sophisticated imaging modes like Doppler ultrasound and contrast-enhanced techniques allow for precise evaluation of vascular relations and pathology in terms of mechanisms of the liver's blood supply and drainage. As the recent imaging literature has elucidated, a multimodal approach can be beneficial in adequately staging diseases such as pancreatic tumors, where overlying structures will frequently determine the clinical presentation.

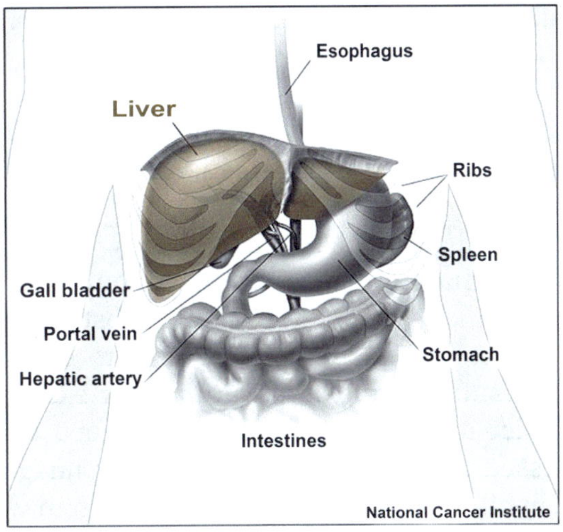

Figure 8.5. Liver and nearby organs.

Source: Don Bliss (2007) Liver and Nearby Organs. National Cancer Institute. https://visualsonline.cancer.gov/retrieve.cfm?imageid=4358&dpi=72&fileformat=jpg.

The pancreas's close proximity to both the liver and duodenum makes surgical planning more complex, and an understanding of the dynamics between the liver and such organs is critical. Thus, the clinicians must be conversant with the identification of the implications of these relations to develop effective treatments, showing the importance of synchronizing ultrasound images with familiarization with the adjacent anatomy in the patient's best interests (Baccari et al., 2016; Focal Spot, 2007) (Figure 8.5).

8.2. Anatomy of the Biliary System

The intricate anatomy of the biliary tracts is central to the whole liver process, ranging from the transport of bile from the liver into the small intestine. The biliary tract comprises the hepatic ducts, gallbladder, and the common bile duct, which collectively are involved in the emulsification and digestion of fats. The right and left hepatic ducts converge to form the common hepatic duct, which comes together with the cystic duct of the gallbladder to form the common bile duct. This is very important in regulating the movement of bile when the body is digesting, so that it may facilitate correct nutrient absorption. Abnormalities of the biliary tree, for example, obstructions or strictures, have the potential to lead to significant clinical complications, for example, jaundice and cholestasis, and thus need to be assessed and treated with diagnostic imaging. When imaging the liver and biliary system with ultrasound, accurate visualization of the biliary structures is paramount. Ultrasound offers measurement of gallbladder and hepatic duct size and patency and detection of gallstones and duct wall thickening. The modality of imaging is particularly valuable in that it does not involve invasiveness or exposure of patients to ionizing radiation. Familiarity with normal vs. pathologic appearance is vitally important for radiologists, particularly in the identification of post-liver transplantation (LT) complications. (Anzidei et al., 2016) describes the significance of imaging modalities in the early detection of vascular and biliary complications following LT. Adequate interpretation of ultrasound findings is important, as incorrect management and compromised patient outcomes can be caused by misdiagnosis. The relationship between the biliary and liver function is also significant, especially against the backdrop of liver disease, which is known to affect biliary drainage. For instance, conditions such as primary sclerosing cholangitis and biliary atresia can lead to progressive injury of the bile ducts that causes bile flow obstruction and subsequent liver damage.

Ultrasound scanning provides a real-time assessment that is extremely helpful in the diagnosis of dynamic alterations of the bile ducts. Proper familiarity with anatomy and potential pathologic alteration of the biliary tree is essential when one is interpreting an ultrasound. As quoted in (Anzidei et al., 2016), it is essential to recognize both the normal anatomical relationship as well as any variation for effective diagnosis and follow-up post-operatively. This underlines the necessity of detailed anatomy knowledge in order to enhance the effectiveness of ultrasound in managing biliary disease (Figure 8.6).

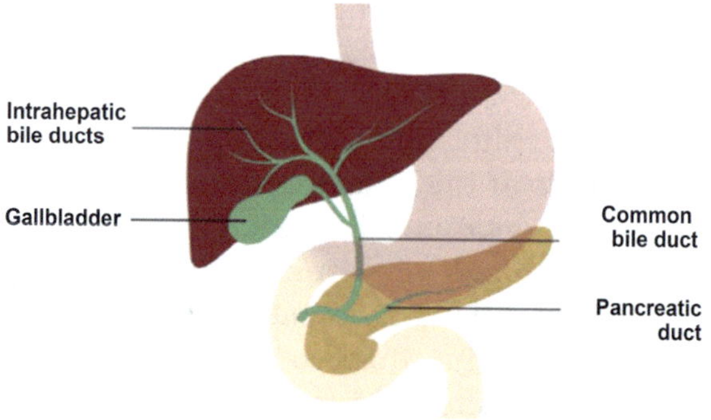

Figure 8.6. Anatomy of the biliary system.

Source: Hartung, P M. and Brown, A. (2024). Abdominal CT: Biliary system and Pancreas. litfl.com https://litfl.com/wp-content/uploads/2023/04/ABdominal-CT-biliary-system-and-pancreas-01.png.

8.2.1. Components of the Biliary Tree

The biliary tree is a critical element of the liver and biliary apparatus and is the conduit of bile drainage from the liver to the duodenum. It is made up of a network of bile ducts that have their origin in the liver, wherein canaliculi merge to form small bile ductules, which ultimately form large bile ducts. These ducts keep connecting and the right and left hepatic ducts are formed, which unite to give rise to the common hepatic duct. This intricate system aids in directing bile, required for the process of digestion and the absorption of fats, into the intestine. The relevance of understanding the segments of the biliary tree extends also to the diagnostic and therapeutic setting, particularly in the case of liver and biliary tree ultrasound, where imaging plays a key role in identifying anatomic variations and pathologies that may obstruct the flow of bile. Ultrasound scanning of the biliary tree is very useful in imaging the structure and function of its components and in the identification of conditions such as biliary atresia or choledocholithiasis. The ultrasound can visualize the intrahepatic and extrahepatic bile ducts to check their size and patency and thereby check the conditions that may lead to biliary obstruction. For instance, dilatation of the bile duct is typically evocative of an obstructive disease. Knowing the histological characteristics of the biliary remnants also comes in handy, especially following surgery for conditions like biliary atresia. Investigations have revealed that meticulous evaluation of biliary remnants can detect patterns of active or inactive lesions, which may influence patients after procedures such as the Kasai portoenterostomy (KHPE) procedure, suggesting the significance of ultrasound in combination with histopathological results (Arva et al., 2018).

The dynamic nature of the biliary tree also leads to a variety of pathologies that must be detected by ultrasound screening. For example, illnesses such as cholangitis, cancer of the bile duct, and strictures demand proper awareness about the anatomy of the biliary system in order to make accurate diagnoses. Ultrasound not only aids in the diagnosis of these diseases but also allows for the planning of follow-up diagnostic tests or interventions. Notably, familiarity with the common imaging characteristics of mesenchymal tissue-related tumors, as reported in recent studies, enhances radiologic accuracy of diagnosis (Ahmed et al., 2017). This implies that integration between anatomical knowledge and imaging diagnostic modalities is pivotal to the management of liver and biliary system disease, and it underscores the role of the biliary tree in liver and biliary system ultrasound (Figure 8.7).

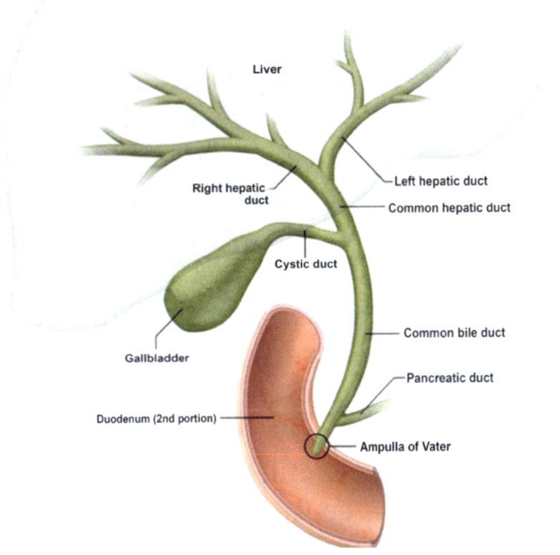

Figure 8.7. Components of the biliary tree.

Source: https://radiologykey.com/wp-content/uploads/2016/09/A303228_1_En_5_Fig1_HTML.jpg.

8.2.2. Function of Bile in Digestion

Bile plays a vital role in lipid digestion and absorption, facilitating it by virtue of its unique biochemical properties. The liver secretes and stores it in the gallbladder, wherein it comprises mainly bile salts, cholesterol, bilirubin, electrolytes, and water. Bile salts, which are synthesized from cholesterol, are required to emulsify fats in the small intestine, breaking them into small droplets that can be metabolized better by digestive enzymes. Emulsification increases the fats' surface area significantly and allows lipases to continue digesting triglycerides to fatty acids and monoglycerides. Not only does the presence of bile ease fat digestion, but it also promotes the absorption of fat-soluble vitamins such as A, D, E, and K, which indicates its priceless position in digestive function. Additionally, the control of bile production and secretion bears a close association with the process of digestion. Once the fats enter the duodenum, they trigger the release of cholecystokinin (CCK), a hormone that leads to gallbladder contraction and bile release into the small intestine. The synchronized effort has the bile ready exactly when it is needed, optimizing the digestive process. In addition, conditions like obstructive cholestasis greatly influence bile flow, leading to reduced fat digestion and absorption. A study notes that the mean duodenal expression of breast cancer resistance protein (BCRP), involved in bile acid transport, was significantly low in patients with obstructive cholestasis, perhaps exacerbating gastrointestinal issues (Adachi et al., 2006). The function of the bile is thus not only a matter of secretion but also an active process with hormonal and physiological feedbacks that significantly contribute to good digestion. In addition, bile structure and viscosity play important roles in the prevention of gallstone formation and efficient digestion. The increased viscosity of gallbladder bile, particularly in patients with cholesterol gallstone predisposition, can obstruct bile flow and lead to complications. Research has established that the viscosity of gallbladder bile is directly related to its composition, while others, such as gallbladder motility, are not significantly influenced by it. This finding underlines the complex interplay between bile composition and digestive efficiency and its potential for influencing biliary health (Althaus et al., 2009). Finally, the function of bile in digestion extends beyond fat emulsification to encompass regulatory, compositional, and mechanical functions, all of which contribute significantly to maintaining digestive health and preventing gastrointestinal disease (Figure 8.8).

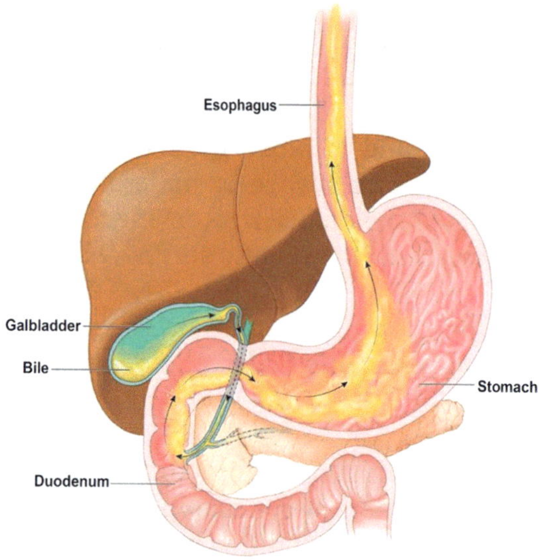

Figure 8.8. Function of bile in digestion.

Source: my.clevelandclinic.org.(2021). Bile Reflux. https://my.clevelandclinic.org/-/scassets/images/org/health/articles/22056-bile-reflux-web.ashx

8.2.3. Pathways of Bile Flow

The biliary channels of bile passage are crucial to understanding the intricate processes of liver function and the biliary mechanism. Bile, a digestive juice secreted by the liver, is produced in the hepatocytes and initially passes through a network of canaliculi before entering the bile ductules. These small ducts coalesce to form large bile ducts that finally coalesce to form the common hepatic duct. At this point, bile can either flow into the gallbladder for storage or continue onward to the duodenum, where fat absorption and digestion depend upon it. Understanding the process is valuable for clinicians, especially during liver and biliary system ultrasonography, as pathology in bile flow can indicate the presence of disease within the liver or the biliary tree. The maintenance of normal bile flow depends on a plethora of factors, including the integrity of bile ducts and the presence of adequate numbers of biliary epithelial cells. In the case of biliary atresia, where developmental bile duct obstruction occurs, histological analysis has revealed significant discrepancies and therefore warrants the explanation of the dynamics of bile flow. For instance, studies have shown that remnants of the bile duct show heterogeneous histological patterns that can direct prognosis and management. Demonstration of active lesions within such remnants, particularly for necroinflammatory changes, could help give clues toward the timing and nature of procedures such as Kasai portoenterostomy and thereby influence long-term results. In these situations, ultrasound scanning becomes an important tool in the visualization of such routes and assessment for any structural defect. Other than the anatomical differences, the chemical composition of the bile plays a crucial role in the avoidance of gallstone formation and effective digestion. Supersaturation of cholesterol in bile has been recognized to be a significant determinant of cholesterol gallstone formation because of the fluctuations in biological conditions within the gallbladder. Findings indicated that higher levels of total biliary protein, together with higher cholesterol, may be significant determinants in the development of gallstones. These findings highlight the importance of bile's biochemical environment in health and disease. For clinical practitioners utilizing the use of ultrasound, being able to recognize the relevance of bile flow and content allows for better diagnosis and treatment planning, thereby enhancing patient care in conditions caused by biliary dysfunction (Figure 8.9).

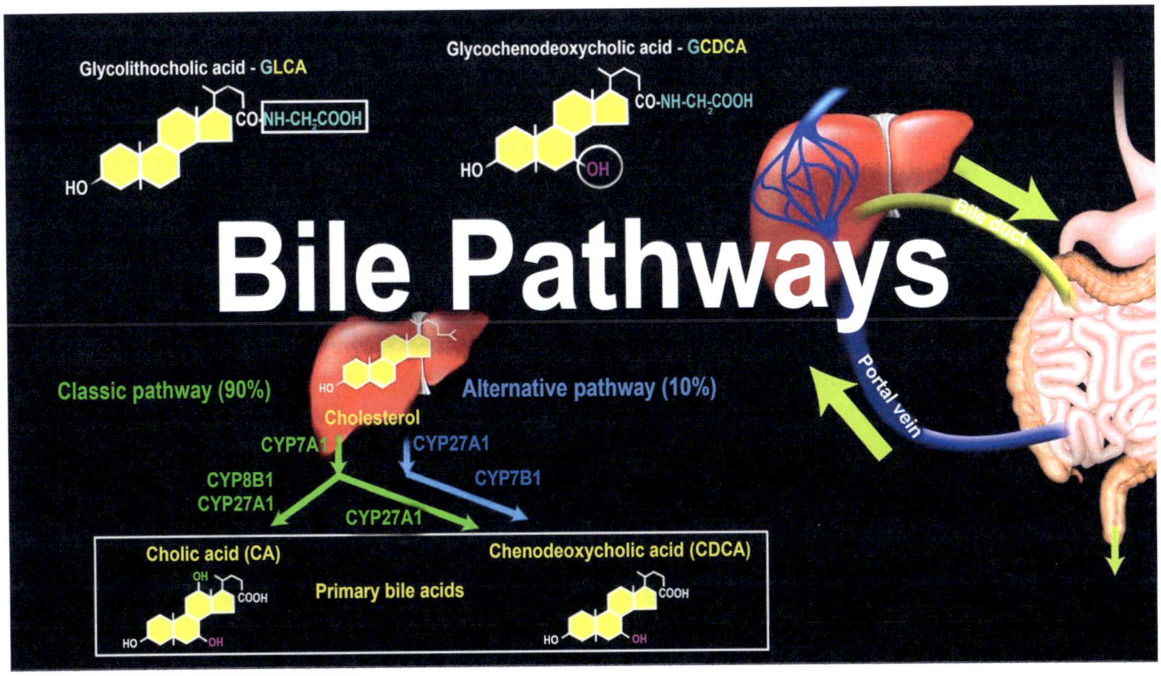

Figure 8.9. Pathways of bile flow.

Source: https://i.ytimg.com/vi/JU-S-R7bQRQ/maxresdefault.jpg.

8.3. Indications for Ultrasound Examination

Application of ultrasound scanning in the assessment of liver and biliary tract illness is often triggered by a wide variety of clinical presentations. Abnormal laboratory findings, such as elevated liver enzymes or bilirubin, which can indicate suspected hepatobiliary pathology, are one of the key reasons for undertaking an ultrasound. Ultrasound provides a low-cost, non-invasive imaging technique for visualizing anatomical structures and potential lesions. It is particularly useful in differentiating between malignant and benign masses, evaluating gallbladder pathology, including cholecystitis, and detecting bile duct obstruction. Additional diagnostic testing may also be directed by ultrasound, hence making it an important component of a proper diagnostic workup for those with hepatic abnormalities. In addition to laboratory results, specific clinical presentations necessitate ultrasound examination. These, such as jaundice, abdominal pain, unexplained weight loss, or fever, particularly along with signs of hepatobiliary distress, require immediate ultrasound assessment. Imaging is of critical importance in the diagnosis of gallbladder disease, including cholecystitis and cholangitis that can manifest with a nonspecific presentation. Besides, ultrasound makes it possible to identify complications of the conditions, such as biliary obstruction and bacterial infection, which allow the clinician to make an informed choice of the best approach to employ in treating such conditions. Given the capacity of ultrasound to define both structural abnormalities and potential fluid collections within the biliary tree and liver, its clinical value extends beyond diagnosis to include treatment planning and prognostication. The inclusion of contrast-enhanced ultrasound (CEUS) is a significant improvement in liver imaging, as it provides further clarity in challenging cases when conventional ultrasound might not be adequate. CEUS is particularly beneficial in children, as it reduces the exposure to ionizing radiation and eliminates the risks associated with iodinated contrast media widely used in other imaging techniques. The current literature offers a growing evidence base for the effectiveness of CEUS in identifying focal liver lesions and assessing vascularity in neoplasms, enhancing diagnostic accuracy. CEUS has been demonstrated to significantly aid decision-making in the clinic, particularly with hepatobiliary infections such as bacterial cholangitis and cholecystitis, in which timely intervention can drastically enhance patient outcomes (Allenspach et al., 2016). CEUS technology development represents the best example of the dynamic nature of ultrasound examination, underlining its increasing use in contemporary medical diagnostics (Cantisani et al., 2016) (Figure 8.10).

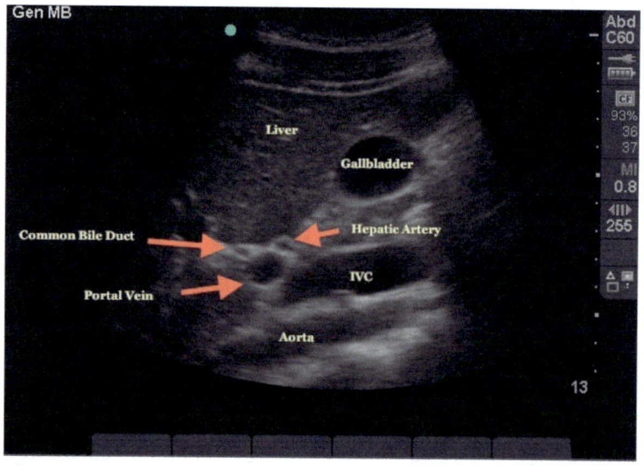

Figure 8.10. Indications for ultrasound examination of the liver and biliary system.

Source: https://coreem.net/content/uploads/2019/05/GB2.png.

8.3.1. Evaluation of Liver Diseases

Liver disease evaluation through ultrasound imaging is now an indispensable aspect of modern diagnosis, giving clinicians a safe and effective means to image hepatic and biliary anatomy. Ultrasound is particularly invaluable since it produces images in real time of blood flow and allows clinicians to screen for several liver conditions, such as steatosis, cirrhosis, and hepatocellular carcinoma. Its greatest benefit is its ability to detect biliary structural pathology and hence aid in the diagnosis of conditions like cholangitis and cholecystitis. As seen in studies, results from ultrasound have been of great importance in decision-making on whether or not to proceed with further diagnostic tests or immediate treatment in patients presenting liver disease-related symptoms. The modality's use is increased due to its capacity for detecting inflammation, structural derangements, or even the presence of neoplasias, thus playing a critical role in the comprehensive evaluation of liver disease. Further, identification of the underlying causes of liver disease is possible using ultrasound imaging because it assists in the identification of features that are associated with hepatic dysfunction. As an example, the measurement of liver enzyme levels in relation to ultrasound findings can be useful in the establishment of infection-related, autoimmune, or neoplastic-related diagnoses. Acute biliary infections, such as bacterial cholangitis, for example, may be localized efficiently by sonography. In a review paper, the utility of ultrasound in diagnosing infection-related complications was established, and it was shown that such detection with ultrasound may necessitate timely interventions. In addition, gallbladder wall thickening or stones can be imaged directly, highlighting the importance of ultrasound as a crucial modality in evaluating complicated biliary disease and guiding future therapy plans accordingly. Ultrasound imaging is a valuable resource in considering liver transplantation, both in preoperative evaluation and postoperative management. The technicalities involved in liver transplant surgery necessitate more advanced imaging modalities to assess potential anatomical or functional defects that would make the operation complicated. After the transplant, the role of ultrasound is expanded to assessing for vascular and biliary complications that are potential. Imaging modalities like ultrasound are responsible for diagnosing complications such as anastomotic leaks or thrombosis that can significantly alter the outcome of the patient. The value of ultrasound in providing rapid assessments in the acute post-transplant environment has been prominent in the literature, making it a first-line imaging method for liver transplantation-related complications, and therefore enhancing the safety and efficiency of the management of liver disease in the practice environment (Anzidei et al., 2016).

8.3.2. Evaluation of Biliary Obstructions

The ultrasonographic diagnosis of biliary obstructions is an important step in the diagnostic algorithm, especially in the detection of underlying pathologies of the biliary system. Ultrasound is particularly valuable since it is devoid of any invasiveness, offers real-time images, and is not based on ionizing radiation. In the evaluation of biliary obstructions, the ultrasonographic techniques focus on identifying dilatations of the biliary tree, which may be suggestive of obstructions. Imaging of structures such as the common bile duct and gallbladder can reveal gross abnormalities, including stones, masses, or strictures. Early diagnosis is crucial because it can influence the direction of treatment, with successful intervention more likely. The dynamic ability of ultrasound allows obstructive changes to be evaluated over time, providing informative information concerning progression and management of biliary illness and hence facilitating early medical or surgical intervention in patient management.

While ultrasound is a first-line imaging tool for obstructions within the biliary tract, it also complements other imaging modalities that could be employed in challenging cases.

Magnetic resonance cholangiopancreatography (MRCP) and computer tomography (CT) scans are generally employed to provide a better picture, especially in the case of equivocal ultrasound results. The multi-disciplinary strategy also determines the etiology of biliary obstruction correctly, which can be a determining factor in the context of the increasing incidence of related malignancies. For instance, pancreatic malignancies or cholangiocarcinoma may manifest as biliary obstruction but always require sophisticated imaging for correct diagnosis and staging. Secondly, endoscopic technological developments such as cholangioscopy supplement traditional practices, in accordance with recent findings of new means of diagnosis (Joshi et al., 2017). Through these, combined with their applications, healthcare professionals may improve diagnostic accuracy, offering better patient outcomes for biliary pathology. Effective management of biliary obstruction relies on precise assessment and timely intervention to allay symptoms and prevent complications from arising subsequently. Having established the presence of an obstruction by ultrasound, other factors are the choice of therapeutic modalities, such as drainage procedures for the biliary tree or surgery when necessary. Data confirm that a multidisciplinary approach, with specialists in radiology, gastroenterology, and oncology, can optimize outcomes (Agarwal et al., 2017). There needs to be a balance between palliative and surgical management in guiding treatment pathways to reduce morbidity and maximize quality of life. Treatment options and imaging modalities are constantly changing, providing good potential for improved assessments and intervention techniques. Thus, the use of ultrasound in the diagnosis of biliary obstruction not only assists with creating diagnostic certainty but also becomes an integral part in creating well-rounded patient management plans for complicated biliary disease (Figure 8.11).

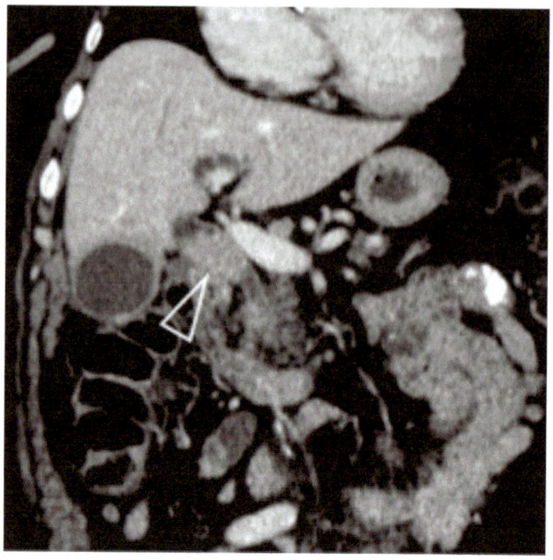

Figure 8.11. Assessment of biliary obstructions.

Source: https://ars.els-cdn.com/content/image/1-s2.0-S2211568413000934-gr1.jpg.

8.3.3. Monitoring of Liver Transplants

Monitoring of liver transplant has radically altered, particularly with the advent of advanced imaging techniques such as ultrasound. In post-operative application, ultrasound is pivotal in ascertaining the viability of the transplanted liver, in identifying complications such as vascular occlusion or biliary issues. Sonographic assessment is non-invasive and allows for real-time imaging, which becomes crucial in the early identification of complications that may arise after surgery. With dynamic imaging of blood perfusion and anatomy of the transplanted organ, ultrasound can help clinicians make proper patient management decisions as well as take timely action if indicated. Early detection of such complications is critical because post-transplant complications can critically affect patient outcome and graft survival. Contrast-enhanced ultrasound (CEUS) has also gained popularity in liver transplant monitoring, expanding the indications for the use of traditional techniques. Though CEUS has been commonly used in adults, its application in pediatric patients is increasingly recognized with the advantage, especially following the European Federation of Societies in Ultrasound and Medicine (EFSUMB) approval. As it spares both radiation and iodinated contrast media usage, CEUS offers a patient-friendly imaging method during the post-transplant period. This aligns with the general goals of enhancing patient care in addition to ensuring the recipients are subjected to the least possible risk while under observation during pivotal phases. With the CEUS application in pediatric liver transplant recipients, hence, pivotal information can be acquired to reduce complications in addition to enhancing liver graft management. Finally, the posttransplant care of liver transplant patients needs to be integrative and involve an interdisciplinary team because the complications that occur postoperatively tend to be multifaceted and complex. The doctors must remain vigilant for complications such as hepatic artery thrombosis and primary graft non-function, particularly in the first few days posttransplantation. These complications justify the need for regular imaging and follow-up to ensure timely interventions. As stated, CRT-associated complications should be preemptively addressed to ensure optimal maintenance of liver function and enhance patient outcomes. Therefore, integrating sophisticated imaging modalities like ultrasound into routine monitoring regimens is essential for maximizing treatment in order to enable healthcare practitioners to maintain high standards at a very critical point during the recovery of patients (Bates &Martin, 2017).

8.4. Ultrasound Procedures and Techniques

Ultrasound techniques are at the core of the assessment and diagnosis of liver and biliary tract disease. The fact that ultrasound is non-invasive makes it a desirable approach for the measurement of liver pathology, including chronic liver disease, cirrhosis, and hepatocellular carcinoma. By emitting high-frequency sound waves, ultrasound generates real-time images of the liver's anatomy and function, allowing clinicians to identify abnormalities in liver parenchyma and biliary ducts. The versatility of ultrasound also allows for bedside examination, which is imperative in critical care settings. With the prevalence of liver disease high in the world, having the capability to perform ultrasound correctly is essential for clinicians to make early and accurate diagnoses, which have a significant bearing on patient management and outcomes. In liver transplantation, ultrasound plays a significant role in postoperative assessment. Radiologists must be proficient at recognizing normal results as well as complications, such as vascular and biliary pathology that may occur after the procedure. The ability to recognize complications in a timely fashion with the use of ultrasound enhances patient safety and can lead to early intervention. Unlike some other imaging modalities, ultrasound has the advantage of portability and immediacy, which are important in caring for liver transplant recipients who may have acute clinical conditions. Besides, the differentiation between anatomical variations of normal tissues and pathological changes relies on a clear perception of surgical techniques of liver transplantation, such as in the case of the detailed interpretation of post-transplantation complications in radiology articles (Anzidei et al., 2016).

Greater advancements in ultrasound technology, including navigational systems, are transforming the specialty of liver surgery. The integration of instrument tracking systems and three-dimensional imaging enhances the accuracy of ultrasound during surgery, particularly in complex conditions with problematic anatomy or tumors that are visually demanding. Initial experience with navigational ultrasound systems suggests significant gains in procedure accuracy, as implied by the successful intraoperative localisation and targeting of liver lesions. Although the Explorer™ Liver guidance system is still in the process of development, its clinical use has been promising in assisting in a high percentage of procedures, along with improving overall surgical outcomes (Clements et al., 2012). Such advancements constitute a forward step towards incorporating more advanced imaging technology, thereby supplementing traditional ultrasound use in the continuously evolving field of liver and biliary system interventions (Figure 8.12).

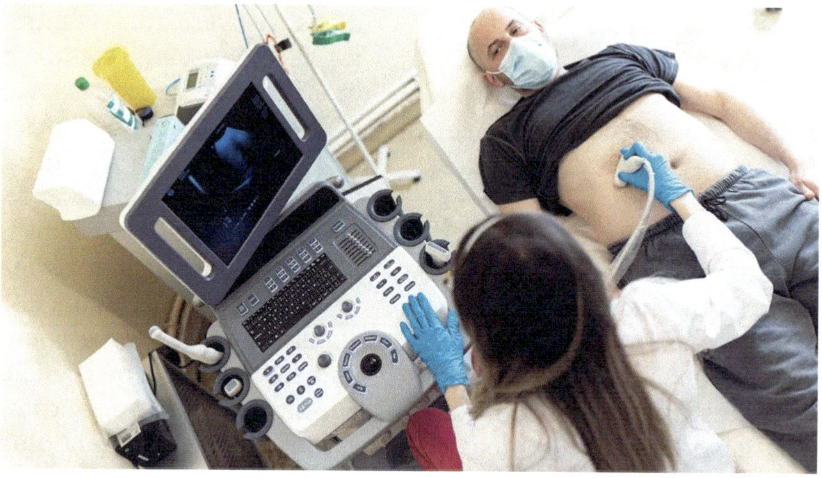

Figure 8.12. Ultrasound techniques and procedures for liver and biliary system conditions.

Source: https://i0.wp.com/post.medicalnewstoday.com/wp-content/uploads/sites/3/2022/06/liver_ultrasound_GettyImages1316611322_Header-1024x575.jpg?w=1155&h=1528.

8.4.1. Preparation for the Ultrasound Exam

Preparation for liver and biliary system ultrasound testing is a crucial element that significantly influences the accuracy of test results. Patients are typically provided with certain instructions to enhance the quality of images and prevent complications from the procedure. At the core of such preparation procedures is fasting, typically lasting for at least six to eight hours prior to the test. This fasting period is important to ensure proper distension of the gallbladder so that visualization of its anatomy and the structures around it is clearer. Patients are also asked not to eat or consume anything that will cause gas several hours before the test, since such may distort the image and hinder the sonographers from collecting accurate data regarding the liver and the biliary status (Gerada, 2012). Consequently, patient education for prep emphasizes taking dietary restrictions in order to obtain optimal diagnostic clarity. In addition to dietary modification, aside from, the timing of the ultrasound examination may also have to be well planned by the patient and healthcare provider. The timing of the test must be during a period when the patient is not experiencing acute symptoms so that there can be some relaxation to facilitate good imaging. The patient's medications should also be monitored, as some medications may affect the result of the ultrasound. For instance, anticoagulant medication may need to be regulated in an effort to minimize complications of the procedure. Patients are encouraged to communicate openly with their medical practitioners about their history and any issues of concern to them since such collaboration is vital in the efficient preparation for the test (Gerada, 2012). Such a wary focus on individual health details ensures that preparatory measures are uniquely tailored to ensure the optimal results for liver and biliary diagnosis. Emotional and psychological preparation is also an essential part of preparation for the ultrasound examination. Fear or anxiety about the procedure from the patient's perspective may stem from fear of what will be discovered or discomfort during the examination. Resolution of these emotional factors is paramount to establishing a favorable experience that promotes cooperation and compliance with the ultrasound. It becomes feasible for practitioners to integrate interventions like pre-procedure education, which entails informing the patient what he or she can expect in the course of the examination and dispelling myths about the procedure. Relaxation techniques and support from relatives could also help reduce anxiety levels. Lastly, creating a supportive environment and ensuring full information before the ultrasound test can enhance patient comfort, satisfy preparation requirements, and improve diagnostic outcomes for liver and biliary systems evaluations (Gerada, 2012).

8.4.2. Types of Ultrasound Techniques Employed

Several diverse techniques are employed within the scope of liver and biliary tract ultrasound to yield the optimal diagnostic information. Conventional gray-scale ultrasound is one of the basic techniques most often employed to visualize the liver and biliary structures. It facilitates estimation of liver size, echotexture, and detection of lesions in the form of cysts and tumors. The technique effectively highlights echogenicity changes that may disclose pathologies and, therefore, is priceless for initial evaluations. Despite its utility, gray-scale ultrasound is not without its limitations, such as the inability to image deeper structures. This calls for the development of newer techniques, including Doppler ultrasound, which maximizes the assessment of blood flow in the hepatic and biliary vasculature and thus provides priceless information about conditions like portal hypertension and vascular occlusions. In addition, three-dimensional (3D) ultrasound has become an essential tool for the study of the liver and biliary tract. This new approach provides a better visualization of the intricate anatomy of the organs, enabling clinicians to examine spatial relationships that two-dimensional imaging cannot detect. Through the imaging of structures reconstructed from various angles, 3D ultrasound is beneficial for surgeons in planning surgical procedures and liver transplantation. With more advanced imaging techniques such as contrast-enhanced ultrasound (CEUS), the diagnostic role is further enhanced, with real-time imaging of perfusion patterns within liver lesions, thereby facilitating benign to malignant lesion differentiation. With the utilization of these advanced ultrasound techniques, accuracy in diagnosis and follow-up assessment of response to therapy in liver and biliary tract diseases is considerably enhanced. Other than the aforementioned techniques, ultrasound elastography has also gained traction as a non-invasive device to quantify liver stiffness, which is an important indicator of cirrhosis and fibrosis. The technique measures the speed of the sound waves traveling through the liver and translates it into clinically valuable information regarding liver health. Liver stiffness increases in a normal manner with progressing fibrosis, which makes the procedure critical in the early detection and treatment of chronic liver disease. Ultrasound-guided interventions such as biopsies and drainage are also made possible using ultrasound imaging, with assurance of safety and accuracy. Imaging protocols for biliary tumors are evolving, led by current international society guidelines, aimed at enhancing preoperative staging and follow-up regimens. Consequently, application of diverse ultrasound methodologies is on the rise, with hopes of improved patient outcomes in liver and biliary well-being management (Gordon et al., 1987; Cannavale et al., 2016) (Figure 8.13).

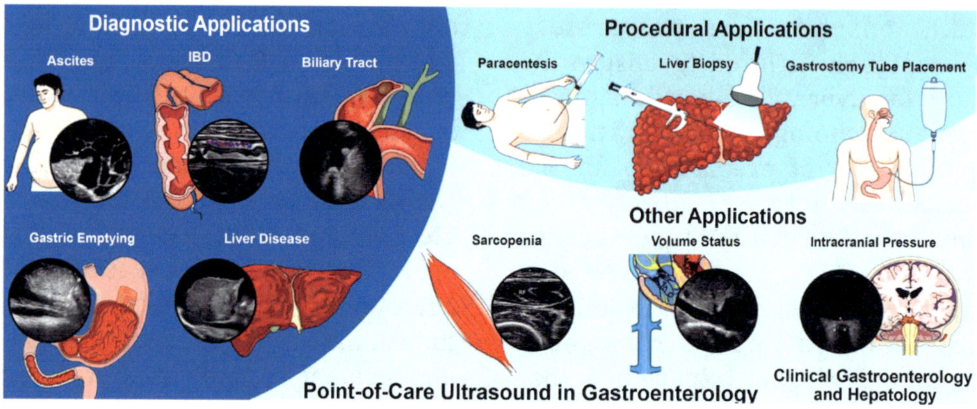

Figure 8.13. Types of ultrasound techniques used for liver and biliary system conditions.

Source: https://www.cghjournal.org/cms/10.1016/j.cgh.2024.09.040/asset/78f9a293-2771-4076-976d-bab89ab8b35b/main.assets/ga1_lrg.jpg.

8.4.3. Interpretation of Ultrasound Images

Interpretation of ultrasound scans is a key skill in liver and biliary system assessment. Ultrasound, with the use of sound waves to create images, enables radiologists to visualize the liver and connected structures in real-time. Subtle interpretation requires a strong familiarity with hepatic anatomy, pathology, and physiological changes caused by various diseases. Radiologists must also be proficient in distinguishing normal anatomical variations from pathological disease, that is, cirrhosis, tumors, or biliary obstruction. Proper interpretation not only assists in guiding diagnosis but also informs further management decisions and therapeutic interventions and, therefore, it is imperative that practitioners remain up to date with the evolving techniques and guidelines. With ongoing developments in imaging modalities, the use of ultrasound together with adjunctive imaging techniques can further enhance diagnostic data, and proficiency in the interpretation of ultrasound is necessary for effective clinical practice.

The use of ultrasound is more than mere visualization; it is a quick and powerful technique for diagnosing complications of liver transplantation. Vascular narrowing and biliary disorders are possible after liver transplantation and should be identified early to prevent added morbidity. Radiologists must be quite familiar with normal surgical anastomoses and the normal appearance post-transplantation so that they do not mistake the latter for an abnormal pattern. The radiologist must be experienced in ultrasound interpretation in order to detect evidence of rejection, biliary fistulae, or vascular anomalies within the graft. Radiologists, therefore, are required to acquire a sound understanding of distinguishing between post-surgical normalcy and complications. This is not only vital for immediate patient treatment but also for improving long-term outcomes in liver transplant recipients, illustrating the significant contribution that proper ultrasound interpretation will have in managing liver and biliary systems (Anzidei et al., 2016). Second, a multimodality imaging approach, with ultrasound, CT, and MRI, can significantly enhance diagnostic capability in complex cases. Even though ultrasound is generally the first choice due to its availability and real-time imaging capability, adjunct modalities provide essential information that can improve diagnoses.

For example, CT and MRI play a key role in the characterization of solid and cystic liver and pancreatic lesions that are typically hard to assess with ultrasound alone. The combination of imaging modalities facilitates a global evaluation that is particularly important in neoplasm or metastasis detection (Baccari et al., 2016). With the integration of a multimodal approach, radiologists can generate more holistic analyses, ultimately yielding improved patient management decisions. This imaging technology partnership is not only responsible for furthering proper diagnosis but also guides therapeutic interventions, as a justification of the preeminent importance of ultrasound image interpretation in the overall scheme of liver and biliary system imaging.

8.5. Pathologies Frequently Identified

Ultrasound scanning is a useful diagnostic adjunct to the diagnosis of common pathologies of the liver and biliary tree. The most prevalent condition found is fatty liver disease, which is the accumulation of fat in liver cells, which will ultimately lead to further liver damage if left untreated. Fatty liver disease is often symptomless and is visible on ultrasound scanning as increased echogenicity. The lack of invasiveness in this imaging technique allows for early detection and monitoring, with significant implications for patient management and outcome. Furthermore, the ultrasound can detect cirrhosis, represented by changes in liver texture and morphology, allowing one to assess the extent of liver dysfunction and associated complications. Another pathology of significant importance typically diagnosed on ultrasound is the presence of gallstones, which can result in bile duct obstruction and associated pain. This condition, cholelithiasis, is benign and can lead to acute cholecystitis if the cystic duct is obstructed by a stone. Ultrasound imaging of gallstones is good because it has the capability to differentiate between echogenic and non-echogenic structures, providing real-time views of bile ducts and gallbladder. Also, when stones are present, ultrasound can detect complications such as perforation or empyema, thus facilitating early surgical plans.

Precise identification of gallstone disease is paramount to avert more serious pathology, so ultrasound is an invaluable modality in biliary pathology evaluation. Besides non-neoplastic disease, ultrasound also has a key role in the evaluation of neoplasms of the liver, both benign and malignant lesions. Hemangiomas, focal nodular hyperplasia, and hepatocellular carcinoma are notable tumors that are frequently seen on imaging evaluations. Ultrasound can characterize these lesions as much as their size, shape, and vascularity, differentiating benign from malignant diseases. The accuracy of ultrasound in detecting changes in the liver's structure is useful in detecting the early development of liver cancer, which is increasingly vital because of the high mortality of advanced malignancies. The clinical relevance of the application of ultrasound for evaluation of liver masses is noteworthy and has the potential to influence treatment decisions and improve patient outcomes, particularly when surgery or additional treatment may be needed (Abela & Borgxuereb, 2013; Berloco et al., 2012) (Figure 8.14).

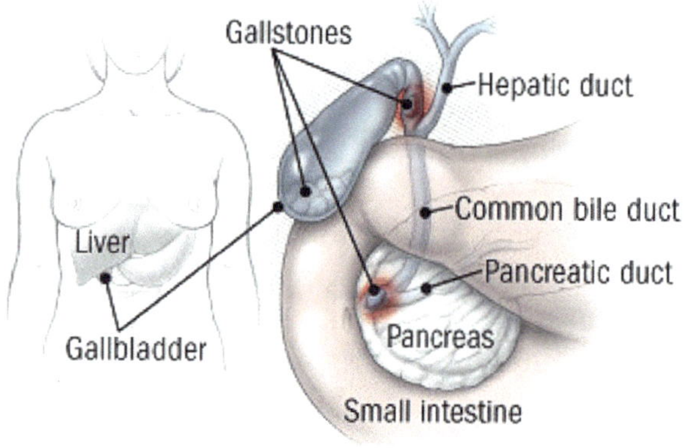

Figure 8.14. Common pathologies detected in liver and biliary system conditions.

Source: https://domf5oio6qrcr.cloudfront.net/medialibrary/12272/conversions/a8db5aab-7103-48e5-a16a-863c083ba029-thumb.jpg.

8.5.1. Fatty Liver Disease

The condition of fatty liver disease, or hepatic steatosis, is a substantial health issue in the field of hepatology and is being increasingly managed using various imaging techniques, more so the use of ultrasound. The condition, denoted by the presence of excessive fat within liver cells, can occur due to several etiological causes, of which excessive alcohol consumption and metabolic syndrome are worth noting. It is crucial to understand fatty liver disease due to its potential to result in severe liver conditions such as fibrosis, cirrhosis, or hepatocellular carcinoma (HCC). Ultrasound plays a crucial role in the diagnosis and detection of fatty liver disease because it is a non-invasive procedure that measures the degree of steatosis on the basis of liver echogenicity. Its application is set against the backdrop of increasing obesity rate and its consequent rise in non-alcoholic fatty liver disease (NAFLD), necessitating proper diagnostic interventions. Application of contrast-enhanced ultrasound (CEUS) adds a high-tech dimension to the assessment of liver conditions, such as fatty liver disease. CEUS utilizes microbubble contrast agents that enhance the visualization of blood flow in the liver, allowing for better distinction between benign and malignant lesions. This technique is of particular interest in the context of fatty liver, in which ordinary ultrasound can identify difficulty in clearly outlining liver lesions in relation to the existing steatosis.

Through the use of CEUS, medical professionals can more accurately categorize liver nodules and evaluate their characteristics in the context of fatty liver disease. There is evidence that CEUS not only assists in the diagnosis of hepatocellular carcinoma but also in monitoring changes of fatty liver disease, thus widening its applicability beyond a sole diagnostic agent to one that informs management (Cantisani et al., 2016). This integrated perspective maximizes clinical decision-making in the presence of hepatic fatty infiltration. Research into the diagnostic accuracy of CEUS, particularly in small liver nodules, is integral to the discussion of fatty liver disease. Recent research based on the American College of Radiology Contrast Agent–Enhanced US Liver Imaging Reporting and Data System (CEUS LI-RADS) reports its efficacy in differentiating benign from malignant nodules in those individuals with liver disease, like fatty liver disease. Findings cite CEUS LI-RADS as having higher specificity in diagnosing small hepatocellular carcinomas, thereby affirming the premise that systematic imaging characterization can avert misdiagnosis and facilitate timely intervention (Huang et al., 2020). Inasmuch as fatty liver disease is at risk for malignancy, use of CEUS in the clinical environment holds the potential for early detection and improved patient outcomes. This capability underscores the need to incorporate sophisticated ultrasound practices in the diagnosis and management of fatty liver disease as part of the overall holistic approach to liver wellness programs (Figure 8.15).

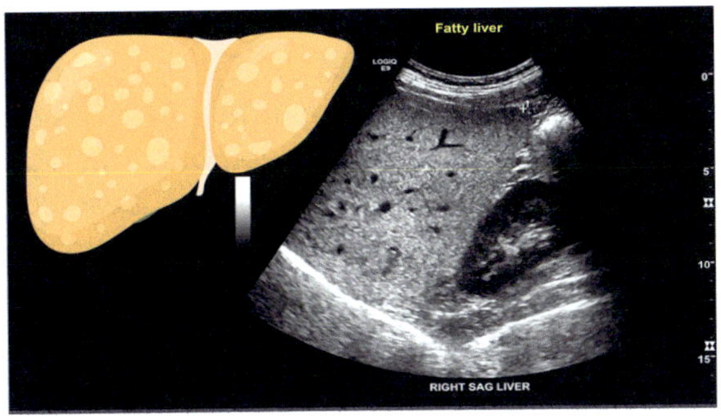

Figure 8.15. Fatty liver disease on ultrasound.

Source: fatty liver. nephropocus.com. https://i0.wp.com/nephropocus.com/wp-content/uploads/2020/08/Figure-1.jpg?fit=1301%2C730&ssl=1.

8.5.2. Gallstones and Cholecystitis

Gallstones are a life-threatening problem in the field of gastrointestinal disease because they have a high prevalence and potential for severe complications. Gallstones are hard formations that form in the gallbladder and are typically composed of cholesterol or bilirubin, which give rise to many symptomatic presentations. Gallstones cause dyspeptic symptoms, biliary colic, and most significantly, cholecystitis, which is inflammation of the gallbladder. As a prevalent gastrointestinal disorder, gallstones underscore the need for efficient diagnostic modalities such as ultrasound, which is a non-invasive and accurate tool for imaging gallbladder pathology, including the presence, size, and content of stones. Due to their potential to complicate into more severe conditions, insights into the pathophysiology and treatment of gallstones continue to be central in the field of gastrointestinal health and diagnostics (Yan & Shen, 2022). Acute calculus cholecystitis most commonly develops following gallstone obstruction of the cystic duct, leading to bacterial invasion and inflammation of the gallbladder. It presents with severe epigastric tenderness, fever, and leukocytosis, indicating an inflammatory response. Ultrasound plays a crucial role in the diagnosis of acute cholecystitis in the form of demonstrating gallstones, thickening of the gallbladder wall, and pericholecystic fluid. The World Society of Emergency Surgery has provided guidelines for various aspects of the management of this condition, such as criteria for diagnosis and timing of surgery (Ansaloni et al., 2017). The guidelines not only emphasize the importance of early detection and treatment but also of personalized clinical judgment, especially in high-risk patients, to enhance patient outcomes and minimize the risk of complications. Gallstone and cholecystitis treatment is primarily surgical, most commonly laparoscopic cholecystectomy, which is still the therapy of choice. The minimally invasive approach benefits from shorterrecovery time and fewer complications in contrast to the open technique. Substitute therapies are provided when surgery is risky, for example, percutaneous drainage or symptomatic management.

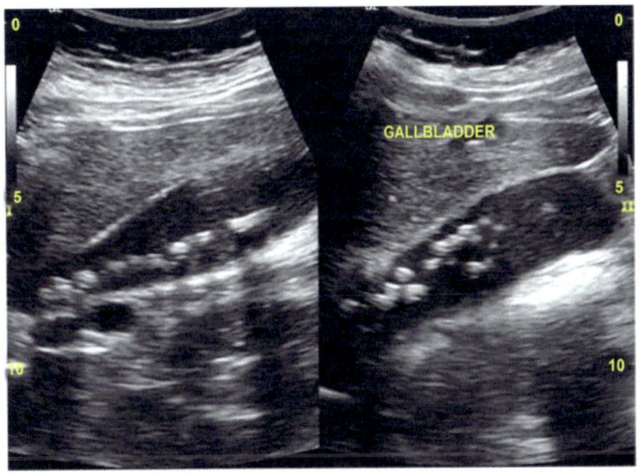

Figure 8.16. Gallstones and cholecystitis on an ultrasound.

Source: https://prod-images-static.radiopaedia.org/images/4480253/d54fddf16670072552675a3e4c026f_gallery.jpg.

The decision-making process of timing and mode of intervention is crucial and must consider the individual health state of the patient and the degree of cholecystitis. With the continuously expanding diagnostic functions through the use of ultrasound technology, the implementation of particular treatment guidelines will become increasingly important to more effectively treat patients under gallstone and cholecystitis care contexts (Yan &Shen, 2022; Ansaloni et al., 2017) (Figure 8.16).

8.5.3. Liver Tumors and Lesions

Identification and characterization of liver lesions and tumors by ultrasound imaging is a significant medical diagnostic field that serves a crucial function in the evaluation of hepatic illnesses. Ultrasound is one of the initial imaging modalities of choice with its broad availability, lack of ionizing radiation, and ability to monitor real-time blood flow. Being non-invasive, it allows clinicians to assess an assortment of lesions ranging from benign adenomas to malignant hepatocellular carcinomas. In addition, the use of ultrasound contrast agents has expanded the scope of traditional imaging, allowing for a greater possibility of distinction between types of liver lesions. Nevertheless, remember that even though ultrasound provides useful information, it is limited in diagnosing certain tumors and lesions and may therefore require the assistance of adjunct imaging techniques in the case of indeterminate findings (Cantisani et al., 2016). Of the homogeneous collection of liver lesions, peliosis hepatis (PH) is one that presents a particular challenge to imaging diagnosis due to its specific morphology. PH is characterized by the presence of many blood-filled cysts in the liver parenchyma, which creates an atypical appearance that will not initially raise suspicion on routine ultrasound examination. The condition could only be apparent in the context of emergent presentations, like following rupture hemorrhage, where acute abdominal pain and bleeding would necessitate investigation. In one case, imaging revealed hypodense areas that displayed characteristic patterns of contrast enhancement on imaging, leading to a diagnosis made by histopathologic examination. These cases underscore the necessity of incorporating careful differential diagnoses in evaluating hepatic lesions because early detection can significantly impact patient prognosis (Crocetti et al., 2015). Management of liver tumors and lesions calls for a multidisciplinary team that combines imaging modalities, clinical examination, and treatment. With improved ultrasound technology, its applications are expanding, particularly with the advent of contrast-enhanced ultrasound (CEUS). CEUS has shown promise in improving the diagnostic efficacy of liver lesions, particularly in children, where traditional contrast media pose a potential risk. The European Federation of Societies in Ultrasound in Medicine (EFSUMB) has recognized the growing evidence in favor of CEUS as a safe and effective method for the evaluation of focal liver lesions. This renders CEUS an effective addition to the imaging repertoire, enabling clinicians to navigate complex clinical situations and lower exposure to more intrusive examinations or radiation, thus optimizing the treatment of hepatic tumors and lesions in diverse patient populations (Cantisani et al., 2016) (Figure 8.17).

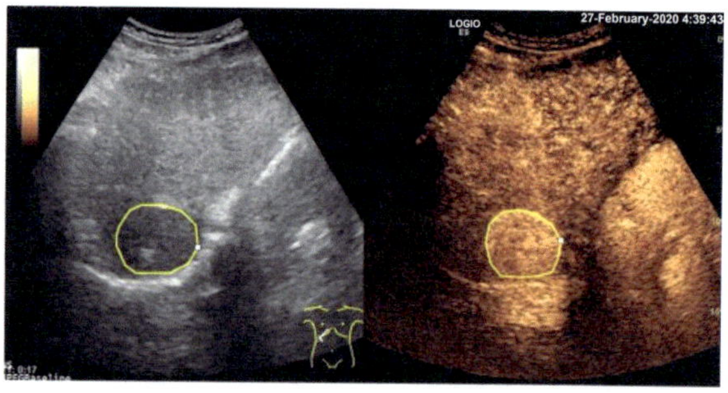

Figure 8.17. Liver cancer ultrasound.

Source: Mitrea, D., Badea, R., Mitrea, P., Brad, S., & Nedevschi, S. (2021). Hepatocellular Carcinoma Automatic Diagnosis within CEUS and B-Mode Ultrasound Images Using Advanced Machine Learning Methods. Sensors, 21(6), 2202. https://doi.org/10.3390/s21062202. https://www.mdpi.com/sensors/sensors-21-02202/article_deploy/html/images/sensors-21-02202-g001.png

8.6. Advantages and Limitations of Ultrasound

Ultrasound imaging has been a useful imaging modality in both the diagnosis and therapy of liver and biliary tract disease due to its numerous merits. Its non-invasive character is one very significant merit, allowing clinicians to perform tests without the hazard that is associated with exposure to ionizing radiation, thus presenting a safer alternative to patients, especially vulnerable populations such as children. This is supported further by the provision of contrast-enhanced ultrasound (CEUS) that facilitates proper assessment of focal liver lesions and is thus particularly helpful in children. In the EFSUMB position statement, CEUS is found to be beneficial in a range of uses while providing an examination experience that is patient-friendly and unencumbered by the complications routinely linked with other imaging modalities (Cantisani et al., 2016). These attributes highlight how ultrasound has emerged as a first-choice imaging modality for liver diagnosis in contemporary medical practice.

Despite its advantages, nevertheless, ultrasound is not without shortcomings. One of the primary drawbacks is operator dependency, which could lead to inconsistency in the results based on the level of experience and expertise of the physician or technician carrying out the scan. Furthermore, the effectiveness of ultrasound is usually compromised in the event of obesity or even heightened gas in the abdominal cavity because these factors compromise the quality of images obtained. Furthermore, even though ultrasound can provide essential information about the liver's structure, it could be inadequate in assessing the etiology of certain lesions or even differentiating between benign and malignant conditions. As highlighted in recent literature, while microwave ablation (MWA) is now a viable alternative treatment modality for metastatic colorectal cancer to the liver, ultrasound's inability to provide broad-based visualization may make it less effective in its use to effectively guide such interventions (Price, 2016). Appreciation of the limitations thereto is thus critical towards optimizing the use of ultrasound in clinical applications. Therefore, upon consideration of these advantages and limitations, it is quite clear that ultrasound is a vital component of liver and biliary system imaging. Its safety, accessibility, and ability for feedback in real-time make it a vital agent in the diagnosis of liver cirrhosis and biliary obstructions. But technology's limitations need to be balanced with a strategy wherein the clinicians know its limitations and use ultrasound combined with other diagnostic methods. Through collaboration between healthcare workers and ongoing education in techniques like CEUS and MWA, practitioners can understand and utilize ultrasound better. This dual-phase approach—leveraging the strengths while surmounting the shortcomings—provides patients with optimal possible precise, and effective treatment options in the evolving sphere of liver and biliary diagnostic (Cantisani et al., 2016; Price , 2016).

8.6.1. Non-Invasive Nature of the Procedure

The non-invasive nature of liver and biliary system ultrasound provides distinctive advantages in the clinical environment, particularly when determining the status of patients with suspected hepatic or biliary pathology. Compared with invasive procedures, such as biopsies or surgery, ultrasound employs high-frequency sound waves to produce accurate images of the liver and associated structures. Not only is this process less likely to be painful to the patient, but it is also less likely to be complicated by the standard techniques of invasiveness. As the demand for safe and efficient diagnostic methods increases, ultrasound has become a cornerstone of hepatobiliary imaging that allows clinicians to diagnose from benign lesions to malignant neoplasms without the morbidity of observing surgical operations. Moreover, the non-invasive nature of ultrasound facilitates playing a significant role in patient access and compliance while conducting assessments of liver status. Because procedures with anesthesia or surgical cuts are likely to discourage patients due to perceived risk, the ultrasound is a reasonable choice that can be made in an outpatient facility. Prompt findings enhance clinical decision-making, which is important in treating diseases like malignant biliary obstruction. Repeatedly and safely exposed to ultrasound are patients, enabling ongoing monitoring of disease progression or treatment response without risking their health from successive invasive procedures, thus contributing to the potential therapeutic alternatives for difficult cases, including those discovered by the advances in minimally invasive techniques for biliary drainage (Hasan et al., 2001). Finally, the incorporation of ultrasound technology as a routine component of regular clinical assessments further evidences its place in the development of non-invasive diagnostic techniques. For instance, as healthcare systems battle the rising global cancer burden, the role of non-invasive technologies like ultrasound becomes increasingly vital in surgical oncology. The development of the international curriculum in oncologic surgery will hopefully incorporate fundamental standards, which will promote the utilization of ultrasound as an affordable, first-line diagnosis in hepatobiliary illness. This drive towards the implementation of non-invasive diagnostics parallels the continued pursuit of patient-care improvement and suggests that ultrasound will continue to gain importance as a quality diagnostic method in liver and biliary system evaluations (Are et al., 2016).

8.6.2. Limitations in Imaging Depth and Detail

The depth and resolution limits of liver and biliary system ultrasound imaging pose enormous obstacles to accurate diagnosis and treatment planning. Standard ultrasound techniques are often unable to penetrate overlying obesity, gas-filled structures, or intervening tissue layers, resulting in degraded image quality. This attenuation of the sound waves renders significant anatomical detail and lesions within the liver or bile ducts opaque to viewing, at risk of delayed treatment or misdiagnosis. Furthermore, structures overlapping one another, such as the diaphragm and organ systems nearby, may complicate visualization and understanding of the pathology at hand. Consequently, doctors may be forced to rely on other imaging modalities, which can increase both time and cost of patient treatment without always providing the needed clarity. Another major limitation arises in the operator-dependent nature of ultrasound technology. Imaging success is largely dependent on the experience and ability of the sonographer or physician performing the study. Technical variation, probe position, and interpretation can lead to variation in diagnostic accuracy and may be responsible for differences in imaging depth and resolution among providers or facilities. This difference can have a negative impact on treatment outcomes, especially in challenging cases that require very detailed anatomical definition, as seen in the shifting trends towards ablation techniques such as MWA and away from RFA in certain contexts, as authors call for an exploration of the nuances of the respective techniques to optimize treatment of colorectal cancer liver metastases (Price, 2016). New technologies such as Near Infrared Fluorescent Cholangiography (NIRFC) with the use of Indocyanine Green (ICG) aim to address some of these limitations, but possess inherent limitations themselves. Although NIRFC has been promising for enhanced visualization of biliary anatomy during laparoscopic cholecystectomy, tissue uptake of ICG and time to fluorescence variability can affect imaging quality and reliability (Armstrong et al., 2017). Moreover, the relative dearth of high-quality, large-scale clinical trials evaluating these technologies' effectiveness underscores the need for ongoing research. Strict testing alone is the only way that the medical community can conclusively decide how best to integrate these new imaging technologies into routine practice for improved patient safety and surgical results for liver and biliary system procedures.

8.6.3. Contrast with Alternative Imaging Modalities

The utility of ultrasound in the diagnosis of the liver and biliary system is often contrasted with other imaging technologies, most notably computed tomography (CT) and magnetic resonance imaging (MRI). Ultrasound is distinctive in that it is non-invasive, does not involve ionizing radiation, and can offer real-time imaging. Such qualities are particularly valuable in the acute clinical setting where quick decision-making is critical, such as during abdominal pain evaluations or cases of liver transplantation. While CT and MRI achieve superior contrast resolution and detailed anatomical evaluation, ultrasound remains the first-line imaging method in most settings, including the outpatient setting. This is even emphasized by its capacity to diagnose diseases such as bile duct obstruction and hepatobiliary disease without the use of sedation, typically required for more invasive techniques like biopsies or contrast-enhanced imaging tests. When a choice between ultrasound and CT, and MRI has to be made, there are some clinical situations to consider. For instance, while restricted in providing full views of complex liver pathology, ultrasound excels in guiding procedures like paracentesis or biliary system drainage based on its ability to image fluid collections and vascular pathways in real time. In liver transplantation, rapid detection of biliary and vascular complications by ultrasound forms an important part of postoperative planning of management. (Anzidei et al., 2016) highlights the importance of imaging modalities in this case, stating that while CT and MRI can provide detailed anatomy, they may not be available at the point of care or acceptable to every patient. Under such a condition, ultrasound's role assumes a large significance, more so in acute cases where delayed results are not possible for proper clinical treatment. Also, the evolving face of imaging technology adds another twist to the comparison between ultrasound and CT, and MRI. Advances in technical aspects of ultrasound techniques, such as contrast-enhanced ultrasound (CEUS), are enhancing diagnostic performance, particularly in the evaluation of treated liver lesions and vascularity that have previously been addressed primarily through MRI or CT. These advances facilitate improved tumor detection and characterization, including in pancreatic neuroendocrine neoplasms that require a multidisciplinary management (Caplin et al., 2017). With continuous progress in imaging modalities, the integration of ultrasound and CT, and MRI allows a comprehensive diagnostic armamentarium such that clinicians can personalize imaging strategies to individual patient requirements and strike a balance of concern for cost, availability, and safety.

SUMMARY

The ultrasound imaging of the liver and biliary system is a breakthrough in diagnostic imaging with important consequences for patient management and treatment. The non-invasive method allows examination of various hepatic illnesses, producing dynamic images that render the clinician's diagnosis of cirrhosis, hepatitis, and hepatic neoplasms more certain. Also, the utilization of ultrasound techniques in the evaluation of biliary obstructions has become pivotal in ascertaining the requirement for surgical intervention. As observed under the results, the use of liver and biliary system ultrasound extends beyond diagnosis; it includes guiding therapeutic procedures, highlighting its relevance in clinical practice and patient care. Also, the application of ultrasound in the context of liver transplantation has been an issue of utmost debate among contemporary medicine. Researchers note that proper utilization of diagnostic imaging would streamline the pre-operative testing process, enhancing the criteria for selecting the potential recipients of the transplant. The continued advancement in ultrasound technologies, including elastography to assess liver stiffness and Doppler ultrasound to examine vascular structures, adds another layer of reliability to such imaging. Of special note, continuing advances in laparoscopic surgery, as seen in recent articles, lend credibility to the application of pre-operative imaging, as accurate assessments help to minimize operative complications and maximize patient outcomes. The integration of these technologies is a great step forward in liver disease management, enhancing ultrasound's integral role in modern medical practice. Briefly, the continuing evolution of ultrasound for the biliary system and liver involves both technical advances and significant improvements in the general strategy for the treatment of hepatobiliary disease. Ultrasound integration into routine daily practice is necessary so that more accurate diagnoses and well-informed decision-making are made. According to the hepatotoxicity-related issues and other complexities of liver disease, as observed in recent case series, restraint in imaging and monitoring remains essential. Secondly, the role of laparoscopic surgery, as described in literature on liver transplantation, is a classic demonstration of the revolutionary character associated with ultrasound-guided interventions, propelling a broader understanding to manage hepatic pathologies. As studies continue and technologies improve, the future of liver and biliary tract ultrasound holds much potential for improving patient care and clinical effectiveness to a greater degree.

The evaluation of the liver and biliary tree by ultrasound is also significant in the diagnosis of many hepatic pathologies and in guiding future management. In liver ultrasound reports, there are some points worth noting, including the evaluation of liver contour and the evaluation of liver masses, which often require distinguishing between benign and malignant lesions. Moreover, ultrasound assists in the detection of liver cirrhosis, characterized by the changes in liver echogenicity, irregularities on the surface, and altered blood flow. The inclusion of elastography in ultrasound devices has contributed to the ability to analyze liver stiffness, providing valuable information on fibrosis stages, an essential aspect in managing chronic liver disease. Therefore, the application of ultrasound as an easily available, non-invasive modality cannot be overstressed in early diagnosis and planning for therapy in cases of liver pathology. Further, the employment of ultrasound in evaluating biliary tree abnormalities is a vital component in managing biliary disorders. Illnesses such as cholangitis, biliary obstruction, and gallstones can be adequately evaluated through ultrasound imaging, which illustrates the anatomy of the bile ducts and adjacent structures. Specifically significant is the identification of dilated biliary ducts, which could indicate obstruction and prompt further examination or intervention. Ultrasound-guided procedures, such as drainage of biliary accumulations or stenting, are the utilitarian application of ultrasound in therapeutic contexts. Safety and reliability of ultrasound in such settings confirm its invaluable position not just for diagnostic assessment but also for delivery of interventional therapy. Overall, ultrasound techniques are reported as having the dual function of diagnosis and treatment of biliary diseases. Aside from direct imaging capability, developments in ultrasound technology point to improvement in liver disease care. The potential of combining artificial intelligence (AI) and ultrasound diagnosis is a promising direction towards greater accuracy and efficiency in the interpretation of liver scans. Additionally, exploration of non-invasive biomarkers through ultrasound may transform the field of monitoring chronic liver disease by reducing reliance on invasive biopsies. Blending of ultrasound technology and new therapeutic agents, such as maralixibat for treating primary biliary cholangitis (Apostol et al., 2019), indicates the active advancement in the treatment of liver and biliary disorders. Agreements among experts have also attempted to enhance practices regarding liver transplant, such as early referral and candidate selection (Burra et al., 2018). Together, the advances and controversy within the field bring into focus the critical role ultrasound plays in influencing patient outcomes in liver and biliary tree diagnosis and treatment planning.

CLOSER LOOK

ELASTOGRAPHY

Elastography is a branch of ultrasound imaging that quantifies tissue stiffness or elasticity in real-time, providing information not possible with standard imaging. It is based on the assumption that unhealthy, abnormal tissue, such as tumors, fibrotic lesions, is mechanistically different, that is, stiffer, than the surrounding normal tissue. By quantifying tissue displacement due to force application (manually, using sound waves, or through physiological pulsation), elastography generates quantitative or qualitative maps (elastograms) to reflect tissue elasticity. The technique has become a precious non-invasive tool in the diagnosis, staging, and follow-up of various diseases like liver fibrosis, breast and thyroid cancers, prostate disease, and musculoskeletal disorders.

There are two general categories of elastography: strain elastography and shear wave elastography (SWE). Strain elastography applies external compression to the tissue and is measured as relative deformation or strain, creating qualitative color maps indicating tissue softness (usually green or red) against stiffness (usually blue). Operator-dependent but valuable in shallow organs like the breast, thyroid, and lymph nodes. Shear wave elastography, on the other hand, is a more quantitative technique that uses focused acoustic pulses to generate transverse (shear) waves within the tissue. The velocity of these waves correlates directly with tissue stiffness—the greater the velocity, the stiffer the tissue. SWE provides objective values in kilopascals (kPa), which is why it is especially useful for tracking and comparing longitudinally and between patients or over time.

Elastography has become the norm in hepatology for assessing liver fibrosis and cirrhosis in patients with chronic liver disease. It reduces the need for liver biopsy by enabling fibrosis staging through painless, reproducible, and rapid assessment. Transient elastography, commonly referred to under the proprietary name FibroScan, is a specific SWE method designed for this purpose. Higher stiffness values may indicate progressive fibrosis or cirrhosis, while lower values are encountered with mild or no fibrosis. Beyond the liver, elastography has been gaining popularity in breast imaging to differentiate between benign and malignant tumors. Malignant tumors tend to be stiffer due to their high cellularity and desmoplastic reaction. Elastography enhances malignancy prediction if added to typical ultrasound characteristics in thyroid nodules. In musculoskeletal applications, elastography evaluates tendons, ligaments, and muscles for scarring, degeneration, or injury and is therefore applied in rehabilitation and sports medicine.

One of the best advantages of elastography is that it is non-invasive, minimizes patient discomfort, and does not involve ionizing radiation. Some restrictions include susceptibility to operator expertise (particularly in strain elastography), reduced effectiveness in obese or ascitic patients, and variability based on technical or physiological differences such as inflammation or congestion. Continuous development in imaging software combined with artificial intelligence is increasing automation, reproducibility, and trust in making a diagnosis. As elastography gets more popular and more sophisticated, it will progressively become more important to diagnostic radiology and point-of-care testing, offering clinicians a useful, in-line means for the evaluation of tissue pathology with improved precision and safety than has been available before.

References

1. Abela, L., & Borg Xuereb, K. (2013). Liver abscess following ingestion of a foreign object. https://core.ac.uk/download/46603960.pdf (accessed on 12th July 2025).
2. Abell, C., Castell, C. von Ritter, Jüngst, D., Fiske, J., Gallinger, S., et al. (1991). Role of high total protein in gallbladder bile in the formation of cholesterol gallstones. https://core.ac.uk/download/12167349.pdf (accessed on 12th July 2025).
3. Adachi, Y., Brendel, C., Zimmermann, C., Beglinger, C., Denk, G. U., Denson, L. A., Dietrich, C. G., et al. (2006). Decreased expression of breast cancer resistance protein in the duodenum in patients with obstructive cholestasis. https://core.ac.uk/download/16432742.pdf (accessed on 12th July 2025).
4. Agarwal, D. M., DeWitt, J., Eagleson, M., Easler, J., et al. (2017). A multidisciplinary approach to pancreas cancer in 2016: A review. https://core.ac.uk/download/129149165.pdf (accessed on 12th July 2025).
5. Ahmed, K., Deshmukh, S. P., Elsayes, K. M., Kang, H., et al. (2017). Imaging features of rare mesenchymal liver tumours: Beyond haemangiomas. https://core.ac.uk/download/155271451.pdf (accessed on 12th July 2025).
6. Allenspach, K., Day, M. J., Hall, E. J., Harris, J., et al. (2016). Bacterial cholangitis, cholecystitis, or both in dogs. https://core.ac.uk/download/36779319.pdf (accessed on 12th July 2025).
7. Almar, E., Arveux, P., Autelitano, M., Baldi, I., Bara, S., Barchielli, A., Benfatto, L., et al. (2019). Treatment challenges in and outside a specialist network setting: Pancreatic neuroendocrine tumours. https://core.ac.uk/download/287859188.pdf (accessed on 12th July 2025).
8. Althaus, R., del Pozo, R., Gruendel, D., Huettl, T., et al. (2009). Relation of gallbladder motility to viscosity and composition of gallbladder bile in patients with cholesterol gallstones. https://core.ac.uk/download/16432736.pdf (accessed on 12th July 2025).
9. Ansaloni, L., Pisano, M., Coccolini, F., Peitzmann, A. B., Fingerhut, A., Catena, F., et al. (2017). *2016 WSES Guidelines on Acute Calculous Cholecystitis*. https://core.ac.uk/download/296795368.pdf (accessed on 12th July 2025).
10. Anzidei, M., Catalano, C., De Vizio, S., Di Martino, M., et al. (2016). Imaging follow-up after liver transplantation. https://core.ac.uk/download/54535527.pdf (accessed on 12th July 2025).
11. Apostol, G., Bacon, B., Bowlus, C. L., Dorenbaum, A., et al. (2019). A randomized, controlled, phase 2 study of maralixibat in the treatment of itching associated with primary biliary cholangitis. https://core.ac.uk/download/323068939.pdf (accessed on 12th July 2025).
12. Are, C., Audisio, R. A., Berman, R. S., Cummings, C., et al. (2016). Global curriculum in surgical oncology. https://core.ac.uk/download/46580365.pdf (accessed on 12th July 2025).
13. Armstrong, G., Smith, A., & Toogood, G. (2017). An overview of near infrared fluorescent cholangiography with indocyanine green during cholecystectomy. https://core.ac.uk/download/83943008.pdf (accessed on 12th July 2025).
14. Arva, J., Bove, K., Chen, Z., Davenport, M., De Jong, J., Feldman, A., et al. (2018). Inflammation, active fibroplasia, and end-stage fibrosis in 172 biliary atresia remnants correlate poorly with age at Kasai portoenterostomy, visceral heterotaxy, and outcome. https://core.ac.uk/download/228066237.pdf (accessed on 12th July 2025).

15. Baccari, P., Cappabianca, S., D'Andrea, A., Falcone, M., et al. (2016). Pancreatic tumors imaging: An update. https://core.ac.uk/download/98333045.pdf (accessed on 12th July 2025).

16. Bates, E., & Martin, D. (2017). Immediate postoperative management and complications on the intensive care unit. https://core.ac.uk/download/111010646.pdf (accessed on 12th July 2025).

17. Benoit, D., De Bus, L., Depuydt, P., Libbrecht, L., et al. (2010). Severe drug-induced liver injury associated with prolonged use of linezolid. https://core.ac.uk/download/55761329.pdf (accessed on 12th July 2025).

18. Berloco, P. B., Di Laudo, M., Frattaroli, F. M., Guglielmo, N., et al. (2012). Laparoscopy in liver transplantation: The future has arrived. https://core.ac.uk/download/154948504.pdf (accessed on 12th July 2025).

19. Bron, K. M., Gartner, J. C., Iwatsuki, S., Malatack, J., et al. (1985). Angiography of liver transplantation patients. https://core.ac.uk/download/12204017.pdf (accessed on 12th July 2025).

20. Burra, P., Caraceni, P., Ferri, F., Giannini, E. G., et al. (2018). Specific issues concerning the management of patients on the waiting list and after liver transplantation. https://core.ac.uk/download/159268374.pdf (accessed on 12th July 2025).

21. Cannavale, A., Catalano, C., Fanelli, F., Fiocca, R., et al. (2016). Updated management of malignant biliary tract tumors: An illustrative review. https://core.ac.uk/download/98341455.pdf (accessed on 12th July 2025).

22. Cantisani, V., Deganello, A., Dietrich, C. F., Duran, C., et al. (2016). Role of contrast-enhanced ultrasound (CEUS) in pediatric practice: An EFSUMB position statement. https://core.ac.uk/download/74320188.pdf (accessed on 12th July 2025).

23. Caplin, M., Falconi, M., Fusai, G. K., Lykoudis, P., et al. (2017). Treatment challenges in and outside a specialist network setting: Pancreatic neuroendocrine tumors. https://core.ac.uk/download/168403284.pdf (accessed on 12th July 2025).

24. Clements, L. W., Jarnagin, W. R., Kingham, T. P., Neese, B., et al. (2012). Image-guided liver surgery: Intraoperative projection of computed tomography images utilizing tracked ultrasound. https://core.ac.uk/download/pdf/82599666.pdf (accessed on 12th July 2025).

25. Crocetti, D., D'Orazi, V., Grazi, G. L., Palmieri, A., et al. (2015). Peliosis hepatis: Personal experience and literature review. https://core.ac.uk/download/54526950.pdf (accessed on 12th July 2025).

26. Fatchett, J. (1997). *Basic Abdominal Sonography*. http://deepblue.lib.umich.edu/bitstream/2027.42/67246/2/10.1177_875647939701300i504.pdf (accessed on 12th July 2025).

27. Gerada, J. (2012). *Gastrointestinal Cancer Screening and Surveillance Programmed: A Worldwide Perspective: Part 1*. https://core.ac.uk/download/46604351.pdf (accessed on 12th July 2025).

28. Gerada, J. (2012). *Gastrointestinal Cancer Screening and Surveillance Programmed: A Worldwide Perspective: Part 2*. https://core.ac.uk/download/46604359.pdf (accessed on 12th July 2025).

29. Gordon, R. D., Iwatsuki, S., Lerut, J., Starzl, T. E., et al. (1987). *Surgical Complications in Human Orthotopic Liver Transplantation*. https://core.ac.uk/download/12204197.pdf (accessed on 12th July 2025).

30. Harrington, D., Lamberton, P. H. L., & McGregor, A. (2017). *Human Liver Flukes*. https://core.ac.uk/download/96882191.pdf (accessed on 12th July 2025).

31. Hasan, I., Lesmana, L. A., Syam, A. F., Tambunan, M., et al. (2001). *Non-Surgical Biliary Drainage on Biliary Obstruction Due to Malignancy*. https://media.neliti.com/media/publications/65934-EN-non-surgical-biliary-drainage-on-biliary.pdf (accessed on 12th July 2025).

32. Huang, J. Y., Li, J. W., Li, T., Lin, Y., et al. (2020). *Diagnostic Accuracy of CEUS LI-RADS for the Characterization of Liver Nodules 20 Mm or Smaller in Patients at Risk for Hepatocellular Carcinoma*. https://core.ac.uk/download/299811580.pdf (accessed on 12th July 2025).

33. Joshi, D., Keane, M. G., Pereira, S. P., Shah, U., et al. (2017). *Novel Biomarkers and Endoscopic Techniques for Diagnosing Pancreaticobiliary Malignancy*. https://core.ac.uk/download/111040563.pdf (accessed on 12th July 2025).

34. *Focal Spot, Summer 1989*. (1989). Bernard Becker Medical Library Archives. Washington University School of Medicine. https://core.ac.uk/download/129069275.pdf (accessed on 12th July 2025).

35. *Focal Spot, Fall/Winter 2003/2004*. (2003). Bernard Becker Medical Library Archives. Washington University School of Medicine. https://core.ac.uk/download/129069889.pdf (accessed on 12th July 2025).

36. *Focal Spot, Winter 2006/2007*. (2007), Bernard Becker Medical Library Archives. Washington University School of Medicine. https://core.ac.uk/download/129069354.pdf (accessed on 12th July 2025).

37. Yan, Q., & Shen, H. (Eds). (2022). Gallstones - Review and Recent Progress. IntechOpen. Doi: 10.5772/intechopen.94688. https://core.ac.uk/download/534897640.pdf (accessed on 12th July 2025).

38. Price, J. (2016). *Microwave Ablation Therapy for Colorectal Liver Metastases*. https://open.bu.edu/bitstream/2144/19441/1/Price_bu_0017N_12297.pdf (accessed on 12th July 2025).

39. Hirai, I., Kimura, W., Fukumoto, T., & Watanabe, T. (2015). *Variations in Portal and Hepatic Vein Branching of the Liver*. https://core.ac.uk/download/72860463.pdf (accessed on 12th July 2025).

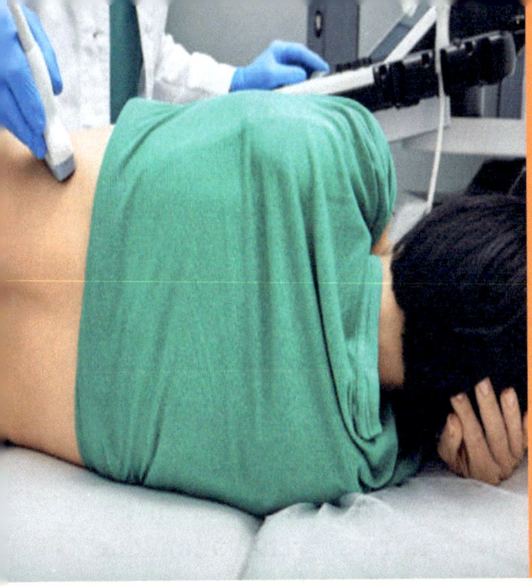

Chapter 9

KIDNEYS AND URINARY TRACT ULTRASOUND

Contents

Introduction

The kidneys and urinary system are accountable for the homeostasis of the body through processes such as the removal of waste, electrolyte regulation, and maintenance of blood pressure. The advancement of non-invasive imaging techniques revolutionized the approach to the diagnosis and management of urinary tract disorders. Among these techniques, ultrasound is an important technique for renal structure and function imaging without its accompanying risks of ionizing radiation and contrast agent, a valuable advantage when applied in pediatric patients and patients with renal insufficiency. Moreover, since urinary tract infections (UTIs) remain prevalent, especially in children, understanding the sequelae of early imaging and diagnosis becomes essential. Early diagnosis not only alleviates present symptoms but also forestalls long-term complications, which emphasizes the need for precise imaging modalities in practice. Ultrasound has emerged as an essential diagnostic tool in assessing conditions such as nephrolithiasis and urinary tract disease. By allowing visualization of the kidneys and ureters under real-time examination, ultrasound helps in the identification of anatomical abnormalities that would expose patients to the risk of recurring infection and stone formation. Not being invasive, the method can differentiate between kidney stones and secondary dilatation of the urinary tract, which otherwise would need more invasive methods like intravenous urography, which involves higher costs and radiation exposure. Therefore, the integration of ultrasound with other imaging methods, such as KUB (Kidneys, Ureters, Bladder), provides enhanced diagnostic precision in the assessment of renal colic patients and can reduce patient management in healthcare facilities. The function of ultrasound is therefore critical in the protection of immediate and long-term patient healthcare outcomes. Besides determining structural abnormalities, ultrasound plays a critical role in comprehending the severity and development of urinary tract infections. Research has made it clear that a high percentage of pediatric UTIs are attributable to intrinsic renal anomalies and thus are in need of proper evaluation using imaging modalities like ultrasound. Specifically, the research has determined that non-E. coli UTIs are typically associated with identifiable renal pathologies that, if left unchecked, may develop into more severe problems such as renal scarring or hypertension. Strategic utilization of ultrasound in clinical protocols can aid in early diagnosis and ensure timely interventions, aligning the practice of healthcare with current guidelines as well as enhancing patient outcomes. Emphasis on the correlation between types of infection and renal function will further enhance comprehensive management strategies concerning the kidneys and urinary tract among children (Figure 9.1).

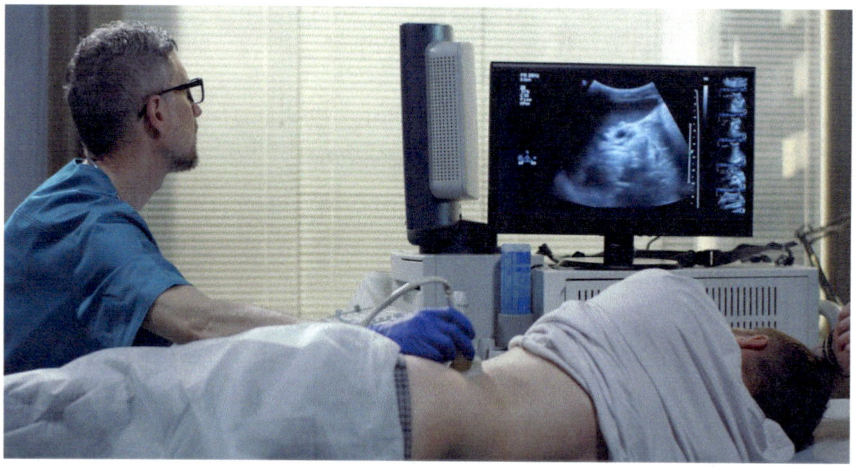

Figure 9.1. Kidneys and urinary tract ultrasound.

Source: Kidney Diseases: What are the Causes, Types and Diagnosis? rizultrasound.com. https://rizultrasound.com/wp-content/uploads/2023/10/Kidney-and-Urinary-Tract-Ultrasound.jpg

Definition of Ultrasound in Medical Imaging

In the medical imaging community, ultrasound technology has emerged as a valuable diagnostic resource and a non-invasive one. Through the application of high-frequency sound waves, ultrasound produces real-time images of internal organs, thereby providing a window into the morphology and functions of many organs. This imaging modality is particularly important in the evaluation of the kidneys and urinary tract since it allows for the evaluation of abnormalities such as cyst, tumor, and obstruction without exposing the patient to ionizing radiation. Its widespread utilization in renal assessment can be attributed to its ability to detect alterations in renal size, echo texture, and fluid retention that result in early detection and treatment of urinary pathosis. As a central component in the diagnostic sequence, ultrasound not only contributes to patient safety but also enhances the effectiveness of clinical examination in nephrology and urology, eventually determining therapy and outcome. Additionally, diagnostic work among patients with hematuria cannot be exaggerated with the use of ultrasound. Since the cause of this symptom may range from as benign as a urinary tract infection to as complex as glomerulonephritis, it is crucial to use proper imaging studies to find the right diagnosis. Ultrasound is a first-line diagnostic test so that the clinician can evaluate the kidneys and the bladder in their entirety. For instance, while gross hematuria will heighten suspicion of a urinary tract disease, the presence of additional clinical findings—proteinuria or hypertension—will mandate investigation of renal function. In the majority of cases, the result of an ultrasound examination can potentially have a significant effect on subsequent clinical management by either confirming a diagnosis or triggering further investigations within a comprehensive plan for clinical evaluation, as detailed in the relevant literature and guidelines surrounding these medical conditions (Horváth et al., 2022).

The use of routine ultrasound protocols is important in ensuring reproducible and consistent results in diagnostic imaging. Such organizations as the American Society of Colon and Rectal Surgeons promote evidence-based guidelines for practice quality enhancement in various specialties in medicine, such as renal imaging (Hall et al., 2020). Adhering to developed standards, medical professionals can guarantee that diagnostic ultrasound is carried out precisely and diligently, preventing variation in interpretation and patient safety optimization. The systematic approach of ultrasound scanning improves not just diagnostic accuracy in renal and urinary tract conditions but also emphasizes the role of continuous professional education and training. Ultimately, the dynamic character of ultrasound technology and its development in renal medicine is a model for the health care advances that most reasonably align with improved patient outcomes and enhanced therapy.

Importance of Kidneys and Urinary Tract in the Human Body

The kidneys and the urinary system are of basic significance in maintaining homeostasis and overall health in the human body. As the body's primary filtration mechanism, the kidneys play a key role in regulating fluid balance, electrolyte composition, and acid-base balance. The filtration system not only aids in the elimination of waste products such as urea and creatinine but also guarantees the return of vital nutrients and minerals into the bloodstream. The urinary system, composed of the ureters, bladder, and urethra, facilitates the storage and excretion of urine, hence preventing the accumulation of toxic substances. Malfunction of either kidney or urinary system will lead to serious health complications, and therefore it is essential that the operation of these systems is under surveillance through regular monitoring and diagnostic examinations, such as ultrasounds, for any abnormality. Prompt diagnosis and treatment of conditions affecting the urinary tract prevent chronic health issues. For instance, bacteria can easily migrate up to the kidneys from the bladder and cause urinary tract infections (UTIs) that will lead to kidney damage if left untreated at an early stage. According to clinical data, delay in the use of antibiotics for UTIs can cause renal structural damage in children, including nephrosclerosis and chronic renal insufficiency, in a significant majority of cases (Zakharova et al., 2025). This highlights the role of health professionals in being proactive in the detection of UTI symptoms and risk factors.

Early diagnosis and treatment of urinary system disease is essential, as it is of importance in sustaining the long-term health of the kidneys and urinary tract, especially in vulnerable groups like children and elderly individuals. Congenital urinary tract and kidney abnormalities (CAKUT) are among the leading etiologies of chronic kidney disease (CKD) in children. Research has determined some genetic factors that are responsible for the manifestation of these anomalies, leading to unusual development and functioning of the kidneys (Kelam et al., 2024). It is important to know the genes that cause CAKUT in order to create the appropriate tools and interventions to prevent or reverse the impact of such conditions. The genetic information can be used to inform the screening as well as treatment decision-making. It is essential that we keep exploring the cellular and molecular mechanisms responsible for kidney development and disease, as this knowledge not only contributes to our understanding of kidney health but also enhances the accuracy of ultrasound diagnosis in finding potential abnormalities before they manifest as severe complications (Figure 9.2).

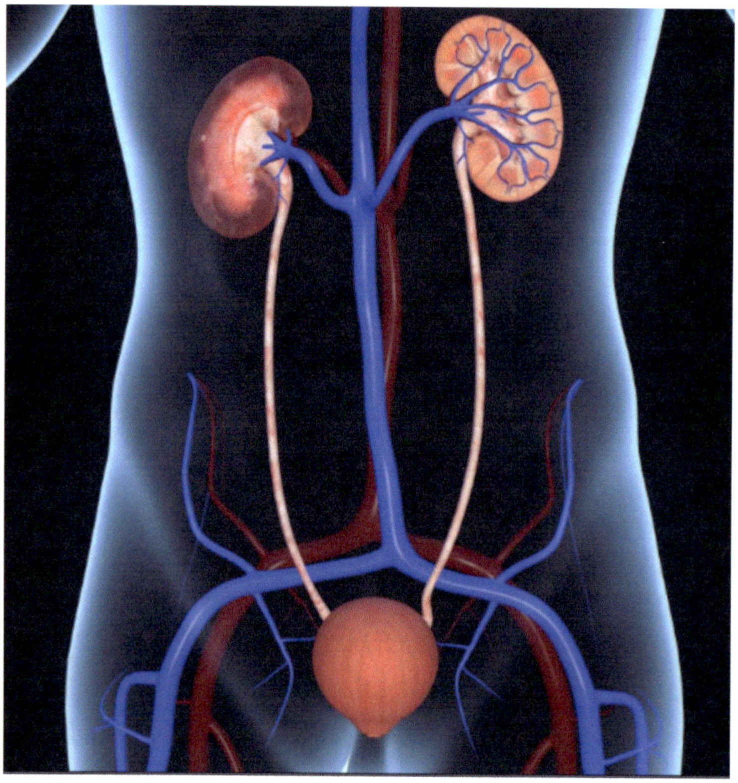

Figure 9.2. Kidneys and urinary tract in human health.

Source:https://media.istockphoto.com/id/499808791/photo/kidneys.jpg?s=612x612&w=0&k=20&c=atUEwUyTmEyxY8XF-5s1oYlwwVpx11sNruf34wACCHw=

9.1. Anatomy of the Kidneys

The kidneys, a sophisticated and essential organ, are responsible for the human body's capacity to achieve homeostasis. Functionally, each kidney consists of three major zones: the cortex, the medulla, and the pelvis. The outermost cortex is filled with nephrons, the functional units that filter blood and produce urine, whereas the innermost medulla has renal pyramids, which drain urine into the renal pelvis. This intricate organization facilitates good filtration and concentration of the waste materials, proving the kidneys' work in keeping electrolyte and blood pressure in balance. Kidneys are also covered with an insulating renal capsule that provides not only structural support but also insulates against infection. Having this anatomy is crucial to the successful application of ultrasound imaging because it provides a visual representation of renal anatomy, which assists in identifying abnormalities on diagnostic tests. Ultrasound imaging has emerged as a valuable tool in assessing kidney structure and function. It employs sound waves to generate images, giving an unobtrusive way of evaluating renal anatomy and detecting pathologies such as hydronephrosis, stones, and tumors. The echogenicity of the kidneys, that is, their ability to reflect back ultrasound, allows physicians to differentiate normal and diseased tissue. Moreover, the recent development of ultrasound technology has provided the opportunity to create multimodal imaging scanners that combine ultrasound with other modalities, for example, impedance tomography, in order to enhance diagnostic accuracy (Głowacka et al., 2024). This conjunction of technologies not only improves visual clarity but also provides the possibility of online evaluation of kidney function, and this is particularly useful in the presence of patients suffering from chronic kidney disease or patients requiring close supervision. Consequently, ultrasound has changed the line of urological diagnostics and has become essential for timely treatment. In specific clinical situations, attainment of the anatomical features of the kidneys will further improve evaluation techniques such as percutaneous cystolitholapaxy, especially with complex urinary tract anatomy. Certain conditions, such as benign prostatic hyperplasia or urethral strictures, may make it difficult with standard techniques of bladder stone removal (Lee et al., 2025). Ultrasound is an essential element of guidance in interventions because it allows for the precise localizing of stones and assessment of neighboring structures. With an appreciation of renal anatomy coupled with ultrasound imaging, health care professionals can tailor techniques to meet individual patient demands, delivering successful treatment along with maximum safety and outcome. The interaction between anatomical information and advanced imaging equipment underscores the central role of ultrasound in urology, enabling widespread patient management and improving the overall quality of care (Figure 9.3).

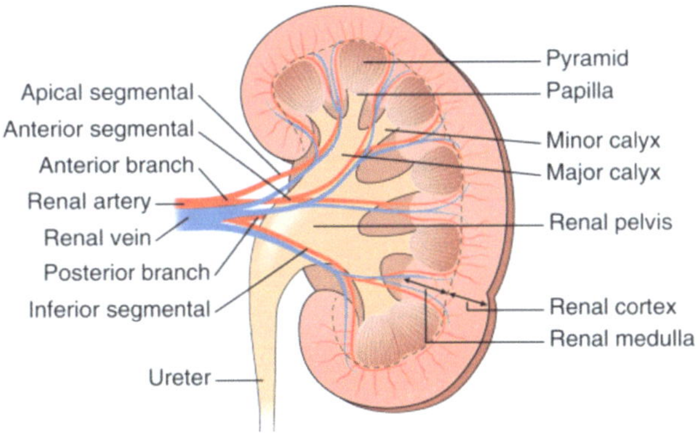

Figure 9.3. Anatomy of the kidneys.

Source: https://ars.els-cdn.com/content/image/3-s2.0-B9780323477949000019-f001-002-9780323477949.jpg

9.1.1. Structure and Function of the Kidneys

The kidneys, vital organs in the urinary system, exhibit a complex structure necessary for their multifaceted functions. Each kidney contains approximately one million nephrons, the microscopic units responsible for filtering blood and producing urine. The nephron is composed of distinct regions, including the glomerulus, proximal tubule, loop of Henle, distal tubule, and collecting duct. The glomerulus serves as a filtration unit, allowing water and solutes to pass while retaining larger proteins and blood cells. This intricate architecture allows the kidneys to not only filter waste products but also regulate water balance, electrolytes, and blood pressure through a series of hormonal responses, underscoring the kidneys' critical roles in maintaining homeostasis. The kidneys' functional efficiency can be assessed through various methodologies, particularly when aesthetically visualized with ultrasound technology. Ultrasound imaging is a non-invasive technique that provides valuable information about kidney structure, size, and potential abnormalities.

It enables the detection of renal stones, tumors, and other structural pathologies that can impede kidney function. In evaluating kidney function, additional tests, such as blood urea nitrogen (BUN) and serum creatinine, offer insight into metabolic waste elimination. As noted in existing literature, while these biochemical parameters indicate kidney function, anatomical representations obtained from ultrasound can enrich clinical assessments, allowing for a more comprehensive understanding of renal health (De Sadeleer et al., 2011).

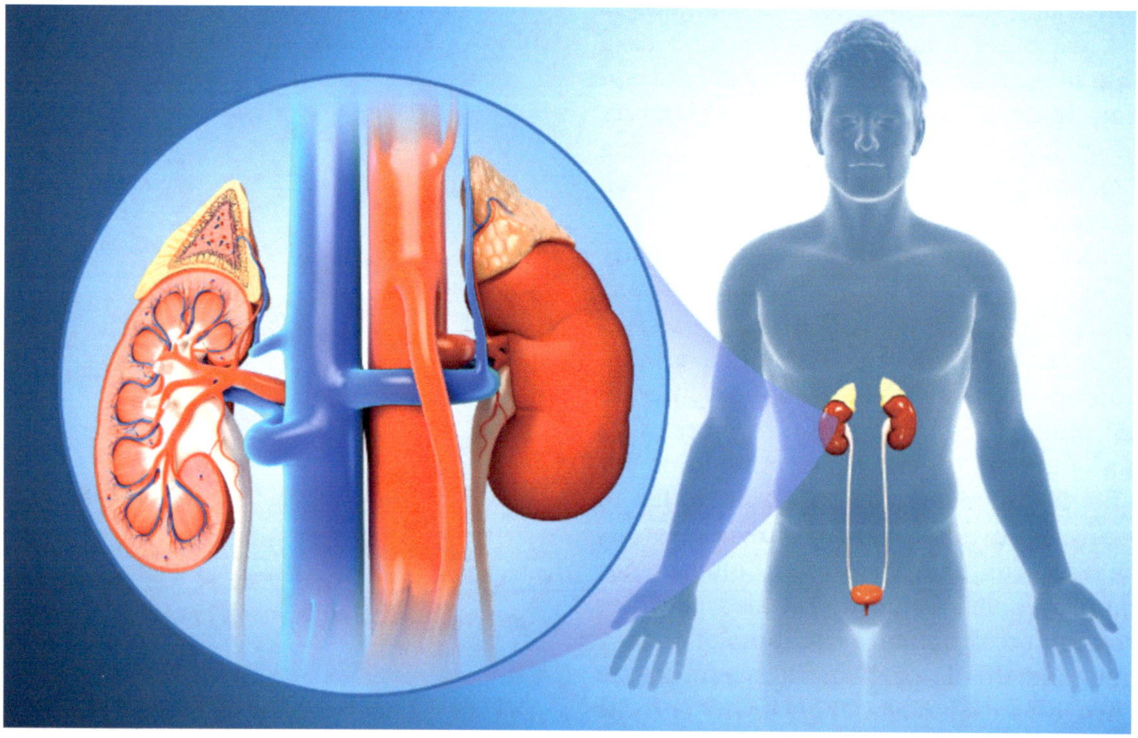

Figure 9.4. Kidney structure and function.

Source: https://external-content.duckduckgo.com/iu/?u=https%3A%2F%2Fwww.verywellhealth.com%2Fthmb%2F2lanqSB2AapNuJPYNv4_xPPVqjc%3D%2F5238x3337%2Ffilters%3Afill(87E3EF%2C1)%2Fmale-kidney-anatomy--illustration-758313113-5aa15ae80e23d90037526254.jpg&f=1&nofb=1&ipt=feea4e16b054b200f64b88ce94c7f9ce68ed9c5b08a678fee50442fb1932b7bd.

Crucially, a deeper understanding of renal vasculature is essential, especially in the context of kidney disease and altered hemodynamics. Abnormalities in intrarenal blood flow can lead to significant complications, including renal vasculopathy and chronic kidney disease. Research has shown a correlation between angiogenic factors, such as endostatin, and renal vasculopathy, offering a potential biomarker for kidney dysfunction (Afeltra et al., 2017). Ultrasound Doppler evaluations can measure parameters like resistive index, providing insights into renal blood flow dynamics. Consequently, integrating functional assessments with imaging techniques enhances diagnostic accuracy, guiding treatment strategies for various renal pathologies and emphasizing the kidneys' vital role in overall health (Figure 9.4).

9.1.2. Location and Relationship to Surrounding Organs

The paired retroperitoneal kidneys have a complex relationship with adjacent structures that is essential for both their function and their evaluation by ultrasound. Located laterally to the spine and bounded by the diaphragm above, the kidneys are approximately at the level of the T12 to L3 vertebrae. This positional anatomy is not only crucial to understand for the appreciation of normal kidney morphology but also for the identification of pathological changes on ultrasound examination. The proximity to nearby organs, say the liver on the right side and the spleen on the left side, also influences ultrasound imaging by commonly requiring clinicians to exclude renal masses from tumors of these overlying organs. Thus, an intimate knowledge of the position of the kidneys in relation to these organs significantly enhances the precision of ultrasound examination. In addition to the liver and spleen, renal blood vessels and urinary tract complicate interrelationships around the kidneys. Renal arteries and veins encircle the kidneys and provide essential blood while assisting in waste expulsion. Knowledge about these vascular relationships is vital, particularly in treatments such as percutaneous nephrolithotomy (PCNL), when accurate placement of the needle in the region of these vessels is hazardous. As emphasized by the most current PCNL research, the integration of high-grade imaging is imperative for effective renal access and minimizing complications with procedures, even showcasing the important role of the surrounding anatomical environment for urological intervention. Here, ultrasound not only serves as an investigative tool but also as a most useful guide to operative planning and patient safety, and illustrates the importance of understanding organ relationships. The close proximity of the kidneys to lower urinary tract structures also highlights the interdependence of renal and bladder function, especially as one would appreciate with conditions such as lower urinary tract dysfunction (LUTD). Ultrasound evaluation of renal function should consider bladder health because the symptoms of incontinence and urgency can be secondary to urinary obstructions caused by renal pathology. Clinical evidence indicates that different imaging modalities, including ultrasound, are capable of determining information about bladder parameters such as wall thickness, which has clinical relevance for urinary abnormalities. Thus, understanding the anatomical position of the kidneys in relation to the organs around them not only aids in diagnostic assessment but also in guiding therapeutic interventions, for which it is crucial that clinicians become familiar with these anatomical details in the context of ultrasound imaging (Aboagye et al., 2019).

9.1.3. Variations in Kidney Anatomy

Anatomical variations of the kidneys play a significant role in interpreting normal renal function and potential pathological states. Of the previously known anatomical variations, the most significant congenital abnormalities are crossed-fused renal ectopia and horseshoe kidneys. Crossed fused renal ectopia, in which both kidneys are fused over the midline, is not only problematic for diagnosis but also offers unique opportunities, such as possibly being a donor organ and therefore aiding in overcoming the long-standing shortage of transplantable kidneys (Abbas et al., 2007). Such anomalies offer potential to nephrologists and radiologists, particularly in interpreting ultrasound images, where abnormal anatomical configurations might influence assessment and management plans. With the exception of crossed fused renal ectopia, the horseshoe kidney is another interesting anatomical anomaly. The kidneys' inferior poles fuse to form a horseshoe shape that defines the condition, which typically occurs in embryonic life. While often asymptomatic, a horseshoe kidney can be incidentally identified in imaging studies, testifying to its clinical relevance (Abdoulaye et al., 2022). Ultrasound is a primary imaging modality in the diagnosis of this renal malformation, enabling practitioners to view structural deformity and evaluate for concomitant complications, including urinary obstruction or infection.

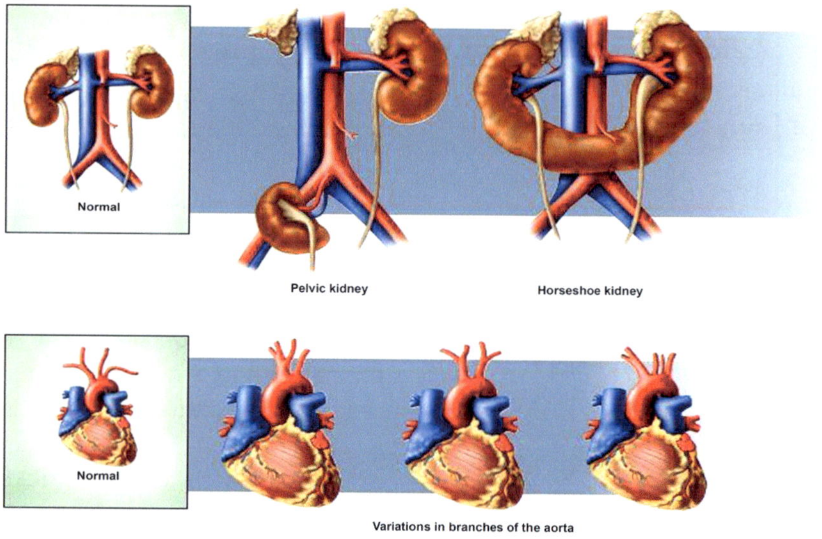

Figure 9.5. Variations in kidney anatomy.

Source: Tyagi S, Chimurkar VK (2021). Congenital Anomalies of Kidney and Urinary Tract (CAKUT)-Literature Review. J Kidney 7:257. doi-10.35248/2472-1220.21.7.257

Knowledge of the implications of horseshoe kidneys is important in delivering comprehensive patient care and in guiding surgical strategies. In addition, anatomical variations of the kidneys can differ substantially among populations and geographical areas and reflect the significance of cultural and geographic factors in medical practice. As an example, congenital renal anomalies could have divergent prevalence rates within different ethnic groups, requiring a divergent approach to ultrasound scans in varied clinical practices. Radiologists need to pay close attention, aware of the fact that some anatomical variations may simulate pathological findings, creating possible misdiagnoses in the case of non-situational consideration. With the understanding of these differences in kidney anatomy, particularly in ultrasound imaging, health care practitioners are then able to enhance diagnostic accuracy and optimize management strategies, ultimately leading to improved patient outcomes in renal therapy (Figure 9.5).

9.2. Anatomy of the Urinary Tract

The urinary system is a multifaceted system responsible for the filtration and excretion of waste products from the body. It is made up of several significant anatomical structures, including the kidneys, ureters, bladder, and urethra. The kidneys, which are bean-shaped organs positioned at the back of the abdominal cavity, play an important role in electrolyte balance maintenance and blood pressure control through urine formation. Every kidney has a complex nephron system where filtration, reabsorption, and secretion take place, and toxins are eliminated while retaining substances that are vital. Understanding the anatomy of the urinary tract is important in medical imaging, particularly in the case of ultrasound technology, since it allows for accurate measurement of both structure and function of these vital organs, emphasized in research highlighting safe and efficient imaging techniques (Aldughiem, 2025).

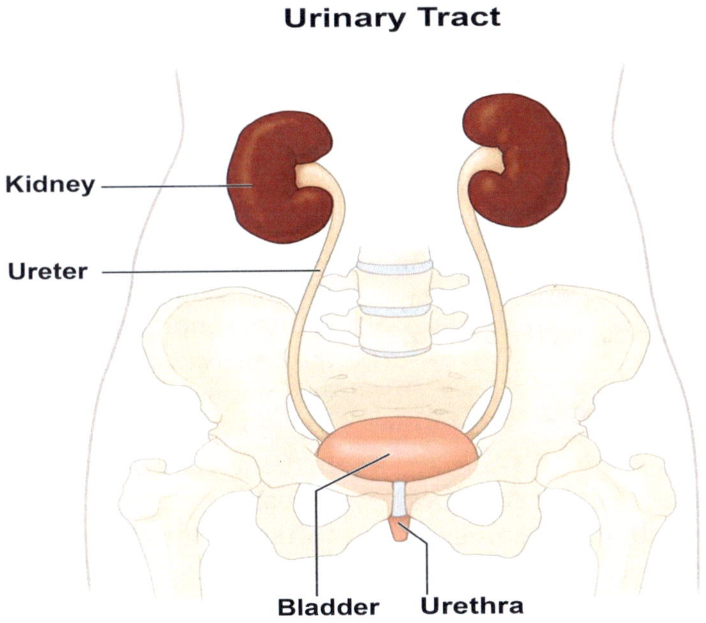

Figure 9.6. Anatomy of the urinary tract.

Source: https://www.niddk.nih.gov/-/media/Images/Health-Information/Urologic/Urinary-Tract-BIG_2064x1895.jpg?imbypass=true.

Ureters are muscular tubes that transport urine from the kidneys to the bladder by peristaltic movements mainly. Measuring roughly 25 to 30 centimeters in length, the tubes pass through the abdominal cavity and slope down into the pelvic region to empty into the bladder. The ureters are also a site of obstruction or stone, which compromises urinary drainage and can be delineated well with ultrasound. The non-invasive imaging mode provides useful information about potential abnormalities, such as a hydroureter or stone in the ureter, which may be caused by various etiologies. In addition, recognition of the anatomical landmarks of the ureters' vicinity is important for accurate interpretation of ultrasound results to enable medical practitioners to make timely diagnoses of conditions associated with urinary tract obstruction (Aldughiem, 2025). Finally, the urinary bladder, which is a compliant reservoir of urine, is located in the pelvic cavity and serves a key role in the storage and voluntary urination of urine. The bladder is structured to accommodate various amounts and is equipped with a muscular wall called the detrusor that tightens when urinating. Familiarization with its anatomy is particularly crucial during the use of ultrasound to diagnose pathologies such as bladder neoplasms, infections, or neurogenic bladder disease. Further, children's urinary systems have some unique anatomical irregularities that require unique imaging techniques to ensure proper diagnosis and treatment. Advanced applications of ultrasound can enhance bladder anatomy and function evaluation, especially in children with congenital urinary tract and kidney anomalies (CAKUT). This emphasizes the need for an extensive knowledge of urinary tract anatomy in the clinical practice of ultrasound (Figure 9.6).

9.2.1. Components of the Urinary Tract

The urinary tract holds several vital structures that enable the storage and expulsion of urine, a critical metabolite of metabolic processes. Beginning from the kidneys, bean-shaped organs cleanse blood, removing waste products and excess water to produce urine. Comprising functional units called nephrons, every kidney performs filtration and reabsorption. The urine produced in the kidneys then drains into the ureters, muscle tubes that pump urine to the bladder through peristaltic contractions. The communication between these components is critical in maintaining homeostasis, as the kidneys filter electrolyte content and blood pressure based on the needs of the body, which can be tracked by techniques such as ultrasound imaging of the structure and function of the urinary tract. As urine enters the bladder, storage and controlled release mechanisms are activated. The smooth muscle-covered bladder enlarges as it fills and, upon micturition, shortens to eject urine through the urethra. It is a highly regulated process of the bladder sphincters to maintain continence until the right time to micturate. Ultrasound scanning is equally valuable in assessing bladder capacity and integrity to enable practitioners to identify any abnormalities, such as bladder stones, hypertrophy, or wall thickness abnormalities. Understanding bladder and urethral dynamics is fundamental in diagnosing conditions that may compromise urinary function or lead to complications such as urinary tract infection or incontinence. In so far as urinary pathologies are involved, ultrasound scanning reveals not only structural abnormalities but also functional data concerning the kidneys and the urinary tract structures. Obstructive uropathy may cause serious complications if left undetected. In this case, the biochemical content of the urine can provide some additional information about the clinical condition; for example, the presence of abnormal material such as cholesterol-containing complexes might be indicative of intrinsic renal disease (Jüngst et al., 1984). The effectiveness of therapeutic interventions, such as that of the herbal drug Canephron N after lithotripsy, points to the importance of the structural but also of the biochemical composition of the urinary system (Vitkovskyy, 2018). Thus, comprehensive ultrasound evaluation along with urinalysis supports understanding of the function and dysfunction of urinary tract components and guides therapeutic approaches and enhances outcomes in patients.

9.2.2. Function of Each Component in Urine Formation and Excretion

The process of urine formation is primarily driven by the intricate functions of the nephron, the fundamental unit of the kidney. Each nephron consists of several key components, including the glomerulus, proximal tubule, loop of Henle, distal convoluted tubule, and collecting duct. The glomerulus plays a crucial role in filtration, allowing water, ions, and small molecules to pass from the blood while retaining larger proteins and blood cells. Following filtration, the proximal tubule is responsible for the reabsorption of 65–70% of filtered sodium and water, along with glucose and amino acids. This selective reabsorption, combined with the secretion of waste products, ultimately influences the concentration and composition of urine. The intricate balance maintained by each component underscores the nephron's critical role in waste excretion and homeostasis in the body. The loop of Henle serves an essential function in creating a concentration gradient in the renal medulla, which is vital for the kidneys' ability to concentrate urine.

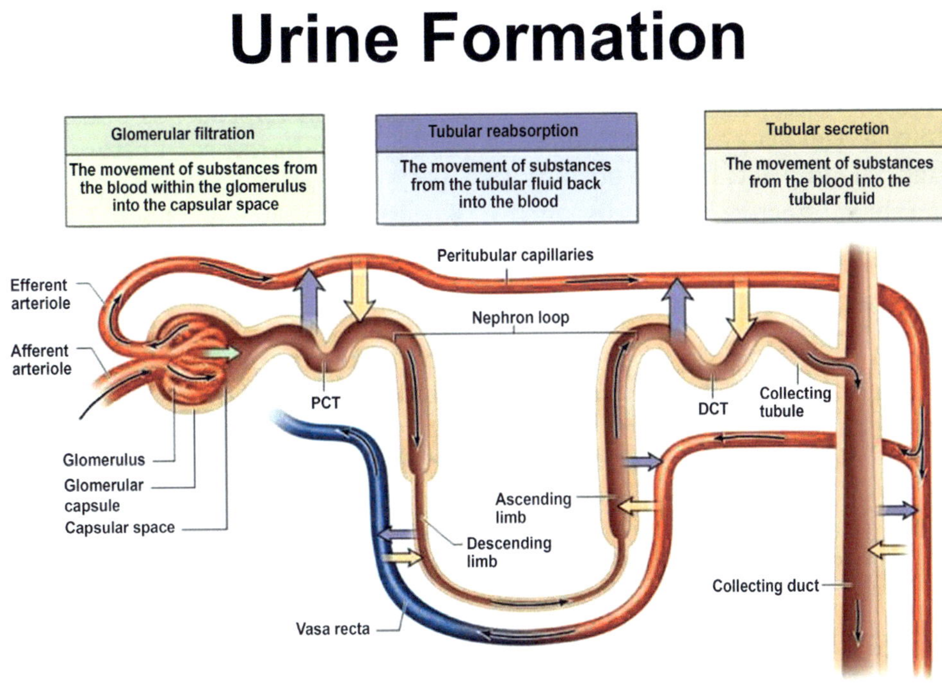

Figure 9.7. Function of each component in urine formation.

Source: https://nurseslabs.com/wp-content/uploads/2017/04/Urine-Formation-Urinary-System-Anatomy-and-Physiology.png.

Through a process known as counter-current multiplication, the descending limb allows water to leave while preventing solute loss, resulting in concentrated urine at the tip of the loop. Conversely, the ascending limb actively transports sodium and chloride ions out of the filtrate without allowing water to pass, further enhancing the osmolarity gradient. Following this, the distal convoluted tubule fine-tunes the composition of urine by adjusting the reabsorption of ions like calcium and sodium, influenced by hormonal signals such as aldosterone. This regulation protects the body against dehydration and ensures effective waste management, illustrating the nephrons' pivotal strategy in urine formation and electrolyte balance. Finally, the collecting duct plays a significant role in the final determination of urine volume and concentration. Hormonal control, primarily through antidiuretic hormone (ADH), adjusts the permeability of the collecting duct to water. When the body is in a state of dehydration, ADH levels increase, stimulating the reabsorption of water back into the bloodstream and concentrating the urine. This mechanism is particularly significant in the context of abnormal conditions such as urinary tract obstruction, where impaired drainage can lead to renal damage (Mohajerzadeh et al., 2024). Furthermore, conditions like autosomal recessive polycystic kidney disease (ARPKD) may complicate urinary function and excretion, underscoring the interconnectedness of kidney health and urine management (Zhou et al., 2024). By understanding the functions of each nephron component, clinicians can better evaluate kidney function through imaging techniques such as ultrasound, enabling effective diagnosis and treatment of urinary disorders (Figure 9.7).

9.2.3. Common Anatomical Variations

Kidneys are susceptible to several anatomical variations that may impact their function and render diagnostic tests such as ultrasounds more complicated. One of these variations is the accessory renal arteries, which is an extremely significant variation. The accessory renal arteries may arise from the abdominal aorta or even the renal arteries themselves, thus leading to variations in renal blood supply. These anomalies must be detected during ultrasounds because they impact surgical planning and imaging interpretation. There has been evidence via studies that there are accessory renal arteries, which present in an appreciable percentage of people, and so it is vital that sonographers are aware of these variations to avoid misdiagnosis or procedure complications. Examination of such variations highlights the intricacies of renal anatomy and the importance of careful evaluation in kidney-focused ultrasound studies. Another such variation is the retroaortic left renal vein, which can be the etiology of clinical presentations like microhematuria. This anatomical variation occurs when the left renal vein falls behind the aorta and, in some cases, can result in vascular compression or pathology. In cryptic urinary symptoms, such as hematuria, the retroaortic left renal vein must be considered in the differential diagnosis. Current literature has shown that such uncommon renal vascular anomalies, while not common, play significant roles in determining patient outcomes. Sonographers should thus be aware of this variation during ultrasound examinations, for early detection to contribute to the identification of the underlying cause of urinary symptoms and help inform subsequent management approaches optimally (Isık et al., 2023). Furthermore, ureterohydronephrosis (UHN) is also another typical anatomical variation that is more likely to be encountered in pregnant women, especially beyond the 20th week of pregnancy. This is a state where the renal pelvis and the ureter become engorged, often due to hormonal and mechanical changes that take place with pregnancy. In ultrasound examinations, grading of UHN is an important diagnostic finding in which results typically correspond to various levels of severity in relation to gestational age. In extreme cases, stenting may be necessary as an intervention, although the majority of patients are receptive to conservative treatment. The prominence and complexity of UHN highlight the necessity to include understanding about typical anatomical variations in everyday ultrasound evaluations because understanding these differences actually enhances diagnosis and treatment of patients (Ciciu et al., 2021).

9.3. Principles of Ultrasound Technology

The principles of ultrasound technology rely on the transmission of high-frequency sound waves and their behavior upon interaction with body tissues. During an ultrasound examination, a transducer is employed to transmit ultrasonic pulses through the skin into other tissues. When the sound waves encounter various interfaces, such as fluid-containing organs like the kidneys or solid structures, they are reflected back or transmitted further. The echo waves rebound back to the transducer and are translated into electric signals. These electric signals are processed to create real-time visual images, allowing clinicians to assess anatomical structures and detect abnormalities, particularly in the urinary tract. The versatility of ultrasound is compounded by its invasiveness and absence of ionizing radiation, making it a very valuable tool in the diagnosis of diseases such as nephrolithiasis and renal pathologies in general (Bove et al., 2013).

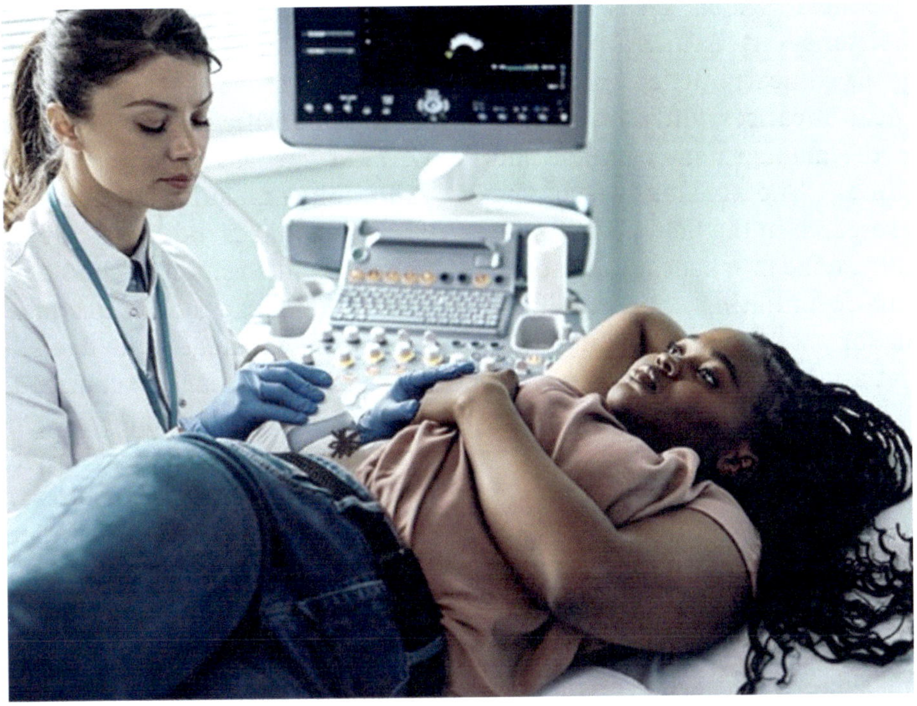

Figure 9.8. Kidney ultrasound process.

Source: Drazen Zigic (2023). www.istockphoto.com https://media.istockphoto.com/id/1495030757/photo/female-doctor-using-ultrasound-during-medical-examination-of-black-woman-at-the-clinic.jpg ?s=612x612&w=0&k=20&c=UNP6BTLPU5fUGIOabHdlliCpAz-sT9s4byowg2tQvJI=

Not only does the technology of ultrasound have diagnostic uses, but it also encompasses a series of advanced techniques that are employed to maximize image acquisition and interpretation. For example, Doppler ultrasound is able to assess blood flow via renal vasculature, information of immeasurable worth regarding perfusion and potential vascular disease. Ultrasound resolution in kidney stone and urinary obstruction assessment is especially important, in which the determination of stone size, location, and composition is mandatorily required for decision making. In addition, new ultrasound technology innovations like three-dimensional imaging and elastography are being used more and more to advance the understanding of renal diseases. These innovations not only aid in clinical decision-making but also open doors to more directed therapies, as evidenced by ultrasound's increasing relevance to urology and nephrology (Calabrese et al., 2016). Also, revised recommendations and guidelines by professional societies place pressure on applying standardized ultrasound practice in order to improve patient outcomes. For instance, the European Federation of Societies for Ultrasound in Medicine and Biology has established protocols to structure gastrointestinal ultrasound examinations, which can be extended to renal examinations as well. These standardized procedures allow practitioners to better recognize normal and pathological findings, which gives way to increased consistency in treating patients. By the synergy of clinical practice guidelines and technological advances, ultrasound is a cornerstone in the management of renal and urinary tract illness. The constantly evolving education and research in the field point to the importance of ultrasound in enhancing diagnostic proficiency and formulating individualized treatment plans for patients with urinary tract disease (Bove et al., 2013) (Figure 9.8).

9.3.1. Basic Principles of Ultrasound Imaging

The fundamental concepts of ultrasound imaging include the use of high-frequency sound waves for the generation of real-time images of internal structures, particularly easy-to-scan organs like the kidneys and urinary tract. It begins with the emission of ultrasound waves from a transducer, which then travel inside the body and reflect from various tissues. These reflected waves, or echoes, are detected by the same transducer and translated into electrical signals. The intensity and timing of the echoes provide valuable information about the size, shape, and composition of the tissues under investigation. Theseare all non-invasive, don't utilize any ionizing radiation, and hence are particularly of interest for repeat assessments, for example, of urinary tract functions or pathology, for example, in pediatric patients with conditions like urinary tract infections (Linden et al., 2024). Advanced imaging technologies, for example, contrast-enhanced ultrasound (CEUS), enhance the diagnostic accuracy of routine ultrasound procedures. In diagnosing conditions such as acute pyelonephritis (APN), CEUS augments traditional grayscale and Doppler imaging with details about renal perfusion and vascularity. This is particularly valuable in pediatric populations, in which limiting the amount of radiation to which the patient is exposed is paramount. Notably, studies have established that CEUS correlates strongly with more traditional imaging techniques like 99mTc-DMSA scans, thereby validating its application in the identification of renal abnormalities without the associated risks of sedation or radiation exposure (Han Lee et al., 2023). These advances point to the importance of enhancing ultrasound technology as more than just a diagnostic tool; it has taken precedence in offering management decision facilitation for renal and urinary tract disorders. Moreover, applying ultrasound imaging when evaluating the kidneys and urinary tract significantly assists in identifying possible complications of conditions like urinary tract infection that may lead to chronic illness. For instance, via the utilization of routine ultrasounds, healthcare practitioners can identify dilating vesicoureteral reflux, which has been associated with irreversible kidney damage. Based on recent findings, approximately 10% of infants with urinary tract infection have renal abnormalities, testifying to the need for frequent ultrasound scans as part of their care process (Linden et al., 2024). Such imaging modalities enable clinicians to establish effective treatment plans, attesting to the use of ultrasound as not only a diagnostic modality but as an essential part of the care continuum of urinary tract pathology.

9.3.2. Ultrasound Modalities Utilized in Renal Imaging

The application of ultrasound in renal imaging is generally categorized into several techniques, each specially designed to respond to specific diagnostic needs. Standard abdominal ultrasound remains the first-imaging modality due to its non-invasive nature and lack of ionizing radiation. It is a technique that allows one to look at kidney size, shape, and anatomy to obtain critical information about conditions such as hydronephrosis and renal tumors. Further, Doppler ultrasonography can assess blood flow in renal arteries with the view to identifying conditions like renal artery stenosis or thrombosis. The versatility of such ultrasound techniques underscores their key role in primary investigation and ongoing management of renal diseases since they can generate immediate images without subjecting patients to the hazards of more invasive methods. Additionally, advancements in technology have introduced specialty uses like contrast-enhanced ultrasound (CEUS). This technique enhances normal ultrasound imaging quality with the use of microbubble contrast agents, facilitating better characterization of renal masses and vascularity. Evidence is available for its effectiveness in detecting conditions such as vesico-ureteric reflux (VUR), which is commonly assessed in children. Studies have demonstrated that CEUS can offer equal results to traditional methods like micturating cystourethrography (MCUG), with the benefits of being real-time and free of ionizing radiation, thus offering a safer alternative in vulnerable patient groups (Biggi et al., 2005). CEUS is thus being increasingly applied in the clinic, opening the door to more patient-friendly imaging strategies. In the evaluation of nephrolithiasis, ultrasound techniques also become helpful, particularly in combination with plain radiography. Although intravenous urography has been a conventional diagnostic tool for decades, it is pervaded by disadvantageous aspects, including ionizing radiation exposure and additional examination time and cost (Ismail, 2001). Compared with ultrasound, however, kidney stones can be detected, and pelvicalyceal system dilation can be assessed and crucial information provided without complication. Research has demonstrated that a combination of kidney, ureter, and bladder (KUB) imaging and ultrasound greatly improves stone detection, particularly when they are localized in the ureter. This synergy highlights the changing game of renal imaging modalities, where ultrasound is increasingly becoming central to providing effective care to patients with minimal risk (Figure 9.9).

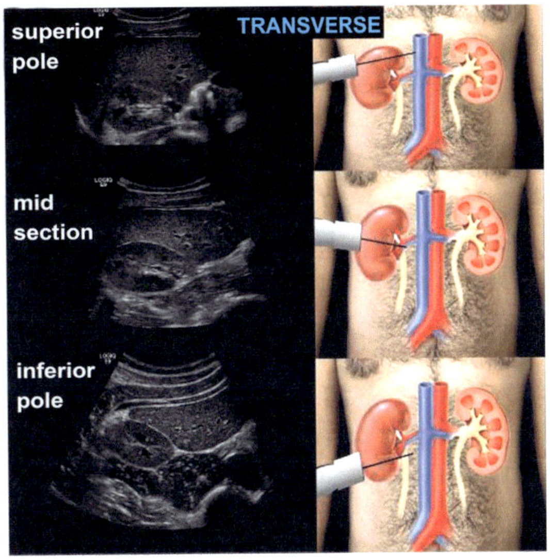

Figure 9.9. Renal ultrasound complete protocol.

Source: Renal Ultrasound Complete Protocol. sonographictendencies.com. https://sonographictendencies.com/wp-content/uploads/2021/03/2.jpg?w=1024

9.3.3. Advantages of Ultrasound over Other Imaging Modalities

The advantages of ultrasound for kidney and urinary tract evaluation are evident when they are compared with other imaging modalities such as computed tomography (CT) and magnetic resonance imaging (MRI). One of the largest advantages of ultrasound is that it is a non-invasive modality that can be used for real-time imaging without exposing patients to ionizing radiation. This is particularly significant for vulnerable groups, including pregnant women and children, as they are more susceptible to the negative effects associated with radiation exposure. Also, ultrasound machines tend to be more portable and cost-effective compared to CT and MRI equipment. This accessibility allows for wider utilization, and emergency assessment can be performed in a variety of clinical settings, ranging from emergency departments to outpatient clinics, thus enhancing patient care and expeditious diagnosis.

Ultrasound also has a unique capability of imaging dynamic physiologic events in real time, making it further distinct from static imaging technologies like CT and MRI. For instance, sonography would provide immediate feedback regarding kidney function and urinary flow, enabling clinicians to see changes with maneuvers or interventions. This dynamic imaging is particularly valuable in the assessment of hydronephrosis or obstructions of the renal tract, where dysfunction is as significant as the anatomic finding. Doppler ultrasound provides this capability with the assessment of the renal vasculature's blood flow and perfusion. Such real-time information is of invaluable utility in clinical decision-making, allowing for timely interventions and improved total patient outcomes. In addition, advances in ultrasound technology, such as techniques like contrast-enhanced ultrasound (CEUS), have significantly expanded its diagnostic use, further solidifying its place in nephrology and urology. CEUS, for example, allows improved visualization of renal lesions and vascular structures with less risk than is typically present in a CT scan with iodine-based contrast agents. Microbubble contrast agents, increasingly utilized in the clinic, allow for ultrasound characterization of lesions non-invasively that would otherwise be indeterminate on conventional ultrasound imaging. This development highlights the evolving function of ultrasound, particularly in male-specific imaging, whereby consensus-based naming and enhanced imaging technologies, as elaborated in (Levi et al., 2019), can enhance diagnostic precision. Overall, the safety and versatility of ultrasound for assessing kidneys and the urinary system highlight its expanded function compared to the traditional imaging techniques, offering patients more individualized and effective types of treatment as referenced in (Sidhu et al., 2018) (Figure 9.10).

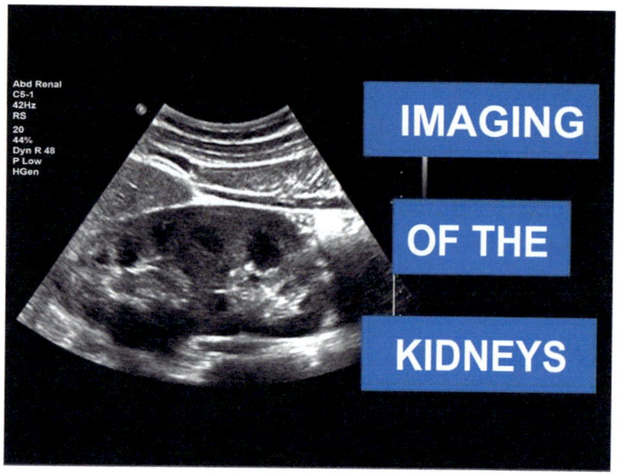

Figure 9.10. Imaging modalities of the kidneys.

Source: https://i.ytimg.com/vi/rGNcOVLKl9g/sddefault.jpg.

9.4. Indications for Kidney and Urinary Tract Ultrasound

The uses of ultrasound of the kidney and ureter are diverse, a testament to its essential place in pediatric and adult medicine. For the most part, this imaging modality is being employed to assess renal stones, hydronephrosis, and congenital anomalies. In children, for instance, the detection and diagnosis of urinary tract obstruction is often necessary; a well-documented case is pelvi-ureteric junction obstruction, frequently diagnosed as an integral part of antenatal screening examination. This early detection underscores the requirement for subsequent imaging to monitor potential complications and guide management decisions, such as whether intervention is required. The non-invasiveness of ultrasound makes it particularly valuable in pediatric presentation, with repeated assessment feasible without patient risk from radiation or nephrotoxic contrast. Ultrasound is thus not only a diagnostic tool but a key element in ongoing patient management. Additionally, a kidney and urinary tract ultrasound is used in acute clinical situations where there is a need to rapidly evaluate. The technique of imaging is commonly used in emergency rooms for patients with flank pain, hematuria, or symptoms of urinary tract infections (UTIs). Ultrasound may be able to visualize obstruction or structural disease of the renal collecting system that would require immediate intervention. Further, its relative ability to differentiate between obstructive and non-obstructive causes of hydronephrosis enhances clinical decision-making and optimizes patient outcomes. The technique is particularly valuable given its availability and efficacy, allowing for quick evaluations that can guide subsequent management strategies, thereby enhancing the delivery of care in emergency situations (Cantisani et al., 2016).

Finally, ongoing improvement in ultrasound technology has broadened its application in the evaluation of kidneys and urinary tracts. Advancements, such as contrast-enhanced ultrasound (CEUS), have expanded its field of diagnostics without the associated danger of traditional contrast agents. Though CEUS is mainstream in adults for a variety of applications, pediatric applications are becoming a worthwhile substitute for invasive techniques or ionizing radiation exposure (Cantisani et al., 2016). This change emphasizes the growing recognition of CEUS as a valuable resource in renal disease treatment among children, particularly in the assessment of focal lesions and other renal pathologies. Lastly, the broad scope of indications for kidney and urinary tract ultrasound illustrates its first-level significance in maximizing patient care among populations and clinical environments to provide immediate and effective renal and urinary tract disease management (Figure 9.11).

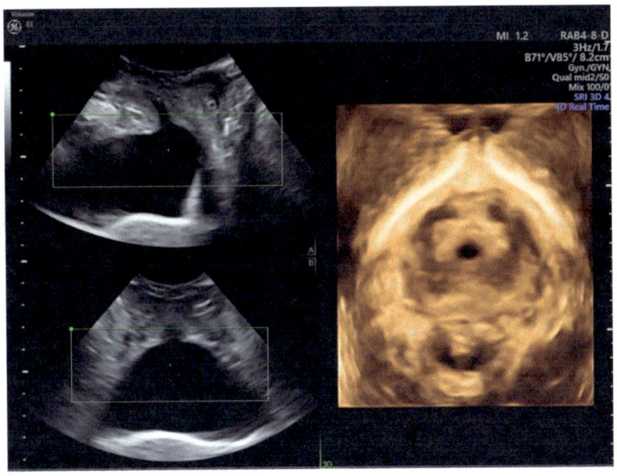

Figure 9.11. Indications for kidney and urinary tract ultrasound.

Source: https://images.takeshape.io/f1ba446a-c0cf-4882-b0c9-50298f143ec2/dev/1ab173bf-2d0e-4e92-a157-1de7bad73fff/622204.

9.4.1. Common Clinical Scenarios Requiring Ultrasound

In nephrology, ultrasound is important in diagnosing various conditions affecting the urinary tract and kidneys. Evaluation of hydronephrosis, where one of the kidneys is swollen as a result of the accumulation of urine, is one of the most common clinical conditions that necessitate the application of ultrasound. The urinary tract obstruction is normally the cause of this condition and must be treated promptly to prevent potential damage to the kidneys. Ultrasound is an innocuous technique through which physicians are able to visualize the renal anatomy along with any associated abnormalities, such as stones or tumors that may be obstructing the outflow of urine. The aspect of providing real-time images without utilizing ionizing radiation renders ultrasound best suited for pediatric presentations, where radiation exposure over the long term is an important concern. Thus, the role of ultrasound in the detection and assessment of hydronephrosis is significant in the decision-making process. Detection of renal masses, either cystic or solid, is another frequent indication for renal ultrasound. Flank pain, hematuria, or renal dysfunction in presenting individuals frequently leads to the utilization of ultrasound as a primary diagnostic test. The modality allows for differentiation between simple renal cysts and more complex masses, facilitating timely interventions. Moreover, ultrasound can also assess the vascularity of a mass, which can be critical in identifying potential malignancies. In cases of suspected renal tumors, ultrasound may guide further imaging or biopsy procedures, streamlining patient management.

Because of its availability and efficiency, ultrasound remains a vital component in the initial evaluation of renal masses, allowing for early detection and ultimately impacting patient outcomes as well as ongoing monitoring following treatment. Ultimately, urinary tract infections (UTIs) are the most common clinical scenario where ultrasound is invaluable, especially in pediatrics. Children with recurrent UTIs are exposed to ultrasound imaging for detecting underlying anatomical malformations such as vesicoureteral reflux or obstructive uropathy. The prevalence of lower urinary tract dysfunction and UTIs among children with chronic kidney disease supports the usefulness of ultrasound for precise evaluation and management. Assessment of the kidneys and bladder with ultrasound might be important to offer details about urinary tract anatomy and function, to guide additional diagnostic and therapeutic management. These observations are particularly relevant to renal transplant patients, who are at heightened risk for UTIs and complications and whose monitoring thus needs to be meticulous. The integration of ultrasound in the UTI diagnostic pathway highlights its crucial role in the effective and efficient management of renal pathologies (Higuchi et al., 2021; Öborn, 2014).

9.4.2. In the Diagnosis of Kidney Stones and Tumors

In nephrology, the ultrasound technology is a milestone in kidney tumor and stone diagnosis, in effect, revolutionizing patient management algorithms. One of the first advantages of ultrasound is that it images renal structures without the use of ionizing radiation or invasive procedures, overcoming the safety implications of traditional imaging modalities like CT scans. As reported by Bigosiński et al. (2022), ultrasound is especially helpful in the differentiation between a range of urological emergencies, including renal calculi detection. Its non-invasive method allows for implementation at the point of care, facilitating timely clinical decision-making for flank pain conditions that may signify tumors or stones. Such urgency is critical in the acute environment where rapid diagnosis can literally make a huge difference in patient outcomes. Further, ultrasound not only allows for the identification of existing pathologies but also identifies underlying conditions that predispose patients to recurrent renal issues. For instance, the radiological findings observed in the case of an ultrasound, such as calyceal dilation, may not only reveal the presence of stones but could also indicate obstructive lesions, thus giving a better general idea of the condition of the patients. In medullary sponge kidney, typically incidental to the diagnosis, ultrasound may reveal cystic formations and calcifications within the renal medulla and thus establish the diagnosis of this rare developmental abnormality (Bigosiński et al., 2022). Such findings are important in that they assist urologists in tailoring treatment plans that might include lifestyle modifications or even surgical interventions to properly manage stones and tumors. The use of ultrasound technology in routine clinical procedures has been found to possess major benefits in the management of renal disease, particularly in the accurate diagnosis of kidney stones and tumors (Mahfoozi & Moslemi, 2011). Studies have indicated that urologist-performed ultrasound has demonstrated a highly sensitive rate of 99.7%, further indicating comprehensive evaluations of patients presenting with corresponding symptoms (Mahfoozi &Moslemi, 2011). This extremely high degree of diagnostic concordance not only enhances patient satisfaction but also makes the process of patient management easy, thereby minimizing the need for unnecessary additional imaging studies. In general, this application of ultrasound in the diagnosis of kidney tumors and stones demonstrates its utility as a first-line diagnostic tool, offering accessibility and economy while significantly improving clinical outcome for those with renal disease (Figure 9.12).

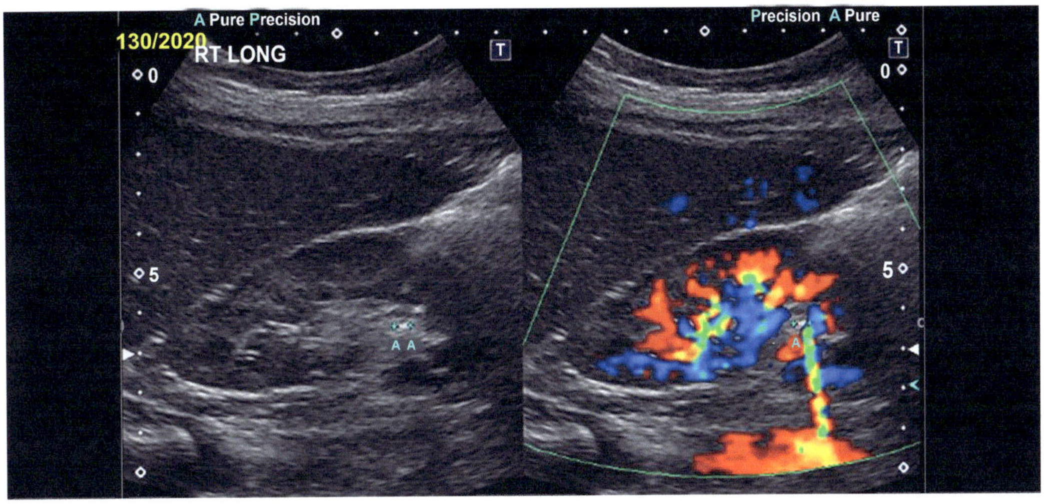

Figure 9.12. Role in diagnosing kidney stones and tumors.

Source: radiologyblog.cincinnatichildrens.org. https://radiologyblog.cincinnatichildrens.org/wp-content/uploads/2021/03/US-kid-stone_915x430.png.

9.4.3. Use in Evaluating Urinary Tract Infections and Obstructions

Assessment of urinary tract infections (UTIs) and obstructions by ultrasound technology is extremely useful in clinical applications. Traditional imaging techniques, such as intravenous urography (IVU), do find application with the help of ionizing radiation and contrast medium, which is inherently dangerous for the patient. Ultrasound, in contrast, focuses on secure, non-invasive methods to study anatomical structures and fluid dynamics of the urinary tract. This imaging modality enables clinicians to visualize beyond obstructions, including tumors or stones, and assess the involvement of adjacent structures in real time. Due to its flexibility, ultrasound is increasingly being recognized as a first-line diagnostic device for conditions leading to UTIs and obstructions in the urinary tract, underscoring its important place in patient care and management. One of the most beneficial uses of ultrasound to diagnose urinary tract issues is that it can reveal the presence of calculi, and hydronephrosis—swelling of a kidney due to urine congestion. Studies have indicated that when ultrasound is combined with kidney-ureter-bladder (KUB) radiography, the rate of detection for urinary stones, particularly in the ureter, where obstructions may lead to acute pain and resultant complications, is boosted. The complementarity of these imaging modalities facilitates clinicians to make suitably informed decisions regarding treatment options, that is, whether lithotripsy or surgery can be undertaken. The effective application of ultrasound in these cases mirrors the need for creative problem-solving in veterinary medicine, as seen by current guidelines for urinary disease management in species (Adams et al., 2016). Further, as new imaging methods become available, the application of ultrasound in routine assessment for urinary tract disease is a demonstration of the shift toward more patient-specific care. The importance of minimizing patient health risks while achieving maximum diagnostic sensitivity cannot be overemphasized. For instance, the findings of studies illustrate that, besides aiding in detecting calculi and obstructions, ultrasound is used to document alterations in urinary patient conditions over time. This constant monitoring is essential in planning particular treatment regimens and forecasting potential complications. In this case, ultrasound is not just a diagnostic tool; it becomes an invaluable assistant to the integrated approach to urinary tract care, having a positive impact on clinical outcomes and enhancing the quality of care as a whole (Ismail., 2001) (Figure 9.13).

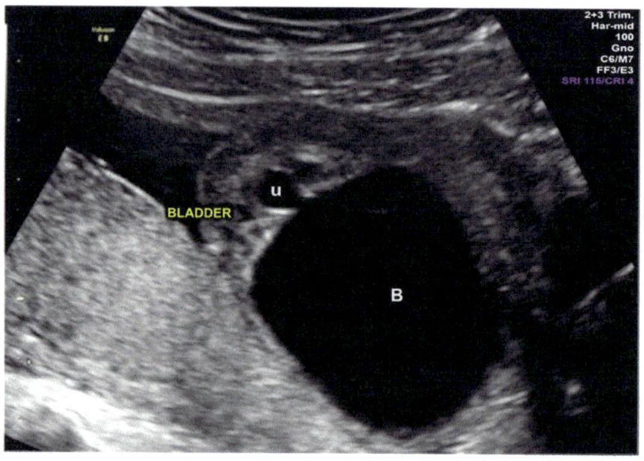

Figure 9.13. Use in evaluating urinary tract infection and obstruction in ultrasound.

Source: Haeri S.(2015. Fetal Lower Urinary Tract Obstruction (LUTO): a practical review for providers. Matern Health Neonatol Perinatol.1:26. doi: 10.1186/s40748-015-0026-1.

9.5. Procedure of Kidney and Urinary Tract Ultrasound

The kidney and urinary tract ultrasound is an imaging procedure that is non-invasive and very important in renal anatomy and disease evaluation. This process involves the use of high-frequency sound waves to produce good images of the kidneys, ureters, and bladder. The patient is typically placed either supine or lateral decubitus position, with a gel applied to the skin for the easy passage of sound waves. The transducer is then rolled across the abdominal region to capture images in multiple directions. This process is particularly useful in that no ionizing radiation is employed, hence the safety of patients, especially vulnerable populations such as children. Images attained assist clinicians in diagnosing conditions such as kidney stones, tumors, cysts, and urinary tract obstructions, hence guiding the next line of treatment. In addition to its role as a diagnostic tool, the kidney and urinary tract ultrasound has a significant place in the evaluation of patients who present with urinary tract infections (UTIs). There is greater interest in using ultrasound for additional evaluation in pediatric patients to prevent possible complications like renal scarring, as per recent studies. The method is an effective screening tool, particularly for children under five years of age with recurrent UTIs, since it is beneficial in establishing anatomical anomalies without having to employ more probing examinations. Moreover, novel techniques such as contrast-enhanced ultrasound have the capacity to diagnose vesicoureteral reflux and are a good alternative to traditional imaging procedures such as micturating cystourethrography. These advances indicate a paradigm shift in the thought process and employment of ultrasound by healthcare professionals in managing urinary tract pathology, retaining its value in maximizing patient outcomes. In general, kidney and urinary tract ultrasound is not only vital in the diagnosis of most renal and urinary illnesses but also reflects advances that enhance patient management. With continued development in ultrasound technology and methods by the medical community, it becomes increasingly crucial to preserve non-invasiveness while at the same time guaranteeing diagnostic integrity. Application of ultrasound for the evaluation of UTI, for instance, highlights its utility and effectiveness in the clinician's daily practice, and challenges traditional methods that are not always optimized in terms of safety and patient convenience. Additionally, additional studies on comparisons of ultrasound effectiveness to other imaging techniques remind us that an explicit understanding of its functionality is essential. In general, this imaging process gives clinicians tools for successful interventions and better long-term management of renal and urinary disorders, ultimately leading to better clinical results for patients (Bove et al., 2013; Biggi et al., 2005) (Figure 9.14).

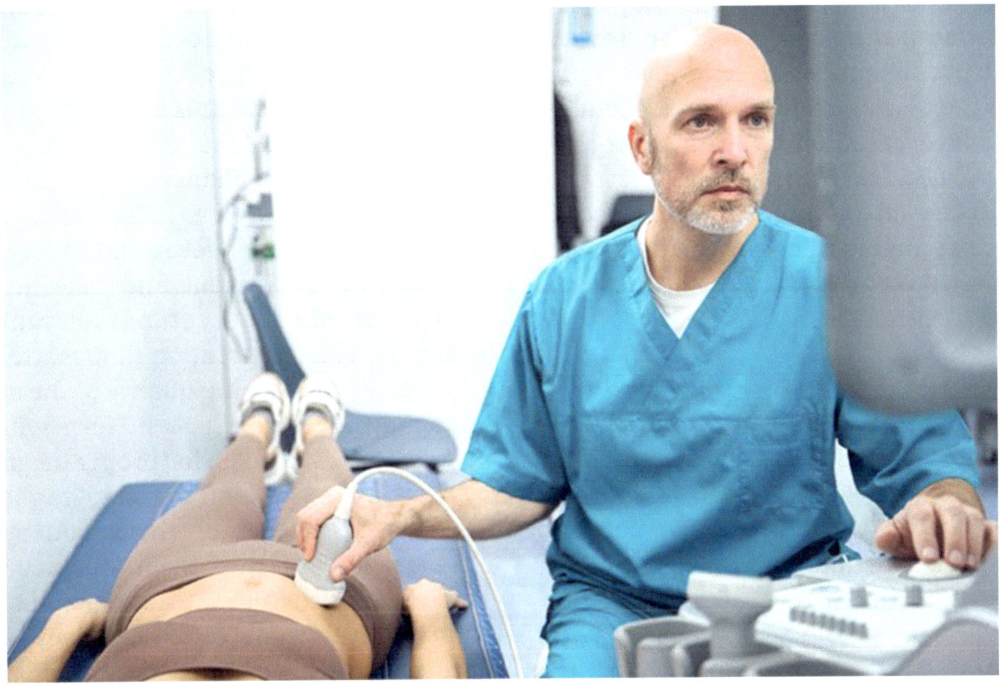

Figure 9.14. Urinary tract ultrasound.

Source: https://external-content.duckduckgo.com/iu/?u=https%3A%2F%2Fwww.ultrasound-scan.co.uk%2Fwp-content%2Fuploads%2F2024%2F02%2Furinary-ultrasound-768x512.jpeg&f=1&nofb=1&ipt=c7c1b98a814ccb5a7e183604396057fe2b3f118c2e652821c3c32028a94dc828.

9.5.1. Preparation for the Ultrasound Examination

Preparation for a kidney and urinary tract ultrasound examination involves careful attention to patient comfort and readiness. Patients should be informed prior to the procedure about the need to either empty or fill their bladder, depending on the type of ultrasound being performed. The bladder should be full to generate more distinct images during the examination, especially when evaluating the kidneys and nearby structures. Therefore, patients are requested to consume a quantity of water prior to the examination and hold off on urination until instructed to do so. Dietary restrictions can also be recommended to reduce gas production in the intestines, further interfering with visual clarity in the ultrasound. More specific instructions on these preparations help enable better imaging outcomes, which are essential in making proper diagnoses and treatment. Besides, patient issues and contraindications must be addressed prior to performing the ultrasound test. Patients must be made aware of any pain that may arise due to the test, alongside the value of ultrasound in assessing renal and urinary pathology. Pre-procedure counseling may further involve disclosing what the procedure will involve, the duration of the test, and what other procedures may be involved based on indications, such as Doppler studies, in case it is required. It is also important to take into account any prior medical conditions that might affect ultrasound results, such as obesity or prior surgery in the renal area.

This kind of thorough preparation not only decreases patient anxiety but also makes workflow easier during the actual examination, thereby maximizing diagnostic effectiveness in total. Finally, effective communication between healthcare providers and patients is important to successful ultrasound preparation. Medical professionals have a responsibility to ensure that the written and oral advice provided is understandable and will foster patient compliance. Additionally, if patients are under medication such as diuretics or herbal supplements, this should be disclosed to them, as this will influence the examining procedure. In other cases, particularly when dealing with conditions such as urolithiasis, information regarding the patients' medical background may guide the need for adjunct treatments, such as medication, which would complement the ultrasound findings in order to make them more useful, as quoted in treatments such as Canephron N in the treatment of urolithiasis (Vitkovskyy, 2018). General preparation, however, is the secret to achieving reproducible and useful ultrasound findings.

9.5.2. Step-by-Step Procedure of Performing the Ultrasound

The initial aspect of conducting a kidney and urinary tract ultrasound is proper positioning and preparation of the patient. The patient will usually be placed in a supine position with the abdomen open to allow maximum access to the renal area. A full medical history should be obtained because this may influence the examination process and reveal relevant factors such as previous surgeries or underlying conditions. Also, the application of a sterile gel on the site enhances transmission of the sound waves, as well as image quality. Clinicians must ensure proper setup and calibration of the ultrasound equipment and take into account frequency and depth settings relevant to kidney imaging. This preparation time matters because it directly impacts the quality of the subsequent imaging process, which in turn will result in quality pictures taken for proper diagnosis. After preparing the patient, the sonographer initiates the actual process of ultrasound by applying the gel and placing the transducer over the particular region of the abdomen. Longitudinal and transverse images of the kidneys are usually acquired, giving critical information about their size, shape, and structure. The sonographer has to systematically move the transducer to capture several planes of imaging to thoroughly evaluate both the kidneys and the nearby tissues. The practitioner needs to be proficient in reading anatomical landmarks in order to successfully recognize and distinguish different structures of the kidney from other intra-abdominal organs. In addition, certain techniques such as breath-holding or changing position can be employed to aid visualization, which would allow for a more detailed scanning of any abnormalities within the renal or urinary tract areas. Finally, the last stages of the ultrasound are taken up reviewing and interpreting the images obtained during the procedure. The sonographer checks the quality of images obtained and ensures that all views necessary for complete evaluation are obtained. Next, an exhaustive report is made, noting observations and identifying any abnormalities such as stones, masses, or cysts with their measurement and location. Such interpretation plays an integral role in determining further diagnostic or therapeutic intervention. Improvements in ultrasound technology and imaging techniques, as cited in recent studies, have also enhanced the safety and accuracy of kidney ultrasounds with minimal complications from more invasive treatments (Lima et al., 2013; Rodrigues, 2017). Therefore, by implementing such a multi-faceted approach, clinicians achieve sufficient proficiency to provide extensive treatment in nephrology and urology (Figure 9.15).

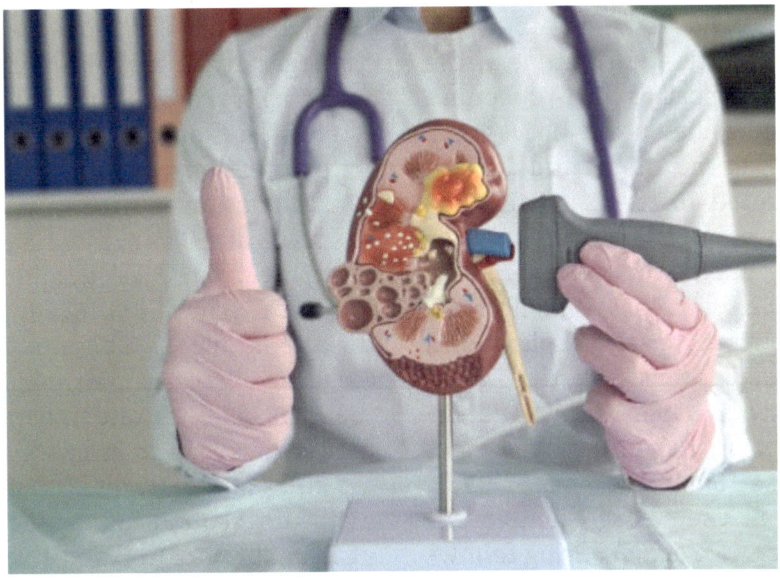

Figure 9.15. The urinary tract process of conducting the ultrasound.

Source: https://media.istockphoto.com/id/1483299804/photo/kidney-ultrasound-doctor-analyzes-the-condition-of-patient-kidneys-with-help-of-kidney.jpg?s=612x612&w=0&k=20&c=Z_TC-JxNJZ4HwlcUzvZBopktca9JzcEVw7fRMJUkVJU=

9.5.3. Post-Procedure Considerations and Follow-Up

Post-procedure care and follow-up are important in handling patients who have had procedures involving the kidneys and urinary tract ultrasound. Following procedures like percutaneous nephrostomy or nephrectomy, close observation is necessary to check for possible complications such as infection and bleeding. For instance, in a patient whose case study consisted of a pyeloduodenal fistula, it was important to monitor post-operative outcomes closely due to her multiple underlying medical conditions, including acute kidney injury and recurrent infection (Salomone et al., 2023). In addition to renal stability, this close follow-up is required to prevent complications associated with prior comorbidities. Furthermore, the patients will need follow-up measures every so often to establish whether the surgical procedure was effective and whether the renal system is healthy. Moreover, another critical aspect of post-procedure care is the need for further imaging and diagnostic studies. Routine follow-up by ultrasound or computed tomography may establish structural changes or complications caused by the surgery, such as hydronephrosis or urinary tract infection. In those with important urinary tract malformations, as shown in a child (Badeński et al., 2020), imaging procedures allowed for the identification of key changes in renal structure. Regular follow-up can include visits every few months following treatment to monitor renal function and detect potential issues early. In addition, these assessments provide very helpful feedback on the effectiveness of intervention and inform any adjustments in treatment modalities that may arise as a direct correlation. Education of the patient is also a key aspect of post-procedure care. Patients who have undergone procedures related to conditions of the kidney and urinary tract are better guided in terms of signs of complications, such as fever, chronic pain, or a change in urinary habits. Providing patients with clear guidance on symptoms to monitor can lead to quicker action if there are complications. The patient in question, for instance, developed ongoing issues after her nephrectomy, and the medical team relied on her ability to detect significant symptoms (Salomone et al., 2023). Involving patients in their care facilitates a team-based approach, not just ensuring follow-up compliance but also empowering patients with the capability to alert concerns instantly. Lastly, a general post-procedure plan involving continuous monitoring, imaging assessment, and patient education is important for effective management and improved outcomes of kidney and urinary tract health.

9.6. Interpretation of Ultrasound Results

Sonographic evaluation, particularly of the kidneys and the urinary tract, is part of urological management and diagnosis of most conditions. Ultrasonography is frequently used since it is non-invasive and no ionizing radiation is involved, making it most appropriate for imaging organs such as the kidneys. Specialized techniques, like Doppler ultrasound, are helpful in evaluating blood flow and can characterize conditions like renal artery stenosis and hydronephrosis. Optimal interpretation depends not only on the imaging technique but also on the clinician's skill to synthesize sonographic information into the clinical context and laboratory results. Besides, although ultrasound is employed as a first-line imaging, its limitations require a comprehensive approach, which may include supportive imaging modalities such as computed tomography or magnetic resonance imaging in challenging cases, thereby enhancing diagnostic yield. One of the areas where ultrasound interpretation becomes particularly critical is the evaluation of urinary tract infections (UTIs) in children. Given the risk of renal scarring from recurrent UTIs, identification of anatomical defects is crucial to prevent permanent damage to the kidneys. Despite this, the evidence suggests that routine imaging on established UTIs in children under five years of age does not always lead to improved patient outcomes. As an example, studies have demonstrated that while ultrasound can diagnose hydronephrosis, it is unable to always predict renal scarring or need for future intervention and therefore raises concern for a balance of benefits and harms of preventable imaging. Literature demonstrates that clinicians need to exercise caution while making ultrasound report interpretations among this population because imaging alone might not be sufficient in informing useful treatment plans; therefore, the necessity of a particular approach based on clinical context (Biggi et al., 2005). The limitations of access to ultrasound in some cases have prompted exploration of adjunct imaging modalities such as fetal MRI for complex conditions. MRI provides a more profound understanding of suspicious or indeterminate findings by ultrasound, particularly in fetal development assessment. The addition of this modality to the evaluation permits clinicians to gain a better appreciation of renal and urinary tract abnormalities, ultimately resulting in more appropriate management. The data imply that MRI provides a better explanation of diagnosis and prognosis for certain malformations on ultrasound. Not only does this integration add more power to diagnosis, but it also makes more effective parental counseling regarding potential outcomes and management options. As ultrasound remains a pillar of urological assessment, continued innovation of the options for proper interpretation will enhance patient outcomes and long-term results (Baldacchino et al., 2016) (Figure 9.16).

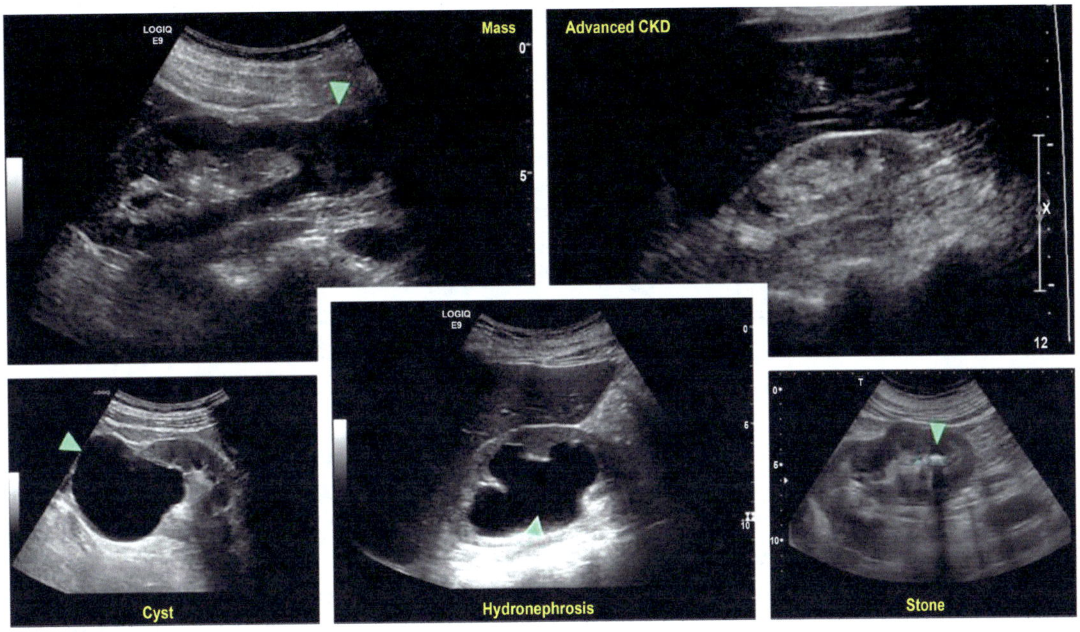

Figure 9.16. Checklist for interpreting a kidney ultrasound.

Source: nephropocus.com. https://nephropocus.com/2022/02/26/checklist-for-interpreting-kidney-ultrasound/#jp-carousel-51757.

9.6.1. Key Findings in Normal Kidney and Urinary Tract Ultrasounds

The ultrasonographic examination of the kidneys and urinary tract is a necessary non-invasive imaging modality, which provides detailed information on structural abnormalities. Important findings in normal ultrasounds include the size, shape, and echogenicity of both kidneys, which, normally, depict a smooth outline and homogenous parenchyma. Normal kidney size is an important parameter for evaluating renal size, as variations can indicate underlying pathology. For instance, multicystic dysplastic kidney (MCDK) presents as an antenatally existing developmental anomaly, characterized by the presence of multiple cysts and potential contralateral renal dysfunction, and thus highlights the importance of thorough ultrasound evaluation in detecting such defects in early stages (Lala, 2017). Moreover, the kidneys should present a clear distinction between cortex and medulla, necessary for pathologies diagnosis, enhancing the clinical perception of any potential anomaly of the urinary system. Besides structural analysis, urinary tract examination is also significant for the identification of anatomical variations or obstruction. The patency of the ureters must be demonstrated by normal ultrasound findings, with neither hydronephrosis nor urinary stasis. The bladder must also exhibit normal capacity and wall thickness, both of which can be quantified on ultrasound. Others, such as ectopic ureters, may also need further evaluation since their diagnosis can directly impact patient management. Isolated BSEUs are particularly challenging for clinicians to manage, with preoperative bladder capacity and other results needing to be precisely established as the foundation for postoperative continence (Charlesworth et al., 2017). Hence, proper assessment of urinary structures by ultrasound not only aids in reaching a diagnosis of intrinsic abnormalities but is also an essential contribution to the planning of clinical intervention. Overall, the most important outcomes of kidney and urinary tract ultrasounds provide valuable information about renal function, making the use of ultrasound a valuable first diagnostic tool. These tests are also supplemented by the ability to detect concomitant anomalies, which significantly influence patient outcomes. Significant parameters such as renal echogenicity, size, and shape are referential markers for the interpretation of renal health, allowing for timely intervention. Both MCDK and ectatic ureters illustrate the way in which abnormal morphology of these structures could lead to severe clinical consequences, further emphasizing the necessity of routine ultrasounds for pediatric and other groups (Lala, 2017; Charlesworth et al., 2017). Last but not least, the combination of structural assessment and functional evaluation highlights the importance of ultrasound in preclinical diagnosis and treatment of renal and urinary tract diseases to determine adequate care and therapeutic management for compromised patients.

9.6.2. Common Abnormalities Detected Through Ultrasound

Ultrasound scanning is not only crucial in the early diagnosis of common kidney and urinary tract abnormalities but also has a profound influence on outcome. The nature of detected abnormalities varies from those occurring at birth, including obstructive uropathy and renal agenesis, to being grouped under the more general term Congenital Anomalies of the Kidney and Urinary Tract (CAKUT). The approximate incidence of CAKUT is to involve 1 to 4 per 1000 pregnancies and accounts for 15 to 20% of all birth defects. Early detection on ultrasound is worth its weight in gold since it allows for the initiation of timely medical or surgical treatment, preventing such complications as severe renal damage and the onset of end-stage renal failure in involved patients. The scenario in this case emphasizes the necessity of employing ultrasound technology to identify irregularities at a stage where proactive treatment can be implemented to avoid devastating long-term consequences (Chaara et al., 2021). Functional defects such as hydronephrosis, along with congenital malformations, are yet another top problem during prenatal ultrasound scanning. Hydronephrosis, as characterized by renal pelvis dilatation due to urine retention, can be caused by a variety of etiologies, including ureteropelvic junction obstruction and vesicoureteral reflux. Diligent evaluation of hydronephrosis by ultrasound is crucial since it can influence decision-making regarding postnatal management strategy. For instance, precise grading of the severity and magnitude of renal dilation informs clinicians about the possibility of renal dysfunction or infection risk after birth. Failing to detect such anomalies has grave implications, including fetal pulmonary hypoplasia and compromised overall fetal development due to abnormally impaired amniotic fluid dynamics (Mileto et al., 2018). Therefore, an awareness of the potential implications of such ultrasound findings is important in optimizing patient care during perinatal life. In general, ultrasound serves not only as a diagnostic imaging modality, but also as an aid to clinical prognostic assessment in cases of renal and urinary tract abnormalities. Sonographic morphology on prenatal scans helps clinicians categorize various anomalies, thereby serving as a guide for the necessity of adequate intervention protocols. The majority of congenital urinary tract anomalies will have an effect on the amount of normal amniotic fluid, and thus an effect on fetal growth and health. By using a multidimensional approach to interpreting the sonographic defects, it is possible for the medical provider to gain a better insight into the pathology involved. A new system—such as the system provided by the Linthicum multidisciplinary consensus panel—effectively categorizes urinary tract dilation based upon associated anomalies. This cautious stratification reflects the importance of prenatal preventive and management strategies in reducing the long-term consequences of such abnormalities on kidney function and overall development (Chaara et al., 2021; Mileto et al., 2018).

9.6.3. Importance of Correlating Ultrasound Findings with Clinical Symptoms

In urinary tract and renal examinations, correlating ultrasound findings with clinical presentation is important for proper diagnosis and best management. Ultrasound is an important imaging modality that provides real-time information regarding the anatomical as well as pathological status of the kidneys and associated structures. If clinical symptoms such as hematuria, flank pain, or abnormalities in urine are correlated meticulously with ultrasound findings, the radiologists can significantly enhance diagnostic accuracy. This concordance becomes highly relevant in distinguishing between benign diseases and more severe pathologies, such as urogenital tuberculosis (UGTB), which can be presented similarly to other lethal diseases, such as malignancy. Thus, a multimodal strategy that blends clinical presentation with imaging is central to facilitate timely treatment and improve patient outcomes, circumventing complications arising from misdiagnosis or delayed treatment (Kearns et al., 2022). Furthermore, knowledge of the clinical context provides insight into interpreting ultrasound results, especially when unusual presentations are encountered. For instance, UGTB, despite its infrequent occurrence in developed countries, may have slippery manifestations that resist initial diagnostic efforts. Radiologists who have a patient's clinical history and associated risk factors at their disposal are better placed to consider differential diagnoses at an early point in the evaluation process. The interfusion of clinical data can highlight possible correlations in ultrasound imaging to facilitate the recognition of individualistic features of infection, structural faults, or malignancy. This synergy of clinical presentation and sonographic findings hence demonstrates the efficacy of diagnostic imaging to allow medical professionals to establish well-informed intervention plans that treat the root cause of the patient's symptom (Lei et al., 2023). Finally, the emphasis on "matching" ultrasound findings with clinical presentations elevates the standards of care in managing urinary tract illness. The practice not only enhances diagnostic precision but also facilitates integrated communication among multi-specialty healthcare teams. By creating a system in which radiologists, urologists, and primary care physicians collaborate, patient assessments become more holistic and complete. The integration of imaging results with clinical presentation allows detection of significant comorbidities and optimization of treatment protocols according to patient-specific needs. This integrated approach emphasizes the growing significance of correlating imaging findings with clinical observations that further guide clinicians towards better care pathways and improve overall prognoses in patients (Kearns et al., 2022).

SUMMARY

In renal health, the role of ultrasound of the kidneys and urinary tract cannot be overstated. The fact that ultrasound can provide real-time non-invasive images establishes it as an invaluable tool in renal evaluation. It makes it possible to identify early on abnormalities such as congenital defects, infection, and other pathological changes without any further invasive procedure. The ramifications of such an early diagnosis are significant, as they allow for timely treatment and control, possibly reversing the course of the disease and enhancing patient outcomes. In particular, in children, ultrasound is not just an imaging tool but also an essential approach in the direction of treatment and future follow-up assessments. Therefore, the position of the kidneys and urinary tract ultrasound becomes central to improving the quality of care and to providing patients with proper and effective interventions. The research demonstrating the prevalence of recurrent UTIs and renal scarring highlights the role of ultrasound in the identification of underlying anatomical abnormalities. For instance, in a specific study, renal scarring was found to develop in patients, although patients were usually normal at the beginning of imaging, highlighting the importance of ongoing monitoring of risk individuals (Naseri et al., 2025). Prophylactic use of ultrasound screening frequently results in the detection of a condition such as vesicoureteral reflux, a common cause of recurrent UTI and resultant renal injury. In addition, it aids in distinguishing between the varied urinary tract abnormalities, which are crucial in compiling a proper management plan. It makes a more accurate correlation between pathology and the appearance on images of ultrasound, thus optimizing the potential benefit of preventive intervention and long-term renal function conservation in susceptible patients. Above all, the application of ultrasound varies from routine screening to investigation of advanced renal anatomical abnormalities, such as renal ectopia. Like in the case of crossed renal ectopia, ultrasound has proven useful in not just describing the occurrence of the condition but also its functional status and associated complications (Al-Mosawi, 2024). This points to the merit in utilizing ultrasound as a first-line investigation that can provide crucial information to guide the following diagnostic and therapeutic interventions. The culmination of the results confirms early and routine ultrasound examination as an integral part of holistic renal health care. Lastly, the integration of ultrasound findings into practice ensures improved care pathways with preservation of renal well-being in all age groups.

Ultrasound technology has proved to be a valuable resource in the assessment of renal health, primarily due to its non-invasive character and ability to provide real-time images of kidney structure and function. The imaging method is optimally useful for the detection of various kidney pathologies, such as hydronephrosis, kidney stones, and tumors. With Doppler ultrasound, clinicians can measure blood flow via the renal arteries and thereby offer measurement of vascular health as well as detection of abnormalities associated with conditions like systemic sclerosis (SSc). Research has shown that Blood uric acid levels are positively correlated with intrarenal arterial stiffness in patients with SSc. This highlights the ability of ultrasound to track renal microvascular injury and to improve the diagnostic accuracy of examinations of clinical practice (Amoroso et al., 2016). Furthermore, Blood uric acid levels have revolutionized the imaging of the kidney since it revealed perfusion of the kidneys, particularly in cases with CKD. This technique can differentiate between the renal cortex and medulla changes in perfusion, which is significant knowledge in understanding the patterns of blood circulation within the kidneys. Research indicates that in CKD cats, the time to peak is increased, and the mean transit time is decreased in the renal cortex compared to normal animals (Daminet et al., 2017). These findings not only highlight the potential utility of CEUS in detecting early CKD but also highlight its revolutionary ability to individualize management in engaged patients. In addition to its diagnostic utility, ultrasound has special relevance to renal health because it acts as a catalyst for therapeutic intervention and disease monitoring. As technology for ultrasound imaging advances, clinicians are able to conduct guided interventions like renal drainages and biopsies, improving patient outcomes through precisely directed treatments. Also, routine ultrasound scans allow continued monitoring of renal function, making it possible to make adjustments to the treatment regimen on time due to changes in kidney function. With the ongoing development of our understanding of renal pathophysiology, the use of ultrasound will inevitably be central to the multidisciplinary strategy for protecting renal function and enhancing patient outcomes.

CLOSER LOOK

CONTRAST-ENHANCED ULTRASOUND (CEUS)

Contrast-enhanced ultrasound (CEUS) is an advanced imaging diagnostic technique that supplements the role of conventional ultrasound with the use of microbubble contrast agents to provide improved visualization of blood flow, tissue vascularity, and lesion characterization in real time. In contrast to conventional contrast media for CT or MRI, CEUS contrast agents are gas-filled microbubbles (usually sulfur hexafluoride or perfluorocarbon gases) coated with a phospholipid or protein layer. These microbubbles are absolutely intravascular and will not diffuse interstitially, thus it is possible to assess the vascular structures and perfusion dynamics accurately. When microbubbles are injected intravenously, they resonate with ultrasound waves and send back the sound energy to the transducer at much higher intensity than normal tissues, providing enhanced images of blood vessels and vascularized tissue. CEUS is increasingly utilized in the characterization of liver lesions, used to discriminate between benign and malignant tumors based on specific enhancement patterns in the different vascular phases—arterial, portal venous, and late. For example, hemangiomas are classically characterized by peripheral nodular enhancement with centripetal fill-in, while hepatocellular carcinoma (HCC) may show early arterial enhancement with washout during the late phase. CEUS is also excellent for the detection and characterization of kidney lesions, evaluation of testicular torsion, bowel perfusion in ischemia, and vascular organ transplantation complications. CEUS may diagnose solid organ injury and intra-abdominal bleeding in the context of trauma without exposing patients to ionizing radiation and is therefore particularly useful in pregnant patients and children.

One of the best things about CEUS is its excellent safety profile. The contrast agents for microbubbles are well tolerated, have minimal possibility of causing allergic reaction, and are non-nephrotoxic, so CEUS is safer for patients with renal impairment or iodine contrast medium allergy. Compared to CT or MRI, CEUS is performed with no radiation exposure and can be repeatedly applied with high frequency for follow-up and monitoring. Additionally, it provides real-time imaging, which is especially useful in the guidance of interventional procedures like biopsies, ablations, and drainages. CEUS is also portable and cost-effective with the added benefit of being ideally suited for bedside use in intensive care, emergency departments, and low-resource settings. While these are benefits, CEUS has limitations. It is dependent on the operator, has a limited field of view, and will not penetrate very deeply within the body in the event of obesity. Further, bowel gas and bone may prevent ultrasound waves from traveling to image some regions. But ongoing technological advancements, such as harmonic imaging and improved transducer sensitivity, are continuing to expand the range and dependability of CEUS. With acquired clinical experience and accumulating evidence, CEUS is being adopted into clinical guidelines and protocols for hepatic, renal, and vascular imaging. As additional studies are performed, new indications are being established, including tumor response to therapy, inflammatory bowel disease assessment, and cardiac perfusion imaging. Overall, CEUS is a safe, broadly applicable, and highly informative modality that significantly contributes to the diagnostic power of conventional ultrasound, providing clinicians with an unparalleled patient-centered imaging tool in real-time.

References

1. Abbas, M., Lee, S. K., Mwipatayi, B. P., Narayan, A., et al. (2007). *Transplantation of Crossed Fused Renal Ectopia*. https://core.ac.uk/download/pdf/82287277.pdf (accessed on 12th July 2025).
2. Abdoulaye, N., Allah-Syengar, A., Ndormadjita, A., Assane, B., Ndiaye, B., et al. (2022). Horseshoe kidney: A case report and review of literature. https://core.ac.uk/download/551548829.pdf (accessed on 12th July 2025).
3. Aboagye, E., Frimpong, A. A., & Frimpong, G. A. (2019). Diagnostic potential of imaging modalities in the assessment of lower urinary tract dysfunctions. https://core.ac.uk/download/322444066.pdf (accessed on 12th July 2025).
4. Adams, L. G., Bartges, J. W., Berent, A. C., Lulich, J. P., et al. (2016). ACVIM small animal consensus recommendations on the treatment and prevention of uroliths in dogs and cats. https://core.ac.uk/download/323070830.pdf (accessed on 12th July 2025).
5. Afeltra, A. M. V., Amoroso, A., Barbano, B., Cianci, R., et al. (2017). Angiogenic and angiostatic factors in renal scleroderma-associated vasculopathy. https://core.ac.uk/download/98348297.pdf (accessed on 12th July 2025).
6. Aldughiem, A. (2025). Imaging diagnosis of major kidney and urinary tract disorders in children. *Medicina, 61*. https://www.semanticscholar.org/paper/a2e4dcaf67d3395e0c4ff5d818255deef72e661d (accessed on 12th July 2025).
7. Al-Mosawi, A. J. (2024). The case forty-one of crossed unfused renal ectopia. *International Journal of Recent Innovations in Medicine and Clinical Research*. https://www.semanticscholar.org/paper/d335783ef79d2b5ddc815053e49e30c325813933 (accessed on 12th July 2025).
8. Amoroso, A., Barbano, B., Barilaro, G., Cianci, R., et al. (2016). Serum uric acid as a marker of microvascular damage in systemic sclerosis patients. https://core.ac.uk/download/74319192.pdf (accessed on 12th July 2025).
9. Badeński, A., Bjanid, O., Badeńska, M., Chmiela, B., Adamczyk, P., Kudela, G., Moskal, G., et al. (2020). A "mysterious ghost kidney stone" in an 8-year-old boy with a solitary right kidney, obstructive megaureter, and ureterostomy: Questions. *Pediatric Nephrology (Berlin, Germany), 36*, 863–864. https://www.semanticscholar.org/paper/aaa57df7d8f500fc09c90a3f2094434b812a1cc4 (accessed on 12th July 2025).
10. Baldacchino, I., Gatt, A. S., & Saliba, I. (2016). *Fetal MRI: An Essential Step in Interpreting Complex Ultrasound Findings*. https://core.ac.uk/download/46604247.pdf (accessed on 12th July 2025).
11. Biggi, A., Fretzayas, A., Gervaix, A., Haberlik, A., Hitzel, A., Hitzel, A., Piepsz, A., et al. (2005). Further investigation of confirmed urinary tract infection (UTI) in children under five years: A systematic review. https://core.ac.uk/download/57941.pdf (accessed on 12th July 2025).
12. Bigosiński, K., Dembowska, A., & Dubaj, M. (2022). *Medullary Sponge Kidney–The Mysterious Name of a Simple Disease*. https://core.ac.uk/download/587245783.pdf (accessed on 12th July 2025).

13. Bove, P., Finazzi Agrò, E., Kim, F. J., Miano, R., Micali, S., Rosa, M., & Usai, P. (2013). Recent findings and new technologies in nephrolithiasis: A review of the recent literature. https://core.ac.uk/download/pdf/54580708.pdf (accessed on 12th July 2025).

14. Calabrese, E., Dietrich, C. F., Dirks, K., Gilja, T., et al. (2016). EFSUMB recommendations and guidelines for gastrointestinal ultrasound–Part 1: Examination techniques and normal findings (Long version). https://core.ac.uk/download/74321241.pdf (accessed on 12th July 2025).

15. Cantisani, V., Deganello, A., Dietrich, C. F., Duran, C., et al. (2016). *Role of Contrast-Enhanced Ultrasound (Ceus) In Pediatric Practice: An Efsumb Position Statement.* https://core.ac.uk/download/74320188.pdf (accessed on 12th July 2025).

16. Chaara, H., Attar, I., Jayi, S., Fdili Alaoui, F. Z., & Melhouf, M. A. (2021). Antenatal diagnosis of renal and excretory tract abnormalities: A report of 36 cases and review of the literature. *Scholars International Journal of Obstetrics and Gynecology*. https://www.semanticscholar.org/paper/cc90ec91fd38615faaa784b7364629534e5dbd15 (accessed on 12th July 2025).

17. Charlesworth, P., Cherian, A., Cuckow, P., Desai, D., et al. (2017). Isolated bilateral simplex ureteric ectopia: Bladder capacity as an indicator of continence outcome. https://core.ac.uk/download/158171009.pdf (accessed on 12th July 2025).

18. Ciciu, E., Pașatu-Cornea, A. M., Petcu, L., & Tuta, L. (2021). Early diagnosis and management of maternal ureter hydronephrosis during pregnancy. *Experimental and Therapeutic Medicine, 23*(1), 27. https://www.semanticscholar.org/paper/4c0dd9d9d53bd1bcaaff8dd12d86007eb662278e (accessed on 12th July 2025).

19. Daminet, S., Duchateau, L., Paepe, D., Saunders, J., et al. (2017). Contrast-enhanced ultrasound examination for the assessment of renal perfusion in cats with chronic kidney disease. https://core.ac.uk/download/158348152.pdf (accessed on 12th July 2025).

20. De Sadeleer, C., Dobbeleir, A., Ham, H., Peremans, K., et al. (2011). Nuclear medicine: Investigation of renal function in small animal medicine. https://core.ac.uk/download/55842771.pdf (accessed on 12th July 2025).

21. Głowacka, M., Błaszczykowski, M., Gauda, K., & Bartnik, G. (2024). Advancing medical diagnostics: A portable ultrasonic-impedance tomograph for non-invasive lower urinary tract monitoring. *Journal of Modern Science*. https://www.semanticscholar.org/paper/dab4d58990f3cf2866a728c867f8c1c7f09edaea (accessed on 12th July 2025).

22. Govindarajan, K. K. (2020). Antenatally diagnosed hydronephrosis and pelvi ureteric junction obstruction from a surgical viewpoint. https://core.ac.uk/download/483636843.pdf (accessed on 12th July 2025).

23. Grech, V. E., Conti, V. S., Torpiano, J. G., Vella, C., et al. (2008). The relationship between infecting organisms and underlying structural anomalies in children with urinary tract infections. https://core.ac.uk/download/46602183.pdf (accessed on 12th July 2025).

24. Hall, J., Hardiman, K. M., Lee, S. H., Lightner, A. L., Stocchi, L., Paquette, I. M., Steele, S. R., et al. (2020). The American Society of Colon and Rectal Surgeons clinical practice guidelines for the treatment of left-sided colonic diverticulitis. *Diseases of the Colon & Rectum, 63*, 728–747. https://doi.org/10.1097/dcr.0000000000001679 (accessed on 12th July 2025).

25. Han Byeol Lee, Seunghyun Lee, Young Hun Choi, Cheon, J., Lee, S., Yeon Jin Cho, Ahn, Y., et al. (2023). Contrast-enhanced ultrasound for the diagnosis of acute pyelonephritis in pediatric patients with urinary tract infection: A feasibility study. *PLOS ONE, 18*. https://

www.semanticscholar.org/paper/dde0569536d3dd95fcc9a29df6aaeb1a370a597d (accessed on 12th July 2025).

26. Higuchi, T., Jain, S. K., Lapa, C., Ordonez, A., et al. (2021). Current and future perspectives on functional molecular imaging in nephron-urology: Theragnostic on the horizon. https://core.ac.uk/download/429115887.pdf (accessed on 12th July 2025).

27. Horváth, O., Szabó, A. J., & Reusz, G. (2022). How to define and assess the clinically significant causes of hematuria in childhood. *Pediatric Nephrology, 38*, 2549–2562. https://doi.org/10.1007/s00467-022-05746-4 (accessed on 12th July 2025).

28. Isık, B., Sarcan, E., Kazcı, O., & Muratoglu, M. (2023). Relationship between retroaortic left renal vein and patients presenting to the emergency department with microhematuria. *Science and Health*. https://www.semanticscholar.org/paper/0b29e4a326d538001dfade5f4625d74dbf50c121 (accessed on 12th July 2025).

29. Ismail, H. S. (2001). Comparative study between ultrasound and KUB and IVU in renal colic patients in Kelantan. https://core.ac.uk/download/132566828.pdf (accessed on 12th July 2025).

30. Jüngst, D., Karl, H. J., Siess, E., Weiser, H., et al. (1984). Urinary cholesterol: Its association with a macromolecular protein-lipid complex. https://core.ac.uk/download/12167328.pdf (accessed on 12th July 2025).

31. Kearns, D., Kemp, B., Kundasamy, P., Lyon, T., et al. (2022). A rare case of disseminated genitourinary tract tuberculosis complicated by emphysematous prostatitis and seminal vesicle abscess. https://core.ac.uk/download/616662409.pdf (accessed on 12th July 2025).

32. Kelam, J., Kelam, N., Filipović, N., Komić, L., Racetin, A., Komić, D., Kostić, S., et al. (2024). Expression of congenital anomalies of the kidney and urinary tract (CAKUT) candidate genes EDA2R, PCDH9, and TRAF7 in normal human kidney development and CAKUT. *Genes, 15*. https://www.semanticscholar.org/paper/22eb46d66fb23c4fbbc8e8ccd3e232b2d95c469a (accessed on 12th July 2025).

33. Lala, N. (2017). Multicystic dysplastic kidney disease at Chris Hani Baragwanath Academic Hospital over a thirty-year period. https://core.ac.uk/download/188774818.pdf (accessed on 12th July 2025).

34. Lee, M. S., Sledge, T. R., Seyer, A. K., Qi, R., & Koo, K. (2025). How I do it: Percutaneous cystolitholapaxy for bladder stones with complex lower urinary tract anatomy. *Canadian Journal of Urology*. https://www.semanticscholar.org/paper/13552a828628c570afb67aded913be6d142f5744 (accessed on 12th July 2025).

35. Lei, J., Lin, W., Wang, Y., Wu, Y., et al. (2023). Can GPT-4V (ision) serve medical applications? Case studies on GPT-4V for multimodal medical diagnosis. http://arxiv.org/abs/2310.09909 (accessed on 12th July 2025).

36. Levi D'Ancona, C. A., Haylen, B. T., Oelke, M., Monteiro, L. A., Arnold, E. P., Goldman, H. B., Hamid, R., et al. (2019). The International Continence Society (ICS) report on the terminology for adult male lower urinary tract and pelvic floor symptoms and dysfunction. *Neurourology and Urodynamics, 38*, 433–477. https://doi.org/10.1002/nau.23897 (accessed on 12th July 2025).

37. Lima, E., Fonseca, J., Vilaça, J. L., Karami, H., Leroy, A., Rodrigues, N. F., Rodrigues, P. L., et al. (2013). Kidney targeting and puncturing during percutaneous nephrolithotomy: Recent advances and future perspectives. https://core.ac.uk/download/55633714.pdf (accessed on 12th July 2025).

38. Linden, M. A., Rosenblad, T., Rosenborg, K., Hansson, S., & Brandström, P. (2024). Infant urinary tract infection in Sweden–A national study of current diagnostic procedures, imaging and treatment. *Pediatric Nephrology (Berlin, Germany), 39*, 3251–3262. https://www.semanticscholar.org/paper/9744f7114f0e8d0ea253b748a023037c6a18f655 (accessed on 12th July 2025).

39. Mahfoozi, B., & Moslemi, M. K. (2011). Urologist-operated ultrasound and its use in urological outpatient clinics. https://core.ac.uk/download/pdf/8541263.pdf (accessed on 12th July 2025).

40. Mileto, A., Itani, M., Katz, D., Siebert, J., Dighe, M., Dubinsky, T., & Moshiri, M. (2018). Fetal urinary tract anomalies: Review of pathophysiology, imaging, and management. *AJR. American Journal of Roentgenology, 210*(5), 1010–1021. https://www.semanticscholar.org/paper/74c2ae935dd7dc417a5a89fe11b459780686ee32 (accessed on 12th July 2025).

41. Mohajerzadeh, L., Jahangiri, F., Salek, M., & Nickavar, A. (2024). Value of urine neutrophil gelatinase-associated lipocalin for prediction of ureteropelvic junction obstruction in children. *Nephro-Urology Monthly*. https://www.semanticscholar.org/paper/03939607e9fc0a56147440197ac9801884f53718 (accessed on 12th July 2025).

42. Naseri, M., Tafazoli, N., Nikrou, A., & Tafazoli, N. (2025). Examining the recurrence of urinary tract infections in children with a history of acute pyelonephritis. *Journal of Pediatrics Review*. https://www.semanticscholar.org/paper/70dcf58152eec1363c63b07368616ddc520184de (accessed on 12th July 2025).

43. Öborn, H. (2014). Lower urinary tract dysfunction in children with chronic kidney disease: Before and after renal transplantation. https://core.ac.uk/download/70341161.pdf (accessed on 12th July 2025).

44. Rodrigues, P. M. L. (2017). Navigation system based in motion tracking sensor for percutaneous renal access. https://core.ac.uk/download/84049522.pdf (accessed on 12th July 2025).

45. Salomone, L., Tinti, F., Lai, S., Pedata, L., Rotondi, S., Tartaglione, L., Luka, K., et al. (2023). #6056 Nephrologic involvement in a surgical complication: When to suspect a pyelo-duodenal fistula. *Nephrology Dialysis Transplantation*. https://www.semanticscholar.org/paper/ad469d5f24734e0680fdb8de0bd42a2b22d94359 (accessed on 12th July 2025).

46. Sidhu, P. S., Cantisani, V., Dietrich, C. F., Gilja, O. H., Săftoiu, A., Bartels, E., Bertolotto, M., et al. (2018). The EFSUMB guidelines and recommendations for the clinical practice of contrast-enhanced ultrasound (CEUS) in non-hepatic applications: Update 2017 (Long version). *Ultraschall in der Medizin–European Journal of Ultrasound, 39*, e2–e44. https://doi.org/10.1055/a-0586-1107 (accessed on 12th July 2025).

47. Steflea, R., Stroescu, R., Gafencu, M., Stoicescu, E., Isac, R., Olariu, I., Micsescu-Olah, A. M., et al. (2024). A pilot comparative study between creatinine- and cystatin-C-based equations to estimate GFR and kidney ultrasound percentiles in children with congenital anomalies of the kidney and urinary tract. *Diagnostics, 14*. https://www.semanticscholar.org/paper/e94ad4684f66e0ed0cd4cfb32e84118c92bea1f5 (accessed on 12th July 2025).

48. Vitkovskyy, V. (2018). Efficacy evaluation of the phototherapeutic drug Canephron N in the complex treatment of patients with urolithiasis using extracorporeal shock wave lithotripsy. https://core.ac.uk/download/301580784.pdf (accessed on 12th July 2025).

49. Zakharova, I. N., Osmanov, I. M., Goryainova, A. N., Tambieva, E., & Shesterikov, N. V. (2025). Urinary tract infection in children. The role of primary health care in the diagnosis and management of urinary tract infection in children: A review. *Pediatrics. Consilium Medicum.* https://www.semanticscholar.org/paper/cf106a25a120cfc1d36dc689774c0463dba63a06 (accessed on 12th July 2025).

50. Zhou, W., Du, Q., Liu, Q., Liu, X., Li, L., & Zhang, H. (2024). A case report of autosomal recessive polycystic kidney disease with noncompaction of ventricular myocardium: Coincidence or different manifestations of ciliopathy? *BMC Nephrology, 25.* https://www.semanticscholar.org/paper/f4c4bb74fe1186a45febb28f5157967dd14e3ae4 (accessed on 12th July 2025).

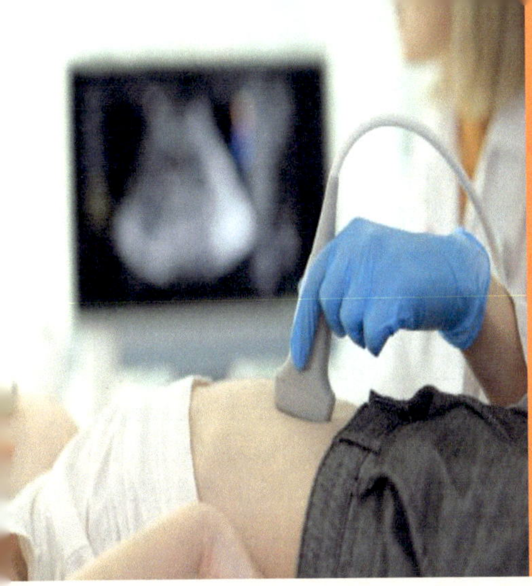

Chapter 10

SPLEEN AND PANCREAS ULTRASOUND

Contents

Introduction

The role of ultrasound imaging in spleen and pancreatic diagnosis becomes increasingly important in contemporary medical diagnostics. As a non-invasive form of imaging, ultrasound has a number of advantages linked to it, including no ionizing radiation, which is particularly important in vulnerable populations such as children. The spleen and pancreas are important organs, the latter playing a key role in immunity as well as blood filtration, and the former being tasked with digestive enzyme secretion and glucose metabolism. Because of the intricate nature of organ sickness, the addition of improved ultrasound imaging, such as contrast-enhanced ultrasound (CEUS), has been able to dramatically enhance diagnostic accuracy and patient safety. This improvement is underscored by mounting amounts of evidence supporting the use of CEUS in children, where radiation exposure concerns remain a concern (Cantisani et al., 2016).

Another driver of improved ultrasound techniques is the development of specifically designed imaging analysis environments intended to streamline and enhance diagnostic processes. The emergence of deep learning technologies has taken medical image analysis to new and improved levels, with more precise and faster interpretation of ultrasound images. The NiftyNet platform, for instance, is a modular deep-learning system specifically targeting the nuances of medical imaging, like segmentation and regression tasks that are critical in organ assessment (Barratt et al., 2017). By exploiting these advanced technologies, clinicians can not just conduct more accurate scans of the spleen and pancreas but also render better visual results for more informed clinical decision-making. This trend towards new imaging technologies is a part of an even broader trend in radiology that aims both for efficiency and accuracy in diagnosis. Furthermore, the advantages of improved ultrasound imaging extend beyond diagnostics; they extend to the field of personalized medicine. In the evolution of healthcare to individualized therapeutic practices, the correct visualization of the pancreas and spleen becomes of paramount importance in tailoring therapeutic interventions to patient-specific disease. Enhanced ultrasound techniques allow for earlier and more accurate identification of anomalies, thus making it possible to perform early and targeted therapeutic interventions, which can significantly improve the prognosis of the patient. The existing research in this domain identifies the need to integrate new imaging modalities and make them accessible and usable for clinical use on a daily basis. Through the development of a general understanding of spleen and pancreas diseases through improved ultrasound imaging techniques, the medical community is capable of delivering improved patient needs and expectations and, ultimately, gastroenterological well-being (Figure 10.1).

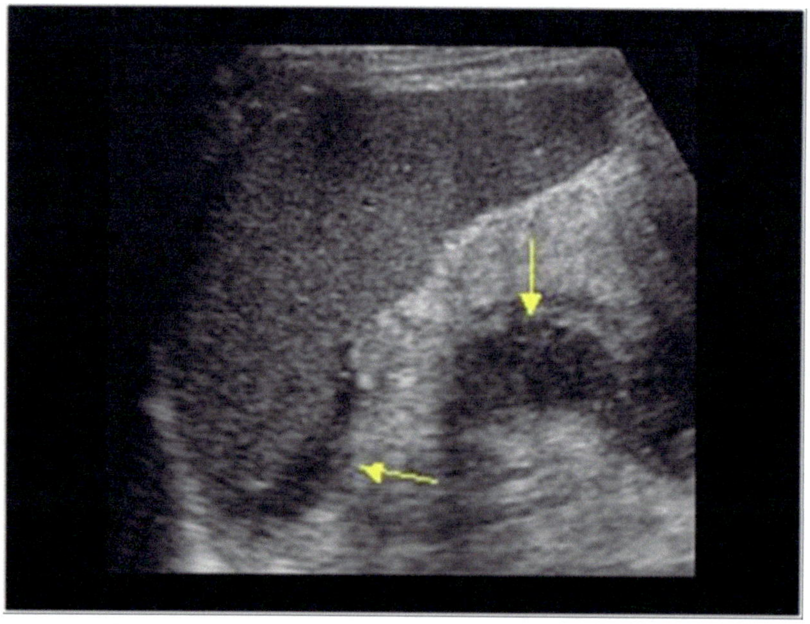

Figure 10.1. Spleen and pancreas ultrasound.

Source: https://external-content.duckduckgo.com/iu/?u=https%3A%2F%2Fwww.ultrasoundcases.info%2Fclients%2Fultrasoundcases%2Fuploads%2Flbox_16694.jpg&f=1&nofb=1&ipt=5090ea18678e8945d74705245620860e82673188a9834286f52bd1cd5cacb5b9.

Definition of Ultrasound Imaging

Ultrasound imaging, a prime diagnostic tool in today's medicine, employs high-frequency sound waves to picture internal organs and structures. This procedure is non-surgical and relies on the echolocation principle, employing the sound waves emitted by a transducer that travel through the body, reflecting off tissues to create real-time images. Ultrasound use is particularly relevant in scanning soft tissues and organs, rendering it ideal for spleen and pancreas evaluation. Unlike other imaging modalities, ultrasound does not employ ionizing radiation, which further underscores the safety profile of ultrasound, particularly in vulnerable patient groups such as pregnant patients and pediatric patients. Additionally, with newer developments in ultrasound technology, for example, Doppler imaging, diagnostic capabilities have improved, enabling clinicians to measure the blood flow in addition to structural defects. In reality, ultrasound imaging is not simply visualization; it helps in the differential diagnostic process. In the assessment of pancreatic and splenic conditions, ultrasound is employed as a first-line modality due to its availability and lower cost. For instance, in pancreatic neoplasms assessment, ultrasound is able to identify cystic lesions and other abnormalities. While ultrasound may satisfactorily provide initial impressions, it typically augments other modalities such as computed tomography (CT) and magnetic resonance imaging (MRI), particularly where definitive diagnoses are required. Research has shown that certain pancreatic lesions, for example, solid-pseudopapillary tumors, occasionally may initially be detected using ultrasound, and subsequent imaging may characterize their nature and subsequent management strategies (Fantin et al., 2016). In addition, the inclusion of tumor markers such as carbohydrate antigen 19-9 (CA 19-9) enhances the diagnostic utility of ultrasound scanning in pancreatic assessments. A raised level of CA 19-9 is a sign of pancreatic cancers and has been proven to be linked with response to treatment, enabling clinicians to monitor disease progression (Andreson et al., 2006). As ultrasound provides the means to guide tissue sampling, its use with such markers facilitates comprehensive examination through preoperative assessment. This biochemistry marker production and imaging shows the complexity of diagnosing pancreatic conditions without exemplifying the multidimensional nature that health care professionals must adopt. Therefore, ultrasound imaging is a cornerstone in the diagnostic armory for spleen and pancreas evaluation, enabling timely and accurate patient management.

Importance of Spleen and Pancreas in the Human Body

The spleen is an immune system organ that serves as a reservoir for lymphocytes and other immune cells. The primary role of this organ is to filter blood, destroy old and damaged red blood cells, and recycle iron for reuse. Apart from its hematologic roles, the spleen also contributes to mechanisms of body defense through the production of antibodies upon encountering pathogens. Its ability to detect and respond against infection makes it vital to the overall health of the body. In the event of splenic deficiency or its removal, patients are prone to infections, particularly of encapsulated organisms. Therefore, it is essential to be aware of the anatomy and physiology of the spleen, particularly when assessing patients using modalities such as ultrasound, which are capable of detecting abnormalities indicating splenic pathology that may jeopardize immune competence (Blair et al., 2015).

The pancreas does possess endocrine and exocrine functions, regulating significant metabolic functions. Its endocrine component secretes hormones such as insulin and glucagon that are critical to maintain glucose homeostasis. The exocrine function of the pancreas aids digestion by secreting enzymes that break down proteins, carbohydrates, and fats in the small intestine. This dual role is inherent not only in metabolic regulation but also in circumventing the digestive challenges created by alternative diets. Pancreatic disease, like pancreatitis or pancreatic cancer, can have serious health effects, including diabetes and malnutrition. Early imaging-based diagnosis can assist in early treatment, thereby mitigating complications associated with pancreatic dysfunction (Ndongo et al., 2010).

The spleen and the pancreas are organs that are non-replaceable, and they play a significant role in human health. Their simultaneous interaction between immune function and metabolic control is a testament to the complexity of body functions. Ultrasound imaging is a valuable diagnostic tool that allows healthcare practitioners to visualize these organs in real time and identify abnormalities that could be indicative of underlying illness. As technology improves with ultrasound, having the ability to examine the spleen and pancreas will enhance our understanding of various diseases, and this will enhance preventative therapy as well as therapeutic interventions. The critical role of such organs in general health requires continued research and clinical scrutiny, indicating the grave implications of early identification and intervention in maintaining body functions (Blair et al., 2015; Ndongo et al., 2010) (Figure 10.2).

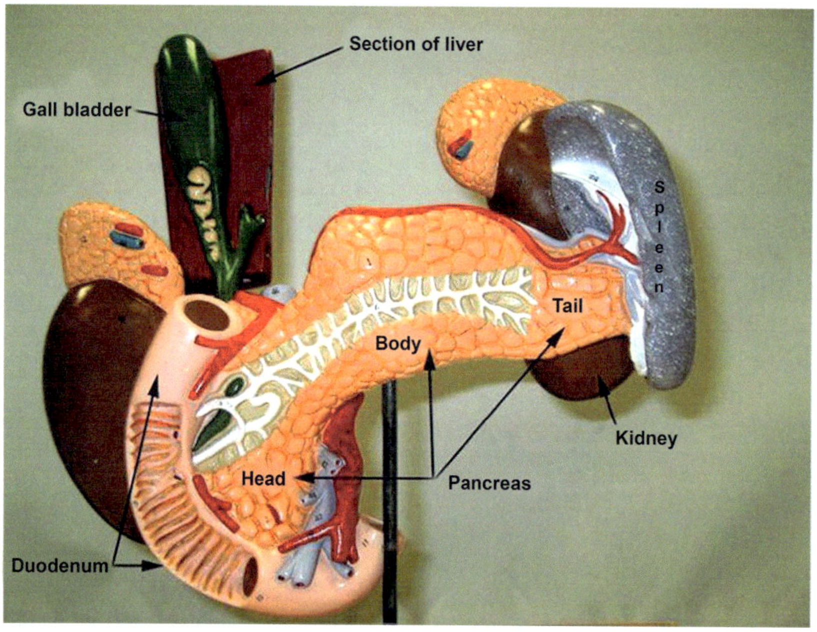

Figure 10.2. Spleen and pancreas in the human body.

Source: http://classroom.sdmesa.edu/anatomy/images/Digestive/pancreaslabel.jpg

10.1. Anatomy of the Spleen

The spleen is an important organ involved in the immune system and blood filtration, located in the upper left quadrant of the abdomen beneath the diaphragm. Understanding its anatomy is paramount for radiologists and clinicians conducting ultrasound procedures. It consists of two important components: the red pulp and the white pulp. The red pulp serves to strain blood, remove old or damaged red blood cells, and the white pulp has lymphocytes, which play a vital role in fighting infections. The unique vascular structure of the spleen aids its double role in that not only does it strain blood, but also quickly reacts to infections by generating immune responses. Anatomical location of the spleen aids in distinguishing it from surrounding organs, such as the pancreas and the kidneys, in carrying out ultrasound studies intended for the diagnosis of splenic or pancreatic pathology. Ultrasound imaging is optimally suited to delineate the structure of the spleen and assess its status. Sonographic features of the spleen include homogenous echotexture and smooth contour, both of which are significant in assessing its health. Size differences, such as splenomegaly, may indicate the existence of infections or hematological disease, warning the sonographer to look for normal versus pathological appearances. In addition, the close location of the spleen to the left kidney and tail of the pancreas necessitates careful examination of these organs when conducting an ultrasound, particularly when pathology would compromise adjacent structures. Ultrasound is also employed to detect abnormalities such as splenic tumors or abscesses, which require accurate anatomical information to design appropriate diagnosis and treatment. Integration of advanced ultrasound technology has also enhanced the diagnostic work concerning spleen examination. For instance, contrast-enhanced ultrasound (CEUS) is being increasingly seen to hold promise for augmenting the diagnostic outcome without the danger of radiation or iodinated contrast, particularly in pediatric patients (Cantisani et al., 2016). The procedure can assess changes in the perfusion and vascular characteristics of the spleen that can provide valuable insight into several diseases. As the science of ultrasound imaging continues to evolve, understanding the anatomical subtleties of the spleen will remain a foundation. Refining new modalities assures thorough evaluations of pancreatic and splenic health, allowing physicians to develop effective treatment plans as tailored as they are patient-centered. The comprehension of the splenic anatomy becomes increasingly important with the evolution of ultrasound technology, which further enhances diagnostic efficacy and therapeutic measures in clinical practice (Adams et al., 2017) (Figure 10.3).

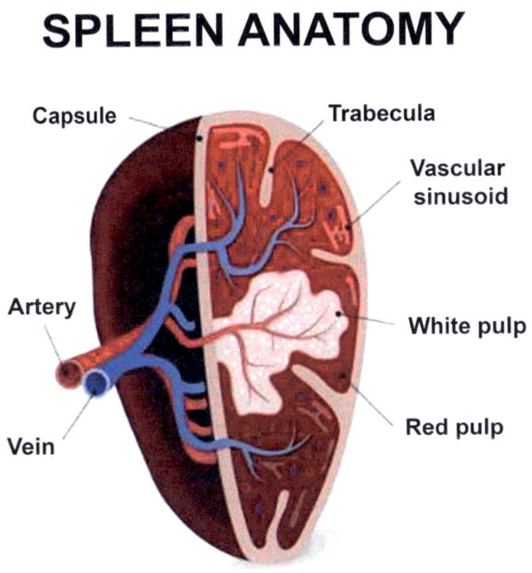

Figure 10.3. Anatomy of the spleen.

Source: https://external-content.duckduckgo.com/iu/?u=https%3A%2F%2Fwww.thoughtco.com%2Fthmb%2FnvjnmvmNJxxL_J8eGmuFKUroogU%3D%2F650x0%2Ffilters%3Ano_upscale()%3Amax_bytes(150000)%3Astrip_icc()%2Fspleen_anatomy-5a7f1d713037130036f0b392.jpg&f=1&nofb=1&ipt=4592f6ed1006c1d0d86c2fd5d310691883a7d18a65dbc6697c04712798cf1eb9.

10.1.1. Location and Size

The location and the size of the spleen and pancreas are two essential factors that determine the effectiveness of ultrasound procedures. The spleen is positioned in the left upper part of the abdomen, very near the stomach and diaphragm, within which it can easily be accessed via ultrasound. The healthy spleen should ideally be between 10 and 15 centimeters long and of varying thickness depending on location, and identification in a healthy individual will therefore usually not be very challenging. Splenomegaly or atrophy would potentially make it more challenging. The relative position of this variable-sized organ to other organs is important in ultrasound scanning since transmission of sound waves through it may affect the image quality produced. An understanding of the normal size and anatomic landmarks of the spleen assists the clinician in distinguishing pathologic processes and making accurate diagnoses on ultrasound imaging. Similarly, the pancreas is centrally positioned within the retroperitoneal cavity and tracks horizontally down through the abdomen from the duodenum on the right to the spleen on the left. It is 12 to 15 centimeters in length and composed of four segments: head, neck, body, and tail. The posterior position of the pancreas to the stomach makes it more difficult for ultrasound imaging because intervening gas can destroy the acoustic window needed for proper imaging. These tumors had an average volume of between 3.3 and 17.0 cm^3, an aspect that shows the importance of accurate measurement of size in therapeutic as well as diagnostic purposes. Accurate interpretation of pancreatic structures' measurements has a significant influence on clinical practice, particularly in developing treatment plans where an understanding of tumor size is essential, as well as how close they are to vital structures (Adams et al., 2017). The use of anatomical data regarding the size and position of the spleen and pancreas enhances the diagnostic power of ultrasound examinations. Ultrasound examinations of the abdomen frequently reveal significant anomalies of these organs, as demonstrated by a retrospective study that revealed a high frequency of findings requiring further investigation (Blair et al., 2015). Further, spatial relations to surrounding vasculature and surrounding organs can impact procedural planning, including therapeutic interventions tailored like ultrasound-guided biopsies or ablations. Understanding not only their normal dimensions but also pathologic alterations as a function of size better prepares the clinician to make rational choices during ultrasound evaluation. Thus, continuous research and clinical experience are pivotal to enhancing our knowledge about anatomical variations influencing ultrasound efficacy in the detection and treatment of pancreatic and splenic pathology.

10.1.2. Structure and Function

The spleen and pancreas share distinct but complementary roles in the human body, with a significant role to play in a number of physiological functions. The spleen, or the body's lymphatic organ, serves a pivotal function in filtering blood, recycling iron contained within hemoglobin, and supporting immunity. Its red and white pulp structure enables it to perform these functions effectively. The red pulp is also responsible for the filtration of aged erythrocytes, but the white pulp contains lymphocytes that are involved in the combat against pathogens. The pancreas, in contrast, has both an endocrine and an exocrine function, regulating blood sugar by secreting insulin and aiding in digestion by producing enzymes. This dual function is inseparable from its anatomy, where clusters of cells known as the islets of Langerhans release hormones into the bloodstream and acinar cells release digestive enzymes into the duodenum. In the past decade or so, advances in ultrasound equipment have made it greatly easier to examine the structure and function of both the pancreas and spleen. Ultrasound imaging is a non-invasive method for imaging such organs, providing information regarding their size, shape, and pathology. For example, echogenicity of the spleen can be indicative of splenomegaly or haematological illness, and pancreatic ultrasound can identify pathology such as tumors or cysts. With techniques such as color Doppler, the assessment becomes better, allowing physicians to examine vascular structures and blood flow within and around such organs. The addition of ultrasound not just aids diagnosis but also allows real-time monitoring of responses to therapy, and is therefore crucial in ideal patient management. As medical imaging develops further, the role of ultrasound in the clinic becomes increasingly useful. Moreover, the application of sophisticated computational algorithms, available in platforms like NiftyNet, is transforming medical image analysis. Through deep learning to automate image segmentation and analysis, clinicians can gain more accuracy in the assessment of spleen and pancreas pathology. Modularity in such platforms allows for bespoke solutions to unique imaging issues, with enhanced efficiency and reproducibility in the diagnostic process. Evidence indicates that such computerized processes can certainly alleviate the workload of radiologists and enhance diagnostic accuracy, for instance, in applications for segmenting abdominal organs or generating simulated ultrasound images. Such technology demonstrates the necessary coordination between structural assessment by ultrasound and advanced computational processing, which also emphasizes the importance of integrating novel methodologies in spleen and pancreas assessment (Adams et al., 2017; Barratt et al., 2017) (Figure 10.4).

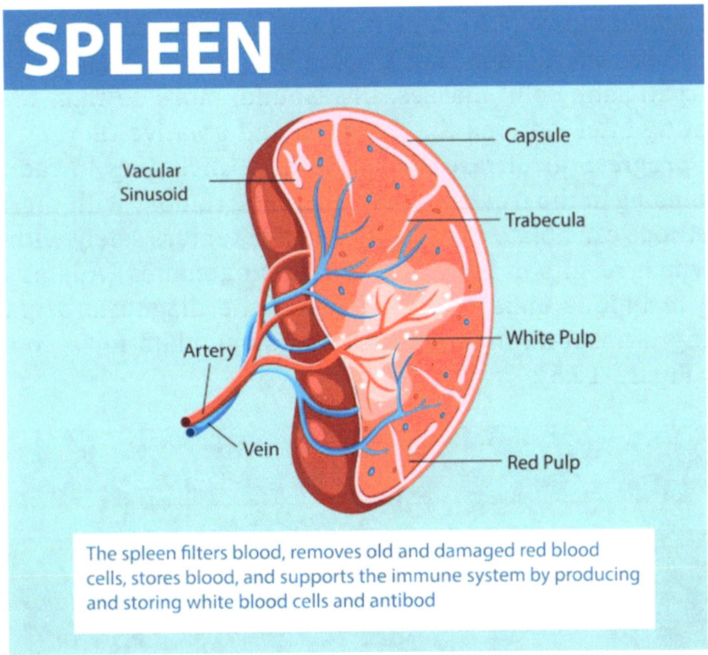

Figure 10.4. Spleen anatomy & function.

Source: https://img.freepik.com/free-vector/anatomy-human-spleen_1308-172081.jpg

10.1.3. Common Pathologies

Awareness of the most frequent splenic and pancreatic pathologies is required to enhance the reliability of ultrasound diagnosis. The spleen can be involved in a myriad of diseases such as splenomegaly, lymphomas, hematomas, and abscesses, which normally need thorough scanning through ultrasound. Splenomegaly or spleen enlargement is usually associated with liver disease, infections, and blood-related diseases. Ultrasound as an initial imaging modality facilitates the assessment of spleen size and echogenicity to differentiate normal from abnormal conditions. Through evaluation of echogenicity and the establishment of any structural abnormalities, physicians are in a better position to make treatment recommendations. For example, the finding of an abscess indicates a concealed infection that can be drained or treated with antibiotics, thus demonstrating the value of ultrasound in both therapeutic and diagnostic scenarios. The pancreas, as with the spleen, is susceptible to all manner of pathologies, most of which include acute and chronic pancreatitis, tumors, and pancreatic cysts. Each condition presents specific sonographic characteristics, and a clear comprehension is justified for accurate diagnosis. Acute pancreatitis is traditionally defined by dilated, hypoechoic glandular tissue, often with peritoneal fluid, readily visualized by ultrasound. Conversely, chronic pancreatitis is defined by a shrunken, calcified pancreas with ductal irregularity, and this must be differentiated from pancreatic neoplasms. Utilizing ultrasound as an iodine-free imaging agent is invaluable, as it allows monitoring and assessment of such conditions in real time without exposing patients to ionizing radiation. This quality is especially useful in the management of chronic diseases that need longitudinal observation and continuous treatment regimen changes. Pancreatic tumors evaluated by ultrasound are important to detect and manage early because lesions have the potential to influence patient outcomes in a significant way. Imaging fusion with ultrasound, computed tomography (CT), and magnetic resonance imaging (MRI) serves as the foundation for accurate characterization and staging of pancreatic tumors, enabling clinicians to differentiate between cystic and solid masses. Ultrasound, more so than the others, serves as an integral part in facilitating interventions like biopsies and ablative therapy owing to its real-time imaging benefit. New progress in ultrasound modalities, including intraductal and transgastric methods, has been promising in the treatment of pancreatic tumors with thermal therapy. Research indicates that these methods can ablate definite volumes of tumors safely with high efficiency within a limited time scale, which results in better therapeutic outcomes (Adams et al., 2017). Besides, a multimodal imaging technique enhances accuracy in the diagnosis of pancreatic lesions with a focus on consolidating ultrasound findings with radiologic data for a comprehensive approach (Baccari et al., 2016) (Figure 10.5).

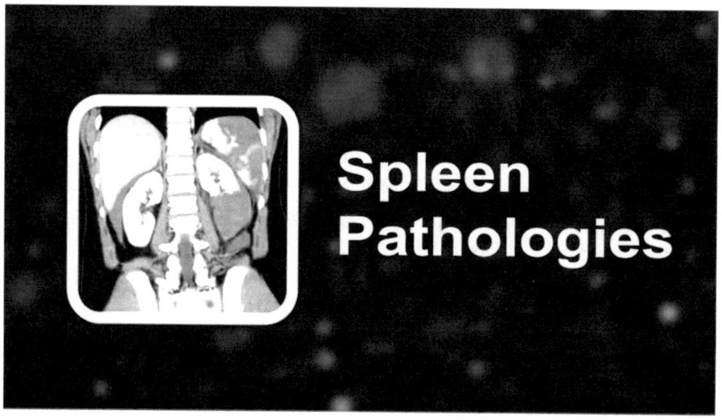

Figure 10.5. Spleen pathologies.

Source: https://external-content.duckduckgo.com/iu/?u=https%3A%2F%2Fembed-ssl.wistia.com%2Fdeliveries%2F7b29e0d23c7a0e17e8a6af191b96463b.jpg%3Fimage_crop_resized%3D640x358&f=1&nofb=1&ipt=3af5710d28cc0a63a2b460e60c92e26a801aa1808c9bea5f6ebf303275b145fe.

10.2. Anatomy of the Pancreas

The pancreas, as an essential organ that is positioned retroperitoneally, has a crucial role to play in double endocrine and exocrine roles. Anatomically, the pancreas consists of four primary components: head, neck, body, and tail. The pancreas head lies in the arcades of the duodenum, and the neck joins the head to the body, which is transversely positioned across the abdomen. The tail of the pancreas extends to the spleen and develops a close anatomical association with it.

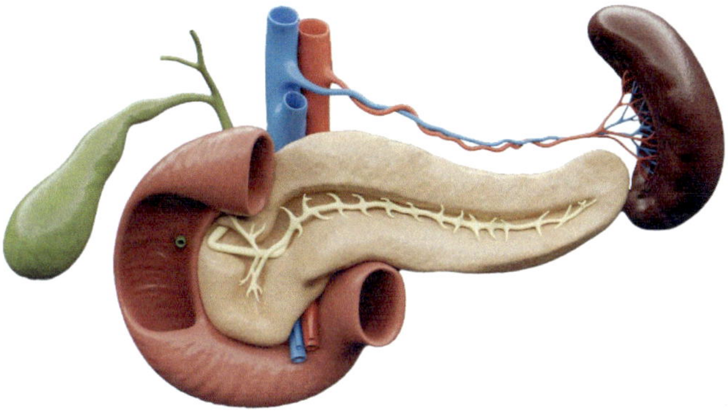

Figure 10.6. Anatomy of the pancreas.

Source: https://img-new.cgtrader.com/items/4051936/3726eed70d/pancreas-cross-section-anatomy-3d-model-3726eed70d.jpg

Familiarity with these anatomical facts is important for imaging in diagnostics, particularly for ultrasound, which is a non-invasive method to visualize these regions. This imaging facilitates clinicians to identify such diseases as pancreatitis, cysts, or tumors, thereby enabling therapeutic interventions related to the health of the pancreas as its intricate anatomy plays a vital part in disease expression and therapy. Ultrasound imaging has emerged as a key element in assessing pancreatic disease because it can depict both organ structure and function. With the aid of high-resolution imaging, one is able to visualize pancreatic lesions, ductal anatomy, and surrounding vascular anatomy. One of the examples of its utility is in the diagnosis of pancreatic tumors, where the dynamic feature of ultrasound is beneficial in determining their size, location, and relationship with adjacent structures, such as major vessels and the duodenum. The potential application of more powerful ultrasound techniques, such as contrast-enhanced ultrasound (CEUS), contributes to the imaging capability even further, enhancing more information in evaluating pancreatic lesions in real-time (Cantisani et al., 2016). With diagnosing and managing clinicians continuing their pursuit of accurate diagnosis, the significance of ultrasound in studying the pancreas cannot be overstated, further underscoring the necessity of strong knowledge of pancreatic anatomy and pathology. Improved ultrasound technology, including intraductal and transgastric approaches for thermal treatment, exemplifies the effect of imaging progress on treatment for pancreatic tumors in a direct manner. Research shows the feasibility of using focused ultrasound applicators within the pancreatic duct or via transgastric routes to deliver effective thermal therapy against cancers (Adams et al., 2017). This approach highlights the significance of precise anatomical data since effective treatment is dependent on good knowledge of tumor size, location, and nearby sensitive tissues in order to prevent unwanted effects. Parametric studies also imply performance, highlighting the need for specialized treatment approaches based on patient anatomy. By integrating such advanced ultrasound methods with fundamental anatomical understanding, doctors are able to achieve better outcomes in the treatment of pancreatic tumors, supporting the significant interplay between anatomy and technology in modern medicine (Figure 10.6).

10.2.1. Location and Size

The anatomic relationship between the pancreas and spleen is critical for ultrasound scanning because their locations are pivotal in both diagnostic imaging and therapy. The spleen occupies the upper left quadrant of the abdomen, generally posterior and lateral to the stomach. The pancreas, on the other hand, extends transversely across the abdomen, located between the duodenum and spleen. This close proximity influences the ultrasound approach, with some familiarity with the surrounding anatomy in order to get optimal images. Localization is especially important when treating these organs for therapy, for example, sonically guided delivery of therapy for pancreatic cancer, which may have to be performed cautiously to avoid major blood vessels and overlying tissue structures, emphasizing the value of accurate anatomical knowledge in both ultrasound and clinical assessment. The size of the spleen and pancreas is mostly unpredictable between individuals and can be a sign of health status.

The normal size of the spleen is typically 7 to 14 centimeters in length, while for the pancreas, it is approximately 15 to 20 centimeters. Any deviation from the normal measurement would suggest pathology, such as splenomegaly or pancreatic atrophy. Ultrasonography is the major imaging method utilized to measure the size of these organs. For instance, studies using newer imaging techniques recognize that individually customized volumetric measurements can yield valuable information about pancreatic tumors that can impact treatment planning (Adams et al., 2017). Continuously offering accurate measurements with ultrasound can assist in detection and follow-up for disease progression, finally allowing clinicians to design individually customized treatment plans based on the size and health of the individual's specific organs. Advances in technology in ultrasound equipment have played a key role in significantly improving the evaluation of the pancreas and spleen, both when they are healthy and ill. The generation of advanced imaging sequences enables clinicians to precisely measure organ dimensions, which ultimately translates into better accuracy in diagnosis. For example, ongoing research demonstrates the efficiency of high-resolution imaging equipment that can differentiate between various types of tissue and observe small changes in the size of the organs over time. These advances are particularly valuable for pancreatic disorder monitoring, allowing for non-invasive, longitudinal assessment of pancreatic size corresponding to other physiological changes (Criscimanna et al., 2014). In such cases, the understanding of the position and size of the pancreas and spleen becomes important not only in diagnosis but also for maximizing treatment interventions and improving patient outcomes through ultrasound-guided procedures.

10.2.2. Structure and Function

The spleen plays an essential role in immunity and homeostasis of blood in that it has a structure and function. It is composed of red pulp and white pulp, which collectively are responsible for filtering the blood and coordinating the immune response. Red pulp clears old or broken down red blood cells, while white pulp includes lymphocytes that initiate immune responses.

This organization allows the spleen to efficiently manage blood and detect pathogens. Ultrasound scanning is a pain-free procedure to evaluate the size of the spleen, its morphology, as well as any pathological changes, helping to understand its role in various hematological disorders. For instance, splenomegaly might be a sign of chronic infections or hematological malignancies, while structural malformations could be related to some immunological disorders, thereby confirming the diagnostic utility of ultrasound in clinical assessment of splenic structure and function. But the pancreas is not only an endocrine and an exocrine organ, but also very closely related to the body's metabolic functions.

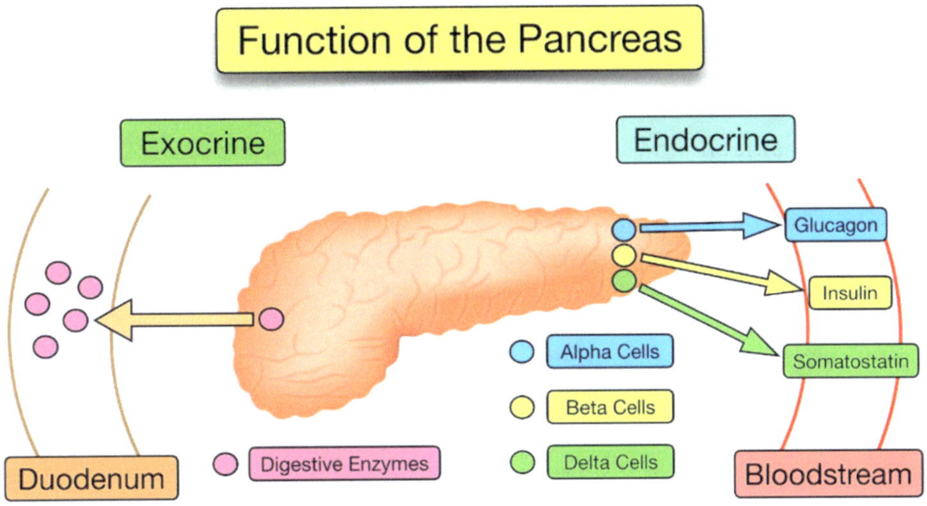

Figure 10.7. Function of the pancreas.

Source: https://external-content.duckduckgo.com/iu/?u=https%3A%2F%2Fimages.squarespace-cdn.com%2Fcontent%2Fv1%2F5e48489da899cd09424943db%2F3e1b4ea6-b4bd-441d-bbd7-29a8d6e3e1da%2Fpancreas-function-digestive-endocrine-insulin.jpeg&f=1&nofb=1&ipt=3da50decb00fb848a147c1e084932fbebd1a3fff24d5ad760d6f67e659c810a9.

The exocrine component secretes digestive enzymes into the small intestine to facilitate nutrient digestion and absorption. The endocrine component, which consists of the islets of Langerhans, secretes hormones like insulin and glucagon directly into the circulation to regulate glucose metabolism. Both functions highlight the pancreas's vital role in digestion and metabolic control. Ultrasound imaging is also capable of detecting structural defects such as pancreatic cysts or tumors, which may impede these essential functions. Notably, recent studies employing ultrasound-based thermal therapy have presented new approaches to treating pancreatic tumors, thus revealing the role of structural assessment in determining the therapeutic pathway of pancreatic pathologies (Adams et al., 2017). Advances in medical imaging, in this case through deep learning-based systems, offer enhanced functionality for the imaging and analysis of organ structure and function, such as the spleen and pancreas. Platforms like NiftyNet offer tailored frameworks for the processing of medical images, such as ultrasounds, allowing for simpler segmentations and regressions to be carried out over the imaging data. With the ability to generate simulated images for diverse anatomical presentations, such technologies simplify image analysis application development focused on intricate medical situations. Researchers are, therefore, able to quickly improve diagnostic methods and treatment planning for diseases involving the spleen and pancreas. Their continued development holds the potential to improve clinical outcomes through enabling precise structural evaluation and thorough functional testing, and thus advance diagnosis and treatment techniques (Barratt et al., 2017) (Figure 10.7).

10.2.3. Common Pathologies

In ultrasounds of the spleen and pancreas, many of the prevalent pathologies represent significant diagnostic challenges and implications for patient management. The spleen, being an organ committed to blood filtration as well as immunity, can exhibit pathology in the form of splenomegaly or lesions indicative of infection or malignancy. For instance, splenic abscesses can result from bacterial infections or secondary to endocarditis-like processes, necessitating accurate ultrasound evaluation to ascertain size, location, and potential interventions. Likewise, conditions such as hypersplenism can lead to cytopenias, further complicating clinical presentations. As the spleen is centrally involved in immunity, the early diagnosis through ultrasound imaging becomes crucial in order to enable appropriate management and treatment plans, hence the justification for learning about common splenic pathologies in the overall context of abdominal diagnostics. The pancreas is susceptible to various pathologies, two of which are the most prevalent: acute and chronic pancreatitis. Acute pancreatitis is typically associated with acute abdominal pain, nausea, and hyperamylasemia and necessitates early imaging to establish severity and complications. Ultrasound can identify fluid collection, necrosis, or even the formation of an abscess, which calls for urgent intervention. For instance, a case report accounts for a patient who initially had abdominal pain, later discovered to have ingested a toothpick, leading to pancreatitis and subsequent abscess formation, bringing into focus the importance of accurate imaging for diagnosis (Abela et al., 2013). Besides, chronic pancreatitis can evolve to pancreatic ductal adenocarcinoma, which often complicates the clinical picture by overlapping symptoms, thus requiring regular follow-up with ultrasound for early detection and treatment of malignancies (Hofstad et al., 2017).

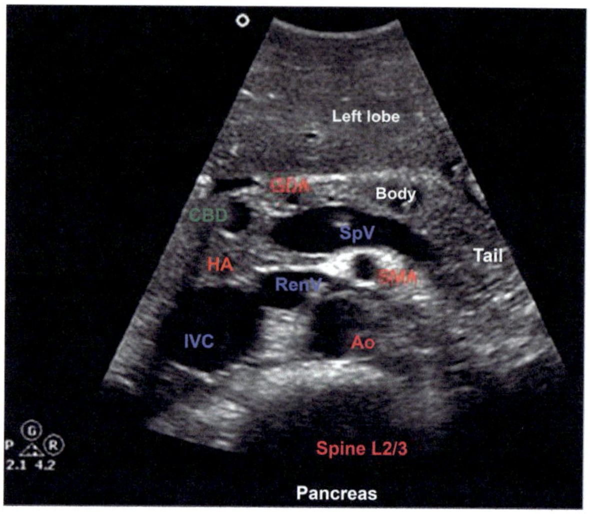

Figure 10.8. Pathologies of the pancreas.

Source: https://external-content.duckduckgo.com/iu/?u=https%3A%2F%2Fradiologykey.com%2Fwp-content%2Fuploads%2F2017%2F02%2Fimage00532.gif&f=1&nofb=1&ipt=4fa8904688488a0970d598f80bf1f151c035416910367c71bcf1a4f30bc01409.\

Also, pancreatic ductal adenocarcinoma (PDA) is an unsuspecting enemy in the realm of common pathologies diagnosed by imaging modalities like ultrasound. As the fourth most common cause of death from cancer, this condition is frequently asymptomatic during its early development, resulting in late diagnoses and prognosis. The complexity of location within the anatomy requires sophisticated imaging modalities to direct surgical methods and improve operative results. Progress in image-guided techniques, combined with laparoscopic surgery, has been promising to improve operative accuracy and reduce rates of complications, particularly where the tumors' definite borders are difficult to delineate (Hofstad et al., 2017). With continued imaging progress, it emphasizes the central role that accurate ultrasound evaluation plays in the management of pancreatic pathologies and refining surgical management (Figure 10.8).

10.3. Ultrasound Technique

Ultrasound is a non-invasive imaging modality that serves a significant role in the assessment of abdominal organs, notably the pancreas and spleen. By utilizing high-frequency sound waves, ultrasound provides real-time imaging that helps to diagnose many pathologies like splenomegaly, tumors, and cysts. Of particular note is the safety profile of the techniques used, with no ionizing radiation exposure, which makes it especially safe for vulnerable groups such as pregnant women and children. Conventional ultrasound methods have evolved wonderfully, improving our capacity to identify and assess lesions in the spleen and pancreas. As technology advances, the sensitivity and specificity of ultrasound in diagnosing abnormalities of the organs continue to increase, thus revolutionizing clinical practice. Perhaps the most significant advancement in ultrasound technology has been the development of contrast-enhanced ultrasound (CEUS), providing enhanced visualization of spleen and pancreatic lesions.

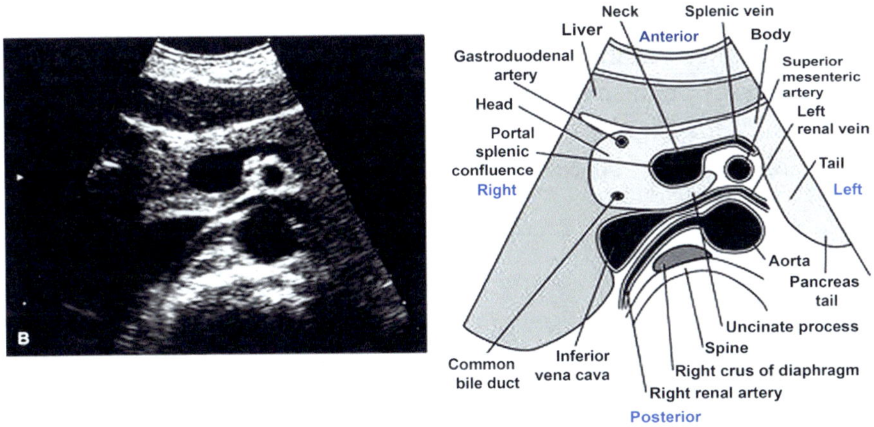

Figure 10.9. Pancreas ultrasound.

Source: https://external-content.duckduckgo.com/iu/?u=http%3A%2F%2Fradiologykey.com%2Fwp-content%2Fuploads%2F2017%2F07%2Fimage00770.jpeg&f=1&nofb=1&ipt=f596b25bcc70b78533253f6a16dcad12b47500f1f2803734c38fc0ec2f2c5b62.

CEUS utilizes microbubble contrast agents that significantly enhance vascular anatomy delineation and characterization of focal lesions. This modality has proven particularly valuable in distinguishing benign lesions from malignant tumors, potentially preventing invasive procedures. For splenic pathology, CEUS has been instrumental in diagnosing disorders such as accessory spleens, which would otherwise be clinically misdiagnosed if they were assessed solely on the basis of conventional ultrasound methods. Application of CEUS simplifies diagnostic pathways, minimizing the occurrence of needless surgical procedures, which is vital in case of diseases such as intrapancreatic accessory spleen (IPAS) versus tumors, as noted in clinical findings (Bellato et al., 2019). Besides, pediatric applications of ultrasound techniques are becoming more popular, highlighting a widening role for ultrasound in the clinical environment among pediatric patients.

Recent research demonstrates the use of pediatric CEUS in the evaluation of various abdominal diseases with special attention given to pathology requiring non-invasive imaging. Prioritizing avoidance of exposure to radiation and iodinated contrast media is according to guidelines currently in place that encourage patient protection and comfort (Cantisani et al., 2016). With increasing evidence in support of CEUS in the pediatric population, it paves the way for enhanced imaging protocols in children. Therefore, the establishment of ultrasound techniques, ie, incorporation of CEUS, not only enhances diagnostic accuracy but also reiterates patient-centeredness in abdominal pathology management, especially of the spleen and pancreas (Figure 10.9).

10.3.1. Preparation for the Procedure

Preparation for the spleen and pancreas ultrasound procedure is necessary to ensure both the validity of imaging results and patient comfort. Intensive patient education is the first step, which entails a full discussion of the purpose and the nature of the procedure. Patient education is instituted in order to minimize patient anxiety. Fasting is typically required for several hours prior to the test to reduce gas in the gastrointestinal tract, otherwise it will obscure the ultrasound images. Further, a complete medical history must be elicited because it may influence the imaging modality or require special precautions during the examination. It is essential that any prior illnesses, for instance, diabetes or previous abdominal operations, are taken into account at this preparatory time to tailor the ultrasound technique accordingly. In addition to patient preparation, there needs to be proper ensuring of equipment and staff available for imaging. The sonographer must be certified and experienced in abdominal exams who is aware of the special requirements for assessement of the spleen and pancreas. The equipment must be calibrated, and the settings must be adjusted based on the body type of the patients and any special clinical questions posed by the referring doctor. In addition, protocols laid down by institutions like the Federation of Societies for Ultrasound in Medicine and Biology create protocols that are standardized and are used to reduce the preparation process by ensuring that all factors relevant to the process are taken care of Brabrand et al. (2015). Through adherence to such protocols, medical practitioners can maximize the effectiveness of the ultrasound, leading to more precise diagnostics. Finally, logistics also need to be accounted for in the preparation of the ultrasound. The scheduling needs to provide sufficient time not only for the scanning process but also for the risk of delays from prior patient schedules. The environment where the ultrasound is performed should be one that provides comfort and privacy so that patients feel relaxed and can actively participate in the process. Having in mind the outcomes of previous research, for instance, the demonstration of immunosuppressive treatment on organ transplantation and its connection with the success of ultrasound diagnostics (Abu-Elmagd et al., 2004), it can be noted that due care in preparation can in numerous ways significantly affect the outcome of the procedure. This systems-orientated approach to preparation ensures that the ultrasound is not just diagnostic, but also part of a continuum of care that continues to put patient safety and satisfaction at its core.

10.3.2. Equipment Used in Ultrasound

Ultrasound technology is largely based on specialized anatomy, primarily the ultrasound machine, which has several essential components. The transducer, commonly regarded as being at the heart of ultrasound, is employed to transmit and receive sound waves. These transducers, which exist in various types such as linear and curvilinear, are chosen based on the specific anatomical area that is to be scanned. For spleen and pancreas ultrasound examinations, curvilinear transducers are utilized as they are able to take enough depth, along with enhancing image definition. The central processing unit of the ultrasound scanner also identifies the information that is obtained from the transducer and produces real-time images through which diagnostic assessments can be made. Besides, technical advancements have brought in the incorporation of 3D imaging technology, such as the advancement of improved understanding of anatomical structures, and a large amount of research is underway to improve diagnostic procedures and patient treatment. By means of a transducer, apart from that, advancement of the multifunctionality of ultrasound equipment comprises the incorporation of contrast-enhanced ultrasound (CEUS) techniques. CEUS employs microbubble contrast agents injectable intravenously that are used to improve visualization of vascular lesions and organs within the pancreas and spleen, where ordinary ultrasound images may be inadequate. Besides enabling more precise diagnoses, the technique reduces the need for invasive procedures. Despite the fact that CEUS has become well established in various pediatric applications, its pediatric application has only been more recently developed, supported by growing evidence of its safety profile and effectiveness in children. The European Federation of Societies in Ultrasound and Medicine (EFSUMB) has facilitated constant development and application of CEUS, hence emphasizing its role in increasing imaging technologies with a decrease in the application of radiation or iodinated contrast media, an essential parameter in children's treatment (Cantisani et al., 2016). Advanced character of ultrasound technology is also found in its use with several imaging packages that aid in the evaluation and interpretation of ultrasound images. Advanced imaging software packages provide the ability to include Doppler imaging, which is very important in the hemodynamic assessment of blood flow through abdominal organs like the pancreas and spleen. Through the assessment of hemodynamics, clinicians are able to detect vascular tumors or occlusions, which influence clinical decision-making to a greater degree. Besides, the computerized nature of present-day ultrasound machines allows for storage, retrieval, and sharing of images between healthcare networks for mutual evaluation by experts. Overall, the technology in ultrasound machines, transducers, CEUS options, and imaging programs as a whole improves diagnostic capacity in spleen and pancreas scans, underlining their utility in the exercise of contemporary medicine (Focal Spot, 2008) (Figure 10.10).

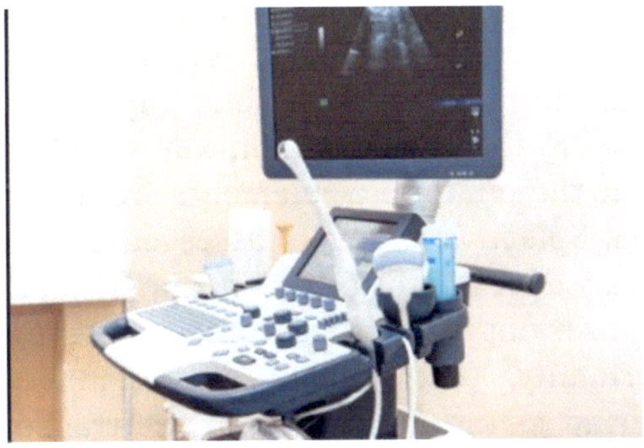

Figure 10.10. Equipment used in ultrasound.

Source: https://external-content.duckduckgo.com/iu/?u=https%3A%2F%2F5.imimg.com%2Fdata5%2FSELLER%2FDefault%2F2022%2F8%2FBB%2FXG%2FRJ%2F50732130%2Fshutterstock-561061939-scaled-500x500.jpg&f=1&nofb=1&ipt=34e53cb0b4726c428fefebb41be134fcfd8ac1754471a4926e32da689f2f3c5d.

10.3.3. Step-by-Step Process of Conducting an Ultrasound

The beginning of an ultrasound examination, particularly to evaluate the spleen and pancreas, begins with patient preparation and education. It is worthwhile to explain the procedure to the patient to alleviate anxiety and enhance compliance. Patients are usually requested to starve for a few hours prior to the procedure since it decreases gas within the gastrointestinal tract, which can impair the images acquired. Once prepared, the patient is then positioned by the sonographer comfortably, either in a supine position, and the abdominal area is covered with water-soluble gel. The gel facilitates better transmission of the sound waves between the transducer and the skin and enables improved image quality. The technical details, including the selection of the appropriate frequency of the transducer, are tested with great care depending on the depth of the structures to be evaluated and the patient's anatomical features. This is an important first step in ensuring that there are clear, diagnostic images of the spleen and pancreas during the ultrasound scan. During the progression of the ultrasound scan, there is an intended scanning technique employed to ensure efficient evaluation of the spleen and pancreas. The sonographer begins by placing the transducer in key positions to look at the anatomical elements from various angles. Spleen is typically assessed by sliding the transducer across the left upper quadrant and observing its size, texture, and echogenic abnormality. Next, the pancreas is inspected, requiring gentle angulation of the transducer to optimally visualize the head, body, and tail. Applying the principles outlined by training standards, such as those of the German Society of Ultrasound in Medicine (DEGUM), ensures that sonographers achieve anatomical identification and image acquisition proficiency. Furthermore, the evaluation adheres to clinical guidelines, reiterating the need for accurate diagnosis and generating valuable images that are central to clinical interpretation (Becker et al., 2014). Upon image acquisition, the next key step is the interpretation and reporting of results. The resultant images are carefully evaluated for evidence of pathology, for example, lesions, cysts, or size and shape distortions that may suggest intrinsic conditions of the spleen and pancreas. Utilization of systematic reporting, as mentioned in recent literature, decreases variability and enhances communication between providers. The integration of rhetorical structure theory (RST) can increase the validity and effectiveness of ultrasound reports, turning spontaneous observations into organized forms that permit comparison and clinical decision-making (Bärenfänger et al., 2019). This phase is key to maximizing the diagnostic value of ultrasound, providing essential information for guiding patient management and determining the role of the procedure in contemporary medical practice.

10.4. Indications for Spleen Ultrasound

Ultrasound scanning is a valuable diagnostic modality for splenic pathology evaluation and the diagnosis of other pathologies. Indications for spleen ultrasound essentially stem from clinical presentation of abdominal pain, palpable splenomegaly, or trauma. Acute abdominal syndrome patients can require a rapid assessment of visceral organs, particularly the spleen, in order to rule out splenic rupture or hemorrhage from blunt or penetrating trauma. Moreover, the non-invasive nature of ultrasound and its capability to provide real-time imaging render it an essential first-line modality in emergency and outpatient settings. By detecting abnormal size, shape, or parenchymal echogenicity, ultrasound can assist clinicians in defining the etiology of splenic disease, which allows for more convenient delivery of timely intervention and management strategies. Chronic illnesses such as hematological conditions can be assessed using spleen ultrasound in order to analyze splenic involvement and provide details of systemic disease severity. Conditions such as lymphoma or leukemia can cause lymphoid hyperplasia, splenomegaly, or the formation of splenic masses, which may be comprehensively described with the assistance of ultrasound imaging. The technique can be employed to analyze the morphology of spleens and any associated abnormalities, such as cysts or infarcts. Furthermore, the use of contrast-enhanced ultrasound (CEUS) is increasingly becoming fashionable among children for the assessment of focal lesions since it minimizes ionizing radiation and iodinated contrast agent exposure, which is aligned with existing medical recommendations to adopt safer imaging for children. With the evolving clinical practice, applications of ultrasound are increasingly on the rise, reinforcing its role in disease management and follow-up of chronic illnesses. In surgery and organ transplantation, spleen ultrasound is very significant in risk stratification and surgical planning. In the case of patients receiving a pancreatic transplant, in whom the spleen may be injured or in the surgical field, sonography can provide valuable preoperative information regarding splenic anatomy and vascularity. Careful spleen imaging is critical in enabling surgeons to identify anatomical variations that may complicate surgery and thus improve overall surgical outcomes. In addition, identification of post-transplant complications such as splenic infarction or thrombosis is critical for graft survival and patient safety. The integration of spleen ultrasound into the routine investigations maximizes the total care management of patients by ensuring maximum treatment is pursued in a timely and efficient manner, hence highlighting the significance of appropriate imaging protocols in the multidisciplinary care setting (Cantisani et al., 2016; Abu-Elmagd et al., 2004) (Figure 10.11).

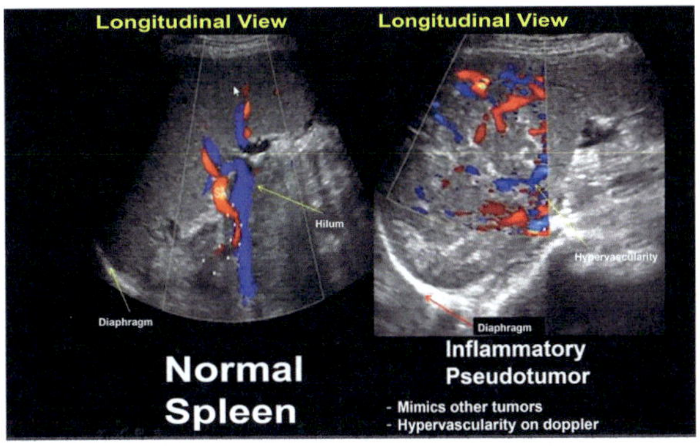

Figure 10.11. Indications for spleen ultrasound.

https://external-content.duckduckgo.com/iu/?u=https%3A%2F%2Fi.ytimg.com%2Fvi%2FCZpeA_lJ6rE%2Fmaxresdefault.jpg&f=1&nofb=1&ipt=ba9b2b4d8fafad12d60c8553af7c0c2ed3d337b4f72ad1a0fc81a73cb8e9b1f5.

10.4.1. Evaluation of Splenomegaly

Evaluation of splenomegaly forms a critical component of ultrasound scanning because the spleen is a central organ for hematopoiesis and immunity. Splenomegaly or enlargement of the spleen is usually found with varied pathologies ranging from infections to hematological malignancies. In ultrasound scanning, the size of the spleen is evaluated by measurements, and the morphology of the spleen is examined to separate benign from malignant causes for the enlargement. Abnormalities such as distortion of form, echogenicity, or findings with association, such as free fluid presence, are highly significant predictors that dictate further diagnostic management. This non-invasive procedure not only provides key information about splenic health but also assists in the evaluation of treatment response, and thus is a useful tool in clinical practice, considering the setting of splenomegaly's impact on overall patient health. Advanced ultrasound techniques significantly enhance the evaluation of splenomegaly, with facilitation of characterization of the underlying lesions. B-mode ultrasound, supplemented with color Doppler (CD) and power Doppler (PD), is a satisfactory technique for the evaluation of splenic pathology. The modalities can elucidate the vascular nature of splenic lesions, the determinants of the likelihood of malignancy. Specifically, lesions with tortuous internal vessels on CD or B-Flow technology have been associated with higher malignancy risks, while larger lesion size or distorting the splenic capsule is also problematic. Such improved imaging technologies combined allow doctors to prioritize their differential diagnosis, leading to more precise and intense therapeutic interventions in patients with splenomegaly and subsequently enhancing clinical outcomes. The use of ultrasound in pediatric patients with splenomegaly cannot be overemphasized, particularly in view of the historic concern regarding radiation-induced exposure by other imaging devices. The recent advancement in contrast-enhanced ultrasound (CEUS) has offered a cost-effective and effective substitute that enables thorough investigation of splenic disease without the side effects of ionizing radiation or iodinated contrast media. As regarded by the European Federation of Societies in Ultrasound and Medicine (EFSUMB), CEUS has gained wider acceptance in evaluating various abdominal diseases, and its value is better evidenced by clinical practice and evidence-based medicine. Moreover, as the technology continues to evolve and is implemented on pediatric cases, clinicians are presented with a great option for the assessment of splenomegaly in children, where a sensitive and non-invasive diagnostic process is required for their ailment (Cantisani et al., 2016) (Figure 10.12).

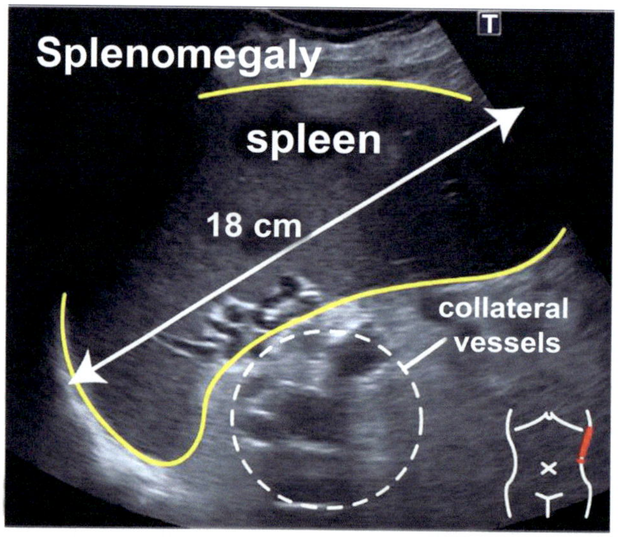

Figure 10.12. Evaluation of splenomegaly.

Source: https://external-content.duckduckgo.com/iu/?u=https%3A%2F%2Fwww.radiology.expert%2Fcontent%2Fimages%2Fmodules%2Fultrasound-abdomen-general%2Fen%2Fresized%2FRadiologyExpert_English_class_ultrasound_abdomen_general_fig44_Splenomegaly_MET_860x0.jpg&f=1&nofb=1&ipt=c7c8a01382089011f47ef7827e6b1954d691114e427057ca651f462477b3a6d9.

10.4.2. Assessment of Trauma

Trauma assessment, particularly in abdominal trauma, is needed to properly manage patients with potential injuries to organs like the spleen and pancreas. Ultrasound and other newer imaging modalities have come to play very important roles in the management of trauma due to their ability to provide rapid, accurate diagnosis with minimal risk to the patient. Use of contrast-enhanced ultrasound (CEUS) has become more popular, especially in children, where it is essential to keep the exposure to radiation to a bare minimum. Although use of CEUS in children has traditionally been considered off-label, cumulative evidence shows its effectiveness in the evaluation of focal lesions and possible traumatic injury, with an important bearing on patient outcomes (Cantisani et al., 2016). Hence, the integration of CEUS into routine trauma assessment is a forward-thinking move toward maximum diagnostic specificity without putting the patient at risk. The epidemiological context and nature of injury in trauma assessment cannot be overstated. The endemicity of trauma injuries, particularly in developing countries, makes it all the more essential that there is a systematic approach towards the prevention of injuries and the management of the patient. For instance, a study conducted in Yaoundé, Cameroon, identified that road traffic accidents accounted for nearly 60% of the injuries and disproportionately occurred among young men. Such demographic trends call for specific interventions and tailored ultrasound assessment to address the unique challenges of certain populations (Ndongo et al., 2010).

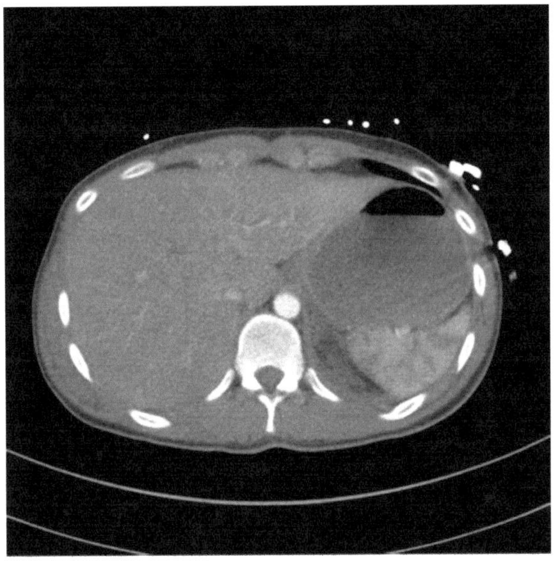

Figure 10.13. Assessment of trauma.

Source: https://external-content.duckduckgo.com/iu/?u=https%3A%2F%2Ftse1.mm.bing.net%2Fth%2Fid%2FOIP.igMkHmw8jPafaE6hf3V4YgHaHa%3Fr%3D0%26pid%3DApi&f=1&i pt=0587ea1b2adebf9ef457a51f0a6c01711006cdeb23b1c80b21056d7e767ce22d.

Appreciation of the mechanisms of such injuries contributes to the development of prevention strategies and improving trauma care management, ultimately ensuring better survival rates and the quality of care for victims. Cooperation between radiologists, trauma surgeons, and emergency medicine specialists is also crucial in ensuring optimal trauma evaluation techniques. Effective coordination and communication may enhance the accuracy of ultrasound scanning, facilitating early diagnosis of spleen and pancreas damage. In trauma, early detection of splenic laceration or pancreatic damage can radically alter management, for example, in determining whether surgical intervention is necessary. By enabling multidisciplinary efforts and the use of advanced imaging modalities like CEUS, trauma centers are able to manage complex abdominal injuries more effectively while staying abreast of the highest levels of patient safety and care (Cantisani et al., 2016). Technological innovation in ultrasound technology and its applications within trauma settings will be instrumental in reshaping how physicians interact with patient assessment and treatment within the increasingly demanding field of emergency medicine (Figure 10.13).

10.4.3. Detection of Tumors

Identification of tumors of the pancreas and spleen is now more sophisticated due to advancements in imaging modalities, with a case in point being ultrasound. Ultrasound is a cost-effective, non-invasive method that employs sound waves to create images of structures within and is particularly useful for the assessment of soft tissue pathology.

Identification of tumors such as pancreatic ductal adenocarcinoma in the case of pancreatic pathology has been especially difficult due to the anatomical location of the organs and the surrounding tissue. Recent technological advancements in ultrasound have enabled more precise diagnostics through the use of contrast-enhanced ultrasound (CEUS). CEUS enhances the definition of vascularity and tissue perfusion, thereby enabling differentiation between malignant and benign lesions.

The role of ultrasound in the detection of tumors at an early stage can be important, as early diagnosis is crucial for proper management and effective treatment strategies, in turn, resulting in better patient outcomes. In addition to ultrasound, magnetic resonance imaging (MRI) has been found to be a valuable modality in the detection and imaging of pancreatic tumors. MRI provides better soft tissue contrast resolution, which helps radiologists in differentiating cystic from non-cystic lesions effectively. Of particular importance is pancreatic ductal adenocarcinoma, which is the most common malignancy in the pancreas, but other neoplasms can have a range of imaging characteristics that may confound diagnosis. The versatility of MRI, especially its use of new motion-resistant pulse sequences and respiratory gating methods, increases its dependability for assessing pancreatic masses. In addition, MR cholangiopancreatography is invaluable for a non-invasive evaluation of pancreatic ducts and adjacent structures. By identifying specific imaging characteristics, MRI can significantly narrow the differential diagnosis, ultimately resulting in more effective management routes for individuals with pancreatic disease (Ansari et al., 2015). In pediatric cases, ultrasound application in detecting tumors within the pancreas and spleen also holds immense promise.

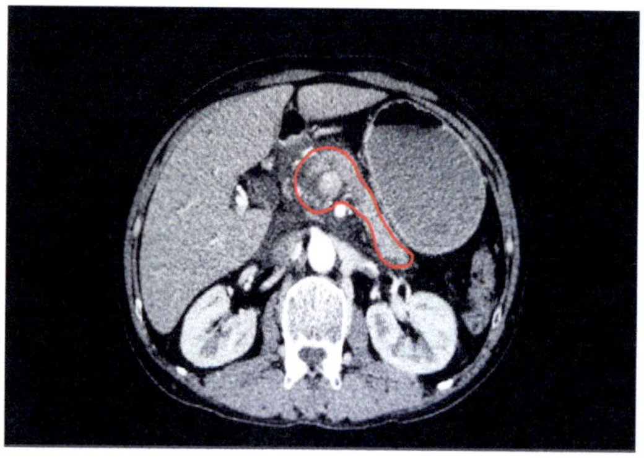

Figure 10.14. The detection of tumors in the pancreas and spleen.

Source: SOPONE/stock.adobe.com. CT of carcinoma of the head of pancreas, pancreatic tumor. https://t4.ftcdn.net/jpg/02/28/14/59/240_F_228145975_TZlad3tTbDyNLHOzUmhPAH90ghosIWCc.jpg

Even though it has traditionally been considered an off-label use, newer research has identified advantages to contrast-enhanced ultrasound in the pediatric population, particularly for the evaluation of focal liver lesions and potentially the splenic and pancreatic exams as well. Not only does CEUS have the advantage of minimizing exposure to ionizing radiation and iodinated contrast, but it is also noninvasive and patient-compatible. The European Federation of Societies in Ultrasound in Medicine (EFSUMB) has embraced the growing evidence base supporting the application of CEUS as a necessary imaging modality in children, encouraging its increased approval and standardization in clinics. This change emphasizes the demand for tailored imaging approaches in diverse populations to enable effective tumor detection and management with lower risks from more invasive techniques (Cantisani et al., 2016) (Figure 10.14).

10.5. Indications for Pancreas Ultrasound

A pancreas ultrasound is a major diagnostic tool utilized to evaluate various pancreatic diseases. High frequency sound waves create real-time images to assist medical experts in identifying abnormalities such as pancreatitis, pancreatic cysts, and tumors. In patients who present with pain in the abdomen, particularly in the upper quadrants, a pancreas ultrasound provides a safe method for evaluating underlying conditions.

Apart from this, it is also a first-line assessment in acute illness, to assist in differentiation between inflammatory disorders or malignancies that may necessitate other forms of therapeutic interventions. Success of such imaging is operator dependent and based on the operator's understanding and knowledge of the pancreas anatomy and good comprehension of the patient's clinical history and symptoms to enable focused investigation and prompt intervention. Thus, pancreatitis and presumptive neoplasia are valuable indications for this imaging method in the clinical setting. Apart from the acute abdomen and the pain of acute abdominal pain, pancreatic ultrasound has a vital function in chronic pancreatitis, where pancreatic ductal anatomy and focal lesions are studied in the center. Patients with long-standing courses of abdominal pain and gastrointestinal symptoms can be assisted using this imaging modality, as it enables the detection of calcifications, stricture of the ducts, and other characteristics common with chronic inflammation. Ultrasound also provides valuable information regarding complications of chronic disease, such as pseudocyst formation that may lead to subsequent clinical complications if left without intervention.

The increasing prevalence of chronic pancreatitis, as is normally related to alcohol and metabolic disease, highlights the benefit of pancreas ultrasound as a normal part of ongoing evaluation. Beyond chronic disease, the ability to longitudinally evaluate changes in pancreatic shape lends credence to ultrasound as a continued patient care and treatment monitoring tool. The benefit of pancreas ultrasound extends beyond the realm of diagnosis; it also provides for guiding therapeutic intervention. For instance, in pancreatic cyst evaluation, ultrasound may be used to distinguish between benign and potentially malignant lesions and hence direct clinical decision-making regarding surgical intervention. The imaging modality also allows fine-needle aspiration biopsies that provide cytological examination of suspicious masses identified during imaging. With the advancement in ultrasound technology, the precision and diagnostic efficacy keep improving. As an illustration, the evaluation and need for interventions through ultrasound imaging are becoming standard for gastrointestinal endoscopic practice with a significant focus on promoting holistic training and certification among clinicians for such practice (Arcidiacono et al., 2019; Bekkali et al., 2023). This new landscape of pancreas ultrasound reiterates its importance not only as a tool for diagnosis but as an integral part of total pancreatic care and management in clinical practice (Figure 10.15).

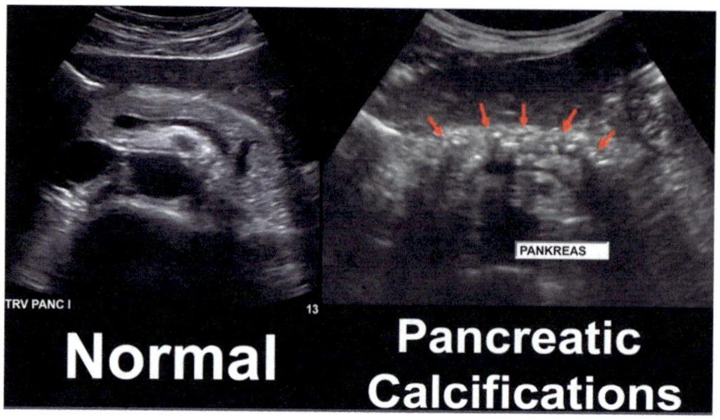

Figure 10.15. Indications for pancreas ultrasound.

Source: https://external-content.duckduckgo.com/iu/?u=https%3A%2F%2Fi.ytimg.com%2Fvi%2FgIOAU51nzqI%2Fmaxresdefault.jpg&f=1&nofb=1&ipt=2881b77b67de97c20a1a65d0ab99a5aa534cfc91b219be4d3806831292f6147a.

10.5.1. Diagnosis of Pancreatitis

Diagnosis of pancreatitis relies on diagnosing pancreatitis, physicians typically rely on the combination of patient history, physical examination, and imaging studies to determine the presence and extent of the disease. Ultrasound is currently a valuable instrument in this diagnosis process, which provides real-time visual representations of the pancreas and surrounding structures. Sonography can detect enlarged pancreatic masses, fluid collections, and potential complications, that is, pseudocysts or abscesses. The availability and non-invasive nature of ultrasound make it extremely useful in the emergency setting. Furthermore, detection of the structural changes in the pancreas may have a significant bearing on the treatment strategy, thus emphasizing the need for accurate imaging in the early phase of the condition. Magnetic resonance imaging (MRI) enhances the sensitivity of diagnosis in pancreatitis, especially for borderline cases. With its better soft tissue contrast resolution, MRI can differentiate cystic from non-cystic pancreatic lesions and image the pancreatic ducts along with associated vascular structures adequately. This ability is useful in the event of abnormal presentation since it helps to distinguish between pancreatitis and other neoplastic pancreatic illnesses. For instance, MR cholangiopancreatography is very effective at imaging the biliary and pancreatic ducts without an invasion. As the literature details, MRIs capacity to define pancreatic lesions affords necessary information, ideally focusing the differential diagnosis and diminishing unwarranted invasive procedures, which is critical to both patient safety and management (Ansari et al., 2015).

In addition, the association between pancreatitis and pancreatic tumor emphasizes precise imaging in diagnosing. Neuroendocrine tumors, presenting with symptoms similar to pancreatitis, complicate the diagnostic course further. The diagnosis of such tumors tends to reveal a range of behavior from benign to malignant, and thus one has to approach the diagnostic work-up with caution. For example, an intraoperative recurrence of a neuroendocrine tumor can mimic the radiographic appearance of post-surgical pancreatitis and can be difficult to diagnose (Adair et al., 2010). Imaging, thus, is not only critical in the process of ascertaining whether or not there is pancreatitis but also in the differentiation of underlying malignancies or complications, and its importance lies in the overall evaluation of pancreatic diseases in the setting of ultrasound examinations.

10.5.2. Assessment of Pancreatic Tumors

Pancreatic tumor assessment has become more sophisticated with the advancement in imaging devices, particularly ultrasound. Ultrasound is an important device used for primary detection of pancreatic masses due to its real-time imaging that can identify features of the tumor, such as size and shape. Also, ultrasound-guided biopsies enhance diagnosis through histopathological examination of suspected tumors. This technique is particularly useful in assessing tumors that are not easily accessible for surgical procedures. As pancreatic cancers are generally associated with nonspecific symptoms, utilizing ultrasound as a first line of investigation allows for timely intervention and treatment plans and ultimately improves patient outcomes and survival. This early assessment opens the way to further therapies, underlining the pressing requirement for precise imaging modalities capable of intraoperative guidance and monitoring of tumor response to therapeutic interventions. New studies have illuminated the new applications of intraductal and transgastric ultrasound-directed thermal treatments of pancreatic tumors. These approaches utilize high-level ultrasound applicators that can be inserted endoscopically to target and ablate tumor tissues with great precision. For instance, research found that tumors of up to 2.5 cm in diameter could be successfully ablated within under 10 minutes using these techniques, which have a revolutionary potential for local treatment of pancreatic tumors (Adams et al., 2017). Moreover, routine volumes of pancreas tumors have shown extremely high response rates to ultrasound thermal ablation, with a high volume percentage of tissue being successfully ablated within brief durations. Such procedural improvements not only advance the therapeutic armamentarium against pancreatic cancers but also mirror the changing horizon of minimally invasive therapeutic modalities to improve the quality of life for those afflicted.

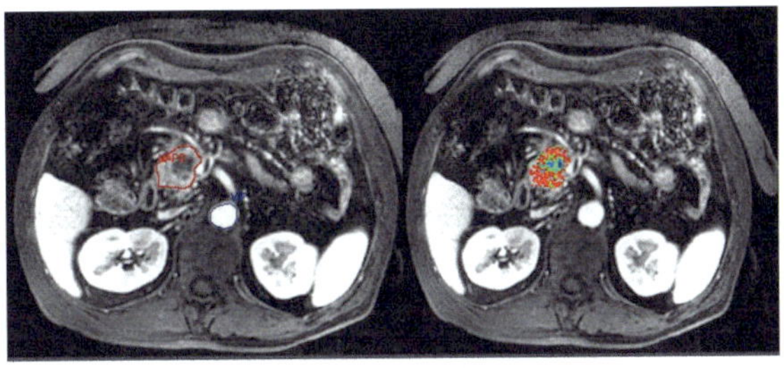

Figure 10.16. Evaluation of pancreatic cancer.

Source: https://external-content.duckduckgo.com/iu/?u=https%3A%2F%2Fels-jbs-prod-cdn.jbs.elsevierhealth.com%2Fcms%2Fattachment%2F303af89e-453b-4580-acd3-0b9a0cdc9015%2Fgr1_lrg.jpg&f=1&nofb=1&ipt=3a672d1e1ffacb15383cdc7a5bac7477645a6e8b51c3aa6e721eb905ee6d6f6e.

Furthermore, distinguishing pancreatic tumors from other processes, including intrapancreatic accessory spleens (IPAS), is paramount to proper management, which is tackled using state-of-the-art imaging modalities. Misdiagnosis can lead to unjustified surgical procedures; hence, a multitude of imaging modalities like CT scan, MRI, and PET scan are utilized in concert for accurate differentiation. A recent experience demonstrated the efficacy of 68-Ga-Dotatoc PET/CT in the detection of non-functional neuroendocrine tumors (NF-NET) along with illumination of pitfalls when differentiating NF-NET from IPAS. In this case, the false-positive uptake led to misdiagnosis, highlighting the need for enhanced imaging protocols in the evaluation of pancreatic lesions (Bellato et al., 2019). Ultimately, the employment of varying imaging technologies not only improves diagnostic accuracy but also informs educated surgical decision-making and effective patient management strategies in pancreatic tumor evaluations (Figure 10.16).

10.5.3. Assessment of Cysts and Abscesses

Assessment of abscesses and cysts in the spleen and pancreas by ultrasound is today an integral component of abdominal imaging. Ultrasound as an initial imaging modality is utilized to evaluate them because it shares some special benefits, including not using ionizing radiation, portability, and having the capability to do imaging in real time. The good resolution of ultrasound can differentiate between simple cysts, which are typically benign and fluid-filled, and complex lesions that may harbor secondary complications such as infection or malignancy. Moreover, the capabilities of ultrasound may often prevent the need for the use of more invasive imaging modalities, and hence it is an appropriate candidate for initial assessment. The interpretation of results is highly important because the management of cystic and abscessal cysts differs widely, depending upon their nature, size, and patient's presenting symptoms. In particular for pancreatic abscesses, proper and early diagnosis by ultrasound is vital for their appropriate treatment. In general, pancreatic abscesses tend to develop as a secondary complication of acute pancreatitis and require prompt intervention in order to prevent further morbidity. Ultrasound not only enables the primary identification of the abscess but can even guide therapeutic interventions such as drainage procedures. The application of contrast-enhanced ultrasound (CEUS) has been proven for its better diagnostic accuracy, particularly in discriminating simple from complicated fluid collections of the pancreas and spleen. CEUS application represents an important progress in the diagnosis of these intra-abdominal pathologies, with an imaging method that has the potential to improve patient outcomes without risk of the intervention linked to radiologic imaging (D'Onofrio et al., 2019). This advancement is a testament to the ongoing improvement of ultrasound technology and its role in clinical practice. In children, ultrasound assessment can take on even more significance due to the need to restrict radiation exposure. With increasing clinical evidence for using CEUS in children, particularly in the assessment of focal liver lesions, it is a possible candidate for further research in other applications, including cysts and abscesses. The European Federation of Societies for Ultrasound in Medicine and Biology recognizes this new trend, campaigning for expanded use of CEUS beyond the liver in non-hepatic diseases, including the spleen and pancreas (Cantisani et al., 2016). Besides enhancing diagnostic capability, this also aligns with the desire to offer safer imaging modalities to the coming generations. As diagnostic imaging technology evolves, the emphasis on the use of ultrasounds in assessing cysts and abscesses serves to advance its acceptability as a first-line imaging tool for both children and adults.

10.6. Limitations of Ultrasound

Ultrasound scanning is now an indispensable resource in the evaluation of abdominal organs such as the spleen and pancreas, but is not without significant limitations. A key limitation is operator dependency, whereby the skill and experience of the technician will influence the quality of images generated. The patients' anatomy, obesity, and the presence of excess gas are reasons for difficulty in complete visualization of structures and, consequently, threats of misdiagnosis or failure to identify major conditions. Moreover, the lack of standardization of ultrasound machines can create inconsistency in image results across institutions, hence making clinical interpretation challenging. Such variation can detract from the value of ultrasound as a useful diagnostic tool, particularly in difficult cases of the pancreas, where visualization clarity is critical to diagnosis and treatment planning. A second significant limitation concerns depth penetration and resolution constraints inherent in ultrasound technology. While ultrasound is optimal for visualizing superficial structures, it is less than optimal for visualization of deeper structures, such as the pancreas. The retroperitoneal location of the pancreas is prone to cause problems for unobstructed imaging, in that tissue interferences in the immediate vicinity can hide minute lesions or pancreatic cancers. Second, contrast resolution is likely to be lower in ultrasound compared to other imaging modalities such as computed tomography (CT) or magnetic resonance imaging (MRI), which can provide greater detail and clarity. This is a limitation with the potential to compromise the diagnostic yield of ultrasound in the assessment of pancreatic pathologies, such as pancreatic ductal adenocarcinoma, where optimal imaging is needed in order to inform clinical decision-making and improve prognostic results (Hofstad et al., 2017). Furthermore, a second important technological limitation is the limited capability of ultrasound in distinguishing or defining lesions or among various lesions in the spleen and pancreas. Compared to advanced imaging modalities capable of giving information regarding the internal structure and vascularity of lesions, ultrasound only provides limited information regarding lesion size and shape. Though newer developments, such as the availability of contrast-enhanced ultrasound techniques, have increased diagnostic capability, these are not yet universally available and could have additional cost and patient risks. Furthermore, the evolving medical imaging landscape, for instance, the advent of platforms like NiftyNet for deep learning in medical imaging analysis, highlights the continued need for better imaging solutions that complement existing modalities without disturbance to provide value on top of these limitations and make the overall assessment of spleen and pancreatic pathologies better (Barratt et al., 2017).

10.6.1. Technical Limitations

Technical limitations involving ultrasound of the spleen and pancreas have a significant impact on diagnosis efficiency and treatment. One of the limitations is the acoustic nature of the abdominal tissue, which may affect the quality of the ultrasound image. Gas in the gastrointestinal tract or extreme body fat may cause attenuation and scattering that hinders visualization of the spleen and pancreas. These challenges are likely to necessitate the use of adjunct imaging modalities or the use of contrast agents to improve image definition and diagnostic precision. Patients with inappropriate abdominal fatness, for instance, may require ancillary imaging modalities in an attempt to get more distinct delineation of such organs, hence rendering the diagnosis more intricate and prone to cause delayed treatment. The complexity of the pancreas and the spleen's anatomical location further complicates these issues. The pancreas lies deeply within the abdomen and is surrounded by critical structures and organs. This anatomical complexity often necessitates specialized knowledge and experience on the part of the operator in order to obtain the optimal imaging results. Tiny or irregularly sized pancreatic tumors, for instance, may not be visualized at all using conventional ultrasound technology. The heat therapy techniques, though promising, have only been proven for tumors of a certain size category, as evidenced by research which has shown that pancreatic tumors under the size of 2.5 to 2.7 cm can be treated more reliably using either transgastric or intraductal approaches (Adams et al., 2017). Tumors that are bigger do not lend themselves easily to the same techniques, and thus, choices are limited for treatment. Lastly, the application of contrast-enhanced ultrasound (CEUS) has introduced opportunities along with challenges in clinical practice, particularly with pediatric patients. Although CEUS has become increasingly popular as a method for enhancing imaging with the safety of not giving radiation exposure, pediatric patient use remains predominantly off-label, thus limiting acceptance on a large scale (Cantisani et al., 2016). This conservative practice is mostly due to the relative novelty of CEUS in these age groups and the need for more research to ascertain standard protocols. Additionally, it is also a fact that even though CEUS can significantly enhance visualization and diagnostic sensitivity, factors such as operator experience and adherence to safety guidelines are paramount to determining its safety and efficacy, thereby emphasizing the repeated emphasis on training and standardization of ultrasound practice.

10.6.2. Patient Factors Influencing Outcome

Patient factors are important in impacting the outcome of spleen and pancreas ultrasound examination and their accuracy and utility. Habitus of the patient is one of the significant factors because obesity can interfere with visualization, making it difficult for sonographers to obtain good images of the pancreas and spleen. The greater abdominal perimeter poses a physical barrier that can attenuate the ultrasound waves and lead to less than optimal imaging and, more significantly, false-negative pathological abnormalities. Habitual variations also mean that alternative transducer settings will be required, further complicating the process of diagnosis. Lastly, image quality from ultrasound is directly linked with patient factors, which highlights the necessity of knowledge by sonographers regarding these factors in interpreting results. A patient history is also important in creating ultrasound findings. Previous abdominal surgeries may form scar tissue, which leads to distortion of the normal anatomy and makes it more difficult to visualize the pancreas and the spleen. Some pathologies, such as pancreatitis or splenomegaly, may also alter sonographic images of these organs, so a familiarization by the interpreting radiologist is required. In addition, concomitant symptoms—such as abdominal pain or tenderness—can affect patient positioning during the procedure and remaining immobile, both considerations for obtaining good ultrasound images. This interaction of history and presentation has a critical impact on the diagnostic utility of ultrasound for these organs and, therefore, requires careful evaluation of the patient.

Another factor that may affect the results of the ultrasound is the timing of the examination relative to eating. For example, ingestion of food may affect the acoustic window and change abdominal organ position as a result of bowel gas. If patients have a pancreatic ultrasound following ingestion of food, it can cause heightened bowel activity, leading to diminished image clarity. Fasting before the test is usually advised to provide optimal visualization and reduce interference due to gastrointestinal contents. The timing cannot be overemphasized; it reflects the demand to adhere to preparatory procedures so as to increase diagnostic accuracy. Pre-procedure advice and patient compliance are therefore important factors in deciding the overall quality of ultrasound reports for the spleen and pancreas.

10.6.3. Comparison with Other Imaging Modalities

In its evaluation of spleen and pancreas ultrasound effectiveness, it is to be compared with the other imaging methods, such as computed tomography (CT) and magnetic resonance imaging (MRI). In this case, the strengths of ultrasound, such as portability, cost, and lack of ionizing radiation exposure, are factors that surface, and which are highly beneficial in vulnerable groups such as children. Similarly, while more effective at delineating intricate anatomic detail, CT scans expose patients to higher doses of radiation and potential effects of iodinated contrast agents. Studies have demonstrated that while required for staging and monitoring of response to treatment, CT has the potential to ignore small lesions at times, particularly in the context of liver disease, thus emphasizing the complementary utility of ultrasound within an integrated diagnostic approach. Among the more recent advances in imaging is contrast-enhanced ultrasound (CEUS), which has brought to focus its possible applications in imaging children. Not only does CEUS increase the diagnostic value of routine ultrasound, but it also lacks ionizing radiation traditionally associated with CT, and the risk of nephrotoxicity with iodinated contrast. Evidence highlights growing validation and utilization of CEUS for the evaluation of various lesions, particularly in pediatric patients, toward more patient-friendly imaging. Therefore, inclusion of CEUS shows a powerful alternative to traditional methods of imaging, being an important breakthrough in ultrasound technology and lesion imaging for the spleen and pancreas. Although ultrasound and CEUS have their advantages, CT is also necessary, particularly in oncological practice, where precise tumor staging and evaluation are critical. However, studies reveal that routine CT may not adequately detect the signs of minute metastatic lesions, making it questionable as a solo imaging technique. For instance, in hepatic tumor patients, the preoperative CT scans failed to identify approximately half of the tumor nodules, which were later found on gross pathology inspection of the resected specimens. This discrepancy serves to indicate that ultrasound should be supplemented with either CT or MRI in order to enhance diagnosis and clinical decision-making. Therefore, a multi-modal imaging technique utilizing ultrasound combined with standard modalities must provide the most comprehensive evaluation of spleen and pancreas disease, consonant with current trends toward less invasive, more effective diagnostics.

SUMMARY

The use of ultrasound scanning for pancreatic and splenic assessment represents a significant advance in diagnostic radiology. It is a non-invasive way of evaluating these two organs, and it can assist medical doctors in identifying numerous pathologies more accurately. Specifically, ultrasound represents a valuable asset in differentiation between benign and malignant tumors, which is critically valuable in determining appropriate management options. Evidence has indicated the challenges in misdiagnosis of intrapancreatic accessory spleen (IPAS) as pancreatic tumors, particularly non-functional neuroendocrine tumors (NF-NET) (Bellato et al., 2019). Thus, optimizing ultrasound procedures may minimize unnecessary surgical interventions, emphasizing the necessity of adopting advanced imaging technologies into clinical practice. Besides, the exploration of new directions for ultrasound-assisted therapeutic strategies may be capable of enhancing therapy outcomes of pancreatic tumors. The availability of technologies such as intraductal and transgastric ultrasound applicators represents a break-through shift in the treatment paradigms. Initial experiences indicate that these methods can produce significant ablation of tumor volumes within clinically tolerable time intervals (Adams et al., 2017). By providing targeted thermal therapy, these technologies have the potential to improve patient prognosis without preserving intervening vital anatomy. Thus, ultrasound in diagnostic and therapeutic use not only enhances our understanding of diseases of the pancreas and spleen but also provides a mode of better control of patients. Lastly, the advancement of ultrasound imaging and treatment is a paradigm shift in the management of conditions of the pancreas and spleen. With increasing accuracy in diagnosis and advancing treatment modalities, better patient outcomes through custom-designed therapeutic regimens should be anticipated. With continuing advancements in ultrasound technology, tighter collaboration among clinicians, radiologists, and oncologists should encourage multidisciplinary solutions for multifaceted issues. Therefore, further research and development in this field are necessary in order to adequately utilize the potential of ultrasound and ensure that patients are being properly cared for within the context of splenic and pancreatic disease.

The application of ultrasound imaging of the pancreas and spleen plays a key role in clinical diagnosis, particularly in pathologies related to these organs. Ultrasound is applied for its noninvasive nature and capacity to provide real-time images, thereby enabling physicians to assess organ morphology and identify abnormalities easily. The spleen, with functions such as filtration of blood and support of immune responses, can also develop other conditions, such as splenomegaly or masses of the spleen, all of which carry patient management considerations. Concomitantly, pancreatic evaluation is required, especially with the rising prevalence of pancreatic disorders. The early identification of lesions, cysts, and inflammatory conditions by ultrasound is of large therapeutic importance. Overall, the key issues highlighted via observation of ultrasound of spleen and pancreas are the functionality of the technique to enhance diagnostic reliability with facilitating prompt clinical intervention. With respect to pancreatic examinations, ultrasound has been viewed as a first-tier imaging modality, particularly for conditions like pancreatitis, obstruction of the pancreatic duct, and tumors. Recent advances in the field of ultrasound offer enhanced high-resolution function, which fortifies the technique's potency in detecting minimal lesions that may be indicative of malignancy or chronic inflammation. From existing literature, imagery of the pancreatic duct and surrounding vascular structures is enhanced, hence complementing detailed evaluations. True correlation of imaging findings with surgical outcome continues to be an area of guided research. Moreover, in instances of vascular complications or significant anatomical abnormalities, the use of improved operative maneuvers such as the modified Appleby procedure highlights the window for improved patient results, leading to margin-negative resections even among patients with locally advanced pancreatic disease (Lamb et al., 2016). Apart from its diagnostic capabilities, ultrasound is also used to monitor treatment responses and to evaluate post-operative conditions for pancreatic and splenic illness. Ultrasound's real-time function allows repeated measurements without exposing patients to radiation, which makes it an extremely useful tool in longitudinal studies and follow-up imaging. For instance, for complications following surgery, such as abscess or necrosis, ultrasound may provide immediate information that necessitates altering patient management strategies. Moreover, the continuous advancement in technology widens the application of ultrasound, such as potentially generating 3D reconstructions providing detailed information about organ morphology and function (Criscimanna et al., 2014). The focus on developing finer ultrasound methods indicates a determination to enhance the care outcomes of patients by facilitating earlier detection and more efficient treatment of spleen and pancreas-related ailments.

CLOSER LOOK

SPLEEN ULTRASOUND

Spleen ultrasound is an accessible, non-invasive imaging technique that may be used to assess the spleen in real-time for size, shape, texture, and blood supply. Located in the left upper quadrant of the abdomen, the spleen plays a vital role in hematologic and immune processes as a blood filter as well as a site for lymphocyte production and storage. Ultrasound is often the first modality for splenic pathology examination due to its being safe, portable, nonionizing, and capable of delivering immediate clinical data at the bedside. It is particularly useful in children and pregnant women, trauma cases, and routine abdominal examinations.

The standard ultrasound protocol of the spleen is in the left upper quadrant longitudinal and transverse planes, either in the left intercostal spaces or subcostal approach, depending on patient anatomy. The normal spleen should be a homogenous echogenic organ with a smooth outer border. It is typically very slightly more echogenic than the liver and kidney in echotexture. The normal adult spleen measures up to 12–13 cm long, but measurements depend on age, gender, and habitus. Splenomegaly is one of the most common indications for splenic ultrasound and is defined as a craniocaudal length of more than 13 cm. Causes of splenomegaly include infections (such as mononucleosis or malaria), hemologic disorders (such as leukemia or lymphoma), portal hypertension, liver cirrhosis, storage diseases, and inflammatory disease.

Ultrasound can also be used in the identification of splenic infarcts as wedge-shaped, hypoechoic areas due to regional ischemia. Trauma survey is also a valuable application, specifically in the Focused Assessment with Sonography in Trauma (FAST) assessment, where perisplenic fluid collections, subcapsular hematomas, or splenic lacerations may be detected. In such situations, detection of intraperitoneal bleeding early can be lifesaving. In addition, splenic cysts, abscesses, hemangiomas, and primary or metastatic tumors can be assessed by ultrasound. A simple cyst will be anechoic with hyperechoic walls and posterior acoustic enhancement, whereas abscesses might be complex with internal echoes or septations. Malignant lesions, that is, metastasis or lymphoma, will typically be hypoechoic or heterogeneous masses and may require further evaluation with contrast-enhanced studies or biopsy.

The Doppler ultrasound can be applied to evaluate the splenic artery and vein, particularly in suspected thrombosis of the splenic vein or portal hypertension-related congestion. Splenic hilum imaging helps to identify patterns of flow as well as detect any vascular insufficiency. Although ultrasound is compromised by limitations such as not being able to image obese patients, bowel gas artifacts, and only being able to visualize deep lesions in part, its value lies in it being a rapid, cost-effective, and reproducible test. New technology, including contrast-enhanced ultrasound (CEUS), also enhances splenic imaging by maximizing lesion detection and characterization.

References

1. Abela, L., & Borg Xuereb, K. (2013). Liver abscess following ingestion of a foreign object. https://core.ac.uk/download/46603960.pdf (accessed on 12th July 2025).
2. Abu-Elmagd, K., Basu, A., Bond, G., Khan, A., et al. (2004). Pancreatic transplantation at the University of Pittsburgh. https://core.ac.uk/download/12205623.pdf (accessed on 12th July 2025).
3. Adair, A., Oniscu, A., & Wigmore, S. J. (2010). Post-surgical pancreatitis masquerading as recurrent neuroendocrine cancer. https://core.ac.uk/download/28977847.pdf (accessed on 12th July 2025).
4. Adams, M. S., Diederich, C. J., Salgaonkar, V., Scott, C., et al. (2017). Theoretical investigation of transgastric and intraductal approaches for ultrasound-based thermal therapy of the pancreas. https://core.ac.uk/download/323063407.pdf (accessed on 12th July 2025).
5. Anderson, J. S., Bekaii-Saab, T. S., Brambs, H. J., Burris, H. A., Ebrahimi, B., Glenn, J., Gogas, H., et al. (2006). Prognostic and therapeutic significance of carbohydrate antigen 19-9 as tumor marker in patients with pancreatic cancer. https://core.ac.uk/download/16432407.pdf (accessed on 12th July 2025).
6. Ansari, N. A., Buonocore, V., Gigli, S., Maccioni, F., et al. (2015). Role of magnetic resonance imaging in the detection and characterization of solid pancreatic nodules: An update. https://core.ac.uk/download/154949520.pdf (accessed on 12th July 2025).
7. Arcidiacono, P., Braden, B., Bun Teoh, A., Burmeister, F., et al. (2019). What should be known prior to performing EUS exams? (Part II). https://core.ac.uk/download/588394970.pdf (accessed on 12th July 2025).
8. Baccari, P., Cappabianca, S., D'Andrea, A., Falcone, R., et al. (2016). Pancreatic tumors imaging: An update. https://core.ac.uk/download/98333045.pdf (accessed on 12th July 2025).
9. Bärenfänger, M., Carlson, J., Edwards, L., Faggioni, A., Feng, X., Hernault, R., Joty, S., et al. (2019). Ultrasound reports standardization using rhetorical structure theory and domain ontology. https://core.ac.uk/download/199215715.pdf (accessed on 12th July 2025).
10. Barratt, D. C., Cardoso, M. J., Doel, T., Eaton-Rosen, Z., et al. (2017). NiftyNet: A deep-learning platform for medical imaging. https://core.ac.uk/download/159081199.pdf (accessed on 12th July 2025).
11. Becker, J. C., Domagk, D., Friederichs, H., Heinzow, H., et al. (2014). Teaching ultrasound in a curricular course according to certified EFSUMB standards during undergraduate medical education: A prospective study. https://miami.uni-muenster.de/Record/0a1907fe-f3a4-4e6d-a905-0f532e3e4dc2 (accessed on 12th July 2025).
12. Bekkali, N., Carroll, N. R., El Menabawey, T., Henry, J., et al. (2023). UK and Ireland Joint Advisory Group (JAG) consensus statements for training and certification in diagnostic endoscopic ultrasound (EUS). https://core.ac.uk/download/587633910.pdf (accessed on 12th July 2025).
13. Bellato, V., Caronna, R., Cerasari, S., Chirletti, P., et al. (2019). Intrapancreatic accessory spleen false positive to 68Ga-Dotatoc: Case report and literature review. https://core.ac.uk/download/231747695.pdf (accessed on 12th July 2025).

14. Ndongo, B, C., Mballa, E.G. A., Hyder, A. A., Juillard, C., et al. (2010). Patterns of injury and violence in Yaoundé, Cameroon: An analysis of hospital data. https://core.ac.uk/download/323075033.pdf (accessed on 12th July 2025).

15. Blair, W. H., Chen, R. X., Sturges, B. K., Taylor, A. R., et al. (2015). Effect of screening abdominal ultrasound examination on the decision to pursue advanced diagnostic tests and treatment in dogs with neurologic disease. https://core.ac.uk/download/323069729.pdf (accessed on 12th July 2025).

16. Brabrand, K., Cantisani, V., Correas, J. M., Cui, X., et al. (2015). EFSUMB Guidelines on Interventional Ultrasound (INVUS), Part II: Diagnostic ultrasound-guided interventional procedures (Long Version). https://core.ac.uk/download/480425559.pdf (accessed on 12th July 2025).

17. Bron, K., Dekker, A., Iwatsuki, S., Kowal, C., et al. (1984). Accuracy of computerized tomography in determining hepatic tumor size in patients receiving liver transplantation or resection. https://core.ac.uk/download/12203985.pdf (accessed on 12th July 2025).

18. Cantisani, V., Deganello, A., Dietrich, C. F., Duran, C., et al. (2016). Role of contrast-enhanced ultrasound (CEUS) in pediatric practice: An EFSUMB position statement. https://core.ac.uk/download/74320188.pdf (accessed on 12th July 2025).

19. Criscimanna, A., Heuck, A., Moore, A., Orabi, A. I., Williams, A. J., Attili, A. K., Saluja, A. K., et al. (2014). A non-invasive method of quantifying pancreatic volume in mice using micro-MRI. https://core.ac.uk/download/20536001.pdf (accessed on 12th July 2025).

20. Czinyéri, J., Garami, M., Kovács, G., Müller, H., et al. (2001). Thrombotic thrombocytopenic purpura, Moschcowitz syndrome. https://core.ac.uk/download/11855967.pdf (accessed on 12th July 2025).

21. D'Onofrio, M., Giannotti, G., Grecchi, A., Rizzo, S., et al. (2019). Clinical use of contrast-enhanced ultrasound beyond the liver: A focus on renal, splenic, and pancreatic applications. https://core.ac.uk/download/217598870.pdf (accessed on 12th July 2025).

22. Fantin, A., Sperti, C., Dalla Bona, E., Pozza, G., Valmasoni, M., & Beltrame, V. (2016). Solid-pseudopapillary tumor of the pancreas: A single center experience. https://core.ac.uk/download/80155265.pdf (accessed on 12th July 2025).

23. Hofstad, E. F., Langø, T., Mårvik, R., Sánchez-Margallo, F. M., et al. (2017). Laparoscopic pancreas surgery: Image guidance solutions. https://core.ac.uk/download/322428869.pdf (accessed on 12th July 2025).

24. Lamb, K. M., Latona, J. A., Maley, W. R., Pucci, M., et al. (2016). Modified Appleby procedure with arterial reconstruction for locally advanced pancreatic adenocarcinoma: A literature review and report of three unusual cases. https://core.ac.uk/download/46976111.pdf (accessed on 12th July 2025).

25. *Focal Spot, Spring 2008*. (2008). Bernard Becker Medical Library Archives. Washington University School of Medicine https://core.ac.uk/download/129069364.pdf (accessed on 12th July 2025).

26. Stevenson, W. S. (2024). Ultrasonographic evaluation of splenic nodules and masses with B-Flow interrogation correlates with cytologic or histopathologic characterization as benign or malignant. https://core.ac.uk/download/618318363.pdf (accessed on 12th July 2025).

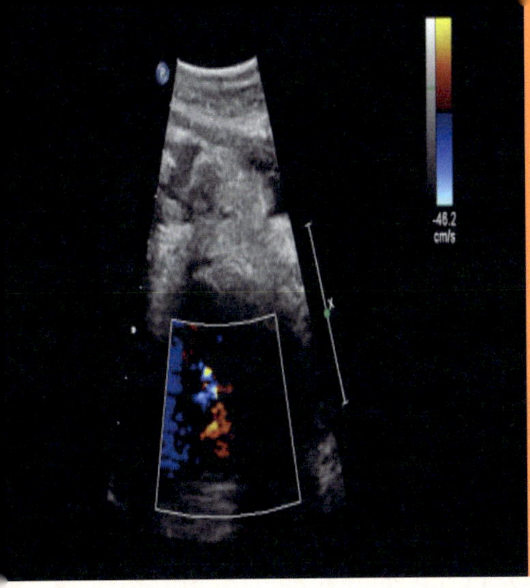

Chapter 11

AORTA AND INFERIOR VENA CAVA (IVC) ULTRASOUND

Contents

Introduction

The circulatory system of humans has a rich network of blood vessels, the aorta and inferior vena cava (IVC) being two of the most important ones among them. The aorta is the largest artery of the body, originating in the left ventricle of the heart and extending down to supply oxygenated blood to various organs and tissues. On the other hand, it is the responsibility of the IVC to return deoxygenated blood from the body below back into the heart, and this is important in the prevention of blood circulation. Ultrasound scanning of the vessels provides an innocuous method of assessing their function and structure, as well as for finding out any possible abnormalities or diseases influencing cardiovascular health. Through imaging study integration, clinicians can make appropriately informed decisions regarding patient management and treatment selection. Ultrasound of the aorta and IVC has become significant not only for diagnosis but also for preoperative assessment. Familiarity with the subtler details of the anatomy of structures that enclose the vessels is critical; abnormalities such as in renal vessels can affect surgical intervention and results. For instance, the presence of more than one renal artery or renal vein drainage variations could make surgical interventions cumbersome and necessitate customized techniques. In looking at literature that points to such vascular anatomical variations, it is obvious that detailed knowledge of vascular anatomy matters in clinical practice and in taking care of patients. This emphasizes the value of ultrasound not only as a diagnostic tool but as an integral component of preoperative preparation and risk assessment. The advent of newer ultrasound modalities further enhanced the ability to image the aorta and IVC in detail, ultimately changing clinical practice for cardiovascular disease. Improvements in image quality have provided more accurate diagnoses of such disorders as an aortic aneurysm or caval thrombosis, with potentially fatal consequences if left undiagnosed. As ultrasound abnormalities become more recognized by skilled interpreters, they can better tailor treatment to correct particular abnormalities. Furthermore, educating doctors in recognizing the relevance of anatomical variations—such as studies on renal vessel variations—will facilitate improved understanding of the interconnectedness of vascular structures and improved patient care. Through this essay, it is hoped to dissect the complexity of aorta and IVC ultrasounds, accentuating their diagnostic importance and relevance in clinical practice, and ultimately guide readers through the intricacies of vascular imaging (Figure 11.1).

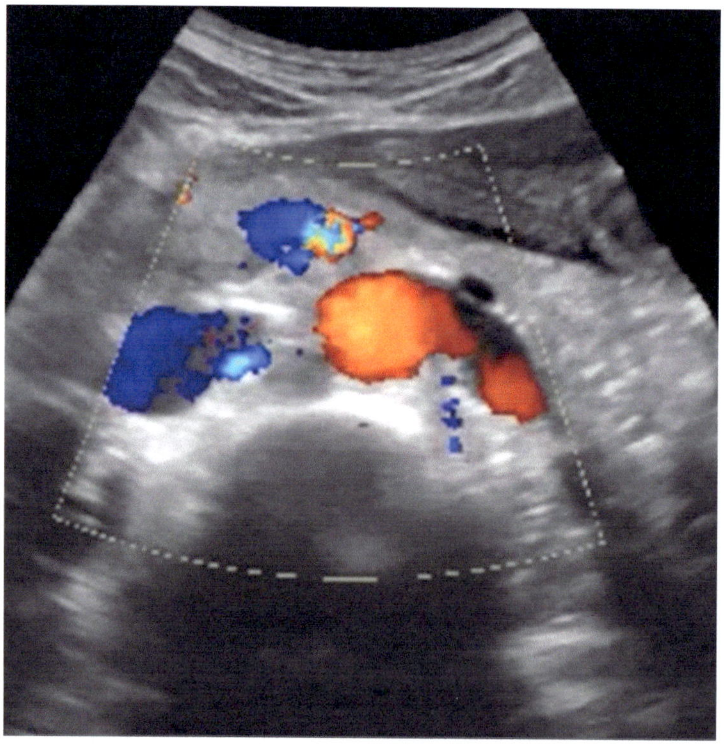

Figure 11.1. Aorta and inferior vena cava (IVC) ultrasound.

Source: sonosim.com/ aorta-inferior-vena-cava-ivc-anatomy-physiology-ultrasound-training.https:// cdn11.bigcommerce.com/s-6er7072zcb/images/stencil/640w/products/168/1233/aorta_ivc_ ultrasound_64954.1652910946.jpg?c=1

Definition of Aorta and Inferior Vena Cava

The aorta, the largest artery of the body, is a vital conduit for oxygenated blood from the heart to the remaining systemic circulation. It originates from the left ventricle, rises, arcs, and descends through the thoracic and abdominal cavities. Its structure is vital in maintaining regular hemodynamic function and comprises three layers, that is, the intima, media, and adventitia. The elastic property of the aorta allows it to accommodate the high-pressure bloodstream developed secondary to cardiac contraction. Elasticity is crucial for effective circulation, as it helps in dampening the pulsatile flow developed by the heartbeat and delivers a steady supply of oxygenated blood to the vital organs. Consequently, learning the anatomy and physiology of the aorta regarding the use of ultrasound examination, wherein it is capable of indicating signs of pathological alteration of its wall, is a must. The inferior vena cava (IVC), on the other hand, plays a significant role in the venous return system by bringing deoxygenated blood from the lower limbs back to the heart. Formed by the joining of the right and left common iliac veins, the IVC ascends with the aorta and empties into the right atrium. The structure is simpler than that of the aorta, with thin walls and a greater lumen. IVC diameter may be a reflection of a patient's intravascular volume status and is thus a region of interest in ultrasound assessment, particularly in critical care and pediatrics. IVC diameter measurement through ultrasound has been shown to accurately predict fluid status and guide clinical decisions, especially in children and neonates. Therefore, accurate interpretation of the IVC during ultrasonography is important in hemodynamic interpretation and the successful management of patient care. Ultrasound assessment of the aorta and IVC offers crucial information about cardiovascular health. New imaging technologies enable doctors to visualize these big vessels in real time, building a dynamic image that can help diagnose diseases such as aortic aneurysm, dissection, and venous thromboembolism. For instance, discrimination of normal anatomical variations versus pathological conditions may be critical in the ability to make swift decisions and take corrective measures. Furthermore, a study explainsthe significant differences and standards of the IVC measurements across different populations, particularly in neonates, where there is limited evidence (Teik, 2015). As described in previous investigations, by knowing these anatomical features through ultrasound, clinical plan and treatment guidelines remarkably become improved for patients presenting with cardiovascular abnormalities (Stümper et al., 1963).

Importance of Ultrasound in Vascular Imaging

Application of ultrasound in vascular imaging, particularly in the aorta and inferior vena cava (IVC), is basically indispensable for non-invasive examinations. Ultrasound allows accurate imaging of the vascular anatomy, making it simpler to detect anomalies such as aneurysms or thrombosis at an early stage. As opposed to the other imaging modalities with ionizing radiation potential or contrast agent requirements, ultrasound presents a safe alternative, especially relevant in patient populations at risk, that is, renal impairment. This aspect is promoted by studies that show the effectiveness of ultrasound in vascular integrity evaluation without compromising patient safety. Furthermore, the general availability of ultrasound and relatively low expense make it a cost-effective choice in emergency centers, as well as outpatient settings, where prompt therapy often is essential to the successful outcome of patients. Doppler imaging, as a recent technological improvement in ultrasound, has significantly improved vascular assessments over the last few years. The Doppler techniques permit blood flow patterns and hemodynamic dysfunction to be evaluated with greater precision. In both IVC and aorta imaging, these technologies enable the detection of stenosis, turbulent flow, and other vascular pathologies that may be predictive of underlying pathologies.

These diagnostic capabilities are vital with the increasing rate of cardiovascular disease, in that early detection significantly contributes to patient prognosis. Secondarily, these imaging technologies are secondary to the trend towards minimally invasive procedural treatment, and they provide guidance and monitoring for procedures like stent placement or thrombolytic therapy by providing real-time imaging during the procedure. In addition, ultrasound use in vascular imaging has implications beyond the diagnostic realm; it plays a crucial role in monitoring for disease course and response to treatment. For intervention patients, follow-up scans are needed to follow up on vascular health over time. This longitudinal approach, which is achieved by non-invasive ultrasound, encourages proactive management practices, thus improving patient care in general. Cardiovascular disease being the leading cause of morbidity and mortality, it is thus important to stress the employment of ultrasound for prevention and management. Clinically, employment of ultrasound simplifies the identification of risk factors for cardiovascular disease, creating public health goals at large. Finally, the ongoing refinement of ultrasound techniques has the promise to further improve the accuracy and utility of vascular imaging to aid health care providers in delivering the optimal outcomes for patients in therapeutic as well as diagnostic contexts, in accordance with findings from current investigations into imaging practice (Figure 11.2).

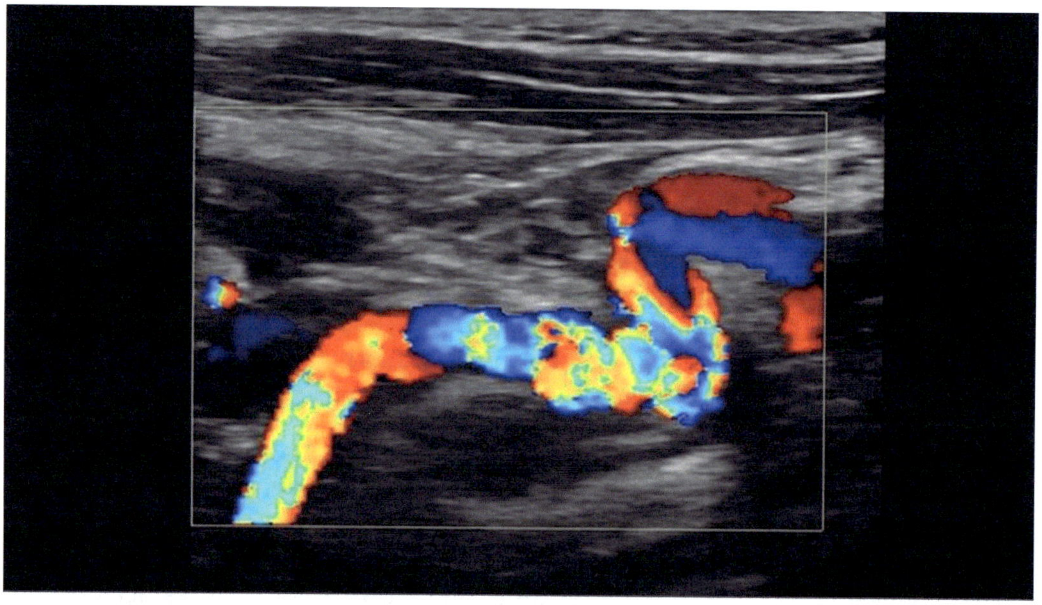

Figure 11.2. Ultrasound in vascular imaging.

Source: Mayfair/ www.radiology.ca (2022). What Is Vascular Ultrasound? https://www.radiology.ca/wp-content/uploads/2022/06/Vasc-US_web.jpg

11.1. Anatomy of the Aorta

The aorta's anatomy is necessary to understand in order to appreciate its function and the potential consequences of some medical conditions. The aorta, which is the largest artery in the body, starts at the left ventricle of the heart and proceeds downward into the abdominal cavity. There are multiple components of the aorta: the ascending aorta, arch of the aorta, descending thoracic aorta, and abdominal aorta. There are several segments, with each acting as a channel for oxygenated blood circulating from the heart to the body's tissues. The aorta's structural complexity which deals with high-pressure blood, requires a strong elastic layer that can be expansive during systole and recoil when diastole occurs, so it can ensure a constant supply of blood. Identification of these anatomic features assists in the assessment of age-related changes, disease processes, and their implications for vascular health in ultrasound examinations. Assessment of the anatomy of the aorta is a significant feature in the diagnosis of vascular disease and any associated complications in aorta and IVC ultrasound. Ultrasound imaging is a non-invasive method to image the structure and disease of the aorta. For example, pathologies such as aortic aneurysms or dissections may be diagnosed from careful assessment of the diameter and contour of the aorta. Furthermore, ultrasound provides real-time imaging that enables clinicians to track over time and modify interventions accordingly. Assessment of the aorta and IVC patency and integrity is important, particularly in surgeries such as organ transplantation, where vascular integrity significantly contributes to the success of the surgery and the fate of the patient, as research on the success of transplantation has identified (Ruemenapf et al., 1998).

In addition, the aorta's relationship with the inferior vena cava is particularly relevant in some clinical situations, including after liver transplantation. Patency of both vessels is significant because disruption or abnormalities in the aorta can have profound effects on venous return through the IVC. For instance, thrombosis of the hepatic artery or complications of primary liver failure can cause difficulties in controlling blood flow dynamics. Specific imaging technologies like angiography are then generally employed to further examine pathways if there are anomalies detected by ultrasound or if results are not conclusive (Bron et al., 1985). By completely understanding the aorta's anatomy and how it coexists with the inferior vena cava, medical practitioners are better equipped to cope with complex clinical conditions and enhance patient care (Figure 11.3).

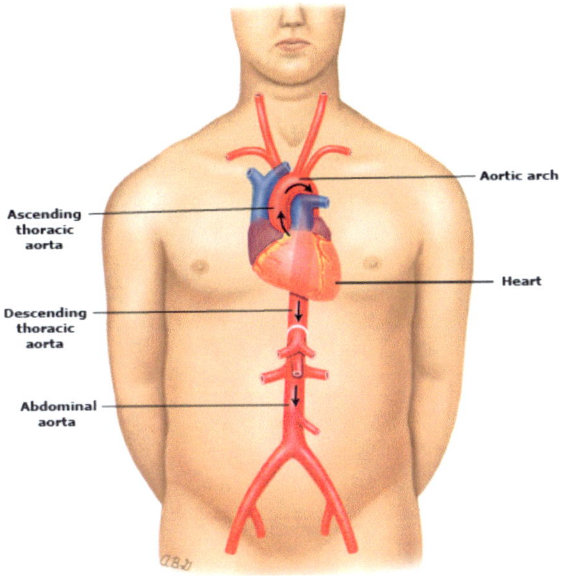

Figure 11.3. Anatomy of the aorta.

Source: https://www.uptodate.com/services/app/contents/graphic/view/PI/74006/AortaanatomyPI.jpg

11.1.1. Sections of the Aorta

The aorta, the largest artery of the body, is composed of several distinct segments that are responsible for delivering oxygen-rich blood from the heart to the peripheral tissues. It is present in four large segments: the ascending aorta, aortic arch, descending aorta, and abdominal aorta. The ascending aorta begins at the left ventricle and continues to the aortic arch. This area is responsible for the supply of blood to the coronary arteries that perfuse the heart muscle itself. Transesophageal echocardiography (TEE) is employed in a routine manner to provide clear, detailed images of these cardiac structures, providing useful information for pathology such as aortic dissection or congenital heart disease where anomalous anatomical positions can render it challenging to evaluate, demonstrating the utility of visualizing such anatomy as an individual in clinical practice in real-time (Stümper et al., 1963). After the ascending aorta, the aortic arch bends and branches into large vessels that supply blood to the head, neck, and arms. The arch is an important junction where several vessels branch off, such as the brachiocephalic trunk, left common carotid artery, and left subclavian artery. High-resolution imaging technologies, including magnetic resonance angiography and ultrasound, are valuable in assessing the integrity of aortic arches, particularly in patients with diseases like vascular occlusions or aortic aneurysms. Being a vital structure that contributes to the distribution of blood flow, assessing the structure and function of the arch plays an important role in clinical diagnosis and intervention planning. In terms of the ability of ultrasound, imaging techniques that enable enhanced visualization and accurate findings are worth their weight in gold, particularly when assessing patency and potential pathology in these critical vessels (Hennessy et al., 2017).

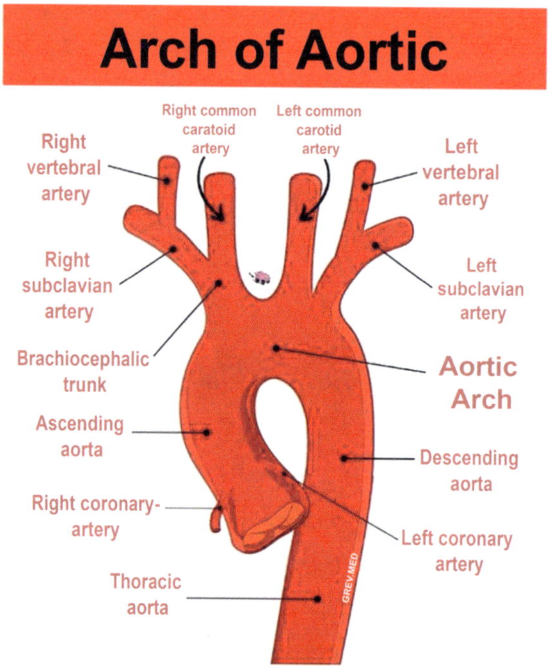

Figure 11.4. Sections of the aorta.

Source: https://external-content.duckduckgo.com/iu/?u=https%3A%2F%2Fi.pinimg.com%2F736x%2F67%2F83%2Fc5%2F6783c5ca5af66520d38153771b9261db.jpg&f=1&nofb=1&ipt=ff8e87c5ef7f28b3f610181bd619ca94bf186afc5607aba7be586d72310fff9d.

Continuing beyond the aortic arch, the descending aorta continues through the thoracic cavity and into the abdominal area, which then classifies it as the abdominal aorta. The thoracic aorta perfuses the organs in the chest, while the abdominal aorta branches off to provide important branches such as the renal arteries and the mesenteric arteries, which perfuse the kidneys and the intestines, respectively. Ultrasonography is particularly valuable in evaluating the abdominal aorta because it is able to detect conditions such as aneurysms or the formation of thrombi through non-invasive means. Besides, it has the capability of doing real-time imaging, and this allows for dynamic assessment of blood supply and vessel structure, the latter of which is vital for preoperative imaging. As a result of its extensive coverage and supply function, assessment of the aorta remains an important component of total vascular imaging in clinical diagnosis and treatment planning (Stümper et al., 1963) (Figure 11.4).

11.1.2. Function of the Aorta in Circulation

The aorta is the principal artery of the body's circulatory system, serving as the fundamental pathway for the distribution of oxygen-rich blood originating from the heart to various tissues and organs.

The aorta starts in the left ventricle and ascends before bending, forming an arch that branches into the carotid arteries and subclavian arteries. This anatomical arrangement enables the aorta to distribute the blood efficiently, serving the upper part of the body, including the head, neck, and arms. In addition, when it travels down through the thoracic and abdominal cavities, it divides into smaller arteries, ensuring even peripheral parts of the body are well supplied with blood. The aorta's ability to accommodate varying blood pressures during the cardiac cycle—expanding during systole and recoiling during diastole—augments its role in maintaining a steady flow of blood, which is critical to organ perfusion and general cardiovascular condition.

The dynamic nature of the aorta is crucial not only for systemic circulation but also for meeting the body's varying demands, particularly during exercise. With increased activity, the heart pumps blood more forcefully, producing higher pressures in the aorta. The increased pressure status enables tissues requiring increased oxygen supply to receive adequate quantities. Aorta elasticity plays an important role in cushioning the pulsatile supply from the heart, converting the intermittent flow into continuous flow. These characteristics are vital in preventing extreme fluctuations in blood pressure that could lead to end-organ damage or compromise perfusion.

The structural integrity and mechanical function of the aorta thus play a pivotal role in the regulation of cardiovascular dynamics under various physiological conditions and reinforce its value both in health and disease. An understanding of the aorta's role is similarly relevant to its clinical significance, particularly to diagnostic imaging like ultrasound. Procedures such as aorta and inferior vena cava (IVC) ultrasound have become the focus in assessing cardiovascular health.

Imaging methods enable the measurement of aortic diameter and elasticity, which are critical indicators of cardiovascular disease, including aneurysm or hypertension. Awareness of the relationship between the aorta and the IVC enables clinicians to assess volume status and cardiac function. For example, Assaad et al. (2017) states that monitoring water accumulation in lungs and its influence on the aorta is essential in formulating treatment protocols for critical patients in the perioperative period.

Moreover, imaging-based early diagnosis of cardiovascular pathologies is essential in adopting intervention strategies in a timely fashion, thereby averting morbidity and mortality in cardiovascular diseases, as observed in Capotosto et al. (2018). Overall, the complex function of the aorta in circulation makes it crucial in both clinical diagnoses and physiological processes (Figure 11.5).

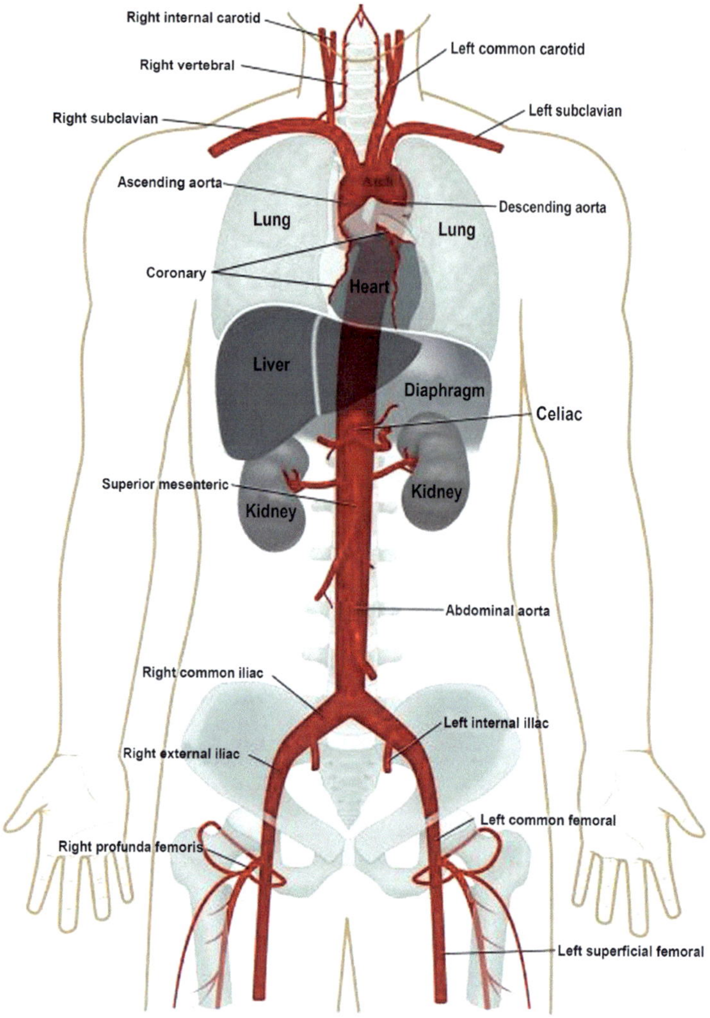

Figure 11.5. Function of the aorta in circulation.

Source: Sankhla N. (2024). Aorta. samarpanphysioclinic.com. https://samarpanphysioclinic.com/wp-content/uploads/2024/05/aorta.webp

11.1.3. Common Pathologies Associated with the Aorta

The aorta, as the largest artery of the human body, is subject to various pathologies that can be harmful to cardiovascular well-being. The most common amongst such pathologies is the aortic aneurysm, which is characterized by dilatation in the aortic wall and can be life-threatening in its rupture if untreated. This condition is likely to arise through the interaction between genetic and acquired factors such as hypertension, hyperlipidemia, and atherosclerosis. Ultrasound is one of the most important diagnostic tools for aortic aneurysms, particularly in an emergency medical setting, where it would enable early detection and management. The urgency associated with an aneurysm of the aorta emphasizes the need for good imaging modalities like ultrasound, which can accurately identify aneurysm diameter and shape, thus affecting decision-making in the clinical setting regarding surgery and ongoing management. Another vital pathology of the aorta is aortic dissection, an emergency complication arising due to a tear in the intima of the aortic wall that allows blood to seep between the layers. It can lead to catastrophic complications, including suspended blood supply to vital organs, stroke, or death. The risk factors for aortic dissection include hypertension, connective tissue disorders like Marfan syndrome, and a history of cardiovascular surgeries. Ultrasound is the most pivotal diagnostic device in the diagnosis of aortic dissection, especially in cases of emergency, as it provides real-time imaging of the aorta and can distinguish between true and false lumens. Further, the rapid evaluation provided by ultrasound may initiate early treatment, either operative or medical management, and thus impact patient prognosis and survival. Nutcracker syndrome also introduces an additional complexity to disease processes in the aorta since it entails compression of the left renal vein, typically caused by an anatomically altered aorta or other vascular elements. This compression has the potential to cause renal venous hypertension, presenting in forms of abdominal pain, hematuria, and proteinuria. As not a primary aortic pathology itself, nutcracker syndrome complicates diagnosis, especially because of its often nonspecific presentation. Doppler ultrasound examination is a first-line diagnostic method in the detection of this syndrome because it provides valuable information about the venous blood flow and whether there is a compressive lesion. Although conservative management options are available, surgical options would be required in some patients, making it critical to have an accurate ultrasound diagnosis in determining the best therapeutic course of action to achieve optimal outcomes in the patient (Dojs et al., 2025) (Figure 11.6).

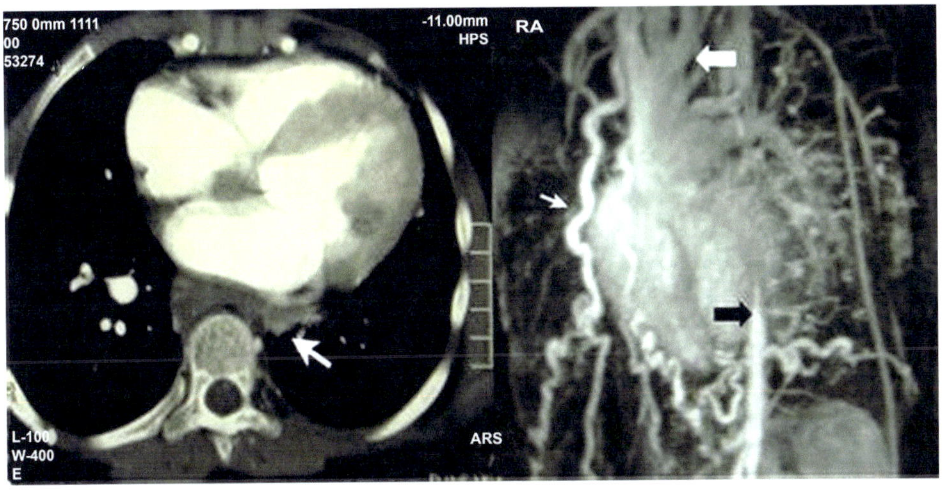

Figure 11.6. Common pathologies associated with the aorta.

Source: Carrel T, Sharipov I, Jalilov A, Sromicki J, Vogt PR. (2022). A case series of rare pathologies of the aorta and the aortic arch in adolescents and younger adults. Front Cardiovasc Med. 9:920614. doi: 10.3389/fcvm.2022.920614.

11.2. Anatomy of the Inferior Vena Cava

The anatomy of the inferior vena cava (IVC) is crucial in correlating with its role in the circulatory system, in this case aorta and IVC ultrasound. The IVC is the largest vein in the human body and plays a role in returning deoxygenated blood from the abdominal organs and lower limbs back to the heart. It typically runs along the right border of the vertebral column, starting at the confluence of the right and left common iliac veins and extending to the right atrium of the heart. Its anatomy is three segments of significance: the abdominal IVC, the thoracic IVC, and the pelvic IVC, with each having variations that complicate diagnostic tests. Understanding such anatomical nuances is essential to clinicians as they read ultrasound images, as they can prevent misdiagnosis during operations such as those on fetuses between 18 to 20 weeks of gestation, in which sonographic features can identify significant congenital anomalies (Richardson et al., 2013).

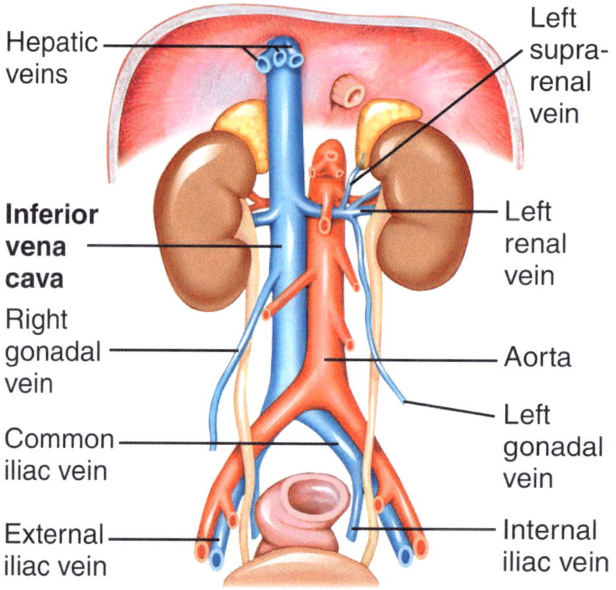

Figure 11.7. Inferior vena cava.

Source: thefreedictionary.com. *https://img.tfd.com/MosbyMD/inferior-vena-cava.jpg*

Moreover, the anatomical aspects of the IVC are often assessed under a number of clinical scenarios, especially in prenatal imaging. The identification of the IVC in fetal sonography is very significant, as any anomaly can lead to severe cardiovascular-related conditions. Sonographers must be familiar with the identification of the course of the IVC as well as with variations in structures that can occur under pathological conditions, as in diseases like tricuspid atresia in right atrial isomerism, where abnormal connections and locations of the IVC can exist (Golbus & Silverman, 1985). The invasive nature of these abnormalities necessitates an intimate understanding of IVC anatomy, which can influence prenatal management and intervention decisions. Accurate identification and assessment of the anatomy of the IVCs can impact patient outcomes, so proficient sonographic ability is important. Advances in ultrasound equipment and technique also contribute to the imaging and assessment of the IVC, enhancing diagnostic accuracy in both prenatal and postnatal contexts. For instance, the inclusion of Doppler imaging enables real-time dynamic evaluation of blood flow within the IVC and awareness of its function. These evaluations not only improve the normal anatomy of the IVC but also detect changes that can be considered as an intervention or further study. In clinical settings, these imaging modalities play a significant role in determining the incidence of structural anomalies, such as those for isomerism and other congenital malformations (Richardson et al., 2013). Detection of the anomalies in utero at 18 weeks of gestation emphasizes the potential for early intervention alongside informed medical decisions, thereby determining the course of subsequent care for the affected individual (Golbus & Silverman, 1985) (Figure 11.7).

11.2.1. Structure and Location of the IVC

The Inferior Vena Cava (IVC) is a significant venous structure and is the principal vessel for returning lower body deoxygenated blood to the heart. Its anatomy begins at the confluence of the right and left common iliac veins, which join together to form the IVC at the level of the fifth lumbar vertebra. This broad, sturdy vein ascends through the belly, positioned behind the abdominal cavity and liver, to become a vital link in the circulatory system. As it ascends, the IVC traverses three regions of anatomy: the abdomen, thorax, and diaphragm, before eventually emptying into the right atrium of the heart.

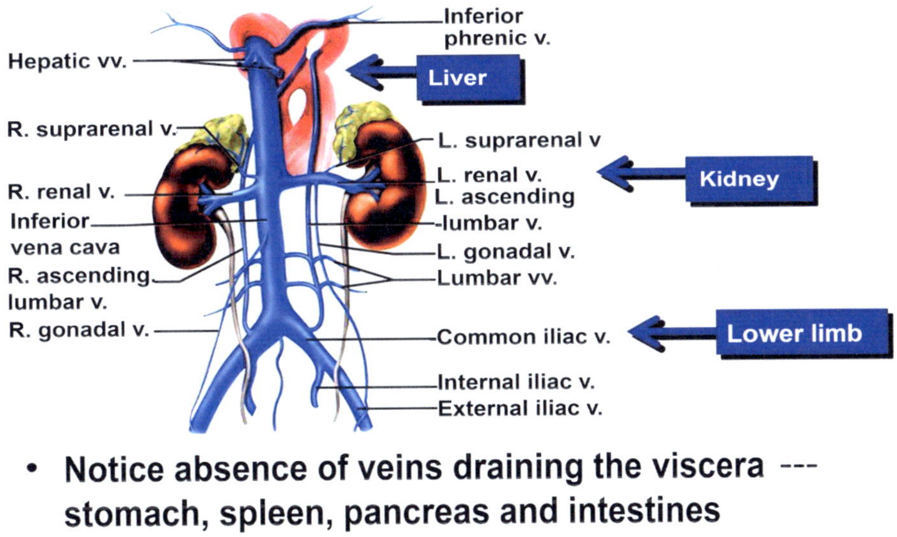

Figure 11.8. Inferior vena cava overview structure.

Source: https://external-content.duckduckgo.com/iu/?u=https%3A%2F%2Fi.pinimg.com%2Foriginals%2F93%2F37%2Fd7%2F9337d75fe42958cb62d937b4449181c5.jpg&f=1&nofb=1&ipt=b29f2e3d09714730a8c6b22ca99c36f7170c87912521b20d083be24a038d0217.

Familiarity with the anatomy and course of the IVC is of crucial significance to clinicians, particularly when interpreting ultrasound scans, as there are huge implications for diagnosis depending on variation. In addition to its anatomical importance, where the IVC is placed is also of special interest when it comes to ultrasound imaging. Its location makes the IVC susceptible to various pathological states, such as thrombosis or compression from surrounding structures that can significantly obstruct venous return. Ultrasound is also an important diagnostic modality for such conditions, allowing real-time imaging of blood flow and vessel integrity. For example, during the ultrasound scan, clinicians can assess the caliber of the IVC and its respiratory reactivity, an important reflection of right atrial pressure. Abnormal reaction in this way can be indicative of underlying cardiovascular disease, reaffirming the IVC's importance in clinical evaluation. Thus, the value of the IVC extends beyond its primitive structure, highlighting its importance in patient evaluation during ultrasound examination. Anatomical variation of the IVC can cause syndromes clinically, most importantly in the case of nutcracker syndrome (NCS), which highlights the complexity of its position and structure. NCS is most commonly ascribed to compression of vessels, particularly where compressive pressure from adjacent vessels is exerted on renal veins. More recent case reports document instances where anatomical deflection, such as an interrupted left IVC with azygos continuation, causes this syndrome. These are optimally diagnosed by high-modality imaging like color Doppler ultrasonography and CT angiography and which highlight the value of these modalities to clinical diagnosis. The relationship between the IVC's anatomy and its location among adjacent anatomical structures contributes to elucidation of the etiology of a majority of syndromes. Greater understanding of these elements facilitates enhancing the evaluation skills during ultrasound examination and supports informed clinical decision-making in the management of venous disease (Abuhamad et al., 2018; Bass et al., 2012) (Figure 11.8).

11.2.2. Role of the IVC in Venous Return

The role of the inferior vena cava (IVC) as a component of venous return is a crucial element of cardiovascular physiology. As the primary route of deoxygenated blood from the lower body to the heart, the IVC provides efficient circulation and maximum venous return under varying physiological conditions. The dynamics of IVC diameter variations are of particular significance in the respiratory cycle due to the fact that expansion and contraction are in accordance with changes in intrathoracic pressure. Familiarity with the variations and ultrasound measurement of IVC diameter has played an important role in calculating central venous pressure (CVP). Studies have also demonstrated that a relationship exists between CVP and IVC diameter, which has given valuable insights into practice in intensive care units. In particular, accurate measurement of IVC diameter is an outpatient technique for determining volume status in patients and hence an important part of cardiovascular examination in most clinical settings. One of the significant characteristics of IVC function is its anatomical variability and points of measurement during ultrasound scanning. Experiments have indicated that the entry point of the IVC into the right atrium best correlates with CVP when determined by transesophageal echocardiography (TEE).

Measurement at this point and other sites of anatomical landmarks is crucial in the understanding of patterns of venous return. The identification of such optimal sites of measurement has not only diagnostic significance but also therapeutic intervention direction, such as central venous catheterization. By examining different anatomic locations (e.g., 2 cm above the diaphragm), physicians can enhance the accuracy of IVC diameter measurements. This identification improves clinical practice and enhances the overall knowledge regarding the IVC's function. The function is to provide cardiovascular homeostasis, especially under states of stress that may threaten venous return. Aside from its essential function in venous return, the IVC participates in many pathological conditions that affect circulatory health. An understanding of its function also involves recognition of complications such as aortocaval fistula (ACF), which, although rare, can alter hemodynamics substantially and present diagnostic challenges. ACF has been found to be present in patients with aortic abdominal aneurysms, producing direct continuity between the aorta and IVC, which alters the venous return dynamics. This makes it a reason for using newer imaging techniques such as CEUS and MRA for the diagnosis of vascular pathology involving the IVC. Early and effective diagnosis is needed, especially in the case of emergencies, where initial treatment could save the patient tremendously. Hence, integration of ultrasound assessment of the IVC into daily clinical practice enables making diagnoses of underlying vascular disease in a timely manner, further increasing the importance of understanding the multi-faceted role of the IVC in venous return and global cardiovascular status (Figure 11.9).

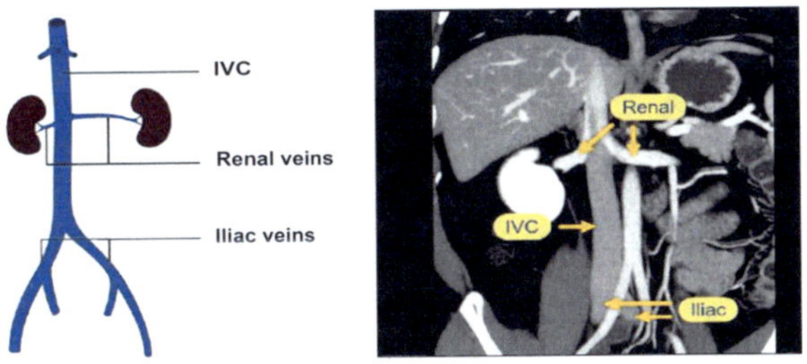

Figure 11.9. Role of the IVC in venous return.

Source: Hartung M. P and Brown A. (2024). Abdominal CT: abdominal veins; litfl.com. https://litfl.com/wp-content/uploads/2023/02/CT-abdomen-Systemic-system.png

11.2.3. Conditions Affecting the IVC

Inferior vena cava (IVC) is a critical structure in venous return, and its physiology can be readily compromised by various anatomical as well as disease conditions. Certain anatomical variations, such as a double or left-sided IVC, can increase difficulties with surgical procedures and result in greater risks on diagnostic imaging studies. As highlighted in an autopsy of a 75-year-old male, a variety of renal vessel variations draining into the IVC were observed, noting anatomical diversity that surgeons must deal with (Jakovcevski et al., 2020). Such vascular anatomy variation may hinder distinct ultrasound visualization of the IVC, which is essential in assessing hemodynamic status and also in the detection of conditions such as thrombosis or compression syndromes. Secondly, extrinsic compression brought about by adjacent structures significantly impacts the function of the IVC.

Pregnancy, tumors, or enlarged lymph nodes can compress the IVC, which can lead to compromised blood flow. The use of ultrasound imaging in such cases cannot be overemphasized; while routine imaging is incapable of revealing the pulsatile flow dynamics in deeply placed vessels, advanced techniques, such as X-ray particle image velocimetry (PIV), offer informative data regarding the behavior of blood flow (Lee et al., 2025). Detection and control of such compressive forces play a significant role not only for diagnosis but also in the management of complications related to the IVC.

Hemodynamic changes caused by various diseases further contribute to the complexity of the IVC condition. For instance, heart failure can elevate central venous pressure, causing IVC distension and thereby making ultrasonographic assessment and interventions difficult. Other diseases, such as cirrhosis, can lead to hepatic venous pressure gradient changes, influencing IVC dynamics. Awareness of these interactions and their implications is essential in developing effective vascular imaging protocols. Consequently, the intricate character of conditions affecting the IVC necessitates an integrated strategy for ultrasound diagnostic processes, informing the demand for continued research into imaging modalities in a bid to improve patient results in vascular health.

11.3. Principles of Ultrasound Imaging

Ultrasound imaging is a workhorse in the assessment of vascular structures, with large roles in imaging of the aorta and inferior vena cava (IVC). With high-frequency sound, ultrasound produces real-time images that enable clinicians to visualize major anatomical landmarks without exposing patients to ionizing radiation. The underlying physiology of this imaging modality is the reflection and transmission of sound waves through various tissues of changing acoustic impedance. This reflection creates echoes that are analyzed to generate two-dimensional images. Most notably, the employment of Doppler ultrasound allows blood flow dynamics to be examined, which is invaluable in assessing conditions such as aortic aneurysms or venous thrombosis. These abilities attest to the value of ultrasound in enhancing diagnostic accuracy and enabling clinical interventions. Evaluation of the IVC by ultrasound is salient in its utility for determining hemodynamic status. The IVC's diameter and dynamics have a close association with blood volume and right atrial pressure, both indicators of a patient's hydration and cardiovascular status.

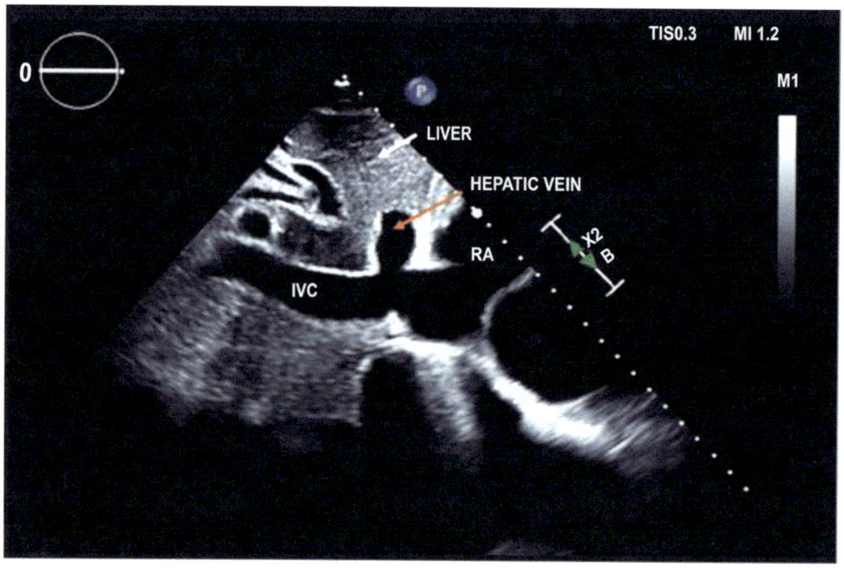

Figure 11.10. Principles of ultrasound imaging of the IVC.

Source: Oesterling A., Gordon A., Babar Fiza B. (2023). Inferior vena cava Point-of-Care Ultrasound. www.openanesthesia.org. https://www.openanesthesia.org/wp-content/uploads/2023/01/12/Inferior-Vena-Cava-Point-of-Care-Ultrasound_figure-2-i81ljh-e1673563114974.png

Due to its lack of invasiveness, ultrasound is an ideal choice compared to more invasive methods. However, although conventional M-mode measurements of IVC diameter are widely applied, they remain susceptible to error, particularly as the veins vary in size with respiration. Improvements in B-mode ultrasound in more recent years have provided more precise assessments of IVC, which allow one to acquire dynamic alterations of size and shape during respiratory cycles. Hence, understanding the advancements and limitations in ultrasound techniques renders IVC examination more trustworthy in the clinical setting (Mesin &Poicastro, 2023). With advancements in ultrasound technology, new uses are continually discovered, with new segmentation and visualization technologies fostering improvements. Automated IVC segmentation through enhancements in image processing algorithms promises to revolutionize vascular structure assessment by clinicians. These types of techniques are capable of giving more standardized and objective measurements, narrowing the possibility of user-dependent errors that may result from manual assessment. Furthermore, the application of B-mode ultrasound techniques possesses colossal advantages in documenting internal jugular vein morphology over traditional techniques. The incorporation of these technical improvements not only enhances diagnostic potential but also holds possibilities for future utilization in alternative clinical conditions. Since non-invasive evaluation remains a high priority in medical imaging, ultrasound imaging concepts will be at the forefront in further enhancing patient care in the fields of cardiovascular medicine (Abuhamad et al., 2018) (Figure 11.10).

11.3.1. Basic Principles of Ultrasound Technology

Understanding the basic principles of the technology of ultrasound is essential to the effective application of this imaging technique to the diagnosis of vascular pathways such as the aorta and inferior vena cava (IVC). Ultrasound is dependent upon the premise of sound waves, whereby high-frequency waves emitted from a transducer travel through the body and reflect off various tissues. These reflected sound waves are, in turn, received by the transducer and converted into electrical signals that form images. The major advantage of ultrasound technology is that it can provide real-time imaging without ionizing radiation, making it a safe option for patients across all age groups. This safety profile is particularly relevant in the case of susceptible groups, like neonates, where recent evidence has documented its validity to quantify the IVC sizes as a marker of intravascular volume status (Teik, 2015). In ultrasound evaluations of the aorta and IVC, it is essential to be aware of the various imaging modalities and parameters for making accurate evaluations. Multiple ultrasound techniques, such as Doppler ultrasound, can provide information regarding blood flow and vessel morphology and enable clinicians to evaluate hemodynamic status in a holistic way. For instance, Doppler imaging has the capability of estimating the velocity of blood flow through vessels and hence enables identification of potential abnormalities such as occlusions or structural defects. Moreover, certain measurements, for example, IVC diameters at different points of respiration, enhance the understanding of preload and volume status in patients. This capability is particularly important because it has been shown through research that normative values of IVC from neonates through adults have been established, hence providing essential reference points for decision-making in the clinical environment (Abuhamad et al., 2018). Use of ultrasound technology in clinical application has significantly enhanced diagnostic performance in vascular assessment, particularly for the IVC and aorta. Through protocols that standardize image acquisition procedures and measurements, clinicians can enhance the reliability of ultrasound findings and facilitate better patient outcomes. For instance, the IVC diameter measurement, a focus of study in recent research, assists in assessing intravascular volume, critical during the management of patients with an array of pathologies. The generation of standardized reference values allows for the assessment of deviations, which can be indicative of issues like dehydration or fluid overload. With ongoing technological innovations, the inclusion of new-generation ultrasound techniques like 3D imaging and computerized measurement remains of immense potential for further streamlining the accuracy and velocity of vascular examination, so ultrasound can remain a cornerstone of modern-day medical diagnostics (Teik, 2015).

11.3.2. Types of Ultrasound Employed in Vascular Imaging

The application of ultrasound in vascular imaging has greatly revolutionized the manner in which clinicians perceive and assess vascular structures, particularly the aorta and inferior vena cava (IVC). Among all the various modes of ultrasound, Doppler ultrasound is an invaluable diagnostic tool. The technique uses the Doppler effect to measure the velocity of blood flow within vessels and detect abnormalities such as stenosis or obstructions. By visualization of flow dynamics, Doppler ultrasound provides critical information on hemodynamic aorta and IVC status and facilitates timely intervention as required. In addition, the ability to quantify flow in real time and with high-resolution imaging significantly contributes to the clinician's ability to understand complex vascular pathologies and tailor treatment plans accordingly. The second important ultrasound imaging modality utilized in vascular imaging is grayscale or B-mode ultrasound, which is primarily structural imaging of the vasculature.

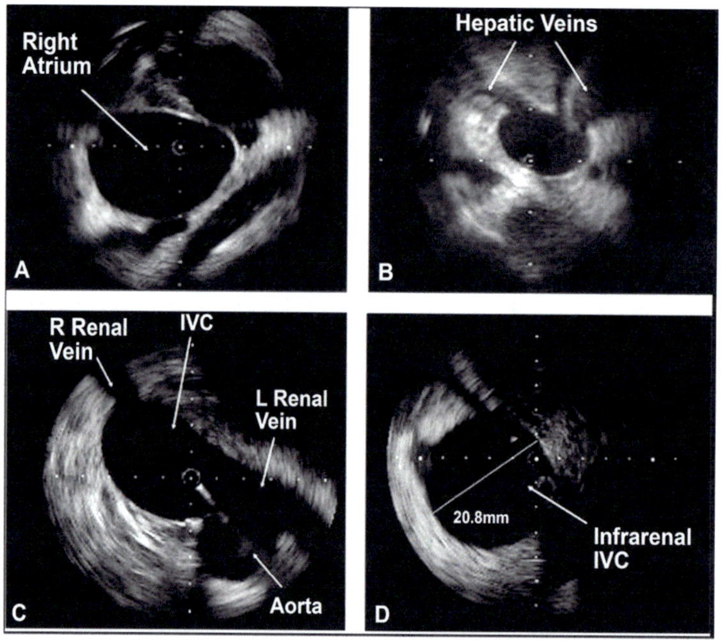

Figure 11.11. Types of ultrasound used in vascular imaging.

Source: Minin, O. (Ed.). (2011). Ultrasound Imaging - Medical Applications. InTech. doi: 10.5772/689. https://www.intechopen.com/chapters/18259

This modality offers an accurate visual description of vessel wall anatomy and is capable of identifying aneurysms, thrombus formation, and other morphological defects. For instance, when evaluating aorta status, B-mode ultrasound is capable of imaging the wall irregularities and the aortic diameter, which can be critical in aortic dissection or aneurysm diagnosis. In addition, the modality is capable of assessing the IVC such that professionals are able to determine correctly its size as well as whether there are any compressions. Utilization of B-mode ultrasound along with Doppler imaging provides an overall understanding of both structural and functional status of the vascular tree, enhancing diagnostic accuracy and patient management. Aside from Doppler and B-mode ultrasound, emerging technologies like CT or three-dimensional (3D) ultrasound are being introduced into vascular imaging as very promising techniques. This technology allows for vascular anomalies to be imaged in a more spatially accurate manner, offering definite advantages over two-dimensional imaging. 3D ultrasound may assist with further comprehension of complex vascular anatomy, such as the aorta and IVC, and is particularly beneficial when planning for surgical intervention. For example, 3D reconstructions may assist in preoperative assessment by rendering the vascular relationship and complications clearer to the surgeon. As highlighted in recent studies, the adoption of future-proof imaging modalities as part of routine practice is important for improved outcomes, particularly in cases where conventional imaging modalities prove to be insufficient (Anwar et al., 2018; Jakovcevski et al., 2020). In general, these developments underscore the landmark development of ultrasound modalities in vascular imaging that enhances diagnostic capability and patient care (Figure 11.11).

11.3.3. Advantages of Ultrasound over Other Imaging Modalities

Ultrasound imaging is advantageous in numerous ways that have made it a sought-after modality for aortic and inferior vena cava (IVC) assessment compared to other modalities. The first major advantage of ultrasound is that it is not invasive, meaning that it minimizes patient discomfort and does not require the use of sedation or contrast agents typically employed in CT and MRI scans. Moreover, ultrasound employs sound waves and is thus safer, particularly for susceptible populations such as pregnant women and children. Because ultrasound offers real-time images, dynamic hemodynamic and vascular characteristics may be assessed, which is significant in pathology such as an aortic aneurysm or IVC thrombosis. In these cases, ultrasound permits immediate clinical decision-making, enhances patient management, yet preserves high diagnostic precision. The second important advantage of ultrasound is that it is cost-effective and accessible. Compared to CT or MRI, which might require specialized machines and longer waiting lists, ultrasound can be rapidly done in various clinical settings, including outpatient clinics and emergency rooms. Because ultrasound is accessible, it ensures timely diagnosis and treatment of vascular illnesses, particularly because cardiovascular ailments are extremely common. Overall, the operating cost of ultrasound is much lower, and health systems are therefore able to utilize resources more meaningfully. While cardiovascular diseases remain the leading causes of morbidity and mortality, upgrading access to effective imaging modalities is the most significant challenge for improving patient outcomes. In this regard, therefore, ultrasound emerges as an effective imaging modality that allows for prompt detection and monitoring of aorta and IVC-related illnesses. Lastly, the ultrasonography imaging is enhanced by the real-time visualization of adjacent structures. This feature is particularly beneficial in the assessment of the aorta and IVC in the context of the intricate anatomy of the retroperitoneal space. In contrast to other modalities, such as CT, that are contrast and ionizing radiation-dependent, ultrasound can be used directly to visualize the vascular structures and the tissues around them, with the potential to diagnose conditions such as idiopathic retroperitoneal fibrosis (IRF) that may encapsulate vital vessels without injurious complications to the patient. The ability to define pulsatile flow in vessels is the sole aspect that distinguishes ultrasound from other techniques, and it is thus a precious tool in understanding hemodynamic changes. Integration of such information into treatment makes a contribution to the diagnostic and therapeutic measures available for management of vascular well-being, demonstrating the potency of ultrasound in contemporary medical imaging (Rees & Twahirwa, 2008; Capotosto et al., 2018).

11.4. Ultrasound Techniques for Aorta Imaging

Ultrasound imaging of the aorta has advanced significantly and has enabled clinicians to have more precision in evaluating this vital artery. Such methods most commonly utilize both 2D and Doppler modes of ultrasound that provide vital information regarding the structural integrity and hemodynamic functioning of the aorta. Optimal visualization of measurements of the aorta occurs with the 2D method, thus enabling aneurysms or dissections to be diagnosed. Conversely, Doppler ultrasound evaluates blood flow kinematics, providing information regarding blood velocity and potential blockages. With advances in ultrasound technology, the use of such methods has expanded to other clinical conditions, offering quick, non-invasive, and real-time diagnostics that are crucial in expediting medical intervention.

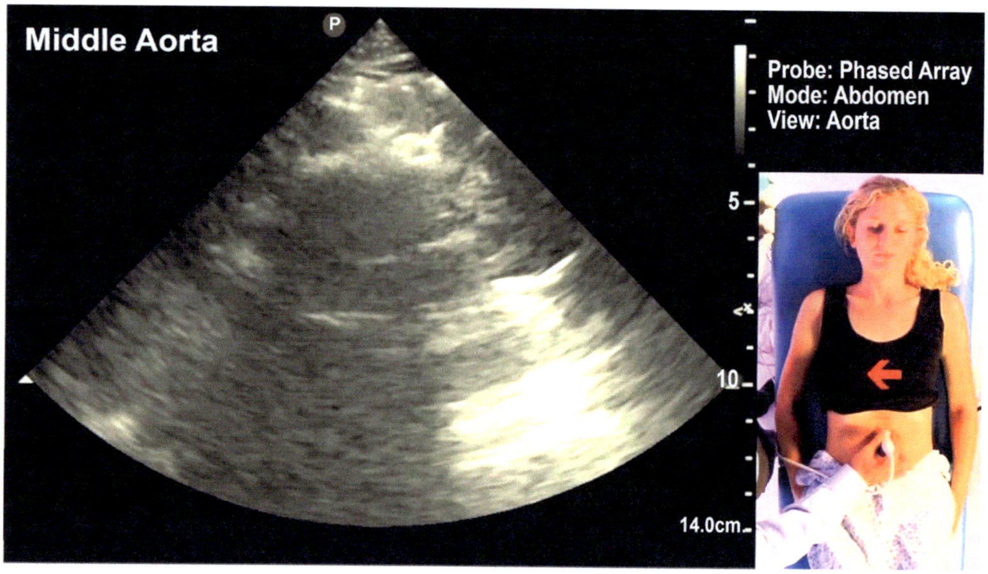

Figure 11.12. Ultrasound techniques for aorta imaging.

Source: POCUS 101. How to Perform Ultrasound of the Aorta -STEP by STEP. https://www.youtube.com/watch?v=p4qTMQZW4sk.

With respect to the inferior vena cava (IVC), ultrasound gives supplementary information that is helpful for general vascular assessment. A stiff and dilated IVC could represent increased intravascular volume, a situation frequently encountered in heart failure patients, and thereby relates IVC measurement to systemic outcomes of health (Albani et al., 2022). Through advanced techniques such as speckle tracking and motion analysis, doctors can quantify the phasic changes in vascular diameter with respiration and thus improve diagnostic sensitivity. These methods also hold promise for broader applications in the assessment of other medical conditions, underlining the necessity of standardized protocols in ultrasound examination to maximize reproducibility and clinical utility. Despite the advances in ultrasound techniques, standardization and accuracy continue to be concerns when one assesses the aorta and IVC in populations with varying characteristics. Variability of operator experience and skills can lead to measurement differences, which is crucial when making clinical decisions. As per studies, a lack of standard procedure prevents reproducibility of results, proving the need for further study and modification of the techniques in ultrasonography (Teik, 2015). Moreover, future studies aiming to test new image-processing algorithms can make vascular tests more consistent and expand their use in various medical situations. While the medical community strives to incorporate standardization in vascular ultrasound, aorta and IVC imaging can become much better, encouraging better patient outcomes (Figure 11.12).

11.4.1. Transabdominal Ultrasound Procedures

Transabdominal ultrasound scans are valuable for the assessment and evaluation of the aorta and the inferior vena cava (IVC), and they offer both non-invasive and comprehensive diagnostic capability. This technique employs high-frequency sound waves to create real-time images of vascular tissue so that practitioners can visualize anatomy and diagnose conditions such as aneurysms or thrombosis accurately. A transabdominal approach, in particular, in evaluating the aorta and IVC, is often preferred as it can provide a good view of these large vessels with a minimally invasive technique. Second, ultrasound technology has been advanced to improve image quality so that diameter measurement and flow patterns are obtainable more easily. Incorporation of these techniques has significantly enhanced the vascular imaging profile to enable early diagnosis and treatment in practice.

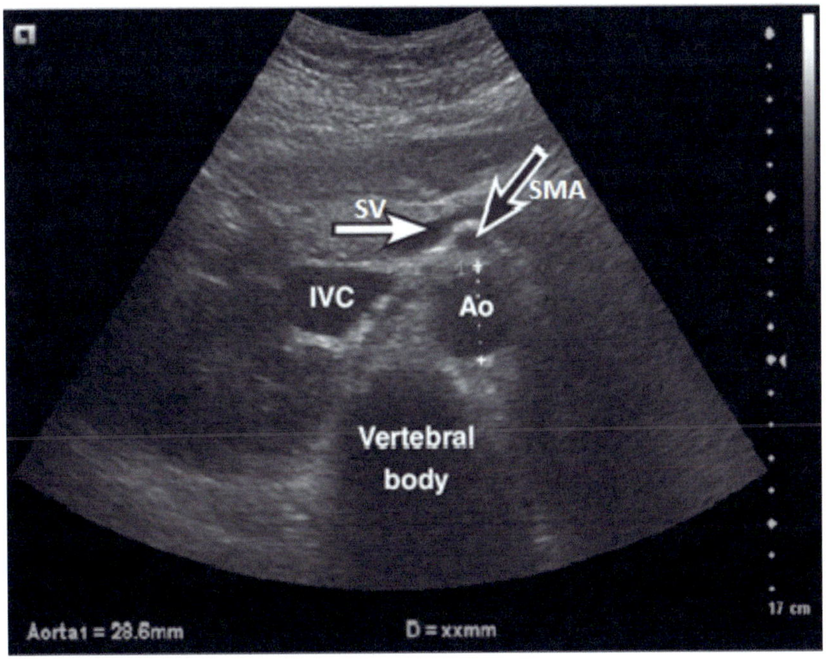

Figure 11.13. Transabdominal ultrasound procedures.

Source: Hwang, James & Kimberly, Heidi & Liteplo, Andrew & Sajed, Dana. (2011). An evidence-based approach to emergency ultrasound. Emergency medicine practice. 13. 1-27; quiz 27.

One of the significant advantages of transabdominal ultrasound to assess the aorta and IVC is that it may direct treatment of other vascular illnesses. For instance, if an abdominal aortic aneurysm (AAA) was detected on ultrasound, follow-up or surgical therapy may be directed on the basis of measurement of the aortas size. Similarly, conditions such as IVC thrombosis are readily diagnosed by ultrasound, allowing treatment to avoid complications such as pulmonary embolism. The absence of invasiveness of ultrasound is particularly valuable in patient groups that are not able to tolerate more invasive imaging modalities, thus improving access to vital diagnostic information. Notably, the increasing use of ultrasound in education emphasizes how crucial it is; the utility of ultrasounds as an educational tool enhances the quality of students learning processes, providing them with the necessary skills useful in real clinical scenarios (Gupta et al., 2011). Transabdominal ultrasound also has crucial diagnostic and therapeutic roles following interventions like EVAR. Complications such as type II endoleaks, the most frequently encountered following such procedures, can be efficiently assessed by ultrasound scanning. An early detection allows for the provision of immediate management strategies, which may include direct percutaneous intervention, such as thrombin injection, thus emphasizing the value of ultrasound in not only diagnosis but also management of post-procedure complications (Gabriel et al., 2018). Thus, transabdominal ultrasound not only allows for initial assessments but also provides life-changing data that dictates real-time treatment. As medical science improves and image study usage becomes more widespread, utilization and evolution of ultrasound modalities remain crucial in maximizing patient care outcomes within vascular medicine (Figure 11.13).

11.4.2. Doppler Ultrasound Applications

Doppler ultrasound has emerged as a primary technology in the assessment of vascular structures such as the aorta and inferior vena cava (IVC). By employing the Doppler effect, this imaging method provides the capability for the non-invasive measurement of blood flow velocity and direction in these structures. Such capability's clinical utility is emphasized in applications including cardiovascular diagnosis and management of fluid status in critically ill patients. Accurate measurement of IVC diameter and respiratory variation in it can provide key information regarding right atrial pressure and central venous pressure, both of which are pivotal factors in fluid management decision-making and the prognosis of heart failure patients. Therefore, Doppler ultrasound techniques focused on these anatomical sites are components of contemporary vascular diagnostics that ensure safety and efficacy at the expense of less invasive procedures. The ability to examine vascular flow dynamics through the application of Doppler ultrasound also assists in recognizing pathological states that can affect the aorta and IVC. For instance, stenosis, occlusions, or development of thrombus can be identified with typical alterations in blood flow patterns. In the case of an increase in intravascular volume, such as evidenced by dilation of the IVC, Doppler ultrasound is a very significant diagnostic tool. Recent advancements in image-processing algorithms have enhanced the technique's accuracy to enable clinicians to quantitatively analyze phasic vascular deformations. The advancement has the potential to make the reproducibility and clinical usefulness of Doppler measurements between and within various patient populations and clinical conditions more standardized, avoiding existing pitfalls in standardization and operator-dependent variability, which are still challenges in practice today (Albani et al., 2022). In addition, use of Doppler ultrasound in emergency departments has significantly transformed critical care practice. Use of this tool in practice enables rapid measurement of important cardiac and vascular parameters, facilitating instant decision-making during resuscitation efforts. In evaluating left ventricular function and in the detection of abnormalities such as cardiac tamponade or right ventricular overload, Doppler ultrasound proves to be very helpful. Studies have shown that even the least specialized practitioners can get a good correlation with expert grading when they apply concentrated ultrasound procedures, which further gives credibility to this modality in acute settings (Franco-Gruntorad & Conorado, 2015). Accordingly, as the field of application of Doppler ultrasound continues to expand, its application in the management of complicated vascular diseases, especially concerning the aorta and IVC, is bound to gain even more prominence in both diagnostic and therapeutic contexts.

11.4.3. Aortic Ultrasound Result Interpretation

Ultrasound findings interpretation is a part of the determination of cardiovascular status, especially in patients who present with an intricate medical history or present with abnormal symptoms. Aortic ultrasonographic imaging provides useful information about the morphology and function of the vessels, enabling clinicians to evaluate potential abnormalities such as aneurysms, dissections, or strictures. The usefulness of ultrasound as an imaging modality that is not invasive offers real-time imaging, particularly useful in the clinical setting. Imaging of the aortic lumen and adjacent structures offers practitioners essential information that guides management decisions, including surgery, drug titration, and monitoring strategies. But explanation of these images requires a holistic impression of the patient's clinical picture because individual findings on ultrasound do not necessarily mirror the underlying pathophysiological processes accurately, and therefore integration of clinical data is required for accurate diagnosis and treatment. Also, the interaction between the aorta and inferior vena cava (IVC) are important consideration during the interpretation of ultrasound findings. Their interdependence is significant in determining preload measurements and hemodynamic stability as a whole. Aortic volume has been found to be directly correlated with global end-diastolic volume (GEDV) by recent research, and thus, aortic measurement must be included while interpreting preload markers obtained with ultrasound. For instance, a larger aortic volume is associated with increased GEDV, suggesting that a proper assessment of the aorta enhances clinical decision making for fluid handling as well as for hemodynamic optimization since aortic volume explains a large proportion of variance in GEDV during ultrasound assessment (Akohov et al., 2019). Understanding of such interactions is important for clinicians who must balance invasive monitoring against the merits of non-invasive technologies like ultrasound. The implications of aortic ultrasound extend beyond structural evaluation to incorporate early diagnosis and management strategies in select clinical situations.

As demonstrated by prenatal diagnosis, the ability to detect congenital cardiac abnormalities through ultrasound significantly impacts management and patient outcomes. The same is true in adult medicine, such that accurate interpretation of aortic ultrasound may guide therapeutic intervention, assist in operative planning, and improve patient prognostication. With the help of the might of high-technology ultrasound, such as Doppler imaging, an improved understanding of blood flow dynamics, as well as associated complications like turbulent flow as it pertains to stenosis or thrombus formation, is made easier. In this case, the use of ultrasound in cardiovascular assessment is not just restricted to visualization but serves to play an important role in personalizing management strategies that take into account subtleties surrounding aortic as well as IVC health (Golbus & Silverman, 1985) (Figure 11.14).

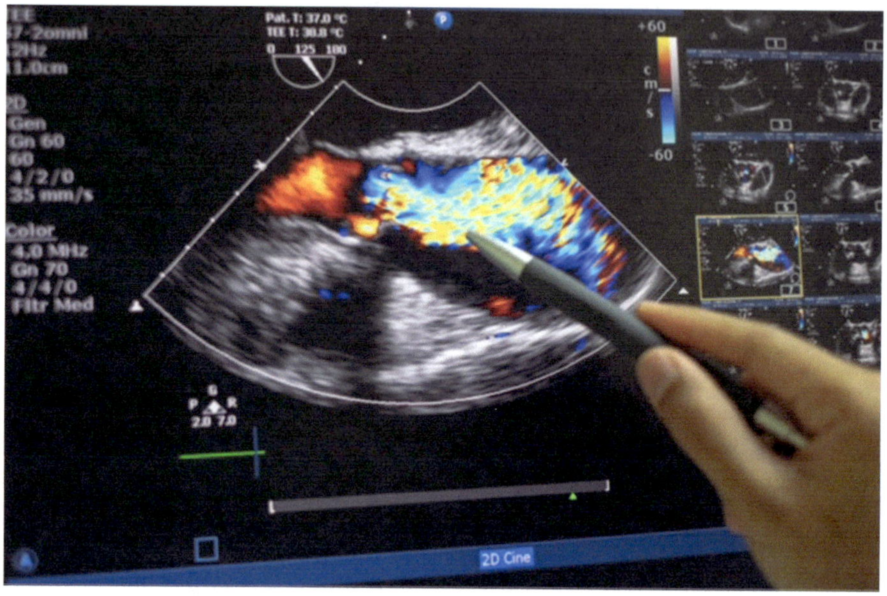

Figure 11.14. The interpretation of aortic ultrasound results.

Source: Pitchayanan *Kongkaew/iStock. https://www.istockphoto.com/photo/echocardiography-gm1188396421-336057621*

11.5. Ultrasound Techniques for IVC Imaging

The use of ultrasound in inferior vena cava (IVC) imaging provides a non-invasive and feasible technique for the assessment of vascular disease, most notably in patients with specific clinical needs. The procedure is especially valuable in cases when standard imaging techniques are hazardous, such as among patients with impaired renal function who are threatened by nephrotoxicity from contrast media. Apart from its safety profile, ultrasound is also aided by its portability, real-time imaging, and ability to assess hemodynamic status through dynamic evaluation of vessel collapsibility and flow patterns, yielding a highly useful tool in the preoperative setting and in emergency situations. With the improvements in Doppler ultrasound methods, clinicians can obtain precise information about the blood flow through the IVC to support the diagnosis of diseases such as thrombosis or venous obstruction, hence preventing delayed interventions that could improve patient outcomes. With the inclusion of new techniques such as echocardiography, IVC imaging can be improved through thorough evaluations of the structural components of the heart as well as neighboring vessels. Though traditionally used for cardiac evaluation, echocardiographic techniques such as cross-sectional echocardiography and Doppler ultrasonography can be adapted for IVC evaluation. These imaging modalities enable detailed visualization of the IVC by obtaining images of the structure from multiple planes, which can elucidate not just anatomical structures, but also functional attributes relevant to venous return dynamics understanding. The synergy of these imaging modalities is significant in the ability to make a diagnosis of collateral circulation, which is a typical response to IVC thrombosis or occlusion. Consequent to this, ultrasound and echocardiographic examinations combined provide a sound paradigm for thoroughly assessing IVC wellness and function. In addition, advances in ultrasound technology have a significant role to play in the usability of the methods in many clinical applications. For instance, ultrasound contrast agents are under research to enhance image quality in venous imaging, a point that is crucial because clear visualization of the IVC is essential to enable appropriate diagnosis and treatment planning. This is particularly the case in patients with severe renal disease, where conventional imaging techniques may be harmful. The application of ultrasound with new agents also bridges the gap of limitations with the conventional ultrasound by offering improved visualization of vascular structures without the associated nephrotoxicity of conventional contrast material and thus enabling more informed clinical choice. With continued advancement in technology, ultrasound techniques still hold the promise to increase diagnostic precision and patient management in vascular imaging, particularly of the IVC and aorta (Figure 11.15).

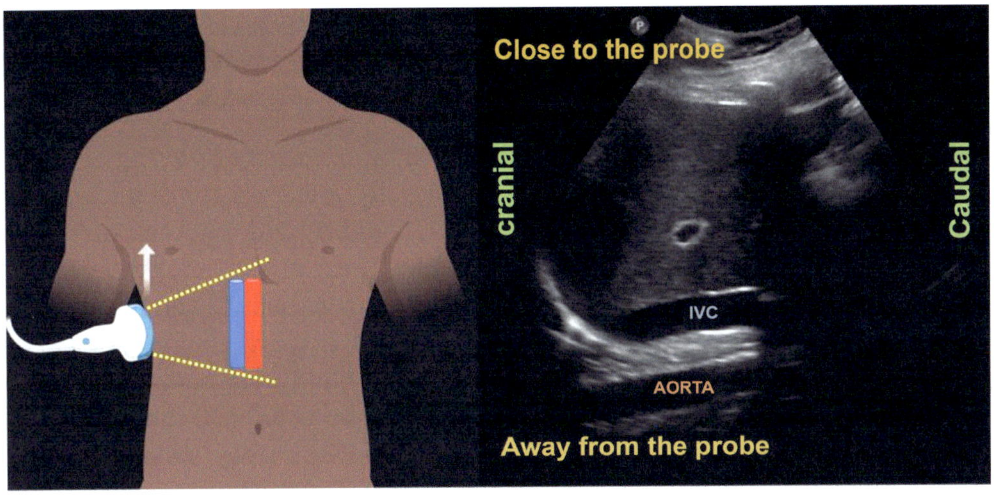

Figure 11.15. Ultrasound techniques for IVC imaging.

Source: Abhilash Koratala (2020). Inferior Vena Cava POCUS: The Basics of Image Acquisition. Renal Fellow Network. https://www.renalfellow.org/2020/03/20/inferior-vena-cava-pocus-the-basics-of-image-acquisition/

11.5.1. Patient Positioning and Preparation

Optimal performance of ultrasound imaging, particularly for aorta and inferior vena cava (IVC) evaluation, relies heavily on optimal patient positioning and preparation. Accurate positioning enables the ultrasound technician to obtain clean images to their maximum capability and facilitates patient comfort while taking the exam. The patient can typically be positioned supine because access to the thoracic and abdominal regions is readily available in this position, and both of these areas have the aorta and IVC. Also, slight accommodations can be made; for example, a left lateral decubitus position will at times assist in better visualization of the aorta and diminish interference from bowel gas. In addition, informing patients that they will have to remain still for the ultrasound is helpful to get good images and avoid duplication, which is time-wasting and adds patient exposure to the test. Equally critical is the preparation time prior to performing the ultrasound. This could be fasting for several hours, which could be absolutely necessary to get good images, particularly of the aorta and IVC. Preparing the patient in this manner avoids an excessive amount of gas and food material within the gastrointestinal tract that could interfere with ultrasound waves. Also, educating patients to wear loose clothing and providing them with a proper gown can make the process more accessible and also aid in their comfort and modesty during examination. Proper preparation sets the stage for a trouble-free process and helps to provide a better experience for the patient according to best practices within clinical settings. This rigorous methodology in positioning and preparation serves to highlight the necessity of an integrated approach in medical imaging, necessary for accurate diagnostic findings.

Education and competency in patient positioning are also vital to the ultrasound practitioner since the skill set will directly affect image quality and patient outcome. For instance, in one of the studies on renal nurse education in performing IVC ultrasound, a structured learning program played an important role in imparting the skills and knowledge that were needed. The program included theory and practice sessions, where the use of proper technique and patient preparation in achieving procedural competence to perform IVC ultrasound was emphasized (Gibson et al., 2018). By highlighting such a scripted approach to training, experts can identify the intricate interconnection between patient positioning, preparation, and successful imaging outcomes. The provision of ongoing feedback also highlights the importance of ongoing skills upgrading, which can further enhance the efficiency of ultrasound procedures on the aorta and IVC (Agnihotri et al., 2016).

11.5.2. Significant Observations and Measurements

In aorta and inferior vena cava (IVC) ultrasound imaging, precise measurement and stringent observation are critical in the assessment of cardiovascular health. The aorta, the biggest artery in the body, is an artery that makes up a midline channel of oxygenated blood from the heart. Parameters of performance, such as aortic diameter and abnormalities such as aneurysms, are fundamental markers of cardiovascular pathology. Besides, Doppler ultrasound can provide valuable information on blood flow parameters like velocity and turbulence, allowing for the detection of the extent of stenosis or other obstructions. In these ways, clinicians are able to obtain an integrated understanding of a patient's cardiovascular state and take early and effective therapeutic interventions accordingly. By contrast, the inferior vena cava also plays a significant role in venous return from the lower body to the heart and is thus also of vital importance to assess.

The findings during IVC ultrasound generally focus on its diameter, respirophasic collapsibility, and whether thrombi are visible or not. These are significant parameters because they measure central venous pressure and fluid status, particularly in patients with evidence of shock or fluid overload. Large measurements, such as the usual IVC diameter (typically <2.5 cm) and inspiratory collapse ($>50\%$), provide non-invasive markers with a high correlation with hemodynamic status. By incorporating these results into practice, the clinicians can enhance body fluid dynamics understanding and thus improve patient management options in critically ill patients. Coupling with more advanced techniques, such as acoustic radiation force impulse (ARFI) elastography, can further improve the assessment of aortic and IVC-related vascular diseases.

ARFI, in quantifying tissue stiffness, provides insight into underlying pathologic changes, possibly connecting observed aortic and IVC dimensions to systemic disease, such as congestive liver or heart disease. This is an expression of the necessity for a global diagnostic approach in which abnormal results in one region can reflect issues in other parts of the body. Here, the investigation of these new techniques is particularly relevant in patient groups with congenital heart disease, where hemodynamic abnormalities are common. By innovation in the field of ultrasound measurements, medical professionals can build a wide-ranging diagnostic map, thus enabling improved patient care and results, as evident through results of studies in patients with such conditions as Fontan circulation and its complications (Pietrobelli et al., 2022; POPP, 2023).

11.5.3. Clinical Significance of IVC Ultrasound Findings

The clinical application of inferior vena cava (IVC) ultrasound results is primarily in its effectiveness to evaluate venous return and intravascular volume status. This is particularly so among specific populations of patients, such as neonates and critically ill adults. Studies have identified that measurements of IVC can be employed as important indicators of fluid status, with important implications for treatment and patient care.

For instance, research demonstrates that accurate measurement of the IVC diameter using ultrasound in neonatal populations has contributed considerably to normative data used by clinicians to facilitate timely intervention. The ability to differentiate normal from abnormal IVC sizes enhances the diagnostic process in the healthcare setting, eventually leading to improved patient outcomes through facilitation of rapid identification of such conditions as dehydration, heart failure, or fluid overload, which can be vital in neonatal and pediatric settings (Teik, 2015).

Apart from its prognostic significance in fluid dynamics, IVC ultrasound findings have extremely significant implications in the broader context of cardiovascular health assessment. The employment of traditional ultrasound techniques and advanced imaging modalities, such as three-dimensional echocardiography, has been utilized in evaluating various cardiac conditions, and the intersection with IVC function cannot be overstated. By adequate assessment of the IVC alongside cardiovascular parameters, clinicians are able to make inferences about the hemodynamics underlying most cardiovascular diseases.

This wide-ranging assessment allows for enhanced risk stratification and management of individuals presenting with symptoms possibly indicating cardiovascular abnormalities. With the healthcare community continuing to advance and adapt these ultrasound tests, their application in secondary prevention and early diagnosis of cardiovascular disease becomes more prominent, highlighting the ongoing relevance of IVC ultrasound findings in routine clinical applications (Capotosto et al., 2018).

In addition, the integration of IVC ultrasound into overall diagnostic protocols is aligned with the changing attitudes in point-of-care ultrasound procedures and telehealth. As medicine progresses towards more convenient and effective diagnostic testing, IVC ultrasound is a minimally invasive but informative test that can be performed rapidly in numerous different environments, including emergency rooms and outpatient clinics. Its ease and non-invasiveness make it an appropriate choice for clinicians who wish to enhance patient care without resorting to more invasive techniques. Standardized protocols for IVC measurement, particularly for neonatal patients, ensure clinicians can apply these results with confidence as knowledgeable support for patient treatment plans. Clinically, the value of IVC ultrasound information is not only in its specific uses but also in how it can revolutionize patient monitoring and management in diverse settings for healthcare (Teik, 2015) (Figure 11.16).

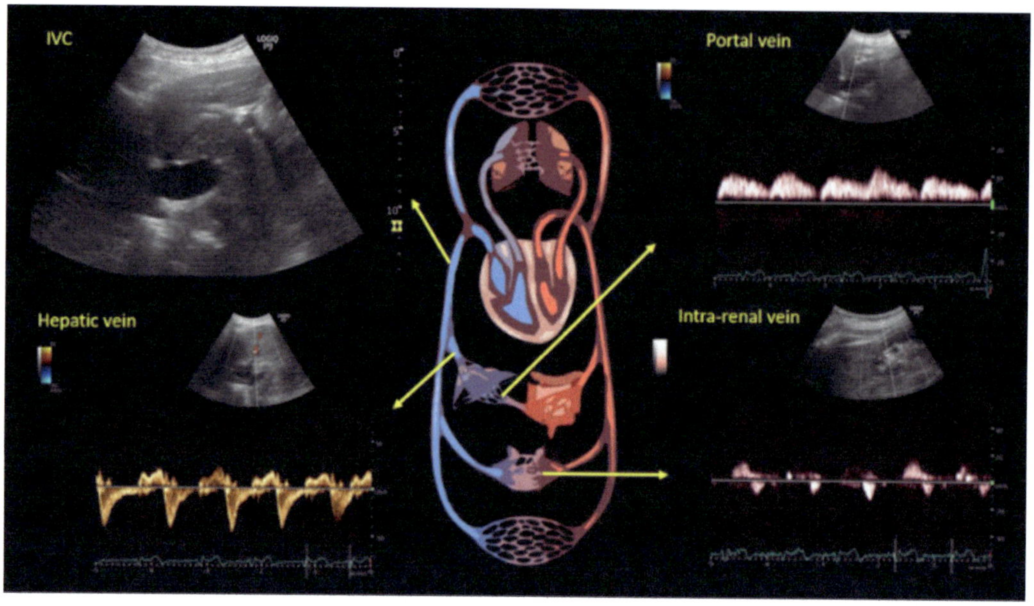

Figure 11.16. Clinical significance of IVC ultrasound findings.

Source: Samant, Samira. (2021). Point-of-care Doppler ultrasound in the management of hyponatremia: Another string to nephrologists' Bow. Clinical Case Reports. 9. 10.1002/ccr3.4687.

11.6. Clinical Applications of Aorta and IVC Ultrasound

Clinical applications of inferior vena cava (IVC) and aorta ultrasound extend into multiple specialties to significantly enhance the capacity for making diagnoses. One of the predominant applications of this technique is in the evaluation of abdominal aortic aneurysms (AAAs). Ultrasound is a low-cost, non-invasive technique by which the morphology and size of AAAs can be assessed, allowing prompt intervention in patients at risk. By facilitating real-time assessment of vascular integrity and perfusion, ultrasound provides surgeons with immediate information that guides intraoperative decision-making. Periaortic structure and aorta anatomy visualization also facilitate comprehensive assessment and, therefore, surgical planning and outcome optimization. In emergency settings, aorta and IVC ultrasound are an important assistant to immediate assessment of traumatic hemorrhage, illustrating the technology's value in acute care settings. Apart from assessment of abdominal conditions, ultrasound of the aorta and IVC is vital in venous disease management particularly that associated with deep vein thrombosis (DVT). Through the ability of ultrasounds to visualize blood movement, clinicians are able to identify thrombi formation in the IVC and its branches, which is important for early diagnosis and treatment. Early management under ultrasound guidance has been linked with reduced complications such as pulmonary embolism. Besides, the dynamic nature of ultrasound allows bedside evaluation, providing critical information about the patient's hemodynamic status. The imaging modality not only contributes to diagnosis but also to monitoring disease progression and response to treatment, enabling a tailored therapeutic approach. The efficacy of ultrasound in various clinical contexts highlights its central role within vascular medicine. Mounting evidence repeatedly highlights the significance of aorta and IVC ultrasound in preventive care, particularly in risk populations for cardiovascular disease (CVD). Early diagnosis of cardiovascular disease can lead to early intervention, improving overall health outcomes. For instance, studies indicate that routine ultrasound assessment can identify asymptomatic CVD patients and facilitate active risk management interventions to prevent complications. In addition, as occupational health is increasingly being recognized as a factor in vascular health, ultrasound can provide useful information regarding the degree to which workplace factors may affect cardiovascular disease. With advances in ultrasound technology, with three-dimensional imaging modalities, physicians are now better positioned to detect subtle alterations in vascular anatomy, and new avenues for early diagnosis and secondary prevention interventions (Golbus & Silverman, 1985; Capotosto et al., 2018). This forward development in the study of ultrasound guarantees to further expand its clinical applications, upholding its value in contemporary medicine.

11.6.1. Diagnosis of Aneurysm and Thrombosis

Aneurysm and thrombosis are diagnosed in the aorta and inferior vena cava (IVC), pointing to the importance of advanced imaging modalities in the modern practice of medicine. Aortic aneurysm is termed as an enlargement of the aorta at certain locations and may be accompanied by dangerous complications such as rupture and thrombosis. Rupture of the aneurysm can lead to acute patient deterioration or death if not detected timely. The use of ultrasound has been found to be immensely helpful as a non-invasive, yet dependable diagnostic agent. Ultrasound has the ability to identify structural changes of blood vessels and ascertain the presence of thrombus formation through real-time imaging. It can serve as an initial line imaging technique in helping identify patients requiring further investigation, thereby actively preventing serious health hazards associated with these conditions. Besides the traditional ultrasound methods, newer modalities such as contrast-enhanced ultrasound (CEUS) are emerging with greater significance as valuable diagnostic tools for vascular disorders, particularly in cases where patients present acutely. CEUS has shown itself to be helpful in providing high-resolution imaging of the vasculature, allowing for assessment of blood flow and identification of thrombi in real time. This technique can be particularly helpful in hemodynamically unstable patients since it makes bedside diagnosis possible without the use of iodinated contrast media. This is valuable in patients with pre-existing kidney impairment, which is frequently seen in vascular disease patients, where conventional CT angiography can be hazardous. With the addition of CEUS to the protocol of diagnosis, health care experts are able to enable efficacious detection and control of aneurysms and thrombosis. Also, there are some factors that highlight the significance of imaging in vascular complication diagnosis and management. For instance, Bron et al. (1985) present instances of how patency examination of the portal vein and IVC through other types of angiographic modalities became essential in determining transplantation viability among liver patients. The need for post-transplantation angiography very distinctly encompasses conditions such as hepatic artery thrombosis and gastrointestinal hemorrhage that demand urgent diagnosis for patient safety. Concurrently, research has proven that detection of complications such as aortocaval fistula (ACF) relies on instant ultrasound and CT scans, as explained in Becker et al. (2018), which proves the necessity for utilization of dual imaging methods for improved patient results. Thus, the addition of diversified ultrasound techniques to the vascular diagnosis paradigm is essential to improve prognosis in aneurysm and thrombosis conditions (Figure 11.17).

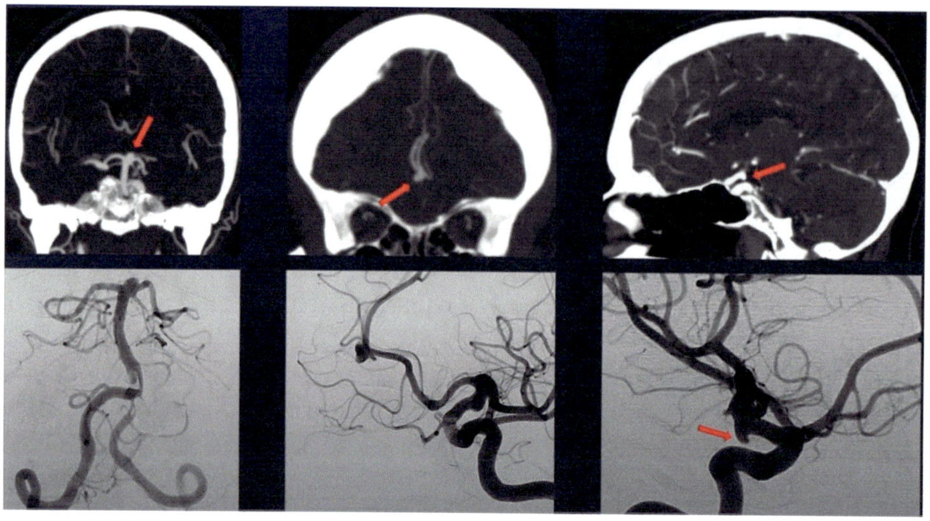

Figure 11.17. Diagnosis of aneurysms and thrombosis.

Source: Brain Aneurysm. Barrow Neurological Institute. *https://www.barrowneuro.org/condition/brain-aneurysm/*

11.6.2. Monitoring of Cardiovascular Conditions

Cardiovascular monitoring is very dependent on the utilization of newer imaging modalities, such as ultrasound. Ultrasound of the Aorta and Inferior Vena Cava (IVC) is a non-invasive modality that provides useful information regarding hemodynamic well-being and vascular integrity. Vascular dimension and function measurements are critical to the diagnosis and treatment of numerous cardiovascular disorders. For instance, a dilated and stiff inferior vena cava is typically a sign of elevated intravascular volume, an imaging marker that can be used to distinguish between high-risk heart failure patients. However, operator skill and the inherent variability that comes with image acquisition and interpretation can compromise the accuracy of ultrasound measurements. With this, the development of standardized protocols and the incorporation of advanced imaging technology are necessary to enhance cardiovascular assessment accuracy and reproducibility. The use of advanced algorithms in ultrasound imaging has the potential to revolutionize cardiovascular monitoring. These processing algorithms for imaging allow improved quantification of vascular deformation because they track wall motion in both longitudinal and transverse planes. Such innovation is instrumental in overcoming the limitations of traditional ultrasound methods, which are prone to operator-dependent variation in measurements. Also facilitated through advanced computational methods real-time assessment capabilities that can make timely provision of feedback regarding a patient's cardiovascular status. This technology not only aids in clinical decision-making but also in making treatment plans tailored to a patient based on real-time data. The potential for implementing such advanced imaging technologies makes it obvious the merit of continuous innovation in cardiovascular monitoring activities. Additionally, monitoring conditions such as pulmonary edema emphasizes perioperative cardiovascular evaluation. Techniques such as transpulmonary thermodilution (TPTD) have been observed to offer valuable adjuncts to fluid status assessment and hemodynamic control during operation. The method enables physicians to monitor lung water buildup, hence better managing fluid treatment by categorizing at-risk patients for pulmonary complications before overt signs. The double function of TPTD to clarify both hemodynamic variables and the pathophysiology of pulmonary edema adds to its relevance. By distinguishing between hydrostatic and permeability-related causes of fluid overload, TPTD is representative of the advances in cardiovascular monitoring that play a direct role in patient outcomes. The integration of imaging modalities such as Aorta and IVC ultrasound with advanced hemodynamic evaluation tools represents a major milestone in effectively managing cardiovascular health.

11.6.3. Role in Preoperative and Postoperative Assessments

The role of aorta and inferior vena cava (IVC) ultrasound in the preoperative assessment is most important in modern-day surgery. This radiologic modality provides doctors with vital information regarding the patient's vascular status, which is extremely beneficial for planning the operation. For instance, the diameter of the aorta and IVC can be followed using ultrasound, providing valuable information regarding hemodynamic compromise intra- and postoperatively. This allows for personalized surgical approaches, especially among high-risk populations such as patients undergoing cardiac reoperations. For example, peripheral cannulation has been shown to reduce cardiac injury and transfusion requirements compared to central cannulation techniques, indicating the importance of accurate vascular assessment prior to intervention (Ata et al., 2020). Thus, a comprehensive preoperative evaluation with ultrasound can decrease risk and enhance the overall safety of surgical procedures. Aorta and IVC ultrasounds, in the postoperative setting, have a similar crucial function in monitoring and evaluation of patients' recovery. IVC diameter measurement, for example, can provide valuable information about a patient's fluid status as well as cardiac function after surgery. Ultrasound helps health professionals to identify possible complications such as thrombosis, fluid buildup, or heart failure, which may compromise recovery pathways. Moreover, with continuous technological advancements, these imaging modalities have grown more advanced and even user-friendly, facilitating early intervention when problems are diagnosed. The ability to view and assess the vascular system dynamically post-surgery can lead to early identification of issues, enabling medical teams to act quickly and effectively to enhance patient outcomes, hence strengthening the patient-centric philosophy's core principle. The integration of advanced imaging modalities such as computer-aided surgical systems also emphasizes the merit of ultrasound in preoperative and postoperative assessments. These systems enhance anatomical detail and relationship visualization, allowing for better surgical planning and execution. In pediatric oncologic surgery, for example, 3D visualization can delineate the anatomy between tumors and neighboring vessels, and this aids surgeons in surgical access planning (Chen et al., 2023). While solitary ultrasound provides significant diagnostic promise, once paired with sophisticated imaging modalities, complications risks in complicated cases can be mitigated, and preoperative evaluations and postoperative monitoring guided by accurate, relevant data. The evolving function of aorta and IVC ultrasound consequently becomes pivotal not only for individual patient assessment but also in impacting overall surgical practice, ultimately improving patient safety and outcomes.

SUMMARY

Finally, the application of ultrasound imaging in aorta and inferior vena cava (IVC) examination is a significant development for non-invasive diagnostic techniques. The technique has been pivotal in evaluating hemodynamics and identifying potential pathologies in patients with diseases such as renal cell carcinoma, where vascular involvement is probable. Several have pointed to its reliability, delivering integral information capable of directing treatment modalities and prognostic assessment. With its increased prevalence and ability to deliver instant output, ultrasound imaging is a cornerstone in contemporary diagnostics, allowing timely interventions and enhanced patient outcomes for complex situations, such as those with tumor thrombus conditions, where surgical treatment heavily depends on accurate imaging data (Bugeja et al., 2013). Furthermore, understanding the normal range of diameters of the IVC for different populations, including neonates, enhances clinical practice by providing comparative markers wherein abnormality can be measured. Current evidence regarding the normal size of the IVC in healthy term neonates demonstrates the utility of ultrasound in pediatric practice and thus broadens the uses of this imaging method (Teik., 2015). Such measurements underlie the detection of deviations implying cardiovascular compromise in infants and may be crucial in neonatal intensive care. By applying standard reference values, clinicians are able to make informed decisions that can form the path for improved prognostic capabilities along with tailor-made therapeutic management. With advancing ultrasonography, sustained improvement and expansion of its uses in the adult and pediatric populations will remain the key. Future research can be directed to develop improved methods and protocols that will maximize the diagnostic utility of ultrasound. Integration of newer technologies, such as 3D imaging and real-time analysis, will add additional useful applications of ultrasound in vascular health monitoring. In the future, as more clinicians implement these practices, the overall quality of care will be improved, and the disease management of both the aorta and IVC will be better. These innovations will continue to make ultrasound an integral tool in modern medicine so that it can remain a critical component in delivering quality patient care in a variety of clinical contexts.

Ultrasound of the inferior vena cava (IVC) and aorta is a useful non-invasive resource in clinical evaluation, particularly in monitoring hemodynamics and volume status in various patient populations. The main focus of this evaluation lies between vessel diameter and outcome in patients. For instance, dilatation and stiffness of the IVC are markers of elevated intravascular volume and are prognostically significant in heart failure patients with potentially poor outcomes. However, variability of measurements and inconsistencies in intra- and inter-operator reproducibility hinder the use of these ultrasound techniques on a broader scale. With the aim to surpass these limitations, new image-processing algorithms have been developed that enhance accuracy in estimates through observation of wall motion and phasic deformation measurement. Such enhancements can enhance clinical utility across broad settings of medical practice and patient populations, yet they emphasize the necessity of instituting standardized practices in vascular ultrasonography (Albani et al., 2022). Ratio of IVC to aorta is an intriguing advance in the non-invasive assessment of dehydration, especially in children. Through studies, it has been indicated that this measure holds the ability to identify severe dehydration from normal hydration status among children suffering from acute diarrhea, gastroenteritis, or vomiting. A systematic review and meta-analysis established that the IVC/Ao ratio was highly sensitive and had moderate specificity, and is potentially an effective instrument in clinical decision-making. The outcome is a combined sensitivity of 86% and specificity of 73%, highlighting its usefulness in accurate hydration status estimation. However, the literature indicates that the IVC/Ao ratio may not be sufficient for definite diagnoses, with the necessity of further robust studies with larger, multicenter populations to confirm such findings and optimize clinical practice (Octavius et al., 2023). In addition to optimizing patient outcomes, the inclusion of ultrasound examination of the aorta and IVC in clinical monitoring on a routine basis can facilitate more advanced interpretation of fluid management in various settings. This is particularly relevant in those conditions requiring meticulous fluid monitoring, such as heart failure or severe dehydration. Better measures for the evaluation of vascular measurements could lead to more individualized treatment approaches and better resource allocation within healthcare systems. However, like with any new technology, constant evaluation must be made to establish best practices and standards. Thus, ongoing research, including prospective and institutional collaborative studies, will remain important in advancing ultrasound methods for aorta and IVC assessments toward improvement in clinical outcomes and patient safety concerning volume status and hemodynamics management (Albani et al., 2022).

CLOSER LOOK

IVC (INFERIOR VENA CAVA) ULTRASOUND

Inferior vena cava (IVC) ultrasound is a focused and non-invasive imaging technique that is most commonly used to assess the volume status of the patient, guide fluid resuscitation, and assess hemodynamic stability, particularly in critical illness and emergency care. The IVC is the body's largest vein and serves to drain deoxygenated blood from the abdominal organs and lower limbs back to the right atrium of the heart. Its collapsibility and diameter are regulated by right atrial pressure, intravascular volume, and respiratory phases and therefore represent a dynamic fluid responsiveness indicator. IVC ultrasound is linked to the use of a phased or curvilinear array transducer, generally in the subxiphoid or the right midaxillary line position, and imaging is performed in longitudinal (long-axis) and transverse (short-axis) planes. The IVC appears as an anechoic tubular structure behind the spine and in front of the liver, and its relationship with the hepatic vein is an anatomical marker for accurate placement.

In clinical practice, IVC ultrasound is often used to estimate CVP and to guide fluid therapy in septic, shocked, heart failure, or dehydrated patients. The best-accepted parameter is the IVC collapsibility index (IVC-CI), or the respiratory change in IVC diameter. In spontaneously breathing patients, a very collapsible IVC (that is, >50% inspiration collapse) typically reflects low right atrial pressure and hypovolemia and is likely to have the patient be fluid-responsive. High right atrial pressure can be seen with a plethoric (dilated and non-collapsing) IVC in conditions such as fluid overload, congestive heart failure, pulmonary hypertension, or cardiac tamponade. In mechanically ventilated patients, the IVC acts the opposite way—expanding with inspiration due to positive intrathoracic pressure—so interpretation must be adjusted accordingly.

Quantitatively, an IVC of less than 2.1 cm with greater than 50% collapse with inspiration suggests a CVP of 0–5 mmHg, while an IVC greater than 2.1 cm with less than 50% collapse suggests a CVP of more than 10 mmHg. These are approximations but can guide clinical decision in conjunction with other hemodynamic data and physical examination results. Aside from fluid assessment, IVC ultrasound can detect IVC thrombosis, compression by mass, or atypical venous flow patterns in Budd-Chiari syndrome. In monitoring for trauma or perioperative circumstances, sequential estimation of the IVC can track a patient's response to fluid or blood loss.

However, IVC ultrasound is not perfect and must not be used alone. Quantifiable parameters like intra-abdominal pressure, body habitus, right heart failure, or mechanical ventilation can also affect IVC measurements. Both the operator's skill and the patient's cooperation are also crucial for proper imaging and interpretation. Despite those limitations, IVC ultrasound is an effective point-of-care ultrasonography (POCUS) bedside tool where clinicians can rapidly estimate volume status and make real-time therapeutic choices. With more widespread POCUS training and the increased portability of equipment and artificial intelligence integration, IVC ultrasound will remain an anchor of non-invasive hemodynamic assessment across many clinical settings.

REFERENCES

1. Abuhamad, A., Acherman, R., Adriaanse, R., Adriaanse, S., Aguilera, D., Allan, L., Allan, R., et al. (2018). Fetal intelligent navigation echocardiography (FINE) detects 98% of congenital heart disease. http://deepblue.lib.umich.edu/bitstream/2027.42/146329/2/jum14616_am.pdf (accessed on 12th July 2025).
2. Agnihotri, A. K., Ailawadi, G., Barnhart, G. R., Farivar, R., et al. (2016). Minimally invasive mitral valve surgery II: Surgical technique and postoperative management. https://core.ac.uk/download/323078625.pdf (accessed on 12th July 2025).
3. Akohov, A., Barner, C., Francis, R. C. E., Grimmer, K., et al. (2019). Aortic volume determines global end-diastolic volume measured by transpulmonary thermodilution. https://core.ac.uk/download/286097305.pdf (accessed on 12th July 2025).
4. Albani, S., Albera, C., Antonini-Canterin, F., Bini, R., Ermini, L., Fabris, B., Giannoni, A., et al. (2022). Assessment of phasic changes of vascular size by automated edge tracking—State of the art and clinical perspectives. https://core.ac.uk/download/638765516.pdf (accessed on 12th July 2025).
5. Anwar, S., Anwar, T., Barach, P., Bernhard, D., Bhatla, P., Biglino, G., Biglino, Z., et al. (2018). 3D printing is a transformative technology in congenital heart disease. https://core.ac.uk/download/212858839.pdf (accessed on 12th July 2025).
6. Assaad, S., Perrino, A., & Shelley, B. (2017). Transpulmonary thermodilution: Its role in assessment of lung water and pulmonary edema. https://core.ac.uk/download/82958547.pdf (accessed on 12th July 2025).
7. Ata, E. C., Erkanlı, K., Paslı, S., Türkoğlu, M., et al. (2020). Peripheral vs. central cannulation in cardiac reoperations: Technical considerations and outcomes. https://core.ac.uk/download/336859863.pdf (accessed on 12th July 2025).
8. Bass, J., Beinart, R., Zhao, C. L., de Schepper, S., Fitoz, S., Qian, G. N., Gupta, A., et al. (2012). Posterior nutcracker syndrome associated with interrupted left inferior vena cava with azygos continuation and retroaortic right renal vein. https://core.ac.uk/download/pdf/8718405.pdf (accessed on 12th July 2025).
9. Becker, C., Bhatia, M., Khabiri, E., Platon, A., et al. (2018). Contrast enhanced ultrasonography versus MR angiography in aortocaval fistula: Case report. https://core.ac.uk/download/159153756.pdf (accessed on 12th July 2025).
10. Bjordal, S. G., & Brotons Paya, C. (2023). Bruk av håndholdt ultralyd av intensivsykepleiere: En systematisk litteraturoversikt. https://core.ac.uk/download/578702641.pdf (accessed on 12th July 2025).
11. Bron, K. M., Gartner, J. C., Iwatsuki, S., Malatack, J., et al. (1985). Angiography of liver transplantation patients. https://core.ac.uk/download/12204017.pdf (accessed on 12th July 2025).
12. Bugeja, S., Galea, J., German, K., Zammit, A., et al. (2013). Surgical excision of renal cell carcinoma with caval and intra-atrial tumor thrombus extension using deep hypothermic circulatory arrest. https://core.ac.uk/download/46602405.pdf (accessed on 12th July 2025).

13. Capotosto, L., De Sio, S., Massoni, F., Ricci, A., et al. (2018). Early diagnosis of cardiovascular diseases in workers: Role of standard and advanced echocardiography. https://core.ac.uk/download/141696274.pdf (accessed on 12th July 2025).

14. Chen, Y., Dong, Q., Hao, X., Niu, H., et al. (2023). Application of computer-assisted surgery system based on artificial intelligence in pediatric precise oncological surgery. https://core.ac.uk/download/568374235.pdf (accessed on 12th July 2025).

15. Dojs, A., Jakubowicz, M., Kuchenbeker, N., Mierzwińska-Mucha, J., et al. (2025). Nutcracker syndrome – Pathophysiology, diagnosis and treatment options: A literature review. https://core.ac.uk/download/656518366.pdf (accessed on 12th July 2025).

16. Faridaalaee, G., & Naghipour, B. (2016). Correlation between central venous pressure and inferior vena cava sonographic diameter; determining the best anatomic location. https://core.ac.uk/download/483638133.pdf (accessed on 12th July 2025).

17. Franco-Gruntorad, G. A., & Pérez-Coronado, J. D. (2015). Utilidad de la ecografía en reanimación. https://core.ac.uk/download/pdf/81185087.pdf (accessed on 12th July 2025).

18. Gabriel, M., Juszkat, R., Kubiak, K., Żabicki, M., et al. (2018). Percutaneous direct thrombin injection with hydro dissection to manage type II endoleak after endovascular abdominal aortic aneurysm repair. https://core.ac.uk/download/187426542.pdf (accessed on 12th July 2025).

19. Gibson, N., Rippey, J., Rosman, J., Steinwandel, U., et al. (2018). Educating renal nurses–inferior vena caval ultrasound for intravascular volume assessment. https://core.ac.uk/download/195697758.pdf (accessed on 12th July 2025).

20. Golbus, M. S., & Silverman, N. H. (1985). Echocardiographic techniques for assessing normal and abnormal fetal cardiac anatomy. https://core.ac.uk/download/pdf/81145316.pdf (accessed on 12th July 2025).

21. Gupta, A., Dean, A. J., American College of Emergency Physicians Emergency Ultrasound Guidelines, Gregg, A. R., Kirkpatrick, A. W., Abuhamad, A. Z., Kimura, B. J., et al. (2011). An integrated ultrasound curriculum (iUSC) for medical students: 4-year experience. https://core.ac.uk/download/pdf/8545333.pdf (accessed on 12th July 2025).

22. Hennessy, M., Kasthuri, R., Kingsmore, D. B., Mark, P. B., et al. (2017). Ferumoxytol-enhanced magnetic resonance angiography for the assessment of potential kidney transplant recipients. https://core.ac.uk/download/83960454.pdf (accessed on 12th July 2025).

23. Jakovcevski, M., Jeremic, D., Kovacevic, M., Minic, G., et al. (2020). Concomitant multiple anomalies of renal vessels and the collecting system. https://core.ac.uk/download/268451898.pdf (accessed on 12th July 2025).

24. Lee, S. J., Park, H., & Yeom, E. (2025). X-ray PIV measurement of blood flow in deep vessels of a rat: An *in vivo* feasibility study. https://core.ac.uk/download/148823847.pdf (accessed on 12th July 2025).

25. Mesin, L., & Policastro, P. (2023). Processing ultrasound scans of the inferior vena cava: Techniques and applications. https://core.ac.uk/download/590967082.pdf (accessed on 12th July 2025).

26. Octavius, G. S., Wibowo, J., Widjaja, M., Imanuelly, M., & Heryadi, N. K. (2023). Inferior vena cava to aorta ratio in dehydrated pediatric patients: A systematic review and meta-analysis. https://core.ac.uk/download/591484874.pdf (accessed on 12th July 2025).

27. Pietrobelli, A., Luciani, G. B., Saccomani, M. D., & Prioli, M. A. (2022). Liver stiffness evaluation using acoustic radiation force impulse elastography in pediatric and adult patients with congenital heart disease. https://core.ac.uk/download/534906630.pdf (accessed on 12th July 2025).

28. Popp, C. (2023). Using personalized cardiovascular models to identify new diagnostic predictors for pre-eclampsia. https://core.ac.uk/download/578082714.pdf (accessed on 12th July 2025).

29. Rees, J., & Twahirwa, N. (2008). Unusual presentation of idiopathic retroperitoneal fibrosis: Case report. https://core.ac.uk/download/47254891.pdf (accessed on 12th July 2025).

30. Richardson, R. R., Silverman, N. H., Solomon, J. E., Stock, A. A., et al. (2013). Fetal heterotaxy with tricuspid atresia, pulmonary atresia, and isomerism of the right atrial appendages at 22 weeks. https://core.ac.uk/download/323063249.pdf (accessed on 12th July 2025).

31. Ruemenapf, G., Rupprecht, H., & Schweiger, H. (1998). Preaortic iliac confluence: A rare anomaly of the inferior vena cava. https://core.ac.uk/download/pdf/82312732.pdf (accessed on 12th July 2025).

32. Stümper, O. F. W., Sreeram, N., Elzenga, N. J., Sutherland, G. R., Van Praagh, L., Tynan, M. J., et al. (1963). Diagnosis of atrial situs by transesophageal echocardiography. https://core.ac.uk/download/pdf/81967261.pdf (accessed on 12th July 2025).

33. Teik, S. T. (2015). Inferior vena cava diameter measurements from ultrasound in the normal and healthy term neonates within 1 week of life in Hospital USM. https://core.ac.uk/download/159615935.pdf (accessed on 12th July 2025).

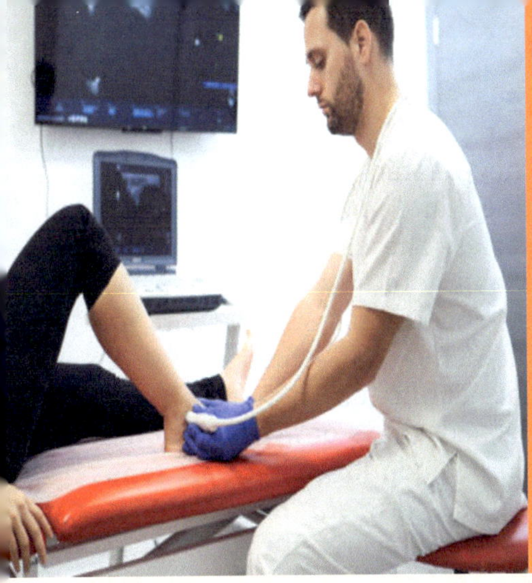

Chapter 12

PELVIS: MALE AND FEMALE ULTRASOUND

Contents

Introduction

The pelvis is a crucial component of the human body because it is a complex structure that supports significant organs, facilitates movement, and carries the load of the upper half of the body. Understanding the pelvis's anatomy is of utmost significance in the practice of medical imaging, particularly in ultrasound, which provides an invasive-free method of seeing this complex region. The pelvis differs between the sexes not just in size and shape but also in terms of function in reproduction. Morphological differences in the pelvis are very important when it comes to diagnostics, especially when it comes to diagnosing conditions that have a direct influence on reproductive health or in cases of trauma. Ultrasound is therefore an essential tool for practitioners because it allows for precise determination that informs treatment protocols as well as surgery. Ultrasound technology uses sound waves to produce clear images of the internal structures of the body and is hence a modality of choice for pelvic examination. This form of imaging is crucial in assessing both male and female patients, providing information on conditions from benign cysts to malignancy-related tumors. In the male patient, pelvic ultrasound tends to be directed towards the prostate gland and bladder, whereas in the female, it is commonly used to examine the uterus and ovaries. The use of ultrasound in routine clinical practice has increased diagnostic accuracy and the ability to follow pelvic disease over time. Further, technological innovation, including 3D imaging and Doppler ultrasound, has expanded the scope of measurement, allowing dynamic imaging of blood flow and structural disease that were previously difficult to localize. The value in realizing the distinctions between female and male pelvic ultrasound cannot be overestimated, for this will decide lines of investigation in diagnosis and planning for management. For instance, assessment in women for pelvic pain tends to go through both the urological and the gynecological causes, whereas in men, the focus could be on the urological cause. In addition, findings on ultrasound must be interpreted in a sensitive understanding of the anatomic and physiological differences beneath. This essay will thus endeavor to examine the nuances and implications of pelvic ultrasound in men and women and to emphasize heightened clinical awareness and improved patient outcomes in the context of pelvic health and disease care. The complexity of the subject, marked by the unique characteristics of male and female bodies, necessitates that the practitioners remain current with regard to the novel ultrasound methods and interpretations in the context of evolving medical knowledge (Figure 12.1).

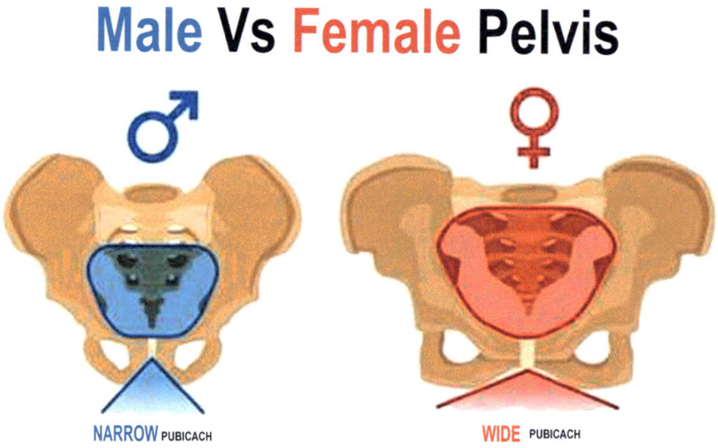

Figure 12.1. Male and female pelvis ultrasound.

Source: Double Brain/ shutterstock.com. https://www.shutterstock.com/image-vector/male-vs-female-pelvis-main-260nw-1069847876.jpg.

Definition of Ultrasound

Ultrasound, a medical imaging modality using high-frequency sound waves, is essential to modern medicine, particularly in obstetrics and gynecology. The non-invasive procedure enables doctors to visualize structures within the body, providing them with valuable information on various medical conditions of the pelvis. The process involves exposure to sound waves that travel through tissues of the body, reflecting off structures such as organs, fluid, and soft tissue. The produced echoes are then digitized to generate in real time images on a screen, allowing dynamic assessment of the pelvic area in both males and females. Unlike other imaging modalities such as X-rays or computed tomography, ultrasound does not require the application of ionizing radiation, making it a safer method, especially in pregnancy. This aspect is specifically relevant in the monitoring of the fetus's well-being and assessment of pelvic pathology throughout the reproductive life course. In pelvic examination, ultrasound has multiple applications, including the identification of anatomical pathologies, masses, and assessment of conditions for infertility. For instance, as has been highlighted in contemporary gynecology, ultrasound can well identify various pelvic pathologies likely underpinning disorders of infertility and therefore guide subsequent management or therapy. Transvaginal and transabdominal ultrasound technologies have enhanced diagnostic potential by facilitating precise imaging of reproductive organs. Specifically, during infertility examinations, ultrasound assists in examining the uterine cavity and ovarian anatomy and therefore aids in the establishment of an accurate diagnosis and treatment regimen. The modality is further a critical factor in the construction of protocols for maximizing reproductive health outcomes and hence forms a fundamental part of clinical practice (Khouri et al., 2004). Furthermore, the development of ultrasound technology continues to change clinical practice engaged in pelvic examination. With advancements such as three-dimensional imaging and Doppler ultrasound, clinicians now have equipment that offers more information and diagnostic accuracy. The integration of these emerging ultrasound technologies allows the comprehensive evaluation of the blood flow through the pelvic organs, the assessment of vascular health of the tissues, which is important in fertility treatment. Further, ultrasound has also been identified as a key component of various birth reform movements to redefine maternity services and foster a more patient-centered strategy to give birth. This is part of a broader pattern in the history of childbirth towards medicalization, which is a response to a demand for safety and efficiency in the practice of childbirth (Henson, 2002). To this end, ultrasound is an essential part of contemporary pelvic care, always guiding the way medical professionals view and approach the conditions of reproductive health.

Importance of Pelvic Ultrasound

The application of pelvic ultrasound extends beyond mere imaging; it is a critical diagnostic tool that contributes to knowledge of pelvic anatomy and potential pathologies in men and women. This non-invasive technique enables clinicians to observe soft tissue organs, examine the status of reproductive organs, and detect abnormalities not apparent by physical examination. For instance, for women patients, pelvic ultrasound is equally crucial in evaluating conditions such as ovarian cysts, fibroids, and ectopic pregnancy, providing critical information to direct treatment. Additionally, in the male patient, a pelvic ultrasound can identify abnormalities such as bladder or prostate enlargement, revealing information that is critical in management. Thus, pelvic ultrasound is a valuable asset in the clinician's toolkit, enabling timely interventions and improving patient outcomes. In addition to its diagnostic function, pelvic ultrasound made a significant contribution to the management of pelvic floor disorders in the daily patient flow. As pelvic floor conditions gain increasing recognition, precise knowledge of normal and pathological conditions through imaging is essential. The use of pelvic ultrasound makes it possible to evaluate dynamic pelvic floor function, which aids in the diagnosis of dysfunctions, for example, prolapse or incontinence. Abramov et al. (2016) points out that the fact that the pelvic floor can be seen in real-time enhances the clinician's awareness and handling of these conditions. Furthermore, the consensus reached by leading organizations is a manifestation of the growing recognition of pelvic floor dysfunction, and it promotes efforts at standardization of the language and communication between medical professionals. Incorporation of ultrasound findings into conservative management plans advances the specialty in a gradual manner toward evidence-based practice that maximizes patient benefit. The educational benefit of pelvic ultrasound cannot be overemphasized because it is also a vital training tool for medical students and physicians from all specialties, including obstetrics, gynecology, urology, and radiology. Exposure to pelvic ultrasound not only aids in the diagnosis and management of patients but also enhances anatomy knowledge and spatial perception, which are two vital elements of every medical specialty. The clinical use of ultrasound techniques encourages the learning process to be more practical, thus boosting critical thinking and clinical decision making. Additionally, with rapid advancement in the area of ultrasound technology, including 3D and 4D imaging modalities, avenues for more accurate diagnosis and therapeutic intervention continue to grow. These educational elements are essential because they prepare the eventual healthcare professionals to utilize pelvic ultrasound in their fields adequately, and that's ultimately going to produce enhanced patient care over time (Figure 12.2).

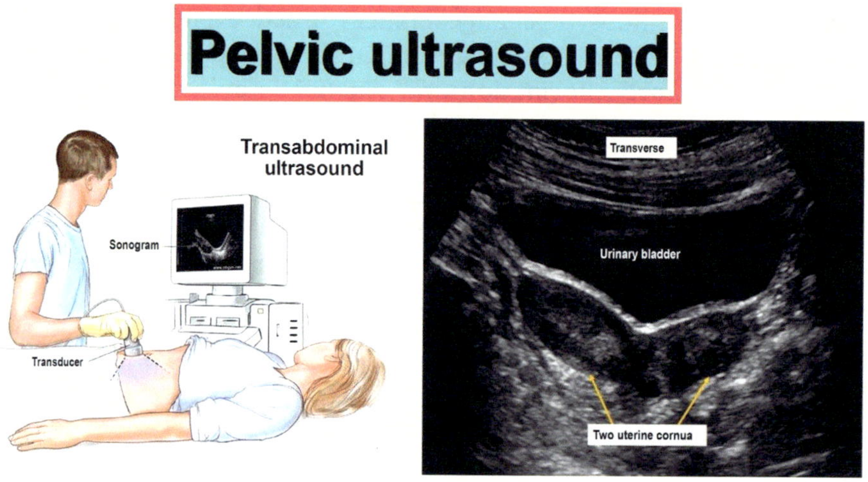

Figure 12.2. Pelvic ultrasound.

Source: Air to air (2022). Pelvic ultrasound (cover image). www.youtube.com/@u-l. https://i.ytimg.com/vi/1XTf3B32RpA/maxresdefault.jpg

Overview of Male and Female Pelvic Anatomy

The male and female pelvis are introduced with considerable anatomical differences, demonstrating their distinct biological roles. The male pelvis is usually described as a narrow, funnel-shaped structure that supports the upper body weight. This shape facilitates increased stability and leads to bipedal walking. The female pelvis is broader and has a larger pelvic inlet, which is crucial for childbirth. The general structure of the female pelvis provides greater room for the passage of the fetus during childbirth, exemplifying a remarkable adaptation in reproductive anatomy. These differences in anatomy emphasize the evolutionary purpose of pelvic anatomy to accommodate diverging reproductive needs, as well as the consequences for the assessment of health and functionality based on various imaging modalities like ultrasound, which play a significant role in the assessment of both male and female pelvic anatomy in clinical practice, in attempts to provide accurate diagnostics and treatment planning. Hormonal influences also have a significant impact on the physiological differences found in male and female pelvic anatomy. In females, the release of estrogen and relaxin during puberty and pregnancy allows for the modification of the pelvic architecture to make it more elastic and accommodating in order to accommodate birth. The hormones allow for the growth and development of the joints and ligaments of the pelvic floor that will result in an overall anatomy optimized for birthing functions. In males, the absence of these hormonal changes creates a more stable pelvic structure, advantageous in supporting the heavier weight of muscles prevalent in the male frame. Understanding these hormone effects creates the appreciation of more functional anatomy encountered with ultrasound imaging. This imaging modality, in addition to yielding structural variation, also helps in the detection of potential pathologies associated with these differences in anatomy, namely in reproductive health.

Postpartum is a period when female pelvic anatomy knowledge is crucial because of the potential occurrence of dysfunctions associated with giving birth. The pelvic floor of the female is a sophisticated one and governs varied functions of the body, that is, urination, defecation, and sexual function.

Postpartum, women may have various pelvic floor dysfunctions, for example, incontinence or musculoskeletal disorders, which can occur directly because of the anatomical changes during delivery. Besides, knowledge of these possible dysfunctions is essential for early intervention. Educational interventions, such as giving the women pamphlets describing pelvic health and treatments available, can empower the women to detect and access early medical care for these complications, therefore preventing long-term effects. Clinicians can effectively assess and treat these postpartum alterations by using ultrasound, ensuring that women have access to full care focused on their anatomical realities (Olson, 2001).

12.1. Anatomy of the Male Pelvis

Anatomy of the male pelvis involves a complex interplay of structures responsible for crucial functions in the reproductive as well as urinary apparatus. The pelvis is made up of numerous bones, namely the ilium, ischium, pubis, and sacrum, which constitute a bony framework to support the pelvic organs. Anatomically, the male pelvis is typically narrower and more robust than that of the female, which is a walking upright feature related to the need for greater body strength. Included in this context are basic structures such as the bladder, rectum, seminal vesicles, prostate gland, and various blood vessels and nerves needed to facilitate reproductive function and urinary upkeep. Understanding the spatial relationships and integrity of these organs is critical in clinical practice, especially in ultrasound scanning of the male pelvis, which enable the evaluation of a vast array of pathologies and conditions of these organs. It is a primary technique in imaging the anatomy and function of the male pelvis. High-frequency sound waves provide real-time images, which are useful in evaluating structures that may be occult in other imaging modalities. The male genitalia are highly amenable to ultrasound, allowing clinicians to visualize seminal vesicles and prostate glands quite effectively. Importantly, ultrasound can diagnose such conditions as cysts, tumors, or congenital abnormalities and thereby allow intervention in a timely manner. As an illustration, the identification of such abnormalities as Zinners syndrome, which is characterized as the coexistence of renal agenesis and seminal vesicle defects, demonstrates the value of ultrasound in identifying rare urogenital anomalies (Garga et al., 2016). Not only does the imaging modality enhance diagnosis, but it also monitors response to therapy. In addition, more recent ultrasound technology also has the capability of further defining pelvic anatomy, including assessing vascular structures relevant to delineating pelvic circulation. Doppler ultrasound, for example, is critical in assessing blood flow to the prostate and in screening for such conditions as prostatitis or prostate cancer. The reliability of ultrasound is comparable to other imaging modalities and justifies its role in clinical practice. Research indicates that MRI skeletal age estimation methods provide useful correlational data to age and developmental abnormalities and provide valuable insight into age estimation within pelvic anatomy evaluation (Tomei et al., 2015). With this, the use of ultrasound in pelvic anatomy evaluation is invaluable to clinical practice and provides a complete characterization of the normal and abnormal presentations in the male pelvis (Figure 12.3).

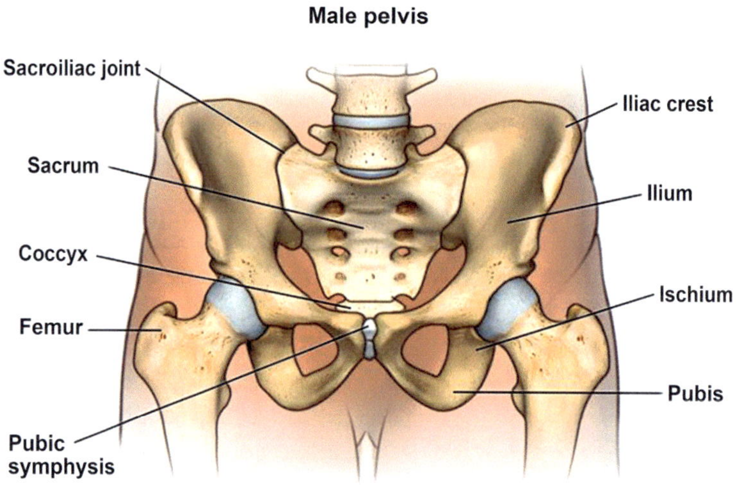

Figure 12.3. Anatomy of the male pelvis.

Source: https://comportho.com/wp-content/uploads/2016/07/322083.jpg.

12.1.1. Structure of the Male Reproductive System

The male reproductive system is an intricate network of highly specialized structures that are engaged in critical activities of sperm production, maturation, and transmission. The testes, which are at the core of the system, have highly coiled seminiferous tubules within them where spermatogenesis occurs. The testes also produce hormones, primarily testosterone, which is responsible for male secondary sexual characteristics and reproductive functions. Surrounding the testes, the scrotum provides not only a protective external environment but also temperature regulation for the best sperm maturation. Temperature regulation is required because spermatogenesis is carried out at temperatures slightly less than the body's core temperature, showing the intimate link between environmental control and reproductive health. Beyond the testes, the men's reproductive tract contains a collection of ducts and glands that permit sperm to be conveyed and matured. The epididymis, a coiled tube above each testis, is where sperm gain motility and are stored until ejaculation. Sperm travel via the vas deferens, which propels them into the ejaculatory duct, mixing with seminal vesicle fluid and prostate gland fluid. These secretions are instrumental in developing semen to provide nutrition and protection to sperm while they travel through the male reproductive tract and into the female reproductive tract. Notably, ultrasound imaging is a valuable asset in the assessment of these structures, giving insight into their morphology and function, particularly when anomalies such as Zinners syndrome are under consideration. Ultrasound is the prime imaging method of evaluation of the male genitourinary tract, providing a non-invasive insight into its complex anatomy. With the use of this modality, the testes, epididymis, prostate, and their corresponding ducts can be imaged, and the detection and identification of pathology can be achieved. Potential pathologies are congenital anomalies, tumors, and infections, which can be identified by size or echogenicity changes. With the use of ultrasound, clinicians can study developmental abnormalities, such as unilateral renal agenesis or seminal vesicle cysts, which are diagnosed as belonging to a syndrome like Zinners syndrome (Kline, 1989). Furthermore, information regarding the structural complexities of the male reproductive system, with the help of ultrasound, underscores the importance of accurate diagnosis and the potential of targeted therapeutic measures. In toto, ultrasound continues to evolve the field's comprehension of male reproductive health and related pathologies, adding to clinical practice valuable diagnostic potential (Kline, 1989) (Figure 12.4).

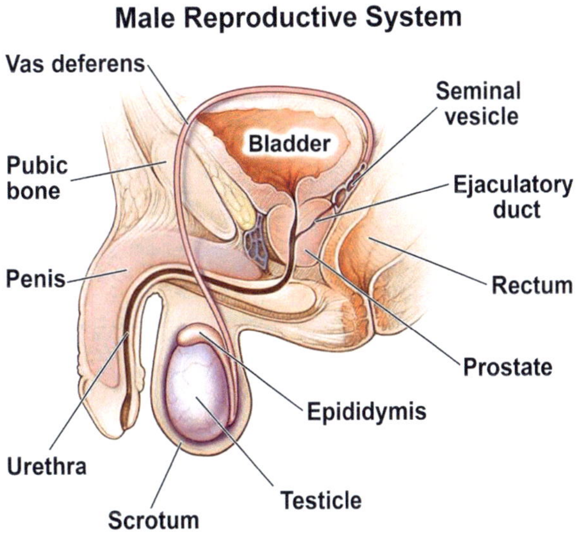

Figure 12.4. Structure of the male reproductive system.

Source: Cleveland clinic (2023). Male reproductive system. https://my.clevelandclinic.org/-/scassets/images/org/health/articles/9117-male-reproductive-system.

12.1.2. Key Organs Visualized in Male Pelvic Ultrasound

The male pelvic ultrasound is a routine test that provides crucial information about a number of anatomical structures in the pelvis. The prostate, seminal vesicles, bladder, and rectum are some of the most important organs that are visualized with this test. The prostate gland, in particular, is relevant not just to reproduction but also to the process of urination. Ultrasound scanning helps us determine the dimensions, form, and abnormality, such as hyperplasia or prostatic malignancies, which is required for the diagnosis of conditions such as Benign Prostatic Hyperplasia (BPH) and prostate cancer. Furthermore, seminal vesicles located behind the bladder are evaluated for their size and any changes that may indicate disorders of the reproductive system. Another fundamental structure that is examined using a male pelvic ultrasound is the urinary bladder. Bladder imaging is used by clinicians to assess bladder wall thickness, volume, and lesions that can lead to inordinate function loss. It's particularly useful to identify conditions such as bladder stones or tumors that result in urinary obstruction and resultant complications. In addition, ultrasound imaging may assist in uncovering the condition of the rectum and facilitate evaluation of potential rectal masses or irregular wall thickening. Both are required for comprehensive male pelvic health examinations, which guide subsequent diagnostic and therapeutic interventions.

In the practice of healthcare in general, an understanding of the anatomical representations obtained from male pelvic ultrasound provides the foundation for effective diagnosis and treatment planning. As further advancements are made in technology for ultrasound, visualization of these vital organs improves to a more detailed level, and the analysis gets more accurate. The integration of ultrasound with clinical skills facilitates the determination of individualized treatment plans with long-term effects in patient care. As can be seen in many studies, including studies of pelvic organ prolapse, good imaging techniques are still the most important tool with which to battle male pelvic anatomy disorders, hence appreciating the necessity for ongoing research and innovation in the medical specialty (Sinex, 2021; De Almeida Joaquim, 2017) (Figure 12.5).

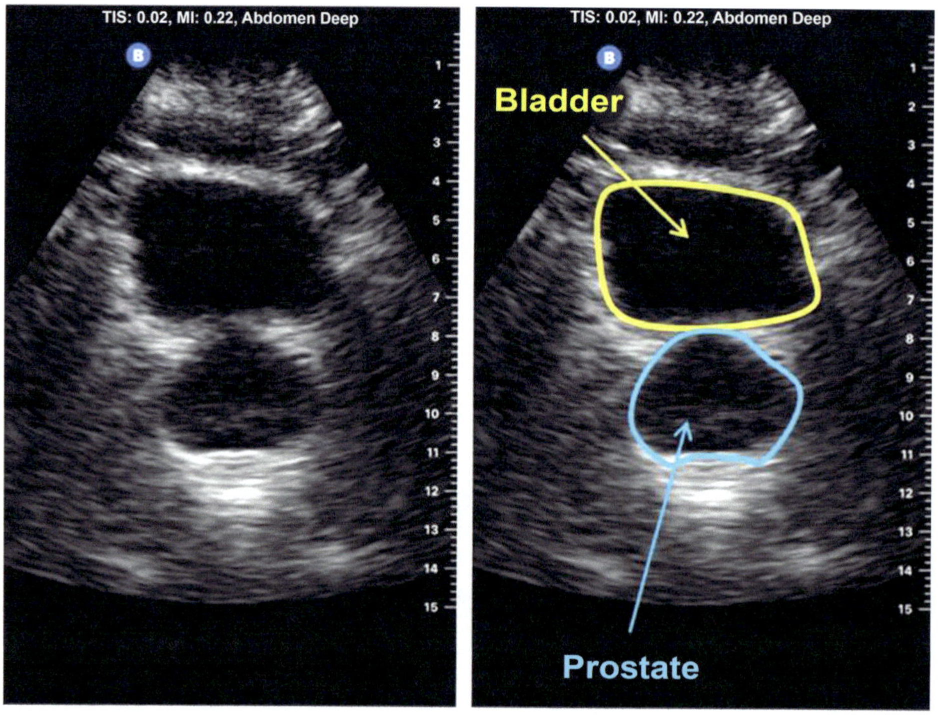

Figure 12.5. Key organs visualized in male pelvic ultrasound.

Source: Wilson, M. A., Brown, D., & Castleberry, L. (2022). Ultrasound of the reproductive system. In Physiology in health and disease (pp. 263–286). https://doi.org/10.1007/978-1-0716-1863-9_10 https://media.springernature.com/lw685/springer-static/image/chp%3A10.1007%2F978-1-0716-1863-9_10/MediaObjects/453410_1_En_10_Fig22_HTML.png.

12.1.3. Differences in Male Pelvic Anatomy Compared to Females

Male pelvic anatomy varies significantly from women's, particularly in reference to the structural composition and function. The male pelvis is narrower and funnel-shaped, and it's designed to accommodate the male reproductive organs and to provide additional musculature support. This is in contrast to the female pelvis, which is broader and basin-shaped to facilitate childbirth. Pelvic inlet and outlet dimensions also vary; the pelvic inlet is wider in females to permit fetal passage during childbirth. These differences in anatomy are essential considerations in pelvic ultrasound imaging because alterations in size and shape influence directly the visibility of internal structures and the interpretation of ultrasound results in clinical settings. In addition, differences in pelvic musculature between men and women are manifested as functional and anatomical variation. The external anal sphincter and pelvic floor muscles are thicker and more powerful in men and conditioned to the respective functional characteristics, that is, bladder and bowel maintenance. The position of these muscles also affects the alignment of the urogenital tract, which is dissimilar from the female. For instance, the position of the prostate and bladder in men needs a unique arrangement of adjacent muscles. Studies using Magnetic Resonance Diffusion Tensor Images have provided an unmistakable image of male pelvis muscles' architecture and direction with evidence of a complex fascicle pattern being accountable for pelvic stability and function, as reported in a study (Cory et al., 2018). Further anatomical variation is revealed by ultrasound examination of the urethrovaginal space, with implications for sexual function and pelvic health. In females, variation in this space has been linked with sexual satisfaction, with an increased thickness of the urethrovaginal space related to the ability to experience vaginal orgasms, again indicating anatomy directly influencing sexual health outcomes. In contrast with male, there is no such directly comparable structure of male anatomy, implying correlational differences in sexual function by pelvic anatomy, according to nature. This makes it imperative to have distinct ultrasound methods unique for the anatomy of each gender when assessing pelvic health, as shown in a number of studies taking into account the functional implications of pelvic structure (Brandetti et al., 2008).

12.2. Anatomy of the Female Pelvis

Female pelvis anatomy is intricate and plays the starring role in a variety of physiological functions, most importantly reproductive. The female pelvis is made structurally wider and more rounded than the male pelvis, which is adapted to childbirth as well as movement. The distinctive female pelvis structure is characterized by the size of the pelvic inlet and outlet, which are required for fetal passage during childbirth. Clinicians must be aware of these anatomical structures in order to utilize ultrasound technology to diagnose conditions that affect the female reproductive health. Pelvic ultrasounds enable the clinician to visualize not just bony frameworks but also soft tissues, like ovaries and the uterus, and thus assess extensively the likelihood of pathological conditions that arise within these structures, which in turn influence maternal and fetal consequences. The variation between the female and male pelvis is more than one of size and shape; anatomical variation has significant clinical significance, particularly in obstetrics and gynecology. For instance, pelvic form can affect delivery and labor, necessitating special prenatal management and observation techniques. Ultrasound scanning is a nonpainful method of assessing the variation, providing for early intervention if necessary. Ultrasound of the female pelvic can detect lesions such as fibroids in the uterus or cysts in the ovaries, which can profoundly affect reproductive health. It is for this reason that thorough understanding of female pelvic anatomy is the foundation of proper interpretation of ultrasound findings. It emphasizes the need for continued refinement of imaging technology and education of healthcare providers so that they can manage the complexity of female reproductive health. Furthermore, more recent studies highlight that the majority of conditions of the pelvis will be improved by an extensive understanding of underlying anatomy for proper management. Interaction among different structures of anatomy, such as pelvic diaphragm and supporting ligaments of pelvic organs, plays a vital role in diagnosing conditions that are characterized by either pelvic dysfunction or pain. This complexity can be observed in conditions like pelvic organ prolapse and abnormal menstrual cycles, which are perhaps due to anatomical imbalance or trauma. As emphasized by studies on athletic pubalgia, pubic joint dynamics fall under diagnosing injured athletic women. With the medical community trying to make ultrasound application more precise, with a focus placed upon depth of anatomical knowledge in order to inform, it allows for a higher detection of variations and abnormalities, leading to improved patient care (Devon et al., 2008; Hamid & Losco, 2014) (Figure 12.6).

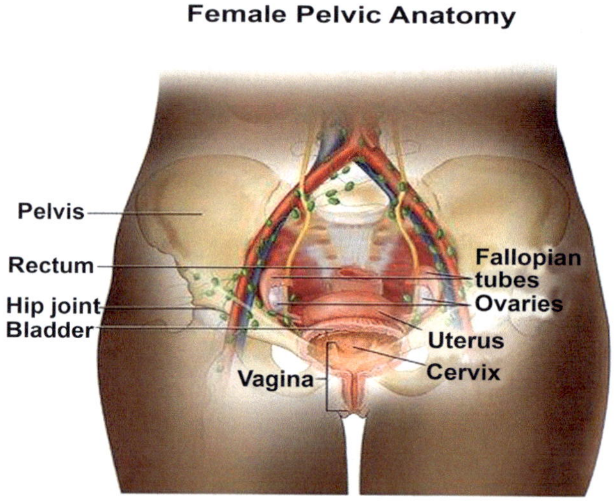

Figure 12.6. Anatomy of the female pelvis.

Source: https://visualsonline.cancer.gov/retrieve.cfm?imageid=13454&dpi=72&fileformat=jpg.

12.2.1. Structure of the Female Reproductive System

The female reproductive system is a highly organized and complex group of organs working together in harmony to facilitate reproduction. At its core are the ovaries, the primary reproductive glands, with the task not only of creating the ova but also of secreting the hormones estrogen and progesterone. Situated at the end of the fallopian tubes, the ovaries play an essential role in the menstrual cycle, as ovulation signals the discharge of an egg into the fallopian tube, where it can be fertilized. The ciliated lining of the fallopian tubes helps to move the egg along the fallopian tubes to the uterus, demonstrating the system's reliance on synchronized biological events to achieve reproductive success. Identifying these anatomical features is significant in the interpretation of ultrasound images, where the visibility of such structures may be the key to a woman's reproductive well-being. Once inside the uterus, the organ's unique structure becomes relevant in the appreciation of female reproductive physiology. Three layers compose the uterus: the endometrium, myometrium, and perimetrium. The endometrium, which develops in preparation for menstruation, plays a significant role in the menstrual cycle. When there is a fertilized egg, it implants in this layer to signal pregnancy. The myometrium, which is the muscular layer, closes the uterus during menstruation and childbirth, showing the active role of the organ. These facts have significant implications when it comes to ultrasound scanning, in that detecting abnormalities in these layers can diagnose conditions like fibroids or endometriosis. The structure of the uterus is hence not only supportive of reproduction but also of interest when it comes to imaging.

Other than the ovaries and the uterus, the female reproductive system consists of the cervix and vagina, both essential to the act of reproduction. The cervix serves as a barrier and passage between the vagina and the uterus, regulating the flow of sperm and menstrual discharge and keeping the uterus shielded from infection. Ultrasound technology is able to see the cervix, particularly during pregnancy, in order to determine its length and health as a predictor of possible complications. The vagina is also a muscular tube and plays a critical role in both sexual intercourse and childbirth, further emphasizing the interconnected nature of these parts. The joining of these parts serves to underscore not only the complexity of the female reproductive system but also the value that ultrasound provides in gaining insight into this system's function and health. An appreciation of these anatomical intricacies thus equips healthcare practitioners with the important information to improve reproductive health outcomes and rectify any issues that are identified (Bumgarner, 2007) (Figure 12.7).

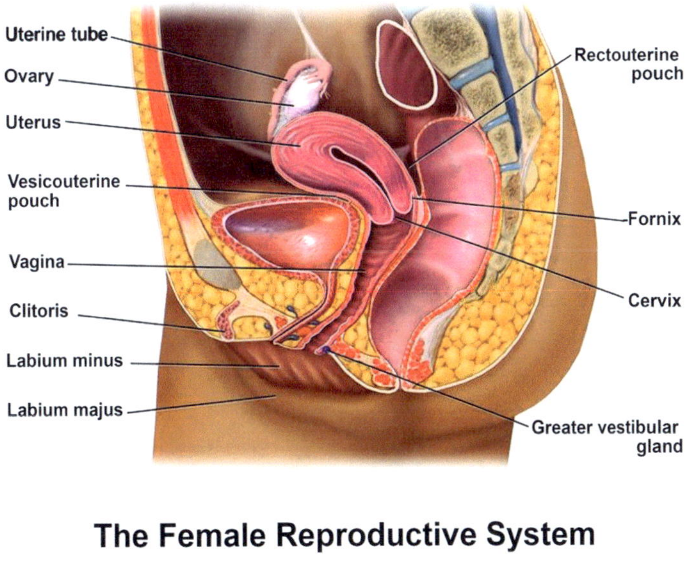

Figure 12.7. The female reproductive system.

Source: https://www.ncbi.nlm.nih.gov/books/NBK554601/bin/FemaleReproSystem_02.jpg.

12.2.2. Key Organs Visualized in Female Pelvic Ultrasound

During a female pelvic ultrasound, several vital organs are scanned, providing valuable information about reproductive and urinary health. The primary structures that are evaluated in the procedure include the ovaries, uterus, cervix, and bladder. Ovaries are evaluated for size, form, and cysts or masses, indicating polycystic ovary syndrome or neoplasms. The uterus is also assessed for abnormalities such as fibroids or endometrial thickening, both of which have the potential to impact menstrual function and fertility. The cervix is also screened for signs of cervical incompetence or lesions that need further assessment. Understanding the normal anatomy and variation of these organs is important to the correct diagnosis and management of many female reproductive disorders. The bladder is another important structure that appears on a pelvic ultrasound and is informative for urinary health. The procedure can detect such conditions as pelvic organ prolapse, bladder stones, or tumors, which are not always apparent with other imaging methods. Since ultrasound employs real-time imaging, dynamic evaluation of bladder filling and emptying can be done, which can help clinicians to diagnose voiding dysfunction or disorders of urinary retention. Second, the use of transvaginal ultrasound imaging provides improved visualization of the pelvic organs, particularly the ovaries and uterus, which enables minimal pathologies to be identified. The addition of such detailed visual assessment may significantly influence treatment planning and clinical decision-making in women's health care. Furthermore, ultrasound is highly utilized in prenatal assessment, where visualization of the pelvic organs plays an extremely critical role in monitoring fetal growth and maternal health. Real-time imaging allows us to check the uterus's structural integrity, as well as an image of the placenta and its position, which may be of relevance to the course of the pregnancy. In others, abnormalities such as gestational trophoblastic disease can also be identified using focused ultrasound examinations. With accompanying clinical presentation, for example, frequency of micturition or bloating, noted in the same studies, ultrasound can result in further investigation, such as MRI, to explore potential underlying pathology (Lee et al., 2013). Therefore, pelvic ultrasound has an additional role beyond screening, becoming an important consideration in the diagnosis and management of complex gynecological and obstetric disorders (Figure 12.8).

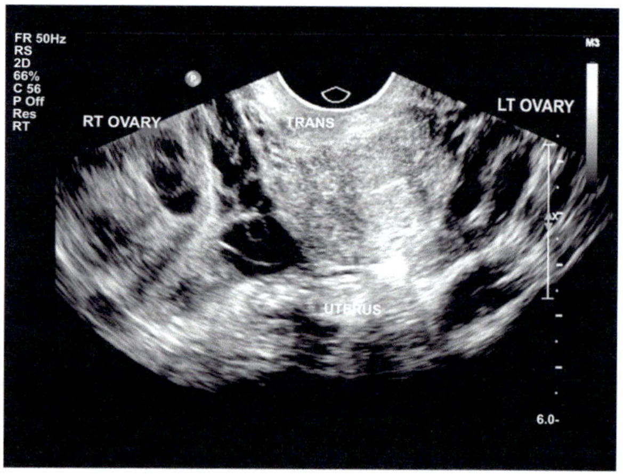

Figure 12.8. Key organs visualized in female pelvic ultrasound.

Source: Annalise Lang, Vi Dinh; Pelvic Ultrasound Made Easy: Step-By-Step Guide. POCUS 101. https://pocus101.b-cdn.net/wp-content/uploads/2020/09/Tubo-ovarian-abscess-pelvic-ultrasound.png.

12.2.3. Differences in Female Pelvic Anatomy Compared to Males

The pelvic structural differences in the anatomy of women and men are substantial and play critical roles in numerous physiological functions and clinical considerations. The female pelvis, for example, is wider and possesses a larger pelvic inlet, which plays a significant role in the passage of the fetus during childbirth. Not only does this anatomical configuration facilitate the passage of the fetus, but also the nearby structures, such as the pelvic floor muscles and pelvic organs, are affected. Conversely, the male pelvis is narrower and shorter, a reflection of its evolution for bipedal walking and bearing weight. These size and shape differences extend into muscle architecture, particularly at the pelvic floor, where sex differences in such activities as exercise or coitus can influence function. It is critical to consider these differences with the aim of optimizing diagnostic imaging protocols, especially in the use of ultrasound techniques based on precise anatomical visualizations. If one considers the anatomy of the female pelvis, a noteworthy consideration is the intricate relationship between sexual function and the urethrovaginal space. Evidence has revealed strong correlations between the anatomy of this area and the likelihood of vaginal orgasm, illustrating how anatomical variation can influence sexual experience (Brandetti et al., 2008). Ultrasound testing illustrates that measurements such as those of the urethrovaginal space may be linked to sexual responsiveness, reinforcing the significance of pelvic anatomy in women's health. These determinants indicate that pelvic anatomy is not merely a structural concern but also a crucial aspect of sexual health and function. Based on these findings, the application of pelvic ultrasound emerges as crucial in the assessment of anatomical variation and its effect on sexual health in females. In addition, understanding the dynamics of pelvic floor muscle architecture further validates the clinical relevance of such variations in anatomy. Superimposition of muscular complexity, particularly of the type that occurs in childbirth, illustrates how external forces may affect female pelvic anatomy to yield complications such as pelvic floor dysfunction. Sophisticated imaging studies, including Magnetic Resonance Diffusion Tensor Imaging (MR-DTI), validate continuation of investigation of pelvic arrangements of muscles and their functional significance (Cory et al., 2018). Through the portrayal of unambiguous muscle architecture, such imaging modalities provide insight into potential mechanisms of injury at the moment of delivery and other activities. The application of such information to clinical practice ensures a better-integrated rendering of diagnoses and treatments for pelvic health disorders, emphasizing the indispensable significance of comprehending the unique complexity of female pelvic anatomy.

12.3. Indications for Male Pelvic Ultrasound

The use of male pelvic ultrasound has become of concern in clinical practice due to its use in the diagnosis of several urological and reproductive abnormalities. The primary indication for employing this imaging modality is to evaluate prostate abnormalities. As prostate cancer remains a serious health concern, clinicians commonly use pelvic ultrasound to assess the size, shape, and texture of the prostate and to look for potential lesions or nodules. Apart from that, this imaging technique maximizes differentiation between benign prostatic hyperplasia and malignancies as it allows for early detection and treatment options. Further, pelvic ultrasound provides informative information about nearby anatomical structures and hence contributes to a complete assessment of any recommended pathologies of the male pelvis, finally improving patient outcomes and directing management. The second significant indication for male pelvic ultrasound is the examination of urinary obstruction and other urological diseases. Some of these patients presenting with symptoms such as hematuria, urinary retention, or flank pain will require ultrasound scans to identify locations of potential obstructions. Pelvic ultrasound is a non-invasive procedure and is able to visualize the kidneys, bladder, and urethra, allowing for immediate interventions. For instance, the modality can be used to detect urinary stones or structural abnormalities such as strictures that are likely to impair the passage of urine. Because these conditions are likely to have severe consequences, including renal damage, detection and intervention at an early stage, facilitated by pelvic ultrasound, are crucial to sustaining renal function, as attested to by the continuing advances in imaging technology. Lastly, pelvic ultrasound is an effective tool for assessing male reproductive status, particularly in the diagnosis of infertility. It can image structures such as the seminal vesicles and testes, and can provide such details on potential anatomical malformations such as varicoceles or congenital malformations. The imaging mode can also be utilized to assess testicular masses that may indicate such conditions as tumors or infection. In sex development disorders (DSD), pelvic ultrasound provides useful information regarding the position and morphology of reproductive organs that helps with general management planning. Hence, its use for male reproductive health is pertinent, aligning with current clinical practice recommendations in support of ultrasound evaluation for the diagnosis and management of male infertility, consonant with the findings of new evidence in this subject (Huysse et al., 2008; Calvo et al., 2016) (Figure 12.9).

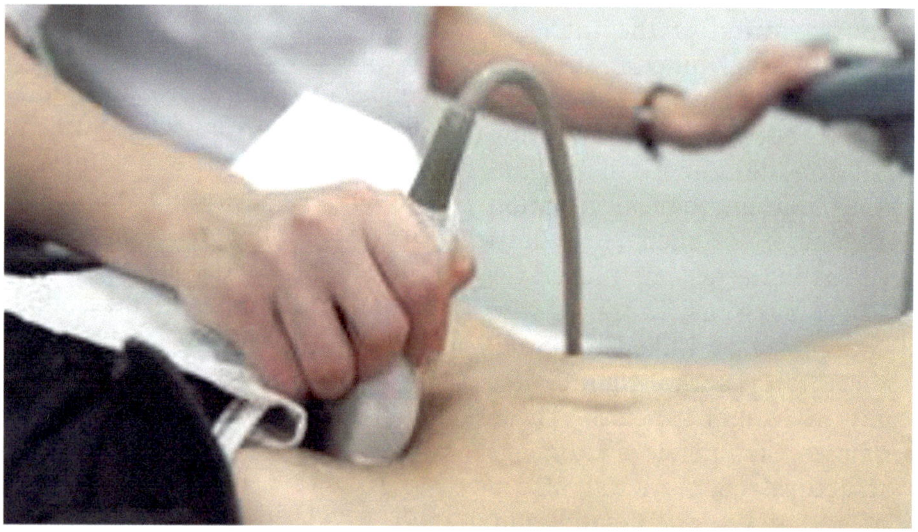

Figure 12.9. Ultrasound of pelvic organs in men.

Source: https://avicennamed.com.ua/wp-content/uploads/poliklinika/xuzi-malogo-taza-muzhchin.jpg.pagespeed.ic.t2fNPbvZuL.jpg.

12.3.1. Evaluation of Prostate Health

Assessment of prostate health is crucial in the practice of male reproductive medicine, as it is susceptible to a range of conditions like benign prostatic hyperplasia (BPH), prostatitis, and prostate cancer. Ultrasound imaging, specifically transrectal ultrasound (TRUS), plays a crucial role in the assessment. TRUS not only provides visualization of prostate gland size and shape but also guidance for biopsy in case of suspected malignancy. This modality of imaging provides high-resolution images that allow clinicians to assess abnormalities effectively, thus early diagnosis and management. Despite the potential of such imaging, gaps in knowledge among primary care physicians can significantly hinder effective management of prostate disorders; a survey showed that most doctors exhibited ignorance of such terms as chronic prostatitis/chronic pelvic pain syndrome

(CP/CPPS) (Calhoun et al., 2009). In addition, an overall assessment of male fertility overlaps considerably with prostate health. Numerous factors of infertility among men can be caused by underlying prostate pathology, and therefore, the prostate must be evaluated extensively in the process of investigating fertility. Extended knowledge regarding a patient's reproductive background and an intensive physical examination provide a basis for determining the possible causes of infertility. This two-fold strategy recognizes each partner's role in infertility and thus underscores the utility of an integrative assessment. Systemized protocols in testing for infertility can assist in more accurate diagnoses and targeted interventions, enhancing treatment effectiveness overall for such couples struggling with fertility. As a basic element in men's overall health evaluation, prostate health testing is thus highly overlapping with issues of fertility (Campana et al., 2015). Lastly, prostate health assessment is an important part of male health care, particularly among pelvic ultrasound. The connection between prostate disease and complicating elements of male fertility highlights the importance of a well-informed and thorough assessment process. Early diagnosis through means like TRUS can lead to timely intervention, which is significant in preventing the progression of more dangerous diseases such as prostate cancer. In addition, the integration of prostate health examination into fertility testing ensures room for early diagnosis of underlying conditions, hence facilitating a full grasp of male reproductive wellness. As the specialty expands, continued education and standard procedures among healthcare professionals continue to be crucial to the improvement of treatment outcomes for men suffering from prostate health issues.

12.3.2. Evaluation of Testicular Conditions

Assessment of testicular status is important in the overall plan for male reproductive health, particularly in relation to the use of ultrasound technology. Ultrasound imaging is a non-invasive tool that permits visualization of testicular anatomy, facilitating diagnosis of many conditions, including tumors, torsion, and congenital anomalies. The bright, high-resolution images derived with ultrasound can significantly contribute to the detection of abnormalities, such as hydroceles and varicoceles that are related to infertility. One of the specific values is in early diagnosis of disorders of the testicles, where early treatment can prevent complications and salvage fertility. Additionally, awareness of specific ultrasound characteristics of different testicular abnormalities assists clinicians in devising appropriate treatment plans based on the requirements of individual patients, thereby improving clinical success in male reproductive medicine. Ultrasound's diagnostic value is particularly pertinent in situations of disorders of sex development (DSD). Such conditions may have varied anatomical changes, making the assessment and management plan for the affected person more complex. Early and accurate imaging can guide surgery, for example, whether or when to perform gonadectomy to avert cancer risks associated with certain intersex syndromes. The availability of laparoscopic procedures has also enhanced the treatment of DSD by providing a minimally invasive operation with very good cosmetic results and fewer postoperative complications. The importance of patient-specific management is highlighted in these cases, with multidisciplinary specialists collaborating to formulate inclusive management plans treating the physical as well as the psychosocial. Thus, ongoing innovation in the subject matter of ultrasound technology continues to be a corner-stone in the effective assessment and management of conditions of the testes, especially in the context of DSD, where standard measures could fall short (Calvo et al., 2016). The second integral component of the assessment of testicular disorders involves the investigation of male infertility, as both partners contribute to fertility issues.

An organized process, including comprehensive history-taking and physical examination of the male, is necessary for the identification of unusual causes of infertility. Ultrasound is a valuable component of this evaluation, allowing identification of conditions such as testicular atrophy or reproductive tract obstruction. Moreover, by gaining a clear insight into the reproductive anatomy of the male and associated pathologies, clinicians are in a position to devise targeted therapeutic approaches capable of increasing fertility. Such an organized method ensures not only that treatment addresses male factors but that the couple as an entity is treated, thus potentially elevating the chances of successful conception. Finally, integrating ultrasound examination into infertility workups highlights the importance of its role beyond mere diagnosis, adding to a better understanding of male reproductive health (Campana et al., 2015) (Figure 12.10).

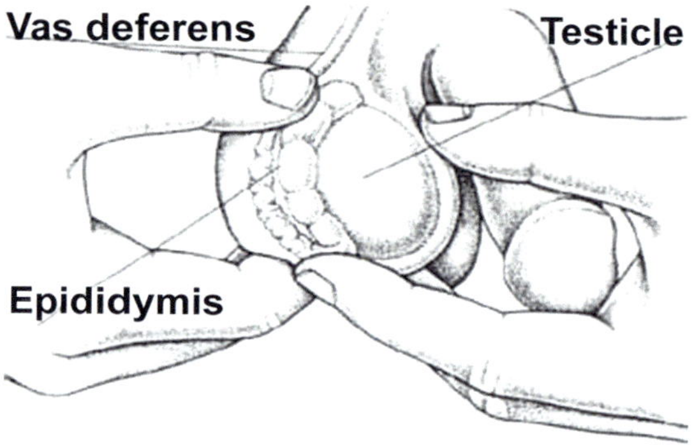

Figure 12.10. Assessment of testicular conditions.

Source: Cincinnati Children's (2022). https://*www.cincinnatichildrens.org/health/t/testicular-self-examination* .

12.3.3. Diagnosis of Urinary Tract Issues

Urinary tract complications should be diagnosed in men and women alike since complications are linked with severe morbidity unless treated. Ultrasound is an innocuous imaging method that gives a complete evaluation of the urinary tract. It can be extremely helpful for illustrating anatomical defects, such as kidney stones, cysts, and tumors, thereby delivering precious information regarding the etiology of urinary symptoms. In addition, the use of ultrasound will enable the assessment of urinary bladder pathology and urinary retention in relation to pelvic floor dysfunction in women. The use of clinical findings combined with ultrasound images enables doctors to make the correct diagnosis and therefore engage in appropriate intervention measures accordingly, as highlighted by the consensus terminology report on pelvic floor dysfunction (Abramov et al., 2016). Additionally, the particular difficulties for urinary tract problems may differ greatly between males and females, calling for specific diagnosis strategies. In women, conditions such as urinary incontinence and prolapse of pelvic organs will complicate the diagnostic evaluation of urinary problems, for which a solid comprehension of pelvic anatomy as viewed on ultrasound will typically be necessary. These imaging modalities help to elucidate the structural interactions between the bladder and surrounding pelvic organs, providing essential information for an integral assessment. In men, disorders such as prostatic hypertrophy can affect urine flow and present unique diagnostic challenges. Sequence imaging patterns on ultrasound can illustrate these gender-specific issues, enhancing diagnostic accuracy and available treatment options for urinary tract presentations (Mu et al., 2015). Lastly, the ideal management of urinary tract pathology is a team approach merging ultrasound data into clinical expertise. Continual advances in the field of ultrasound technology are improving the diagnostic competence of clinicians to allow increasingly precise identification of urinary tract diseases. Aside from that, establishing a standardized language for urinary tract dysfunction, as proposed in Abramov et al. (2016), enables clinicians to communicate patient examination and treatment algorithms. This diagnostic consistency reduces the incidence of misdiagnosis and guarantees patients receive optimal management strategies tailored to their unique clinical presentation. Therefore, the intersection of imaging and clinical information lies at the heart of addressing urinary tract disorders in pelvic health.

12.4. Indications for Female Pelvic Ultrasound

The role of the female pelvic ultrasound is central to the diagnosis of many gynecological pathologies, especially those with pain or abnormalities. Due to the anatomical complexity of the female reproductive organs, ultrasound imaging is an evidence-based method through which essential information about pelvic anatomy, including the uterus and ovaries, can be determined. The most common referral for this research is pelvic pain, which accounts for approximately 72.3% of ultrasound requests based on recent articles. Other significant indications involve assessment of pelvic inflammatory disease (PID), benign ovarian cysts, and other structural disorders. By detecting such conditions, ultrasound not only aids effective diagnosis but also helps to guide the course of further treatment by being a highly valuable tool in gynecological health care (Ameh et al., 2022).

In addition to managing acute conditions, a female pelvic ultrasound also yields valuable information for reproductive health assessment, particularly in fertility assessments. Infertility is often multi-factorial, and ultrasound plays a key role in the detection of potential anatomical disparity. Through diligent visualization, patients' physicians can detect abnormalities such as uterine fibroids, endometriosis, and abnormalities of the fallopian tubes, all of which are potential obstacles to conception. Further, ovarian reserve can be determined by transvaginal ultrasound, providing critical information regarding follicle number and morphology. This function of ultrasound is particularly relevant to women who are being treated with assisted reproductive technology, so that any identifiable deviation is addressed prior to intervention. Indications for female pelvic ultrasound, therefore, extend far beyond diagnosis and include broader aspects of reproductive health and planning for family (Ameh et al., 2022).

Age and overall health are the considerations that must not be excluded in the process of establishing indications for ultrasound. With increasing age in women, the prevalence of some gynecological conditions, such as ovarian cysts and uterine fibroids, is likely to increase. Routine screening is thus often recommended in women who are in particular age groups, particularly 30–50 years. Ultrasound can also assess conditions related to hormonal changes, such as menopause effects and polycystic ovary syndrome (PCOS). Emerging evidence underscores the role of age, height, and sex on specific anatomical measurements in the pelvis in modulating the use of ultrasound as a diagnostic tool. Through the adjustment of the use of ultrasound to population data, clinicians can enhance accuracy and maximize patient care, thereby solidifying the modality's role in integrated women's health care (Figure 12.11).

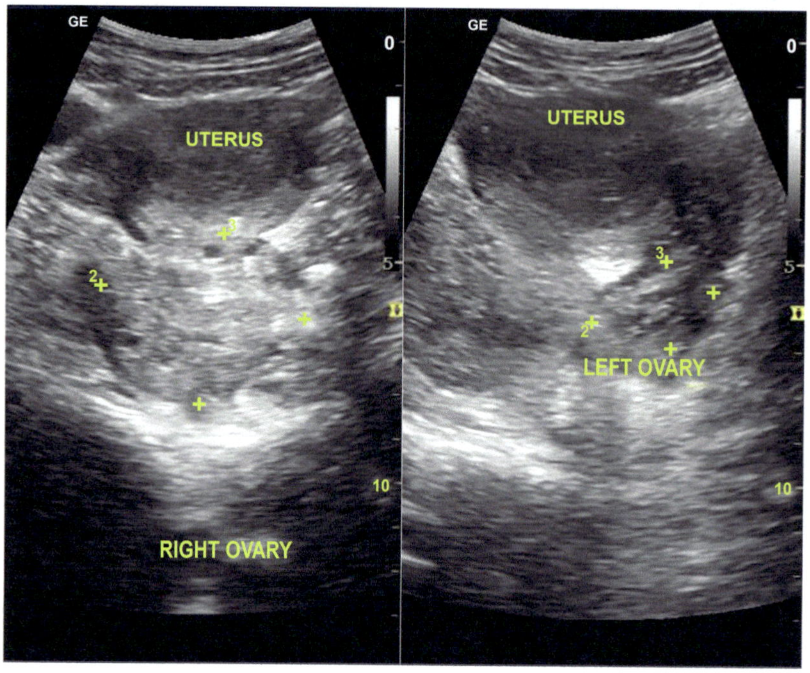

Figure 12.11. Indications for female pelvic ultrasound.

Source: https://www.emdocs.net/wp-content/uploads/2021/06/Screen-Shot-2021-07-11-at-2.19.23-AM.png.

12.4.1. Evaluation of Ovarian Health

Evaluation of ovarian health is significant for diagnosing a host of gynecological conditions, including ovarian cysts, tumors, and polycystic ovarian syndrome (PCOS). Ultrasound scan is a useful, non-traumatic method applied in the evaluation of the dimensions, morphology, and vascularity of the ovaries. Application of the transabdominal and transvaginal approaches allows satisfactory visualization of the ovaries, which facilitates the detection of abnormalities indicative of underlying pathologies. For instance, measurements using Doppler ultrasound can define blood flow characteristics that are useful in differentiating between malignant and benign lesions. These kinds of measurements are very important in clinical practice since they help clinicians make informed decisions regarding patient management and intervention plans. Early detection through ultrasound has the potential to significantly enhance patient outcomes, particularly in malignancies, making imaging vital in reproductive health. Given the complexity of ovarian health, emphasis is put on the implementation of standardised protocols that enhance diagnostic sensitivity without compromising efficiency. Research has indicated that reduced imaging sequences, such as those involving diffusion-weighted imaging (DWI) in magnetic resonance sequences, facilitate higher turnaround times without loss of sensitivity or specificity necessary for proper assessment. For instance, the application of optimized two-sequence magnetic resonance imaging (MRI) has been demonstrated to have similar diagnostic accuracy to conventional techniques at the expense of keeping patients for shorter periods in emergency rooms (Ali et al., 2018). As access to healthcare facilities continues to be under pressure, such innovations have the potential to rationalize workflows in radiology departments, ultimately leading to timely interventions for patients presenting with suspected ovarian conditions. Moreover, the implications of ovarian health examinations go beyond immediate diagnosis to more general reproductive and psychological effects for patients. PCOS and ovarian tumors can impact not just a woman's chances for conception but also her overall hormonal status and mental well-being. Therefore, examinations must have educational elements involved for the implications of ultrasound findings, as well as interventions that may be necessary. Furthermore, ongoing research on ovarian pathologies reinforces the need for enhanced awareness and early detection strategies, particularly in populations that are at increased risk of having ovarian cancer. One should take precautions about these issues because intervention on time can lead to better prognosis as well as a quality life in such patients (Dubreuil et al., 2013). Lastly, evaluation of ovarian function using ultrasound is a core component of modern gynecological practice with significant implications for patient care and well-being (Figure 12.2).

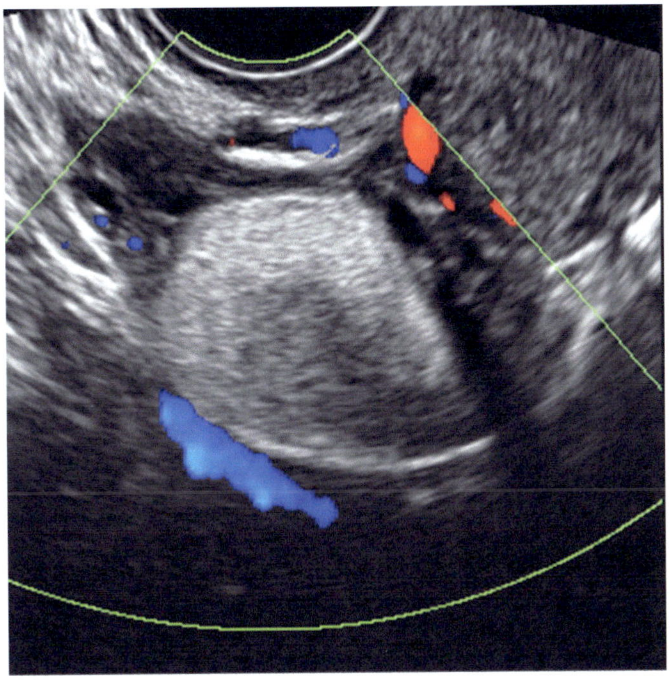

Figure 12.12. Evaluation of ovarian health ultrasound.

Source: Diane M. Twickler and Moschos E. (2010).Ultrasound and Assessment of Ovarian Cancer Risk. AJR. 194 (2). https://doi.org/10.2214/AJR.09.3562

12.4.2. Assessment of Uterine Conditions

Assessment of uterine status is of utmost significance in the overall context of pelvic ultrasound scans, particularly in women. Ultrasonography is a painless imaging modality with the potential to offer complete visualization of the uterus and surrounding structures. This imaging modality is very useful for the detection of several abnormalities of the uterus, such as fibroids, polyps, and congenital malformations. Through evaluation of changes in uterine size, shape, and echogenicity, clinicians can identify pathological processes that may be responsible for symptoms such as pelvic pain or abnormal bleeding. The aversive nature of ultrasound provides an advantage over invasive investigations, making it a useful tool for routine surveys and more advanced diagnostic assessments. Besides, the ability to apply ultrasound in real-time facilitates guided intervention upon necessity, improving patient care outcomes and the efficacy of clinical practice. Clinically, an understanding of the connotations of uterine status necessitates correlational examination between the results from ultrasound and clinical symptoms. As revealed in studies, pelvic pain remains the prevalent reason for ordering ultrasounds among women, embodying a significant proportion of diagnostic queries (Ameh et al., 2022). The majority of these presentations are connected with pathology such as pelvic inflammatory disease (PID) and adnexal masses, and this underlines the importance of thorough evaluation. The correlation between clinical presentation and imaging findings not only assists in diagnostic assessment but also influences treatment protocols. For instance, identification of endometrial pathology might provoke further evaluation or intervention, while benign appearances might lead to conservative treatment protocols. This targeted assessment ultimately enhances the clinician's ability to provide individualized care based on patient presentations. Additionally, ultrasound application in assessing uterine condition also includes monitoring the development and structural integrity during pregnancy. As depicted in various studies, the biomechanical environment of the uterus also contributes significantly to fetal movement, which ultimately affects fetal skeletal development and overall health (Nowlan, 2015). Abnormal fetal movement may indicate potential underlying pathology in uterine or placental well-being, necessitating thorough investigation by ultrasound. This broad-based approach not only explains the relationship between fetal well-being and uterine pathology but also enhances knowledge of prenatal growth. Through routine screening and targeted investigations, health workers are able to actively manage risks associated with uterine anomalies and, in so doing, secure better outcomes for the mothers and their developing fetuses (Figure 12.13).

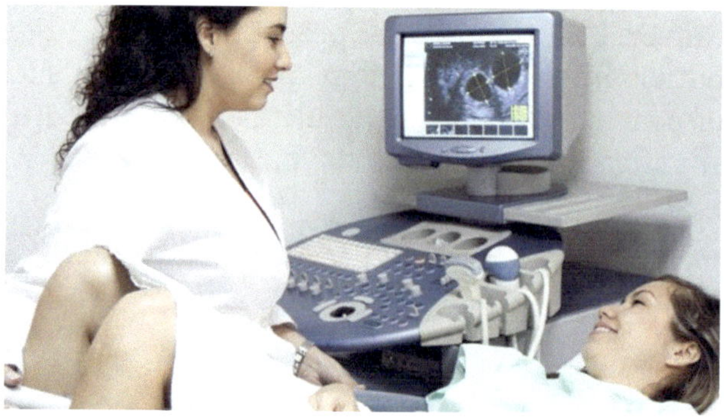

Figure 12.13. Assessment of uterine conditions.

Source: https://www.indoreinfertilityclinic.com/wp-content/uploads/2013/10/transvaginal_ultrasound_shutterstock.jpg.

12.4.3. Diagnosis of Pregnancy-Related Issues

Pregnancy-related conditions are also diagnosed more effectively today with advances in ultrasound technology, today a standard procedure in prenatal examinations. Of particular interest is the pelvic region, where critical fetal and maternal anatomy is located. Pregnancy-related defects, such as proximal focal femoral deficiency (PFFD), can be detected from standard ultrasounds. Notably, PFFD is a highly rare condition that may present with a variety of presentations, such as hypoplasia of the femur or absence of the femur. Prenatal ultrasound detection of these deformities in early stages is important not only for their treatment but also for counseling the prospective parents on potential interventions and preparation for the child's management. An awareness of the nuances in diagnosing the conditions enhances the ability of health professionals to provide appropriate support throughout pregnancy and following delivery (Aikten et al., 2016).

Secondly, fetal motion biomechanics have a critical role to play in diagnosis, in addition to fetal development. Fetal motion is said to start as early as week seven of gestation, with varying motions that are crucial for normal skeletal formation (Aikten et al., 2016). Ultrasound scanning measuring fetal movement patterns may be an indicator of potential developmental disorders, such as developmental dysplasia of the hip or arthrogryposis, these being conditions that can occur inappropriately or with restriction from a suboptimal intrauterine movement. By such observation of these movements using ultrasound, experts can quantify the physical volume of the womb, like amniotic fluid volume and baby position that significantly influence freedom of movement and subsequent development of the skeleton (Nowlan, 2015). This type of diagnosis emphasizes the interconnectedness between fetal movement and structural development.

Lastly, the integration of new imaging techniques with traditional ultrasound enables an enhancement in diagnostic capability for pregnancy issues. Technologies such as 3D and 4D ultrasound are capable of producing high-resolution images that help to depict fetal movement and anatomical detail, and hence allow more accurate assessment of fetal health. These technologies are capable of identifying subtle anomalies that do not obviously appear on usual 2D images. Therefore, health care workers are capable of providing a more tailored intervention and prescribing necessary treatment earlier. Moreover, the continued investigation into ultrasound practice can potentially enhance the diagnostic reliability and provide an environment where possible complications can be foreseen and resolved proactively, thus improving the outcomes for both infants and mothers (Aikten et al., 2016).

12.5. Methods Applied During Pelvic Ultrasound

The application of ultrasound imaging of the pelvis has come a long way through many imaging modalities, crucial for both male and female diagnosis. Transabdominal and transvaginal ultrasound are the two primary methods utilized to image pelvic organs. Transabdominal ultrasound is a broad view that allows clinicians to evaluate organs like the bladder and the uterus, while transvaginal ultrasound enhances specificity and resolution for pelvic organs like the ovaries and the prostate. This technique involves positioning a transducer within the vagina, which provides a nearer proximity to the anatomy of interest and increases the sensitivity in registering abnormalities. The combination of these techniques not only augments the diagnostic accuracy but also helps in quantifying conditions such as fibroids, ovarian cysts, and prostatic enlargement, proving the utility of pelvic ultrasound in clinical evaluation. Over the last few years, sophisticated imaging techniques have revolutionized pelvic ultrasound's diagnostic features. Three-dimensional (3D) ultrasound technology has become an important tool, providing volumetric analysis of organs of the pelvic cavity, most importantly in obstetric applications. The method records multiple two-dimensional (2D) images, which are reconstructed into a volume in three dimensions, enabling a detailed examination of anatomy. Moreover, the addition of Doppler ultrasound permits inspection of blood flow within pelvic organs, vital for the diagnosis of such as ectopic pregnancy or tumor-related vascular complications. Such advancements reflect the dynamic nature of pelvic imaging and the necessity to adopt new modalities to improve patient care and refine clinical assessment. The significance of accurate anatomical imaging cannot be overstated in cases of pelvic floor dysfunctions, particularly during delivery and resulting damage. Evidence has shown how pelvic floor muscles like the external anal sphincter tend to come under duress during childbirth and result in long-term complications if not properly tested (Cory et al., 2018). The non-invasive imaging modalities, such as Magnetic Resonance Diffusion Tensor Imaging (MR-DTI), have been proposed as add-ons to ultrasound to aid in the determination of muscle integrity and structure. Visualization of such anatomical features allows clinicians to formulate targeted management strategies for patients with pelvic floor dysfunction. Thus, the integration of emerging imaging techniques with traditional ultrasound enhances not only diagnostic accuracy but also pelvic health knowledge, optimizing treatment in worried patients (Figure 12.14).

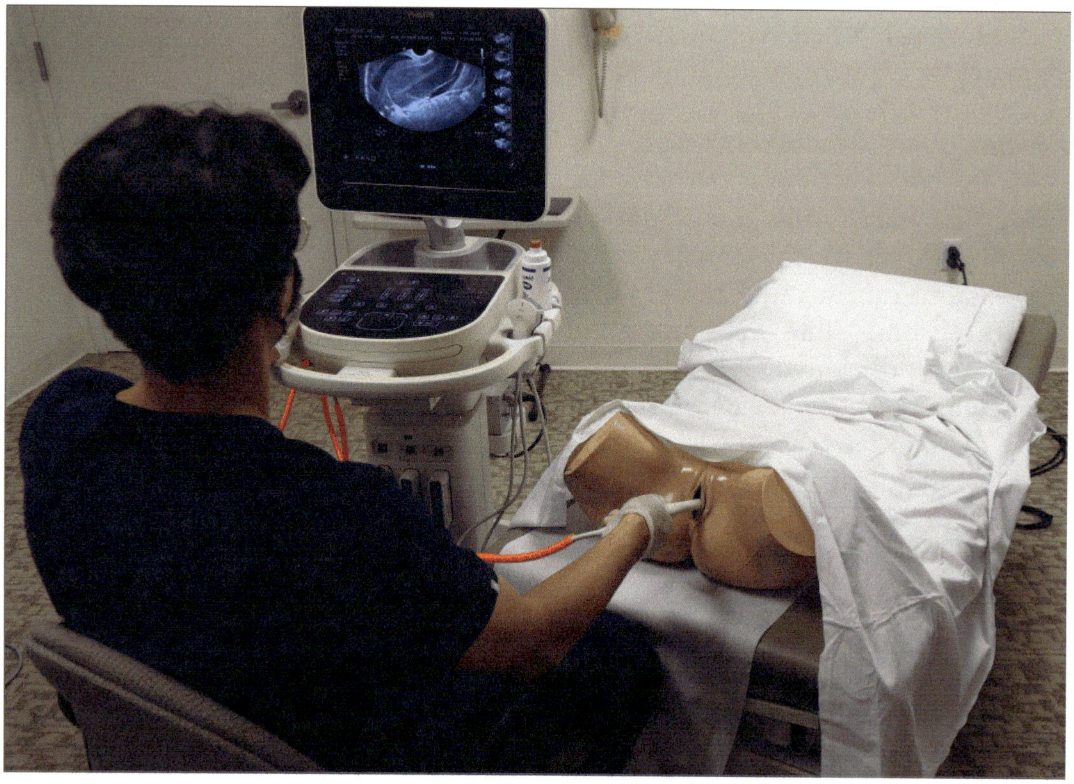

Figure 12.14. Techniques used in pelvic ultrasound.

Source: Annalise Lang, Vi Dinh. Gynecology/Pelvic Ultrasound Made Easy: Step-By-Step Guide. POCUS 101 https://pocus101.b-cdn.net/wp-content/uploads/2020/09/Ultrasound-Machine-and-Patient-Positioning-for-Gynecology-Pelvic-Ultrasound.png.

12.5.1. Transabdominal Ultrasound

Transabdominal ultrasonography is perhaps the most significant imaging modality in assessing pelvic structures in both women and men. Ultrasonography is a minimally invasive technique that employs high-frequency sound waves to acquire real-time images of pelvic organs, which are extremely helpful in visualizing their morphology as well as function. The transabdominal approach is particularly beneficial when conventional transvaginal or transrectal routes are not feasible or viable, such as in early pregnancy assessment or for patients with complicated anatomical access. Importantly, the abdominal wall must be well prepared to enable improved transmission of ultrasound waves, which is typicallyachieved through the administration of water orally to the patient prior to the scanning to distend the bladder, thereby enabling better visualization of pelvic structures. The preparatory element underscores the importance of cooperation and patient awareness of the process involved in obtaining a quality imaging outcome. Transabdominal ultrasonography is an essential part of examining conditions such as bladder pathologies and male prostate disease. Diagnosis and characterization of bladder hernias, for example, which occur at an incidence of approximately 1–3% of all inguinal hernias, are routinely done with this modality. Over the age of 50 years, the patients also have a higher incidence of such hernias, most often caused by conditions like obstruction of the urinary outlet and chronic distension of the bladder, compromising bladder function and integrity (Autieri et al., 2015). Sonographic identification of fluid accumulation or mass lesions in the bladder on ultrasound may alert practitioners to underlying pathology requiring further intervention. Therefore, this imaging technique not only assists in diagnosis but also plays an important role in directing therapeutic interventions specifically customized for a patient's individual needs. In women, transabdominal ultrasound is essential for diagnosing and managing several gynecologic conditions, including congenital anomalies like Müllerian duct abnormalities. These are the most frequent congenital genital malformations and have a very broad spectrum of clinical presentations, ranging from mild to severe, and therefore should be evaluated carefully using imaging studies. The best example is Herlyn-Werner-Wunderlich syndrome, which is uterus didelphys with hemivagina obstruction which usually leads to severe gynecological and renal complications. Accurate and timely diagnosis of such disorders using transabdominal ultrasound can prevent late sequelae such as infertility or long-term pain (Hosseini, 2023). Effective incorporation of skilled image acquisition and interpretation is important in the effective management of these complex issues, elucidating the importance of transabdominal ultrasound as a useful commodity in pelvic exam (Figure 12.15).

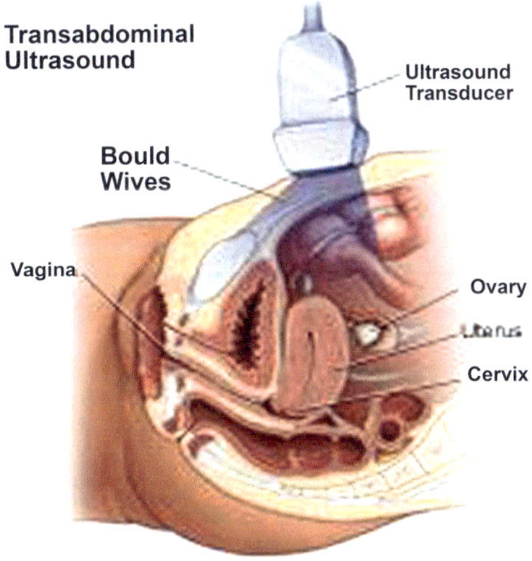

Figure 12.15. Transabdominal ultrasound.

Source: Pelvic Ultrasound. www.hopkinsmedicine.org. https://www.hopkinsmedicine.org/-/media/images/health/2_-treatment/gynecology/getimage-(9)/getimage-(9).png?h=200&iar=0&mh=360&mw=520&w=200&hash=94913919204845A71B0269C945C366F5.

12.5.2. Transvaginal Ultrasound for Females

Transvaginal sonography (TVUS) is now an essential imaging modality in gynecological practice, offering a very effective though non-invasive means of imaging female pelvic structures. TVUS significantly enhances the assessment of many disorders of reproductive health, including ovarian cysts, fibroids, and intrauterine pathology. With the use of a specialized transducer introduced within the vagina, doctors can obtain high-resolution images of the uterus and ovaries in order to better detect pathologies that would not be revealed under abdominal ultrasound. Moreover, the high-resolution images produced by TVUS allow for more accurate measurements and assessments, thereby improving clinical decision-making protocols for potential therapies. With advancing technique, it is being used increasingly in outpatient settings, enhancing comfort and access to basic diagnostic procedures for patients. Transvaginal ultrasound not only restricts to imaging anatomy but is also critical in evaluating fertility.

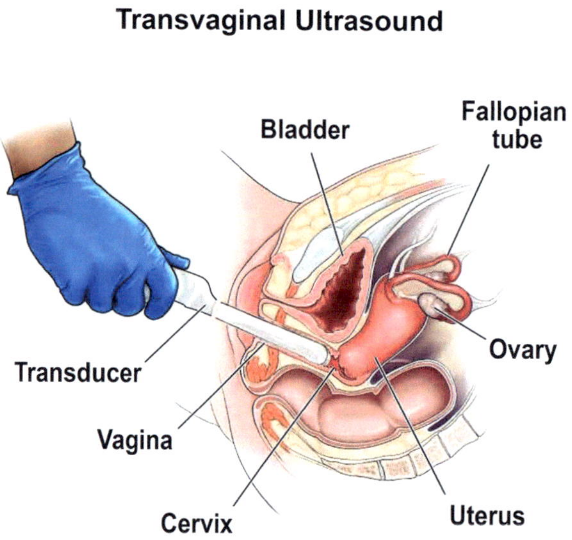

Figure 12.16. Transvaginal ultrasound.

Source: Cleveland Clinic (2022). Transvaginal Ultrasound. my.clevelandclinic.org https://my.clevelandclinic.org/-/scassets/images/org/health/articles/4993-transvaginal-ultrasound.

By providing crucial information about follicular development, endometrial thickness, and uterine anomalies, TVUS is critical in the evaluation of women with issues of fertility. Furthermore, transvaginal ultrasound has been proven to be feasible as an adjunct to multi-modal approaches such as the One-Stop Fertility Clinic model (Khouri, 2004). The model allows for simultaneous assessments through the integration of pelvic ultrasound, hysteroscopy, and culdoscopy within a single outpatient visit. These partnerships aim to streamline patient management without compromising lengthy assessments done in a more comfortable setting. The increasing acceptability and feasibility of TVUS in outpatient practice are indicative of its applicability in patient-focused care and reproductive medicine. Furthermore, findings from more contemporary research reiterate the utility of transvaginal ultrasound in defining and diagnosing pelvic pathology that can affect reproductive health. Notably, pelvic measurement correlations with other factors such as age and height have been valuable in shedding light on anatomical differences that may determine surgical methods and treatment interventions (Aguado del Hoyo et al., 2022). Accurate measurement and interpretation of anatomy through TVUS have become required steps for personalized interventions and improved clinical outcomes. Therefore, the role of transvaginal ultrasound in gynecological practice is not only limited to diagnostic situations; rather, it is a fundamental component in the overall management of women's health, particularly regarding reproductive disorders. In view of continued research and shift in imaging modalities, TVUS will undoubtedly be an invincible cornerstone of feminine pelvic exams (Figure 12.16).

12.5.3. Scrotal Ultrasound for Males

Scrotal ultrasound is a valuable diagnostic imaging tool in contemporary urology for the evaluation of a variety of male reproductive abnormalities. As a non-invasive imaging tool that employs high-frequency sound waves, it provides superior visualization of the scrotal contents, such as the testes, epididymis, and surrounding structures. It is especially invaluable for testing for testicular torsion, varicocele, and tumors. In addition, its use extends to the diagnosis of sex development disorder (DSD), where proper imaging is necessary for management guidance. Scrotal ultrasound's capacity for quick assessment renders it not only valuable in emergency presentations, but also valuable in the outpatient setting, where the potential for clinicians to deliver timely and accurate diagnoses essential for effective patient care is enhanced. The frequency of germ cell tumors (GCTs) highlights the role of ultrasound of the scrotum in the detection of testicular masses that could be malignant or benign. Since such tumors constitute a significant percentage of childhood malignancies, especially in males, early detection by the right imaging can mean a lot in terms of treatment. Scrotal ultrasound can permit lesion characterization, enabling cystic versus solid masses to be discerned—information critical to surgical planning and subsequent care.

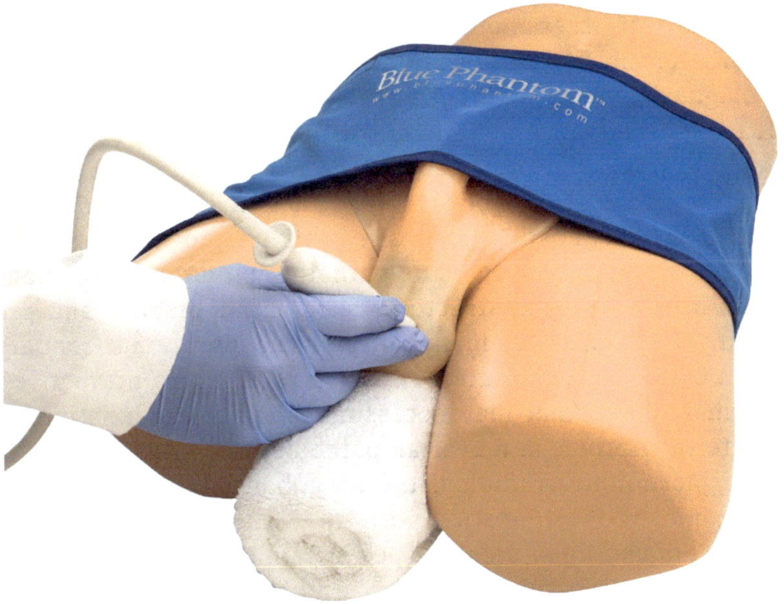

Figure 12.17. Scrotal ultrasound for males.

Source: Scrotal ultrasound training model. https://adam-rouilly.co.uk/wp-content/uploads/adamrouilly/product-images/blue-phantom-product-images/ABP092/ABP092-1.jpg.

It has been demonstrated that routine screening methods, including ultrasound, can lead to early interventions that can improve prognosis. In the pediatric population, for instance, those who come with tumors because of abnormal migratory patterns of the germ cells, being aware of their clinical profiles becomes all the more important and points to the employment of ultrasound as an initial-line method of diagnosis in traumatic or pathological conditions of the testes (Singh, 2014). In addition to neoplasm diagnosis, scrotal ultrasound is also important in directing therapeutic interventions, such as aspiration of hydroceles and epididymal cysts. The procedural application of scrotal ultrasound not only assists with diagnosis but also with surgical planning since the imaging provides surgeons with a map of the anatomical structures encountered during surgery. Most importantly, the effectiveness and safety of minimally invasive procedures such as laparoscopy have been shown to reduce postoperative complications compared to standard surgery in cases of conditions leading to testicular anomalies (Calvo et al., 2016). This complementarity between ultrasound and procedure intervention is essential in the effective management of intersex disorders alongside associated conditions. Through the integration of ultrasound data with clinical histories and physical examinations, healthcare providers can develop holistic management plans specifically suited to the individualized needs of male patients, ultimately leading to improved urologic clinical outcomes (Figure 12.17).

12.6. Interpretation of Ultrasound Results

The interpretation of pelvic ultrasound images is a technical and clinical process. Ultrasound plays a significant role in the assessment of many conditions of the male and female pelvis, especially in the emergency setting when urgent assessment must be achieved. The imaging of soft tissue anatomy, blood flow, and organ morphology without harm is enabled by non-invasive ultrasound technology, facilitating easy diagnosis of ectopic pregnancies, ovarian cysts, and testicular torsion. According to (Ali et al., 2018), the advancement in ultrasound technology has enhanced its usefulness, as there is better diagnostic performance as well as less interpretation time, hence enabling clinicians to intervene on time. The evolving arena of ultrasound modalities, including Doppler imaging, also increases the diagnostic potential of this imaging tool, allowing detailed vascular assessments that are critical in suspected acute pathology situations. For the male pelvis, ultrasound interpretation classically deals with structures such as the bladder and prostate. One common application is assessing the prostate for malignancy or lesions, often secondary to benign prostatic hyperplasia or cancer. Correct interpretation relies on recognizing normative anatomical variation and detecting abnormal results that may necessitate further examination. Similarly, in pelvic ultrasound in females, uterine fibroids and ovarian pathology are under close scrutiny. With the addition of advanced imaging techniques, radiologists have enhanced capabilities to assess such conditions effectively. The development of diagnostic algorithms, which are highlighted in Devon et al. (2008), has improved the understanding of complex pelvic pain syndromes and paved the way for improved management using a combination of surgical and non-surgical interventions. Good ultrasound interpretation is more than the mere identification of abnormalities; it constitutes a full evaluation that considers a patient's clinical history, presenting symptoms, and potential differential diagnoses. For instance, when assessing athletic pubalgia, a prevalent condition in high-level athletes, imaging diagnostic procedures ought to be supplemented with a full understanding of the anatomical and physiological pathways involved. The ability to identify subtle changes in anatomy, as highlighted in Devon et al. (2008), has direct implications for treatment trends, enhancing the approach to both conservative treatment and surgical intervention. Therefore, interpretation of ultrasound is an important competency that combines technical knowledge with a generalist clinical perspective to deliver optimal patient outcomes in pelvic health.

12.6.1. Normal Findings of Male Pelvic Ultrasound

Normal male pelvic ultrasound findings are critical in establishing baseline anatomy and detecting potential pathologies. In most instances, the ultrasound allows one to see such vital structures as the prostate gland, seminal vesicles, bladder, and elements of the urinary tract. The prostate, on the other hand, must be a well-circumscribed, symmetrically lobed organ located just beneath the bladder. Distinct echogenic patterns like sharp boundaries and homogeneous texture are major characteristics confirmed by ultrasound. In healthy individuals, the seminal vesicles should also be bilaterally appearing with clear echogenicity that contrasts them from surrounding tissues. The ultrasound can well detect abnormalities in size or contour that may indicate underlying pathologies like prostatitis or malignancy, and hence the role of periodic screening in clinical practice. A pelvic ultrasound scan of the urinary bladder obtains important information about bladder shape and function. A normally filled bladder is thin-walled, smooth, and anechoic and is easily separated from surrounding structures. Ultrasound studies are able to detect potential abnormalities, such as wall thickening or masses within the bladder, that are indicative of such conditions as bladder stones or tumors.

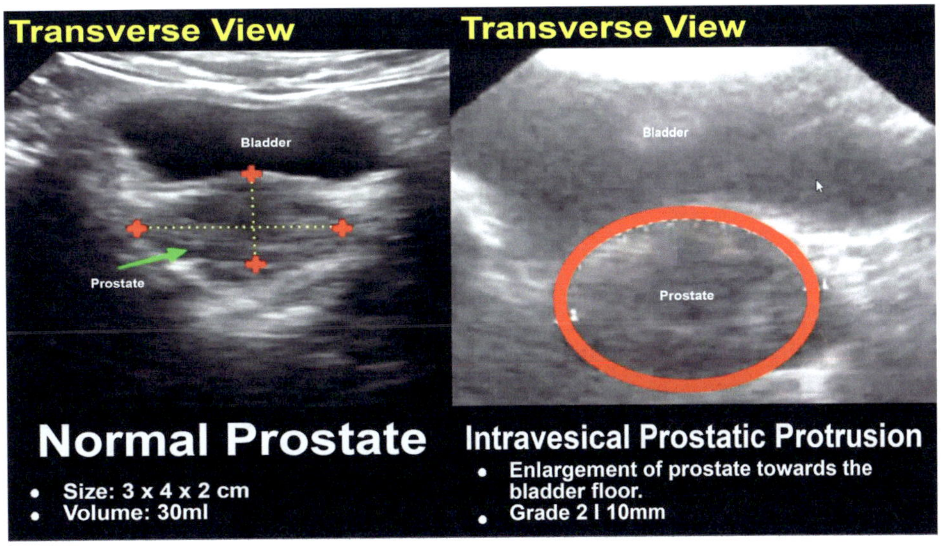

Figure 12.18. Normal findings in a male pelvic ultrasound.

Source: Dr. Sam's Imaging Library. Prostate Ultrasound Normal Vs Abnormal Image Appearances. https://www.youtube.com/@DrSamsImagingLibrary

Moreover, the assessment includes measurement of post-void residual volume to determine bladder function, particularly valuable in symptomatic patients with urinary complaints. Having such normal bladder results allows clinicians to differentiate between benign and those requiring diagnostic workup. However, correlation of ultrasound findings with patients' history still remains significant for accurate diagnosis as well as effective treatment planning, highlighting the essential role of ultrasound in urologic evaluation. In addition, ultrasound is an essential method of assessing the vascular anatomy of the male pelvis. Normal Doppler ultrasound examinations can show clear patterns of flow of the internal pudendal arteries, which supply blood to the genitals, and on erectile function testing. Normal vascular integrity will show no signs of thrombosis or severe stenosis. These measurements substantially contribute to the diagnosis of diseases like erectile dysfunction, where vascular etiology is typically suspected. Moreover, diseases like varicocele can be diagnosed by virtue of the dilation of the pampiniform plexus, which would otherwise lie beyond normal venous drainage patterns. Incorporating anatomical and vascular measurements in ultrasound scans, clinicians gain an overall impression of male pelvic health, which ultimately guides clinical management. Therefore, identification of normal appearances is necessary for accurate diagnosis and targeted therapeutic measures in male pelvic ultrasound examinations (Figure 12.18).

12.6.2. Normal Findings in Female Pelvic Ultrasound

Normal female pelvic ultrasound appearances are of extreme significance in assessing reproductive and urinary health. A normal pelvic ultrasound of a well-conducted study should reveal the anatomy of the uterus, ovaries, fallopian tubes, and bladder. The uterus should appear as a homogenous organ with a smooth endometrial echogenicity with a hyperechoic line in the center, representing the endometrial cavity. Routine ovarian follicles appear as small anechoic structures in the ovaries, as evidence of normal functioning reproductive machinery. In addition to the detection of normal anatomy, ultrasound also has the ability to evaluate for disease, helping practitioners form proper treatment plans on suspicion of disease, such as polycystic ovarian syndrome or uterine fibroids. Second, ultrasound assessment of the pelvic organs not only serves a diagnostic purpose but also yields details regarding physiological changes that may occur in a woman's reproductive cycle. For instance, many females can exhibit various phases of follicular development, which can be visualized through the dynamic changes in ovarian shape over the course of a menstrual cycle. This can demonstrate the ovarian reserve and health, and associate sonographic findings with potential fertility. Besides, normal findings are also accompanied by a well-circumscribed pelvic floor anatomy, an important factor in urinary issue prevention, such as incontinence, which can be exacerbated by structural abnormalities. As such, ultrasound scans have a two-pronged purpose for both diagnosis and overall reproductive health evaluation. Beyond analyzing reproductive organs, a female pelvic ultrasound is beneficial in determining bladder integrity and conducting checks for common urinary tract abnormalities. The bladder on sonographic appearance is in a normal condition as an anechoic structure and distended, with normal wall volume and thickness. The irregularity of walls or the presence of masses is suspicious of pathologies that should be assessed further. Another important aspect is an evaluation of potential fluid collections or cysts within the pelvis due to other medical issues. Thus, identifying normal findings in female pelvic ultrasound not only helps to establish the status of health but also provides a foundation for the detection of possible complications, ultimately enhancing patient outcomes in gynecological and urological situations.

12.6.3. Shared Abnormalities and Their Significance

The pelvis is an important anatomical area that contains several organs and is thus prone to a variety of common abnormalities amenable to diagnosis by ultrasound. Ovarian cysts in women and seminal vesicle cysts in men are common findings on pelvic examination. These abnormalities have important clinical consequences and may cause complications such as pain, infection, or infertility. Such ultrasound detection of anomalies not only assists in making an early diagnosis but also guides clinical management schemes. For instance, identification of an abnormal cyst may require additional tests to rule out malignancy or assess other conditions present, highlighting the importance of ultrasound monitoring of pelvic health (Ali et al., 2018). Aside from cystic lesions, congenital abnormalities of the genitourinary tract are also notable features of pelvic ultrasound scans. Conditions such as renal agenesis or positional defects of the bladder can occur in males and females and have had diverse impacts on urinary function and health. Specifically, loss of one kidney, which is often discovered incidentally on a routine scan, can have a profound impact on renal function and render patients vulnerable to urinary tract infection or hypertension in adult life. Early detection by ultrasound permits anticipatory management, which may be ongoing surveillance or operation if needed, thus highlighting the imaging role in preventing long-term damage (Gheissari et al., 2011). Furthermore, pelvic ultrasound plays a pivotal role in diagnosing abnormalities like fibroids, endometriosis, and other pathological processes that can affect female reproductive health. Fibroids are benign muscle tumors of the uterus, which are prevalent and are sometimes found with heavy menstrual bleeding, pelvic pain, and complications during pregnancy. Evaluation of such abnormalities typically consists of a critical assessment of their size, location, and symptomatic significance. Accordingly, sonographic findings are part and parcel of formulating proper treatment strategies, from medication to surgery, targeting relief of symptoms as well as enhancement of quality of life. The cascading effects of these prevalent abnormalities go beyond the realm of salient clinical considerations to touch on psychological wellbeing and family planning choices and therefore underline the holistic significance of pelvic ultrasound in medicine (Ali et al., 2018).

SUMMARY

The evaluation of male and female pelvic anatomical structures by ultrasound imaging emphasizes the clinical relevance of such an imaging modality. The various ultrasound techniques offer imaging of key pelvic organs such as the bladder, prostate, uterus, and ovaries to facilitate abnormality detection and diagnosis. In men, ultrasound plays a vital role in the diagnosis of such conditions as prostate enlargement or cancer, and for women, it plays a vital role in evaluating reproductive health and in diagnosing conditions like fibroids or ovarian cysts. Real-time imaging capability of pelvic ultrasound significantly contributes to the speed at which clinical decisions can be made by healthcare providers without risking patient safety. The performance of pelvic ultrasound is also evidenced by its non-invasive nature and lack of ionizing radiation, making it a preferred choice for routine assessment in clinical practice. The variation between male and female pelvic ultrasound protocols highlights the need for special training among ultrasound technologists to ensure proper attention to detailed anatomical variation. Moreover, technological advancements in ultrasound, such as contrast-enhanced ultrasound and 3D imaging, are offering enhanced visualization capability, enabling precise evaluation of pelvic pathologies. Advanced imaging techniques are not only essential for diagnosis but also for the direction of therapeutic intervention to promote better patient outcomes in pelvic well-being. With the expansion of literature on pelvic ultrasound techniques, it is important to have more studies carried out to enhance methodologies and individualize them to specific patient populations. More training of experts in the field and the inclusion of emerging technologies will most likely enhance the diagnostic effectiveness of pelvic ultrasound. Further study of the male and female ultrasound uses will provide a better understanding of sex-specific health issues, thereby enabling gender-specific healthcare solutions. Ultimately, results achieved from pelvic ultrasound imaging can be a determining factor in the enhancement of clinical outcomes in a large patient population, again underscoring the requirement for ongoing education and research in this important medical imaging field.

The pelvis is a critical anatomical structure in both males and females, playing a significant role in numerous physiological functions as well as fostering reproductive health. Through ultrasonography, the variations between the male and female pelvises are made apparent, with the female pelvis usually wider to accommodate birth. The male pelvis is thicker but narrower. It is necessary to comprehend these variations while interpreting the ultrasound images. Moreover, the dynamic motion of pelvic organs as induced by adjacent structures is indispensable in the diagnosis of many conditions. Conditions with pelvic inflammatory disease, ovarian cysts, and masses require proper imaging modalities to differentiate between normalcy and pathology. Because the pelvis is a nidus for a variety of medical conditions, the role of ultrasound in making timely and accurate diagnoses cannot be overemphasized. Apart from structural differences, functional pelvic characteristics also direct ultrasound testing. In males, ultrasound can be employed to make diagnoses in prostatitis and testicular torsion, conditions with significant implications for reproductive function. For females, ultrasound is crucial for inspecting reproductive organs, making diagnoses like fibroids or polycystic ovarian syndrome. Another important application of ultrasound technology is the assessment of foetal health in the woman's pelvis; foetal movement visible in utero, beginning as early as seven weeks of gestation, is crucial for monitoring and assessment of overall development and detection of abnormalities (Nowlan, 2015). The health of the pelvic floors and their role in these evaluations affirm the importance of knowing both anatomy and function in ultrasonography. Ultrasound technology advancements have also enhanced diagnostic activities concerning pelvic disorders. Improved resolution imaging improves soft tissue structure visualization with precision in the delineation of potential pathologies. Furthermore, the incorporation of 3D imaging modalities has significantly contributed to the investigation of complicated pelvic anatomy to aid in diagnoses that prove challenging using typical 2D approaches. The identification of pelvic dynamics differences, particularly in athletes with injuries such as athletic pubalgia, indicates the necessity of using a multi-factorial assessment technique (Devon et al., 2008). The developments demonstrate the importance of the use of ultrasound as a less invasive alternative to other diagnostic modalities, ultimately promoting improved patient results and sooner intervention for different pelvic-related disorders.

CLOSER LOOK

TRANSABDOMINAL ULTRASOUND

Transabdominal ultrasound is a widely used, non-invasive imaging technique employing high-frequency ultrasound sound waves to visualize organs and structures of the pelvic and abdominal cavities via the anterior abdominal wall. The method utilizes a curved (or convex) transducer positioned against the skin surface, usually after application of a conductive gel to eliminate air spaces and allow sound wave conduction. Transabdominal ultrasound is a cheap and easily accessible technology, used commonly in emergency, outpatient, and inpatient settings for the evaluation of abdominal pain, masses, organomegaly, vascular disease, and pregnancy. Its use is favored by its lack of ionizing radiation exposure, combined with its real-time imaging capability, ease of portability, and low cost.

Transabdominal ultrasound in practice imaging visualizes the large abdominal organs such as the liver, gallbladder, pancreas, spleen, kidneys, bladder, and abdominal aorta. It is pivotal in the diagnosis of gallstones, liver cirrhosis, splenomegaly, kidney stones, hydronephrosis, abdominal aortic aneurysms, and ascites. The scan will usually start in the epigastric area and systematically progress through the quadrants. For optimal imaging, patients are usually asked to fast for 6–8 hours to reduce bowel gas and gallbladder distension. A full bladder is usually required in pelvic exams, particularly in gynecologic or early pregnancy investigations, since it acts as an acoustic window for improved visualization of the adnexa and uterus.

Transabdominal ultrasound is usually the first line of imaging in gynecology and obstetrics for the evaluation of pelvic anatomy, uterine fibroids, ovarian cysts, and embryological development of early pregnancy. It finds special utility during the first and second trimester of pregnancy, for fetal biometry, detection of cardiac activity, identification of placental position, and assessment of amniotic fluid volume. Although transvaginal ultrasound has superior resolution for pelvic anatomy due to its proximity, transabdominal scanning is applied in initial assessments, for large masses, and when a broad field of view is needed. In urology, it is employed to find bladder tumors, prostate hypertrophy (indirect), and post-void residual volumes. It is also used extensively for the follow-up of liver lesions, monitoring renal function, and guiding needle placement in interventional procedures such as paracentesis or biopsies.

Although it possesses numerous advantages, transabdominal ultrasound is not without limitations. Its quality can be compromised by patient body habitus, bowel gas, and operator skill. Deep or hidden structures, like the pancreas in an obese patient, can be hard to visualize clearly. In addition, overlying gas-filled bowel loops can impede sound waves, decreasing the diagnostic yield. However, advances in technology transducers, harmonics, and image processing continue to raise resolution and diagnostic capability. In addition, portable and handheld ultrasound equipment have broadened the availability of transabdominal imaging to resource-scarce and point-of-care settings.

References

1. Abramov, Y., Almeida, F. G., Berghmans, B., Bo, K., et al. (2016). An International Urogynecological Association (IUGA)/International Continence Society (ICS) joint report on the terminology for the conservative and nonpharmacological management of female pelvic floor dysfunction. https://core.ac.uk/download/293861075.pdf (accessed on 12th July 2025).
2. Aguado del Hoyo, A., Bravo Arribas, C., De León Luis, J. A., García-Tizón Larroca, L., et al. (2022). Effects of sex, age and height on symphysis–ischial spine distance measured on a pelvic CT. https://core.ac.uk/download/580467840.pdf (accessed on 12th July 2025).
3. Aikten, J., Alanay, A., Amstutz, C., Ashkenazy, M., Bevan-Thomas, R., Bronstein, M., et al. (2016). Prenatal diagnosis of proximal focal femoral deficiency: Literature review of prenatal sonographic findings. https://core.ac.uk/download/54529276.pdf (accessed on 12th July 2025).
4. Ali, I. T., Chang, S., Khosa, F., Klass, D., et al. (2018). Faster magnetic resonance imaging in emergency room patients with right lower quadrant pain and suspected acute appendicitis. https://core.ac.uk/download/160736740.pdf (accessed on 12th July 2025).
5. Ameh, P. O., Joseph, D. S., Joseph, D. Z., Laushugno, T., et al. (2022). Pattern of pelvic ultrasound request and findings in Abubakar Tafawa Balewa University Teaching Hospital (ATBUTH), Bauchi. https://core.ac.uk/download/524772369.pdf (accessed on 12th July 2025).
6. Armour, J., Boyd, R., Cunningham, C., Darwin, C., Department of Health and Human Services, Dunsworth, H. M., Fausto-Sterling, A., et al. (2020). Expanding the evolutionary explanations for sex differences in the human skeleton. https://core.ac.uk/download/322809885.pdf (accessed on 12th July 2025).
7. Ather, M. H., Ettinger, S., Hoffman, S., Martin, R. A., McLoughlin, M. A., Ross, L. A., Scott, R. C., et al. (2019). Endoscopic laser-ablation for the treatment of orthotopic and ectopic ureteroceles in dogs: 13 cases (2008–2017). https://core.ac.uk/download/213444929.pdf (accessed on 12th July 2025).
8. Autieri, D., Axer, S., Basilico, G., Bertoglio, F., et al. (2015). Topic: Rare and special cases, the real "strange cases." https://core.ac.uk/download/54524712.pdf (accessed on 12th July 2025).
9. Bonifacino, A., Carico, E., Giarnieri, E., Giovagnoli, A., et al. (2017). Clinical-pathological features of an occult mixed mucinous male breast cancer: A case report. https://core.ac.uk/download/153369666.pdf (accessed on 12th July 2025).
10. Brandetti, F., Carosa, E., Di Stasi, S. M., Gravina, G. L., et al. (2008). Measurement of the thickness of the urethrovaginal space in women with or without vaginal orgasm. https://core.ac.uk/download/pdf/53823740.pdf (accessed on 12th July 2025).
11. Bumgarner, A. (2007). A right to choose? Sex selection in the international context. https://core.ac.uk/download/62548099.pdf (accessed on 12th July 2025).
12. Calhoun, E. A., Clemens, J. Q., Kusek, J. W., Litwin, M. S., et al. (2009). Primary care physician practices in the diagnosis, treatment, and management of men with chronic prostatitis/chronic pelvic pain syndrome. https://core.ac.uk/download/323079649.pdf (accessed on 12th July 2025).

13. Calvo, A., Caprio, M. G., Escolino, M., Esposito, C., et al. (2016). Laparoscopic approach for gonadectomy in pediatric patients with intersex disorders. https://core.ac.uk/download/80338153.pdf (accessed on 12th July 2025).

14. Campana, A., de Agostini, A., Bischof, P., Tawfik, E., et al. (2015). Evaluation of infertility. https://core.ac.uk/download/pdf/85214735.pdf (accessed on 12th July 2025).

15. Cory, E., Ledgerwood-Lee, M., Mittal, R. K., Reisert, J., et al. (2018). Connectivity of the superficial muscles of the human perineum: A diffusion tensor imaging-based global tractography study. https://core.ac.uk/download/323065402.pdf (accessed on 12th July 2025).

16. De Almeida Joaquim, T. A. (2017). Designing technologies for intimate care in women. https://core.ac.uk/download/188733503.pdf (accessed on 12th July 2025).

17. Devon, O., Horner, M., Jain, N., Lauencin, M., et al. (2008). Understanding sports hernia (athletic pubalgia)–The anatomic and pathophysiologic basis for abdominal and groin pain in athletes. https://core.ac.uk/download/46965603.pdf (accessed on 12th July 2025).

18. Drennan, M. J., & Murphy, B. M. (2006). A comparison of the productivity of suckler cows of different breed composition. https://core.ac.uk/download/45656706.pdf (accessed on 12th July 2025).

19. Drennan, M. J., McGee, M., Murphy, B. M., O'Mara, F. P., et al. (2008). Post-weaning growth, ultrasound and skeletal measurements, muscularity scores and carcass traits, and composition of progeny of five beef suckler cow genotypes. https://core.ac.uk/download/45656404.pdf (accessed on 12th July 2025).

20. Dubreuil, A., Clements, A. B., Khan, A. J., Majmudar, B., Piura, B., Tam, C., Calista, D., et al. (2013). Sister Mary Joseph's nodule at a university teaching hospital in northwestern Tanzania: A retrospective review of 34 cases. https://core.ac.uk/download/pdf/18410880.pdf (accessed on 12th July 2025).

21. Garga, U. C., Mehra, S., & Ranjan, R. (2016). Zinner syndrome—A rare developmental anomaly of the mesonephric duct diagnosed on magnetic resonance imaging. https://core.ac.uk/download/pdf/82721525.pdf (accessed on 12th July 2025).

22. Gheissari, A., Lusch, A., Stocks, A., Shokeir, A. A., Ayede, A. I., Becker, A. M., Agunloye, A. M., et al. (2011). The role of routine post-natal abdominal ultrasound for newborns in a resource-poor setting: A longitudinal study. https://core.ac.uk/download/pdf/8606642.pdf (accessed on 12th July 2025).

23. Hamid, R., & Losco, G. (2014). Pelvic organ prolapse-associated cystitis. https://core.ac.uk/download/29410932.pdf (accessed on 12th July 2025).

24. Henson, M. L. (2002). *Medicalized Childbirth in the United States: Origins, Outcomes, and Opposition*. https://core.ac.uk/download/232714688.pdf (accessed on 12th July 2025).

25. Hosseini, A. (2023). A case report of Herlyn-Werner-Wunderlich syndrome. https://core.ac.uk/download/588468461.pdf (accessed on 12th July 2025).

26. Huysse, W., Sundaram, M., Verdonk, P., Verdonk, R., et al. (2008). Imaging findings after meniscal repair with degradable polyurethane scaffold: Preliminary results. https://core.ac.uk/download/55868375.pdf (accessed on 12th July 2025).

27. Karlan, B. Y., Mansfield, B. C., Miller, B. E., Chalas, E., Bigsby, G. E., Bertenshaw, G. P., Barter, J. F., et al. (2010). Validation of a multivariate serum profile for epithelial ovarian cancer using a prospective multi-site collection. https://core.ac.uk/download/pdf/289269.pdf (accessed on 12th July 2025).
28. Khouri, A. (2004). Evaluation of diagnostic culdoscopy in women with infertility. https://core.ac.uk/download/326710925.pdf (accessed on 12th July 2025).
29. Kline, R. C. (1989). *Equine Reproduction and Genetics*. https://core.ac.uk/download/286359847.pdf (accessed on 12th July 2025).
30. Lee, A., Romero, J. Y., Dewar, R., Natural, R., & Tatishchev, S. (2013). Primary diffuse large B-cell lymphoma of the uterus manifesting as a leiomyoma: A unique presentation with review of literature. https://core.ac.uk/download/pdf/26926544.pdf (accessed on 12th July 2025).
31. Lei, J., Lin, W., Wang, Y., Wu, Y., et al. (2023). Can GPT-4V (ision) serve medical applications? Case studies on GPT-4V for multimodal medical diagnosis. http://arxiv.org/abs/2310.09909 (accessed on 12th July 2025).
32. Mu, Z. H., Wang, D. X., Wu, H., Xu, Y., et al. (2015). A case of Prune Belly syndrome. https://core.ac.uk/download/pdf/82691610.pdf (accessed on 12th July 2025).
33. Nowlan, N. C. (2015). Biomechanics of fetal movement. https://core.ac.uk/download/76995826.pdf (accessed on 12th July 2025).
34. Olson, R. (2001). Potential dysfunctions occurring in the postpartum years. https://core.ac.uk/download/235074289.pdf (accessed on 12th July 2025).
35. Sinex, D. C. E. (2021). Shifting and Shaping Perceptions: Towards the Characterization and Literacy of Female Pelvic Organ Support. https://core.ac.uk/download/479151697.pdf (accessed on 12th July 2025).
36. Singh, D. S. (2014). Clinical profile of children with extracranial germ cell tumors. https://core.ac.uk/download/288215544.pdf (accessed on 12th July 2025).
37. Tomei, E., Zaccagna, F., Rodacki, K., Marinelli, E., Martino, M., Semelka, R. C., et al. (2015). Accuracy of MRI skeletal age estimation for subjects 12–19: Potential use for subjects of unknown age. https://core.ac.uk/download/54248856.pdf (accessed on 12th July 2025).

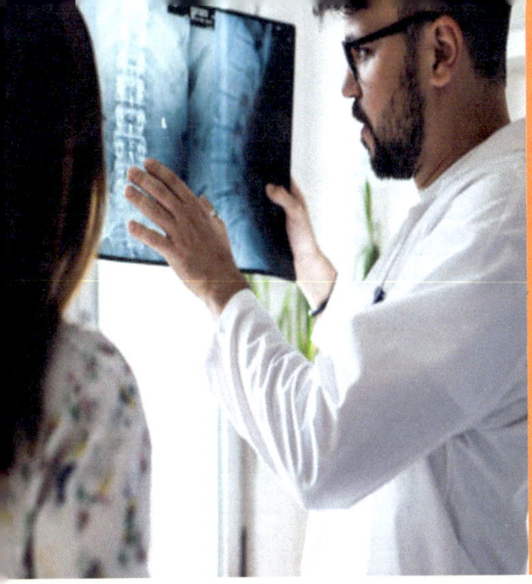

Chapter 13
MUSCULOSKELETAL (MSK) ULTRASOUND

Contents

Introduction

Clinical application of musculoskeletal ultrasound (MSK ultrasound) has revolutionized the diagnosis and treatment of numerous musculoskeletal disorders. This method is distinct compared to other imaging modalities in that it does not emit ionizing radiation and has the ability to generate real-time images of joints, muscle structures, and soft tissues. Anatomical abnormalities can thus be detected by practitioners, as well as functional impairments and even therapeutic interventions directed accordingly. The utility of MSK ultrasound also exists in conditions such as tendinitis, bursitis, and joint effusions, where it provides valuable information to assist with clinical decision-making. In addition to its diagnostic application, MSK ultrasound allows for guided injection and aspiration, thereby increasing procedural success and patient safety. One of the most significant uses of MSK ultrasound is for the management of gout, an acute inflammatory arthritis with crystal deposition of monosodium urate. The ability of ultrasound to identify specific abnormalities associated with gout is particularly striking, as it maximizes diagnostic accuracy and long-term surveillance. As an example, ultrasound can clearly visualize the tophi, or tissue deposits of urate crystals, and evaluate the degree of joint destruction. Clinical symptoms closely relate to the findings of ultrasound, its importance underlining both in acute gout and in chronic management. Furthermore, the technology allows for monitoring changes in the natural history of the disease, and it is, therefore, an important device to use both in research and practice (Finucci et al., 2015).

As ongoing innovations in technologies enhancing the effectiveness of musculoskeletal imaging continue to emerge, the advent of computer-assisted orthopedic surgery (CAOS) systems has garnered increasing attention. The systems employ imaging techniques, including ultrasound, to provide precise navigation in orthopedic surgery. With the application of advanced algorithms and imaging modalities, CAOS systems augment traditional surgical methods with improved precision and patient results. Indeed, ultrasound is becoming an integral part of CAOS, enabling surgeons to visualize anatomical features in real-time during intricate procedures. This synergy between ultrasound and surgical robotics is bringing about a new era of orthopedic surgery, which facilitates improved diagnosis and management of complex musculoskeletal disorders. With increased research in the application of ultrasound in CAOS systems, its application in musculoskeletal medicine is also expected to increase in the future (Kalová et al., 2019) (Figure 13.1).

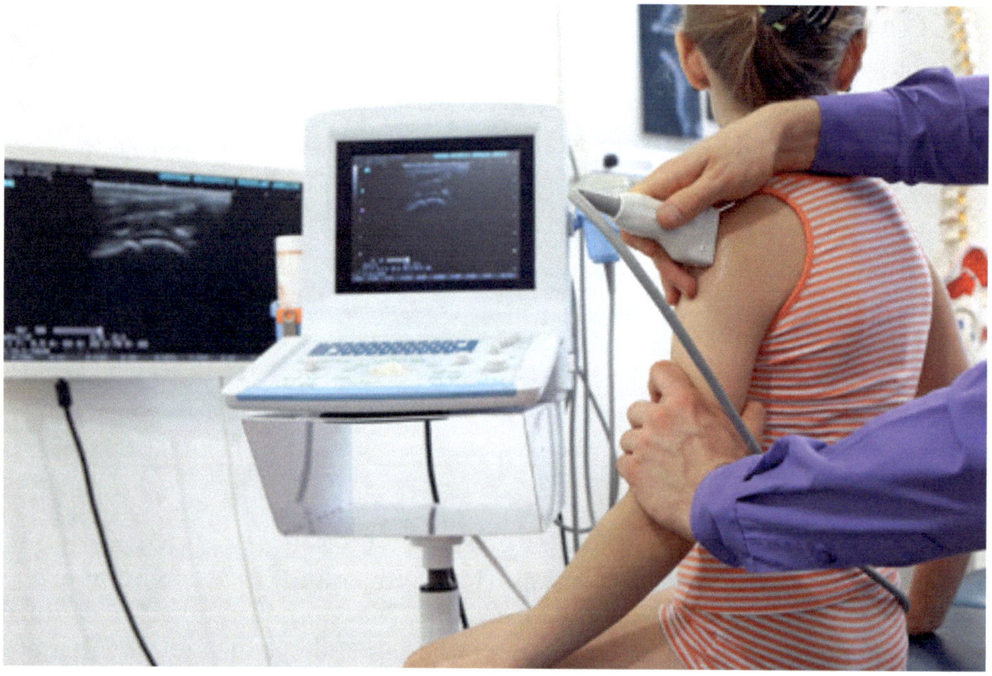

Figure 13.1. Musculoskeletal (MSK) ultrasound.

Source: https://external-content.duckduckgo.com/iu/?u=https%3A%2F%2Fhanhamclinic.co.uk%2Fwp-content%2Fuploads%2F2023%2F11%2FDIAGNOSTIC-MSK.jpg&f=1&nofb=1&ipt=ca8fdd73ddce33219e70219ebf0252609860be38d2e6734572e94be829c25490.

Definition and Purpose of MSK Ultrasound

Musculoskeletal (MSK) ultrasound is a new-generation imaging technology that allows for pain-free evaluation of a wide variety of musculoskeletal pathologies. MSK uses high-frequency sound waves to create real-time images of tendons, muscles, ligaments, and joints. MSK ultrasound enables clinicians to visualize structures with clear force, thus diagnosing injuries such as tendon rupture, bursitis, and arthritis. Additionally, it is now more widely used for its ability to guide therapeutic injections or aspirations with precision. The dynamic visualization feature makes it possible to assess joint motion and soft tissue function, which allows a comprehensive assessment that fixed imaging equipment like X-rays or MRIs may fail to achieve. Therefore, MSK ultrasound is an essential component of a clinician's diagnostic tool set since its application goes beyond mere visualization to include guiding treatment and continuous monitoring of musculoskeletal wellness. The changing role of MSK ultrasound mirrors its increasing importance to all medical specialties, solidifying its position in orthopedics and rheumatology, among others. As clinical ultrasound (CUS) guidelines for health system development have come into focus, the necessity for standardized methods and training has become clear. For instance, ensuring competency and quality assurance mechanisms for using ultrasound assures valid and reliable diagnoses of musculoskeletal pathology. Adhering to these guidelines, the quality of care for the patient improves. With continuing technological advancements, investment in quality education and infrastructure in equipment continues to be of top priority towards maximum use of CUS in institutions. The progressive character of this development reflects the necessity for making MSK ultrasound an integral part of daily clinical practice, making it even more important in personalized medicine and precise diagnosis (Abo et al., 2018). For operation, MSK ultrasound also plays a significant role in computer-assisted orthopedic surgery (CAOS). With the advancement of ultrasound computer-assisted orthopedic surgery (UCAOS) systems, physicians are now able to maximize the precision of musculoskeletal interventions. Such systems leverage the use of ultrasound imaging for real-time feedback, which results in more accurate navigational surgery compared to conventional imaging technologies such as MRI or CT scans. The addition of UCAOS allows for real-time assessment of joint and soft tissue anatomy intraoperatively, minimizing the risk for complications and optimizing surgical success. With continuous research in this area, the future for the application of ultrasound technology in the development of orthopedic procedures is promising and thus indicates the varied use in the broader context of musculoskeletal care management (Kalová et al., 2019).

Historical Development of Ultrasound Technology

In the medical imaging field, the historical development of ultrasound technology is a prodigious achievement. It originated at the dawn of the 20th century when researchers started experimenting with sound waves for various purposes, such as sonar for World War II. The realization that high-frequency sound waves were capable of visualizing internal body structures marked the beginning of a revolution in medical diagnosis. By the late 1950s, the initial clinical uses of ultrasound were being used successfully, particularly in obstetrics and gynecology. The ability to view soft tissue without the use of ionizing radiation was revolutionary, eventually leading to increased use across a range of different medical specialties. With increased technology in ultrasound, newer techniques such as pulsed-wave Doppler and harmonic imaging have made imaging and diagnosis superior, opening doors for its application in musculoskeletal (MSK) assessment. The application of ultrasound in musculoskeletal imaging represents a significant advancement in diagnostic capability. Musculoskeletal ultrasound was initially considered to be an ancillary tool, used primarily to examine superficial structures such as tendons and ligaments. However, with technological advances, the capability of ultrasound began to expand. As resolution improved and more advanced imaging methods were introduced, practitioners could observe deeper structures more clearly. Not only did this increase the diagnostic capabilities for various ailments—like sports trauma and inflammatory ailments—but also opened the door to examination of ultrasound-guided procedures. Techniques such as MRI-guided focused ultrasound surgery (MRgFUS) are an example, continuing to illustrate the intersection of therapeutic and diagnostic modalities as well as further consolidating the treatment for musculoskeletal disorders. MRgFUS derives its basis on non-ionizing energy, which remains at the heart of the continued advancement of ultrasound technology in MSK applications (Albisinni et al., 2015). In addition to technical advancement, the establishment of standardized guidelines for the application of clinical ultrasound (CUS) has been deemed essential in its appropriate application in all health care systems. Protocol creation in areas such as training, competency testing, and quality control is crucial in attaining the use of ultrasound in routine practice. As greater reliance on CUS in different fields of medicine is being seen, a systematic approach ensures that the professionals are well prepared to optimize the use of this technology. Interdisciplinary work has resulted in developing platforms that focus on education and best practices, which ultimately enhance patient care in musculoskeletal settings. As ultrasound technology advances further and gains wider proliferation, the use and implementation of these guidelines will enable healthcare professionals to be in a position to apply ultrasound not just in diagnosis but as part of an essential tool in therapeutic interventions. Hence, embracing ultrasound technology throughout history is a reflection of a broader movement towards sophistication and reliance on non-invasive imaging technologies by doctors (Abo et al., 2018) (Figure 13.2).

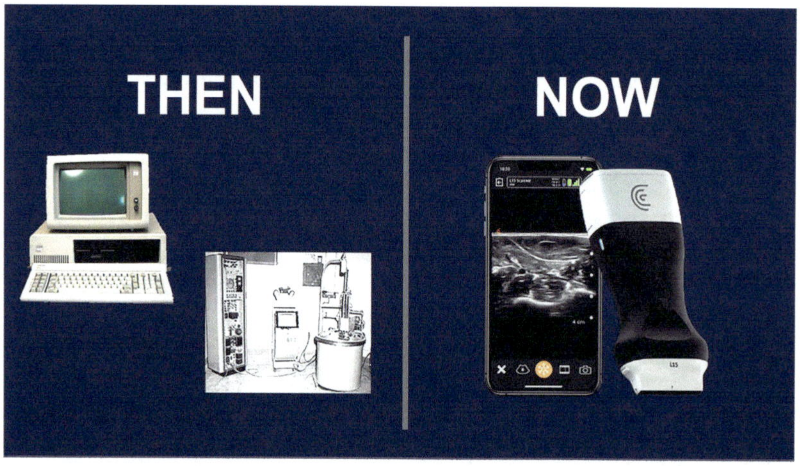

Figure 13.2. Historical development of ultrasound technology.

Source: A Brief History of Medical Ultrasound. clarius.com (2020). https://clarius.com/wp-content/uploads/2020/01/2020.01.03-A-Brief-History-of-Medical-Ultrasound.jpg

Importance in Modern Medical Diagnostics

The significance of musculoskeletal (MSK) ultrasound in modern medical diagnostics cannot be overstated, particularly in its ability to provide real-time imaging of soft tissues. This technological advancement allows clinicians to visualize muscles, tendons, ligaments, and joints, leading to improved diagnosis and management of various musculoskeletal disorders. Unlike other imaging modalities, ultrasound is non-invasive and does not involve ionizing radiation, making it a safer option for patients, particularly for populations requiring frequent imaging, such as athletes and the elderly. The dynamic nature of ultrasound enables practitioners to assess not only the structure but also the function of musculoskeletal components during movement, which is essential for accurately diagnosing conditions like tendon tears and joint effusions. In addition to its diagnostic capabilities, MSK ultrasound has proven invaluable in guiding interventional procedures. For example, it enhances the accuracy of injections into joints or bursae, facilitating the treatment of pathologies that would otherwise require more invasive surgical intervention. Ultrasound guidance minimizes the risk of complications and maximizes the effectiveness of therapeutic agents, leading to better patient outcomes. Moreover, the technology supports dynamic assessments, enabling doctors to observe how musculoskeletal structures respond to movement or stress over time, which is critical for developing effective rehabilitation strategies. This integration of diagnostic and therapeutic functions underscores the importance of ultrasound as a multifaceted tool in modern medicine, bridging the gap between imaging and treatment. As medical technology progresses, the incorporation of complementary techniques, such as MRI-guided focused ultrasound surgery (MRgFUS), further amplifies the potential of MSK ultrasound in clinical practice. MRgFUS combines advanced imaging modalities with therapeutic ultrasound, allowing for targeted treatments of various musculoskeletal disorders. With this minimally invasive approach, clinicians can achieve precise therapeutic effects while minimizing collateral damage to surrounding tissues. The continuous evolution of ultrasound technology exemplifies a promising trajectory in musculoskeletal diagnostics and treatment, offering new avenues for managing complex conditions. As practitioners gain insights into ultrasound's evolving capabilities, its role in comprehensive musculoskeletal care will only become more pronounced, ultimately enhancing patient outcomes and fostering innovative treatment pathways (Focal Spot, 1979; Albisinni et al., 2015).

13.1. Principles of Ultrasound Imaging

The foundational principles of ultrasound imaging lie in the generation and reception of sound waves. High-frequency sound waves, typically in the range of 2 to 18 MHz, are emitted by transducers and penetrate biological tissues. These sound waves experience reflection and refraction as they encounter boundaries between different types of tissues, resulting in echoes that are subsequently captured by the transducer. The time it takes for these echoes to return to the transducer is used to create detailed images of the internal structures, providing exceptional resolution in soft tissue visualization. This non-invasive imaging technique has gained prominence in musculoskeletal (MSK) applications, enabling clinicians to assess joint, tendon, and muscle pathologies with remarkable precision while avoiding ionizing radiation typically associated with other imaging modalities, underscoring its vital application in both diagnosis and treatment strategies for MSK disorders (Albisinni et al., 2015). In addition to its diagnostic capabilities, ultrasound imaging encompasses therapeutic applications, specifically in guided interventions such as injections or aspirations. Utilizing real-time imaging allows practitioners to visualize target structures during procedures, thereby enhancing accuracy and reducing the risk of complications. The ability to guide needles precisely into affected areas is particularly significant in conditions like tendonitis or bursitis, where drug delivery directly to the pathological site can improve treatment outcomes. Moreover, ultrasonography can facilitate the assessment of joint effusions, such as in arthritis, by enabling both diagnosis and therapeutic drainage. The integration of these ultrasound-guided techniques into MSK practice enhances the clinician's ability to provide comprehensive care, ensuring that interventions are performed safely and effectively, significantly improving patient satisfaction and outcomes (Patience et al., 2018). As the field of musculoskeletal ultrasound continues to evolve, the importance of training and mentorship becomes paramount.

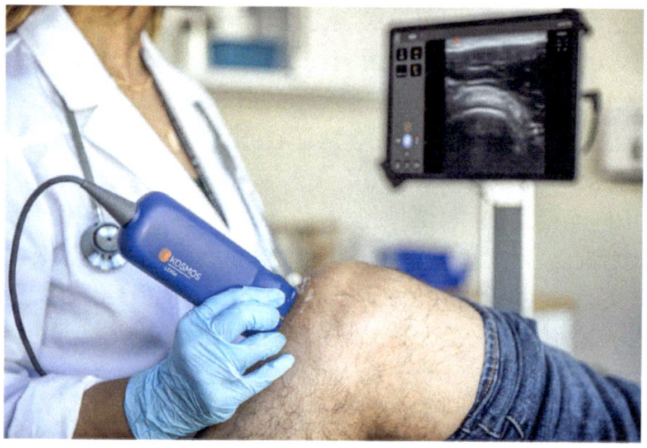

Figure 13.3. Principles of ultrasound imaging of musculoskeletal (MSK).

Source:. EchoNous.Musculoskeletal (MSK) Ultrasound. echonous.com. https://echonous.com/wp-content/uploads/2023/11/T1_MSK_00961-Edit-1024x683.jpg

Despite the growing prevalence of ultrasound in podiatry and MSK practices, there remains a significant lack of standardized training programs and mentorship opportunities. For instance, survey data indicate a substantial proportion of practitioners utilize ultrasound without formal education, which raises concerns about the quality and safety of imaging practices. Importantly, developing a structured training framework could enhance skill acquisition, ensure safe practices, and foster confidence among practitioners. Efforts such as integrating ultrasound training into existing curricula and establishing mentorship programs with experienced sonographers and clinicians are essential. This proactive approach will undoubtedly contribute to the professional development of podiatrists and other MSK specialists, ultimately leading to improved patient care and outcomes in the clinical setting (Patience et al., 2018) (Figure 13.3).

13.1.1. Basic Physics of Ultrasound Waves

The fundamental principles underlying ultrasound waves are rooted in physics, where sound energy is transformed into mechanical waves that propagate through various media. Ultrasound operates at frequencies higher than the audible range, typically exceeding 20 kHz. By harnessing piezoelectric crystals, ultrasound machines generate these high-frequency sound waves, producing a sound that can penetrate biological tissues. When these waves encounter different structures within the body, such as muscles, tendons, and ligaments, they reflect back at varying degrees. This reflection forms the basis for echogenicity, which is vital in distinguishing between various types of tissue during a musculoskeletal ultrasound examination. By carefully analyzing these returning echoes, clinicians can obtain critical information regarding the anatomy and pathology of musculoskeletal structures, thereby facilitating timely and accurate diagnoses. When ultrasound waves travel through biological tissues, their interaction is influenced by several physical properties, including density and elasticity. These properties dictate how sound waves are transmitted, absorbed, and reflected, ultimately affecting image quality and resolution. For instance, while muscles generally exhibit high acoustic impedance and provide clear images due to their density, fat and air can lead to decreased resolution due to their differing acoustic properties. The difference in the speed of sound through various tissues must also be taken into account, as it affects the accuracy of depth perception in ultrasound imaging. Understanding these nuances allows healthcare providers to optimize ultrasound parameters—such as frequency and gain settings—tailored to specific evaluations of musculoskeletal conditions. Such optimization is essential in enhancing diagnostic precision and ensuring that subtle pathological changes are captured effectively. Additionally, the exploration of ultrasound waves in MSK ultrasound is closely tied to the principles of the Doppler effect, which enables the assessment of blood flow and tissue dynamics. As sound waves encounter moving structures, such as blood cells, their frequency shifts, allowing clinicians to evaluate not only the quality of tissue but also its vascularization, which is vital in conditions like tendinopathy or muscle tears. The Doppler assessment enhances the functional diagnostic capabilities of ultrasound, broadening its utility beyond mere structural evaluation. Advances in Doppler technology have further refined this capability, allowing for the visualization of perfusion and pathology that might otherwise go undetected. Consequently, the integration of Doppler capabilities in musculoskeletal ultrasound fosters a comprehensive understanding of both the static and dynamic features of musculoskeletal disorders, becoming instrumental in formulating effective management strategies for patient care.

13.1.2. Types of Ultrasound Transducers Used in MSK

Ultrasound transducer choice is critical to ensuring optimal quality of images from musculoskeletal (MSK) ultrasound examinations. Transducers can be divided based on frequency ranges, which play a significant role in the resolution and penetration of the ultrasound beams. Superficial tissues such as muscles, ligaments, and tendons are scanned with high-frequency transducers, most typically between 7.5 and 15 MHz. They also provide increased axial resolution, enabling practitioners to visualize greater detail and pathological changes. Lower-frequency transducers, however, typically between 2 and 5 MHz, are utilized for deeper structures such as larger muscles and joints since they penetrate tissues more effectively but sacrifice some resolution. Proper selection of the type of transducer directly impacts the diagnostic image quality and resulting musculoskeletal pathology management. The configuration of another very important aspect of ultrasound transducers employed in MSK practice dictates their versatility in various clinical situations. Linear transducers are commonly employed for the formation of high-resolution images of superficial tissues and are therefore appropriately suited to investigate locations like the shoulder or knee. Curvilinear transducers offer larger fields of view and are generally employed in the event of larger structures, like hips or abdominal organs. In MSK ultrasound, the transducer must be positioned accurately to minimize artifacts and maximize diagnostic utility. Well-practiced technique in transducer positioning and handling steps is essential in preventing pitfalls such as anisotropy and acoustic shadowing that can compromise diagnosis. Understanding these design nuances and their effects on imaging is crucial for MSK professionals to ensure efficacious evaluations of musculoskeletal illnesses (Maliborski & Serafin-Krol, 2017). Lastly, the evolution of ultrasonographic technology in the transducers has also introduced the integration of newer technology designed to enhance the diagnostic function of MSK ultrasound. As an illustration, some newer transducers are now able to perform advanced modalities of imaging, such as Doppler imaging, which can provide useful information regarding blood flow and vascularity around musculoskeletal structures. In addition, handheld and portable ultrasound scanners are transforming the field of MSK imaging with the capability of conducting real-time scans in a variety of environments from clinics to outpatient units to sports events. In addition to being beneficial for timely decision-making in practice, these also pose issues of work-related musculoskeletal discomfort (WRMSD) to sonographers since ergonomics in the usage of these devices could impact practitioner well-being (Sommerich et al. 2016). As the field evolves, understanding the implications of transducer technology on both patient care and sonographer health will be increasingly important (Figure 13.4).

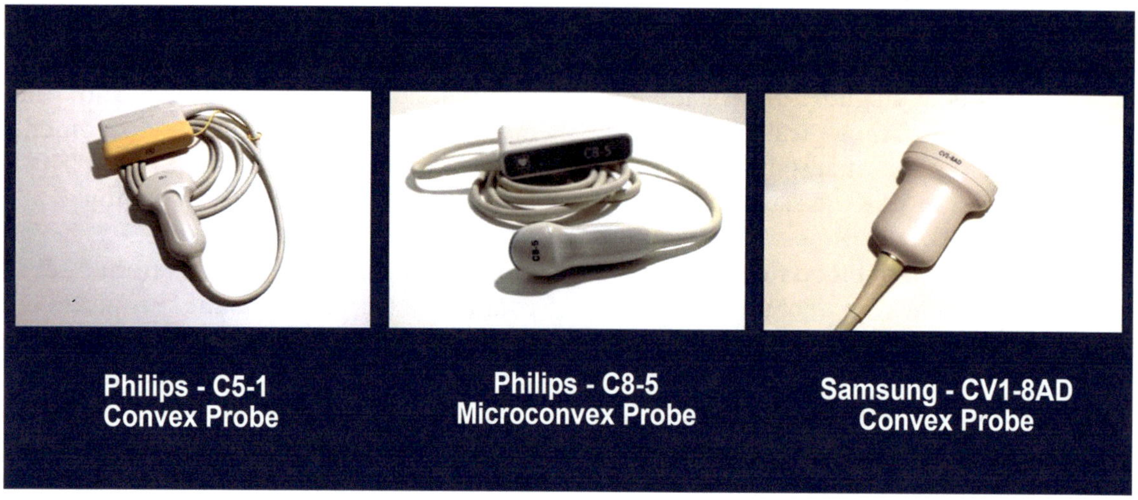

Figure 13.4. Types of ultrasound transducers used in MSK.

Source: LBN Medical (2025). Choose the Best Ultrasound Probe: Guide to Ultrasound Transducer Types. lbnmedical.com. https://lbnmedical.com/wp-content/uploads/2024/06/Convex-probes.png

13.1.3. Image Formation and Interpretation

Creation of an image in musculoskeletal (MSK) ultrasound basically relies on sound wave propagation and reflection principles. When high-frequency sound waves are emitted from a transducer, they meet various body tissues. The echogenicity of the tissues—defined by how much they reflect sound waves—is reflected through the level of brightness on the ultrasound image. Soft tissues such as muscles and tendons reflect sound waves in a different manner to denser tissue types such as bone. This difference in reflection allows for the meaningful interpretation of anatomical and pathological information within the musculoskeletal system. MSK ultrasound thus serves as a keystone tool for clinicians, allowing a non-invasive visualisation of conditions such as joint effusion or tendon rupture, thus facilitating early and accurate diagnosis. MSK ultrasound reporting is based on a large knowledge base of normal and abnormal anatomy. The clinician should be proficient in detecting variability in tissue properties so that normal structures can be distinguished from those engaged in injury or disease. Being able to quantify cartilage thickness, as in one review, shows the ability of ultrasound to detect subtle change over time. Here, the efficacy of a symptomatic slow-acting drug for osteoarthritis (OA) was assessed using femoral hyaline cartilage thickness measurement, proving the high-resolution capability of ultrasound (Barbulescu et al., 2019). Such high-level imaging not only helps monitor treatment efficacy but also enhances the clinician's capability to make evidence-based decisions regarding patient care. Moreover, combining ultrasound with other imaging modalities may enhance the diagnostic process to a large degree. Although ultrasound is sufficient for the detection of musculoskeletal system lesions in most instances, there are certain situations under which more advanced imaging techniques such as MRI or computed tomography

(CT) may become necessary. For example, if ultrasound findings are not conclusive as well as unrelated to clinical symptoms, the occurrence of diseases like metacarpo-/metatarsophalangeal joint injuries in horses should be studied further with more sophisticated imaging equipment (Bergman et al., 2011). This collaborative approach to imaging helps achieve the whole picture of the sub-jacent pathologies and prevents diagnostic mismatches, thus contributing to the role of image formation and interpretation as essential components in the larger context of musculoskeletal ultrasound (Figure 13.5).

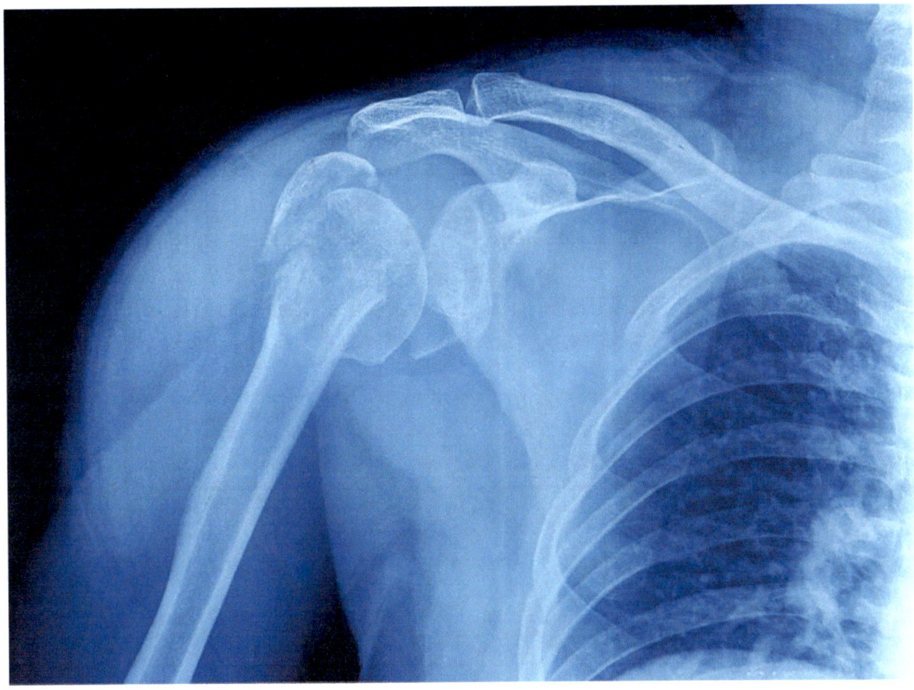

Figure 13.5. Musculoskeletal radiograph interpretation.

Source: Yok_onepiece/shutterstock.com. Shoulder X-ray. https://www.shutterstock.com/image-photo/shoulder-xray-showing-closed-comminution-fracture-1585665940

13.2. Indications for MSK Ultrasound

The application of musculoskeletal (MSK) ultrasound has grown in importance when diagnosing a variety of disorders of the musculoskeletal system. It is one of its significant applications in the assessment of soft tissue injuries, including ligament sprains or tendon ruptures. Unlike other imaging modalities, for example, MRI, with ultrasound, there is real-time imaging that allows dynamic assessment of structures in motion. This characteristic is particularly beneficial in sports medicine, where professionals might have to evaluate the functionality of tendons during specific movements. Studies have shown that MSK ultrasound can detect partial and complete tears in tendons with great accuracy, which improves diagnosis and helps develop the best treatment methods for musculoskeletal trauma patients. In addition to soft tissue injury, ultrasound can also be a valuable means of evaluating inflammatory conditions such as bursitis and tendonitis.

Due to its ability to produce high-resolution images of adjacent tissue, physicians can visualize synovial tissue and monitor for evidence of inflammation that is less obvious with other imaging modalities. Such capability allows monitoring and diagnosis of conditions like rheumatoid arthritis and gout more efficiently, for which prompt detection and treatment can significantly alter the patient outcomes. Also, the absence of ionizing radiation exposure with ultrasound makes it an ideal imaging technique for repetitive follow-up examinations. The therapeutic effect of MSK ultrasound is also emphasized by the prospect of employing it to guide interventional therapies, such as injections or aspirations, for improved therapy. New techniques, including quantitative ultrasound (QUS), are expanding the scope of MSK ultrasound and enhancing its diagnostic capability. QUS has been discovered to be employed in characterizing nerve fascicles by quantifying structural components such as collagen and myelin content. It enables a targeted evaluation of peripheral nerves, specifically valuable in the diagnosis and treatment of neuropathies or compressive syndromes, as for example, carpal tunnel syndrome. The addition of advanced ultrasound techniques not only provides further diagnostic information for the clinician but also allows for individualized treatment based on specific pathological findings. With the continually changing character of the musculoskeletal ultrasound specialty, these advanced uses are expected to enhance the quality of care being provided for patients with disparate musculoskeletal conditions (Albisinni et al., 2015; Andre et al., 2019) (Figure 13.6).

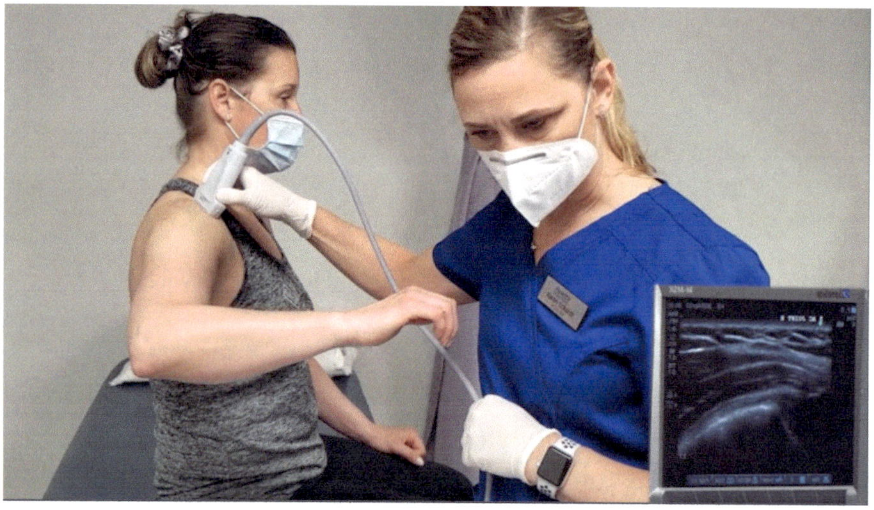

Figure 13.6. Indications for MSK ultrasound.

Source: Panetta Physical Therapy. Musculoskeletal Ultrasound Examination (MSKUS). https://www.panettapt.com/diagnostics/musculoskeletal-ultrasound-examination-mskus/

13.2.1. Assessment of Soft Tissue Injuries

Assessment of soft tissue trauma is significant in musculoskeletal ultrasound because the trauma impacts the quality of life and functional ability of the patients. Soft tissue structures like ligaments, tendons, and muscles can be evaluated through ultrasound imaging to determine their condition and functional ability. The musculoskeletal ultrasound's ability to be flexible allows professionals to obtain real-time images, which helps for immediate diagnosis of injury, such as tears, inflammation, or degenerative wear. Moreover, as podiatrists and physiotherapists become more integrated into their practices, learning how this technology can enhance the accuracy of diagnosis and guide treatment planning, and how this, in turn, enhances patient outcomes in the management of soft tissue injury, is vital (Patience et al., 2018). In addition to increased diagnostic capabilities through ultrasound, it can also be used to identify the best plans of management for soft tissue trauma. According to this, ultrasound allows the clinician to visualize the degree of the injury and surrounding conditions, and adopt a more holistic attitude towards therapy. This imaging technique has been shown to be particularly successful in enabling methods like corticosteroid injections and other interventions for tendon pathology. It is reported in existing research that numerous healthcare practitioners apply the use of ultrasound as a means of enriching their decision-making and therapeutic capacity, an indication of the technology's increasing impact on the evaluation and treatment of musculoskeletal disorders (Auckland University of Technology et al., 2018). Such real-time imaging of soft tissue structures means that clinicians have at their disposal an incredibly useful aid for individualizing rehabilitation planning for their patients. Lastly, the integration of musculoskeletal ultrasound within soft tissue injury assessment bears witness to the need for expert education and guidance among healthcare professionals. While several practitioners report applying ultrasound for effective purposes, challenges such as lack of adequate training and access to advanced hardware remain (Patience et al., 2018). Elimination of these hurdles is essential to unlocking maximum gain from the use of ultrasound in clinical practice, notably in terms of elevating competence within podiatry and physiotherapy. When clinicians become more skilled with musculoskeletal ultrasound, the potential for improved patient care increases, leading to more accurate assessment, effective intervention, and ultimately better outcomes for individuals who suffer from soft tissue injuries (Auckland University of Technology et al., 2018) (Figure 13.7).

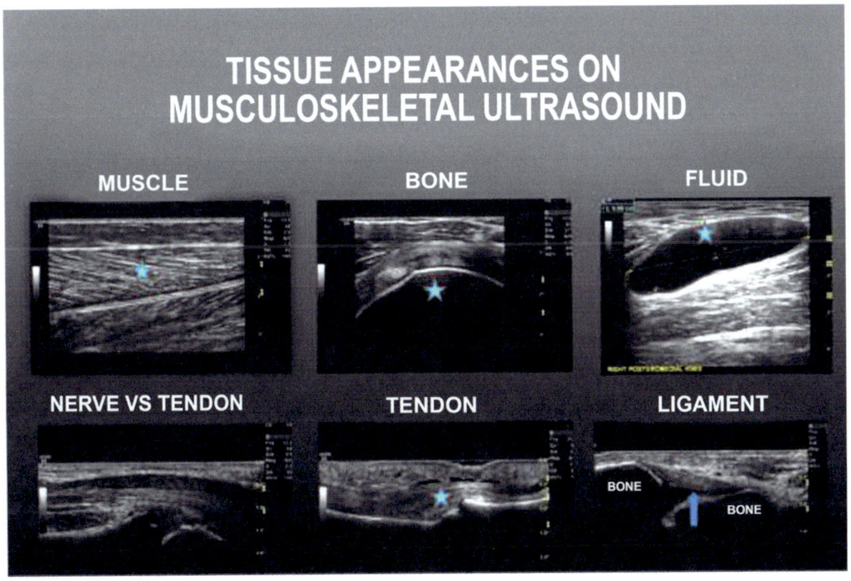

Figure 13.7. Assessment of soft tissue injuries for MSK ultrasound.

Source: What do different tissues on ultrasound look like? https://theultrasoundsite.co.uk/ultrasound-case-studies/starting-article-2-different-tissues-ultrasound-look-like/

13.2.2. Evaluation of Joint Conditions

Joint condition assessment has been significantly improved by the advancement of high-resolution imaging modalities, most particularly musculoskeletal ultrasound (MSK US). This is a non-invasive, real-time imaging of joint structures, providing invaluable information regarding soft tissues, including tendons and ligaments, and joint effusions and pathologies. One of the biggest advantages of MSK US is that dynamic movements can be visualized, and that is imperative when diagnosing conditions such as rotator cuff syndrome and bursitis. The anatomical resolution seen with ultrasound enhances the clinician's ability to determine the exact structures involved in the pathology, thus allowing for proper diagnoses and treatment planning. These skills make the role of MSK ultrasound as a guide to therapeutic intervention and, as a result, to improve outcomes in joint disease treatment stand out. Furthermore, the effectiveness of surgical or conservative treatment can be established with the aid of ultrasound, most importantly for follow-up of degenerative diseases like osteoarthritis. In studies, for example, symptomatic slow-acting antirheumatic drugs in the treatment of osteoarthritis, ultrasound has been shown to provide quantitative cartilage thickness measurements, which are crucial in measuring treatment effectiveness. Visualization of changes in the structural integrity of cartilage over time allows clinicians to provide correct treatment adjustments and long-term management. By upgrading the traditional clinical exams with ultrasound imaging, an enhanced understanding of joint health can be achieved, and early intervention prior to the development of severe degeneration can be facilitated, thereby enhancing patient care. Furthermore, incorporating musculoskeletal ultrasound into traditional evaluation procedures improves the clinical assessment protocol through the addition of a multi-dimensional analysis of joint pathology. Individual investigations have demonstrated the correlation of ultrasound results and radiographic findings, determining its role as a valuable diagnostic method. For instance, ultrasound assessment of femoral hyaline cartilage thickness has revealed striking changes over treatment periods relative to initial values, determining its relevance in monitoring osteoarthritis advancement. A combination of ultrasound with clinical assessment forms a robust foundation for the assessment of joint status, thereby improving the treatment strategy. This enhanced diagnostic capability ultimately follows in accordance with goals for personalized medicine, allowing for individualized treatment regimens based on patient-specific pathology and response, illustrating the revolutionary impact of musculoskeletal ultrasound in the evaluation of arthropathies (Figure 13.8).

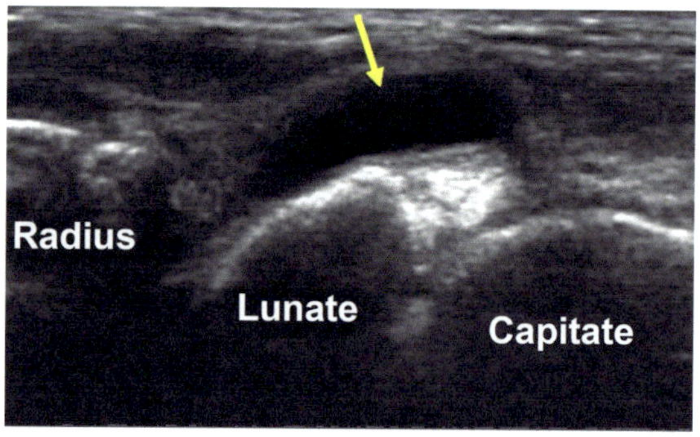

Figure 13.8. Evaluation of joint conditions using MSK ultrasound.

Source: Jacobson JA. Wrist and Hand Ultrasound. In: Fundamentals of Musculoskeletal Ultrasound. Elsevier; 2018

13.2.3. Guidance for Interventional Procedures

The control of interventional treatments in musculoskeletal (MSK) ultrasound is a significant development in medical interventions, particularly as healthcare professionals strive to enhance the precision of treatment and diagnostic techniques. As advanced imaging technologies, such as MRI-guided focused ultrasound surgery (MRgFUS), are incorporated into healthcare, medical practitioners are better positioned to treat a range of MSK conditions effectively. Such sophisticated technology facilitates non-invasive treatment that can significantly alleviate patient discomfort and optimize procedural accuracy. Combining non-ionizing imaging modalities not only ensures improved visualization of target tissues but also permits real-time monitoring, hence optimizing patient outcome and reducing the risk for complications. As technology advances in this field, it is essential that the professionals handling such advanced methods are appropriately trained in them so that they can appropriately utilize them in different clinical applications (Albisinni et al., 2015). The success of interventional procedures hinges on robust methodological designs that critically compare heterogeneous techniques. Current developments in procedural protocols show that comparing old and established protocols, such as fluoroscopy, with newer MRI-guided regimens provides interesting contrasts for workflow efficiencies and patient safety. In controlled trials, the application of MRI-guided protocols has been shown to have comparable procedure times with, if not greater than, established protocols, indicating a vast potential for enhanced clinical practice (Cox et al., 2015). On top of that, the ergonomic assessments done in such studies emphasize the necessity of maximizing the workspace for clinical professionals, ultimately reducing their risk of musculoskeletal injuries. This multi-disciplinary approach, which integrates findings from various fields, makes MRI guidance a viable alternative worthy of more research into MSK interventions. Recognizing the unique challenges interventional procedures pose is essential to the development of MSK applications of ultrasound. While it is worth introducing new guidance systems like MRI for benefits, practitioners must be aware of the technical demands and potential complications in such methods. Mass training programs must be introduced that not only address the technical demand for performing MRI-guided interventions but also consider the factor of cognitive load and psychological readiness for optimal performance. User experience and process ergonomics are core to clinical success and need to take precedence in protocol development. In such a manner that MSK ultrasound technologies' full capabilities can be unleashed by the healthcare community, ultimately becoming pioneers towards safer and more effective patient treatment (Albisinni et al., 2015; Cox et al., 2015).

13.3. Benefits of MSK Ultrasound

One of the major advantages of musculoskeletal (MSK) ultrasound is that it is non-invasive, permitting patient comfort with the provision of diagnostic information. In contrast to traditional imaging methods such as magnetic resonance imaging (MRI), MSK ultrasound does not require the application of contrast agents or exposure to ionizing radiation. This aspect is particularly useful in pediatric patients and in those patients who have limitations on the use of radiation exposure. The safety profile of ultrasound makes it more useful and applicable both for initial assessment and follow-up examination. Also, the real-time imaging offers a method of dynamic musculoskeletal structure evaluation. The clinicians are able to observe motion and activity, which are essential in order to determine function and sites of pain onset, and thus enable individualized treatment plans based on the real-time observations conducted through the ultrasound. The addition of MSK ultrasound to clinical practice can significantly impact the quality of diagnosis and patient participation in their own health care. Cost-effectiveness is also one of the significant advantages of MSK ultrasound, particularly during an era of tightened healthcare budgets. Ultrasound is a less costly method compared with MRI and CT scanning, both when considering the equipment cost as well as operational costs involved in the imaging. This cost-effectiveness makes it available for use in most disparate healthcare settings, such as outpatient clinics, and accessible to more patients. In addition, the rapidity of ultrasound technology gives the advantage of quicker diagnosis and follow-up. Results are most often given to patients during the test, reducing the clinical process and waiting times related to other imaging methods. Consequently, the economic benefits coupled with the quick availability of valuable diagnostic information position MSK ultrasound as a realistic choice for the management of musculoskeletal disorders, eventually enhancing patient care and utilization of resources in clinical practice. The therapeutic applications of MSK ultrasound further emphasize its benefits, particularly in the guidance of intervention.

MSK ultrasound can also be applied to facilitate procedures such as joint aspirations and injections, enhancing the accuracy of the procedure. As it provides real-time images, it minimizes complications and enhances the effectiveness of treatment by allowing medical professionals to precisely visualize the target area. As attested to in recent literature, the use of ultrasound guidance for procedures in conditions such as medial collateral ligament injury has been very favorable, allowing for better rehabilitation outcomes and quicker recovery. This union of diagnostic and procedural potential is a testament to the versatility of MSK ultrasound and its role within clinical practice. Through the integration of ultrasound into diagnostic as well as treatment regimes, physicians can deliver a more comprehensive care that considers the multiple requirements of musculoskeletal disorder patients, making it a more efficient rehabilitation and symptomatic relief process (Zhang et al., 2025; Manske et al., 2024) (Figure 13.9).

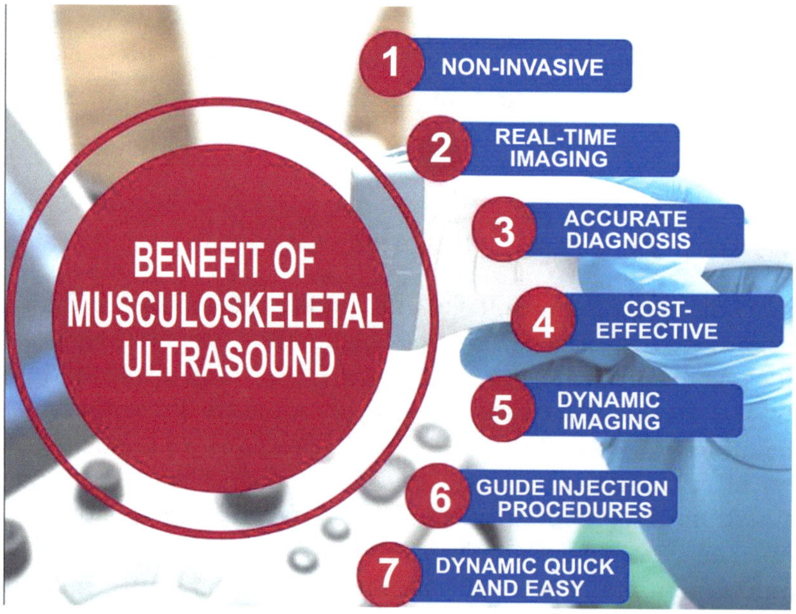

Figure 13.9. Benefit of musculoskeletal ultrasound.

Source: Sameer Gohir/ jointinjectionclinic.co.uk. https://jointinjectionclinic.co.uk/wp-content/uploads/2024/01/Colorful-Minimalist-Linear-Steps-Circular-Diagram-1.webp.

13.3.1. Non-Invasive Nature of the Procedure

The non-invasive nature of musculoskeletal (MSK) ultrasound is one of the key attractions in current therapeutic and imaging modalities. Because it employs sound wave technology for image formation, the process does not require the application of ionizing radiation, unlike many other imaging modalities such as X-rays and computed tomography (CT) scans. This characteristic not only minimizes patient exposure to dangerous radiation but also makes repeated assessments without the risk factor possible. Real-time imaging of MSK ultrasound further adds to its utility in enabling clinicians to visualize dynamic joint and soft tissue motion. The non-invasive nature of this imaging modality is thus a primary consideration in maintaining patient safety and comfort as well as accurate diagnosis and treatment planning. The application of non-invasive tools extends beyond diagnostics to sophisticated interventional techniques, such as ultrasound-guided injections. These interventions are supported by the accurate localization of anatomical structures by means of MSK ultrasound's high-resolution imaging ability. For instance, the administration of a corticosteroid injection to an inflamed joint can be administered with improved precision, thus reducing the risk of complications. Besides, ultrasound-assisted interventions give the clinician immediate feedback and, hence, optimize therapeutic outcomes and patient satisfaction. Hence, the non-invasive nature of MSK ultrasound not only assures effective imaging but also allows clinicians to introduce controlled treatments with minimal discomfort to the patient.

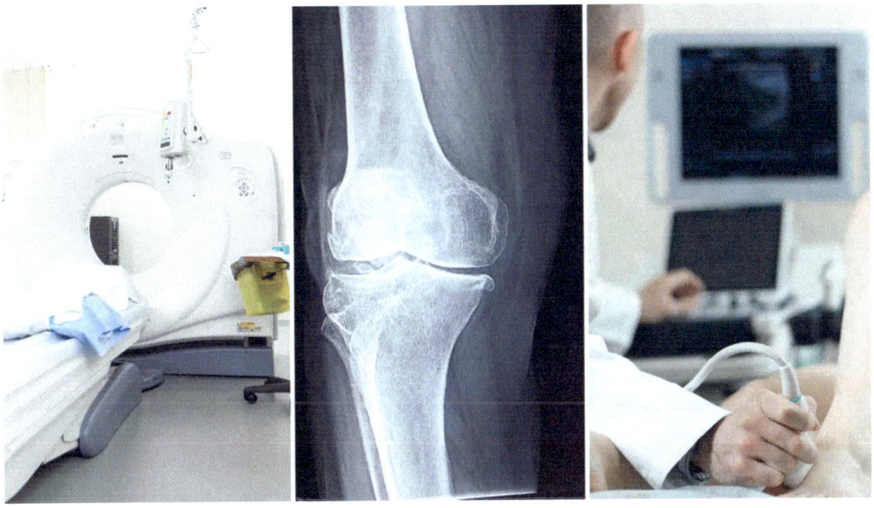

Figure 13.10. The non-invasive nature of musculoskeletal (MSK) ultrasound.

Source: Musculoskeletal Ultrasound. https://www.swflrheum.com/wp-content/uploads/2022/04/Difference-Musculoskeletal-Ultrasound-MRI-XRay.jpg.

Last but not least, the introduction of computer-aided orthopedic surgery (CAOS) systems showcases the growing applicability of non-invasive modalities in MSK therapy. These systems, embedded with ultrasound technology, employ real-time imaging to project surgical procedures with astounding precision. As outlined in more recent studies, the integration of ultrasound into CAOS systems helps allow for better visualization of anatomical landmarks, allowing the surgeon to better navigate complex musculoskeletal anatomy (Albisinni et al., 2015). This exchange between advanced surgery and non-invasive imaging represents a paradigm change, in which traditional invasive tactics are increasingly being replaced with less injurious methods. Ultimately, the non-invasive nature of MSK ultrasound allows for advanced clinical practices to align patient safety and improved treatment outcomes, thereby redesigning the practice of musculoskeletal care (Figure 13.10).

13.3.2. Real-Time Imaging Capabilities

The evolution of real-time imaging capabilities of musculoskeletal (MSK) ultrasound has revolutionized the diagnosis and treatment of musculoskeletal diseases. Unlike other imaging tools such as X-ray and MRI, which provide static images, MSK ultrasound allows for dynamic assessment of mobile soft tissue structures. This real-time capability is particularly valuable in evaluating tendon and ligament injuries, where information regarding functional movement can provide clues about damage severity. For instance, with dynamic imaging, the clinician is able to observe the patellar tendon as the patient performs active motion, detecting subtle deficits that could be missed on static imaging. Consequently, the integration of real-time imaging enhances diagnostic sensitivity, as well as addresses the clinical need for functional assessment in musculoskeletal trauma therapy, thus complementing the role of MSK ultrasound in current practice (Wolfe et al., 2023).

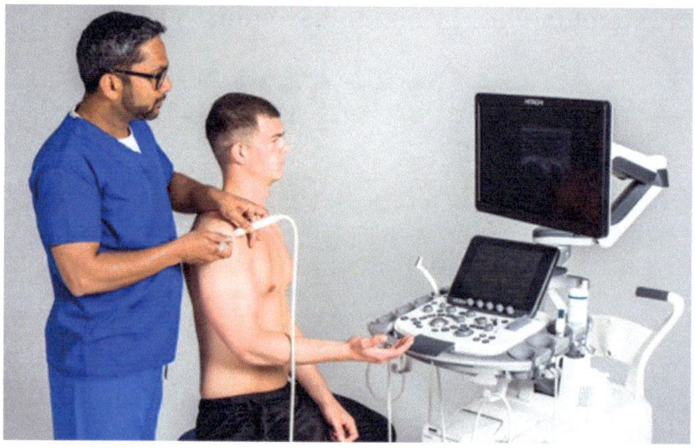

Figure 13.11. Real-time imaging capabilities of musculoskeletal (MSK) ultrasound.

Source: MSK Ultrasound. https://www.proactive-wellbeing.co.uk/wp-content/uploads/2019/10/MSL-ultrasound-therapy-4.jpg.

Real-time imaging has value beyond diagnostics; it is necessary to guide therapeutic intervention. MSK ultrasound makes the precise location of injections in bursitis and tendinitis possible by imaging anatomy in real-time. This makes it possible to reduce the risk of complications from inappropriate needle placement and improve patient safety and comfort throughout the procedure. Also, the clinicians can adjust their techniques based on real-time feedback so that interventions become not only effective but also tailored to the subject's differences in anatomy. This versatility also highlights the benefit of real-time imaging in increasing the effectiveness of diagnosis and treatment since practitioners are able to see the effects of their interventions in real time during procedures, which results in improved patient outcomes (Focal Spot, 1980). Secondly, MSK ultrasound's ability to perform real-time imaging greatly assists patient participation and satisfaction. Compared to the frequently time-consuming methods employed with conventional imaging modalities, MSK ultrasound can be rapidly performed and at the point of care, minimizing patient wait times. While under examination, clinicians can explain results to patients while seeing their own anatomy on-screen, resulting in a natural integration with the healthcare process. This real-time feedback imaging not only demystifies the imaging process for the patient but also allows them to take an active role in their treatment procedures. Thus, the integration of real-time imaging into MSK ultrasound is a landmark development in patient-focused care, representing the trend towards more interactive and reactive paradigms of healthcare that can balance both clinical effectiveness and patient participation (Wolfe et al., 2023) (Figure 13.11).

13.3.3. Cost-Effectiveness Compared to Other Imaging Modalities

Cost-effectiveness of musculoskeletal (MSK) ultrasound is now a critical determinant in the comparison of imaging modalities for the assessment of musculoskeletal disorders. In contrast to conventional imaging technologies such as X-ray and magnetic resonance imaging (MRI), ultrasound is significantly less expensive and more accessible, and therefore an ideal first-line diagnostic tool. This is most relevant in settings where early diagnosis will lead to early intervention, and overall lower healthcare costs. MSK ultrasound makes possible real-time assessment of soft tissue anatomy and immediate diagnostic capability that could potentially avoid more expensive alternatives. Moreover, as healthcare systems move towards value-based care, the ultra-sensitive availability of diagnostic information with not overwhelming expenditure sits well with current healthcare objectives. MSK ultrasound cost reduction is supplemented by the modality's effectiveness in many clinical scenarios, but particularly so when making diagnoses such as rotator cuff calcific tendinopathy. Vintage imaging methods, while beneficial, are more costly and take longer for providers and patients. Research has established that ultrasound has the ability to make quicker diagnoses, which would get patients treated conservatively earlier and avoid costly surgical interventions. For instance, ultrasound-guided aspiration and lavage techniques for rotator cuff calcific tendinopathy can enhance patient outcomes and satisfaction as well as keep healthcare costs affordable, as noted in related research demonstrating the possibility of treating the majority of patients successfully conservatively without undergoing surgery (Derrington et al., 2015). Secondly, the cost-effectiveness of MSK ultrasound goes beyond its fee to how it can help improve clinical decision-making. The real-time imaging capability of ultrasound can make interactive assessment with the patient possible in the consultation, which provides more precise insight into the injury or condition under assessment. Interactivity can be a factor in better treatment decisions, which could lead to reduced frequency of repeat imaging studies, contributing to increasing cost. Within the setting of institutions where the use of sophisticated imaging modalities may be limited, MSK ultrasound stands out not only for its economy but also for its ease and simplicity compared to the other modalities. Therefore, the employment of ultrasound in musculoskeletal diagnosis forms part of a greater trend toward the optimal utilization of accessible resources within the health setting without a reduction in standards of patient care (Focal Spot, 1983).

13.4. Limitations of MSK Ultrasound

The limitations of musculoskeletal ultrasound (MSK US) must be properly known, especially in relation to its growing prominence in clinical practice. A leading concern regards reliance on the operator since the reliability and effectiveness of MSK US largely depend on the expertise and experience of the practitioner. Inadequate training can lead to incorrect interpretation of ultrasound findings, particularly in areas of deep anatomy, and this can result in diagnostic faults. While advancements have been observed in instructional strategies, such as the integration of ultrasound education into medical school curricula, evidence indicates that procedures like arthroscopy are more likely to yield better anatomical learning acquisition compared to ultrasound techniques (Andre et al., 2019). This indicates the necessity for high-intensity training programs that ensure practitioners will be capable of practically implementing MSK US in various clinical conditions, acknowledging one main limitation to its present practice. Another MSK ultrasound weakness is that it has a poor capacity to penetrate deep tissues. Though MSK US is excellent at outlining surface structures due to its high-resolution imaging potential, it is weak at imaging deep muscles, ligaments, and joints. For example, some body morphologies with a significant amount of adipose tissue can attenuate the ultrasound signal significantly, rendering interpretation challenging. Further, effusions like joint or synovial fluid accumulations are capable of masking underlying pathologies when their assessment is not conducted with utmost vigilance. Studies have proved that this limitation is a drawback while clinicians make diagnoses solely based on MSK US, as underlying pathologies are omitted or wrongly interpreted (Andre et al., 2019). This limitation necessitates the use of complementary ultrasound with other imaging methods to ensure complete assessments of musculoskeletal disorders. Lastly, the use of musculoskeletal ultrasound is frequently restricted by its inability to discriminate among types of pathology. For instance, while MSK US may illustrate soft tissue pathology like tears or inflammatory tissues, it typically cannot determine if these changes are due to acute trauma, chronic degeneration, or inflammation. Such ambiguity might lead clinicians to make less-than-ideal treatment decisions based on the findings of the ultrasound alone. With conditions possibly having a similarly equal ultrasound appearance, the specificity limitations point toward the necessity of strong diagnostic certificates through the utilization of more advanced imaging modalities or invasive diagnostic procedures when necessary (Beckers et al., 2012). So, as with MSK ultrasound being a valuable tool in musculoskeletal assessment, it is similarly vital to appreciate its limitations for yielding better clinical outcomes and true diagnoses.

13.4.1. Operator Dependency and Skill Level

Operator dependency is a significant factor in musculoskeletal (MSK) ultrasound, as it has a direct impact on diagnostic performance. Technical skill is not only involved in image interpretation when using ultrasound, but anatomy and pathology of the musculoskeletal system also need to be comprehensively understood. Operator dependency can generate significant image quality, diagnostic accuracy, and overall clinical effectiveness variations in the use of ultrasound as a diagnostic modality. Research shows that more experienced operators make better-quality images, which further helps in more precise diagnosis. This highlights the critical role of standardized education and continuing education in ultrasound practice, enabling practitioners not only to improve their technical skills but also their interpretive skills, ultimately leading to better patient outcomes in different clinical settings, as described in contemporary research of community-based diagnostic services (Sommerich et al., 2016). Operator level of skill is also increased while using advanced technology, such as artificial intelligence (AI). Even though AI is increasingly being utilized in point-of-care ultrasound (POCUS) for automating calculations and image interpretation, it is still predicated on the operator's underlying skill and knowledge. Higher advanced competency is required to effectively select imaging protocols and configure machine parameters for different clinical scenarios. In addition, operators must have the competence to recognize the limits of AI, and more specifically, in challenging cases where image quality can be compromised or where fine clinical judgment has to be exercised. The increased level of complexity with which AI introduces MSK ultrasound further supports the need for operators to be extremely talented and adaptable, as elaborated on in the most recent literature for AI applications in ultrasound technology (Kim et al., 2025). Lastly, establishing an environment of skill and competency in MSK ultrasound is essential to advance patient care. Ongoing professional development by means of targeted training sessions and peer-to-peer communication can augment operator performance, reducing variability inherent in operator reliance. As the discipline evolves, establishing proficiency levels and implementing feedback loops can facilitate ongoing learning and improvement. Also critical will be comprehension of the impact of operator competence and emerging technologies like AI to streamline MSK ultrasound practice and to ensure operators can safely deal with the nuances of musculoskeletal examination. Formal training and standardization are evidently needed in acknowledgment of the challenge and opportunity presented by diverse service models in community diagnostic provision (Sommerich et al., 2016) (Figure 13.12).

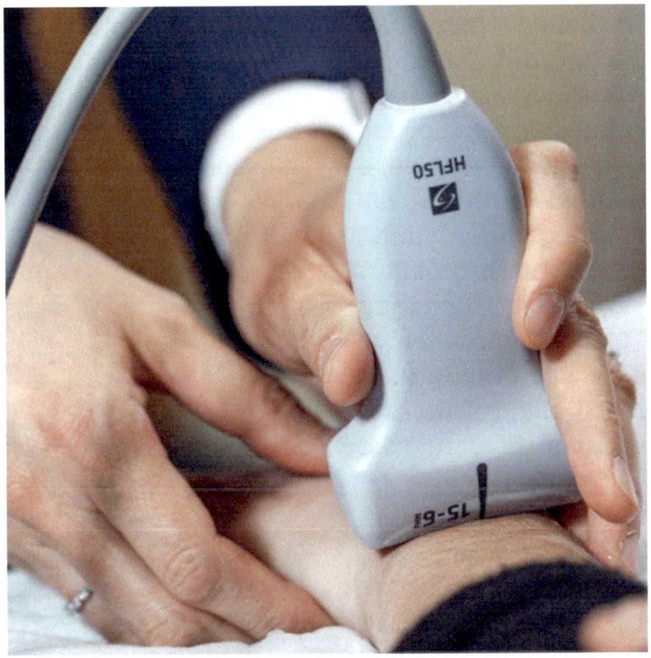

Figure 13.12. Operator dependency and skill level of MSK ultrasound.

Source: https://ysm-res.cloudinary.com/image/upload/ar_1:1,c_fill,dpr_3.0,f_auto,g_faces:auto,q_auto:eco,w_500/v1/yms/prod/a3b05f8e-064f-40e4-a60d-ff74b4130b5d.

13.4.2. Limited Penetration in Obese Patients

The efficiency of musculoskeletal (MSK) ultrasound in obese patients is normally hampered by the attenuated penetration of the ultrasound waves. Obesity creates a hindrance in the successful imaging process because additional subcutaneous fat may potentially reduce the resolution and crispness of the ultrasound images obtained. Attenuation of ultrasound waves by fatty tissue poses a dilemma to clinicians, particularly in distinguishing between pathological and normal anatomical structures. Additionally, the extensive ramifications of these restrictions reach as far as diagnostic precision and treatment effectiveness. As an example, when analyzing synovial joints or soft tissues within obese patients, failure to achieve clear images has the potential to result in an incorrect diagnosis or missed pathologies, eventually complicating treatment methods. Therefore, awareness and overcoming of such limitations become important to clinicians who must have to rely on musculoskeletal ultrasound as the only diagnostic tool in the growing number of obese patients, necessitating the need for ongoing refinement of ultrasound technology and technique overall (Lento & Primack, 2007). Apart from concerns of image quality, operator knowledge and proficiency are also a critical part of managing the challenge presented by MSK ultrasound in the obese population. Skilled ultrasonographers must adapt their style to accommodate the anatomical changes brought about by obesity, including adjusting the frequency of the transducer or the angle of insonation to achieve optimal results. These adjustments can counteract some of the attenuations, although at the cost of higher expertise. Clinicians must also be constantly vigilant so that they can adequately visualize relevant structures, that is, muscles, ligaments, and tendons. This requirement for higher-level skill has the potential to increase the demand for advanced training for clinical professionals, backing the argument that effective utilization of MSK ultrasound in this group of patients relies on technology as well as manpower, highlighting the harmonious balance between operator competence and ultrasound usability in challenging conditions (Lento & Primack, 2007). The development of focused advances in the technology of ultrasound provides promising prospects for MSK image improvement, particularly in the situation of obese patients. Improvements such as high-frequency transducers and advanced software algorithms for enhancing image quality can help to counter some of the difficulties related to increased body mass. The integration of these technologies may lead to enhanced penetration depth and resolution for imaging fat-neighboring musculoskeletal tissues. Also, research on adjunctive methods, such as the use of contrast agents or other imaging methods when ultrasound proves inadequate in a given case, may also be able to provide necessary solutions. With researchers striving for these alternatives, the potential for better diagnostic capabilities remains great, rendering ultrasound an adaptable tool for clinicians working with the diverse and complex cases obesity brings. Ultimately, addressing the limitations of ultrasound penetration in obese patients will not only enhance diagnostic accuracy but also improve overall patient outcomes in musculoskeletal care (Figure 13.13).

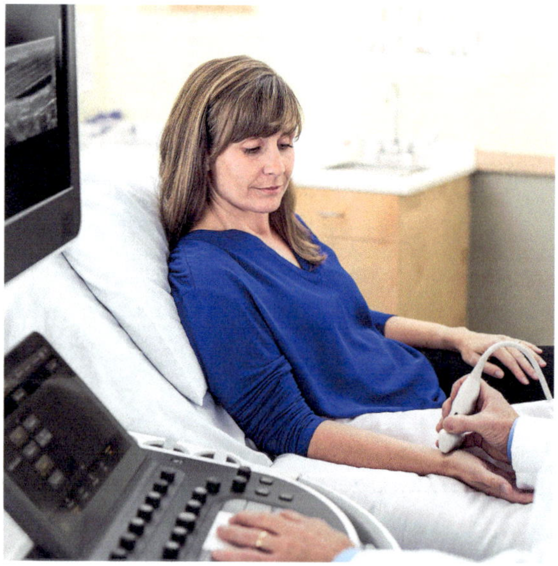

Figure 13.13. Limited penetration in obese patients of MSK ultrasound.

Source: https://images.philips.com/is/image/PhilipsConsumer/01532876320a4197bc8bb27a01471816?extend=-408,0,-1491,0&wid=1024&hei=1024&fit=stretch,1&$jpglarge$.

13.4.3. Challenges in Imaging Deep Structures

Obstacles in imaging deep structures with musculoskeletal (MSK) ultrasound are complex and mainly arise from the limitations inherent in the technology of ultrasound itself. The first major challenge is the depth of penetration of the ultrasound waves, which can make anatomical structures deeply seated hard to see in clear detail. This limitation often necessitates the inclusion of complementary imaging modalities, such as MRI or CT, to reach a complete understanding of the musculoskeletal system. As an additional limitation, ultrasound imaging is also operator-dependent in that the skill and level of experience of the technician or clinician are important determinants of image quality. Thus, intersubject variability can produce inconsistent findings, complicating diagnosis. It demands not only skilled practitioners but also an understanding of the specific protocols necessary to optimize images of deeper structures. Advances in imaging technology serve only to highlight the challenges of imaging deep structures in MSK ultrasound. New developments like computer-assisted orthopedic surgery (CAOS) systems highlight the necessity of including volumetric imaging techniques in overcoming the shortcomings of traditional ultrasound methods. Such systems incorporate existing navigation tools and surgical equipment, making worthwhile possibilities for future advancements in visualization within procedures. An example is employing ultrasound in combination with other imaging modalities to offer a more complete visualization, particularly when aiming at challenging deep structures. Still, notwithstanding such advancements, challenges remain, particularly with respect to protocol standardization across different imaging systems to ensure accuracy and consistency in diagnostics. Integrating CAOS into dynamic environments fueled by imaging modality advances necessitates ongoing research and development to improve these processes to maximize their potential in orthopedic clinics (Kalová et al., 2019). The introduction of artificial intelligence (AI) and deep learning technologies makes things more complicated in imaging deep structures with MSK ultrasound. While deep learning models, especially convolutional neural networks, have tremendous potential for enhancing image analysis, they also present a variety of challenges. The efficiency of the algorithms to classify correctly and detect abnormalities relies on the quality and amount of training datasets available. In the absence of solid datasets that cover various scenarios, like the depth of structural imaging, the application of AI can yield inconsistent or incorrect results. In addition, the integration of AI into existing imaging pipelines must be extensively tested to ensure reliability and safety for use in the clinic (Bejnordi et al., 2017). Thus, while AI has the potential to revolutionize MSK ultrasound, note must be taken of these challenges in order to bring it to fruition successfully.

13.5. Comparison with Other Imaging Techniques

The musculoskeletal imaging landscape has changed considerably, with different methods at the disposal of practitioners. Two of the most prevalent techniques used are magnetic resonance imaging (MRI) and computed tomography (CT), which tend to be the preferred methods because of their high resolution. Yet, musculoskeletal ultrasound has some unique benefits that render it a valuable option, especially for the assessment of inflammatory diseases like gout. Studies have established that ultrasound can effectively image monosodium urate crystal deposition in the joints, a significant diagnostic feature of gout. MRI provides sensitive information about soft tissue anatomy and is helpful in challenging situations, but it is potentially limited by its availability and expense. The portability and relative affordability of ultrasound, combined with its real-time imaging, make it a feasible option for musculoskeletal-condition-specializing healthcare environments (Finucci et al., 2015). Based on the effectiveness of diagnosis, musculoskeletal ultrasound can be identified apart from others due to its unique capability of offering dynamic testing. Compared to static imaging machines, ultrasound allows physicians to visually inspect joint movement in real-time, potentially enhancing the diagnosis of joint effusion and tendinopathy. This dynamic evaluation is particularly valuable for primary care doctors and physiotherapists who may be performing ultrasound examinations in their clinics. Further, the technique has been embraced in New Zealand, where physiotherapists use ultrasound for various applications, from diagnostic purposes to tracking for rehabilitation (Auckland University of Technology et al., 2018). The shift indicates the evolving role of musculoskeletal ultrasound in clinical day-to-day practice, particularly as a tool for direct patient interaction and real-time feedback within treatment protocols. While not without its demerits, musculoskeletal ultrasound also has a number of advantages to it. One of the most prevalent issues is operator dependency of ultrasound examinations; the accuracy of the results will be greatly reliant on the skill and experience of the clinician. This variation can be detrimental to diagnostic reliability, particularly when compared to standardization often observed with MRI and CT scanning. In addition, while ultrasounds can detect a wide range of abnormalities, their effectiveness may be reduced in deeper tissue structures or more complex anatomical sites. Therefore, while musculoskeletal ultrasound is an effective imaging technology within the arsenal for the treatment of musculoskeletal complaints, its application to practice needs to be treated carefully, utilizing its strengths while mindful of its limitations and the setting in which it will most benefit (Finucci et al., 2015).

13.5.1. MRI Versus MSK Ultrasound

The choice between musculoskeletal ultrasound (MSK ultrasound) and magnetic resonance imaging (MRI) is a significant consideration in the evaluation of musculoskeletal disorders. MRI is greatly appreciated for its good anatomical resolution and ability to image soft tissue architecture. MRI finds particular utility in diagnosing conditions with complex presentation, such as ligament injury and cartilage degeneration. Its non-invasive nature and capacity to produce cross-sectional images of the body through various planes give clinicians an overall impression of pathologies beneath. However, high cost, longer scanning times, and fewer MRI machines in clinical environments pose possible limits to clinical practice. This contrasts with MSK ultrasound, which, though operator-dependent, offers real-time imaging and dynamic assessment of musculoskeletal tissues. Because it uses sound waves and not ionizing radiation, MSK ultrasound presents an extremely promising alternative with reduced side effects, thereby solidifying its enhanced popularity as a tool for musculoskeletal assessment.

Used in clinical decision-making, the advantages accruing through the employment of MSK ultrasound cannot be overlooked. The ability to perform guided injections and dynamically investigate abnormalities contributes to its application in real-time imaging. This modality allows clinicians to visualize the region of pathology in real time during the performance of therapies and thereby improve patient outcomes. MSK ultrasound can also be an economically sound option and is often more readily available than MRI, so it is a good first-line imaging for musculoskeletal disorders. Clinical studies have repeatedly demonstrated that MSK ultrasound can offer similar diagnostic accuracy for certain conditions, such as tendon rupture and bursitis, compared with MRI. However, it should be noted here that the effectiveness of MSK ultrasound also lies to a large degree with the operator's skill and expertise, which may result in variations. The influence of these imaging modalities does not end at diagnosis; they also influence patient treatment and management. Emerging technologies such as MRI-guided focused ultrasound surgery (MRgFUS) are making it possible for new therapeutic applications in musculoskeletal disorders. According to emerging studies, MRgFUS combines the sophisticated imaging potential of MRI with the therapeutic advantages of ultrasound to provide minimally invasive treatments for conditions formerly subject to more invasive surgical interventions (Albisinni et al., 2015). This emerging approach in imaging and intervention reflects the changing milieu of musculoskeletal healthcare. As more research keeps us abreast of MRI and MSK ultrasound's comparative advantages, practitioners must know the specific environments in which each modality is optimally used to provide the greatest benefit for patients (Focal Spot, 1997) (Figure 13.14).

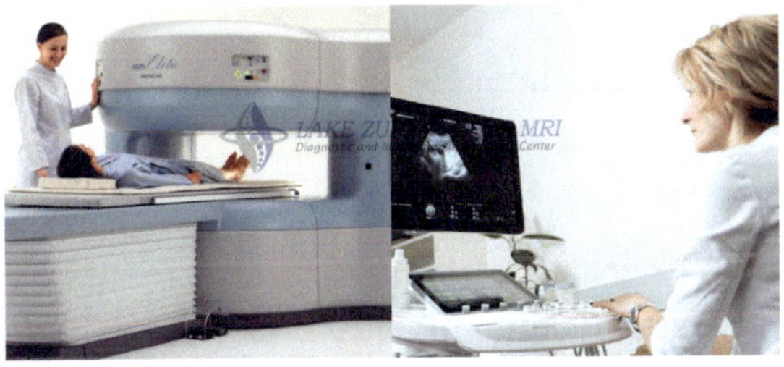

Figure 13.14. Ultrasound vs. MRI for diagnosis.

Source: https://lakezurichopenmri.com/wp-content/uploads/2024/10/Ultrasound-vs-MRI-for-Diagnosis.jpg.

13.5.2. CT Scans and Their Role in Musculoskeletal Imaging

In musculoskeletal imaging, the CT scan has been an invaluable friend, an auxiliary to basic modalities such as X-rays and MRIs. While other imaging modalities can only provide low-resolution longitudinal views, CT scans provide high-resolution cross-sectional views that allow closer examination of complicated structures. This can be particularly valuable for the diagnosis of fractures, abnormalities of joints, and complicated soft tissue disease that are not well visualized with other imaging methods. The accuracy of CT imaging helps clinicians make accurate diagnoses, thereby refining treatment plans based on patient needs. Furthermore, preoperative assessment is based significantly on CT scans since they provide surgeons with the precise information required to schedule complicated orthopedic procedures. Therefore, the addition of CT imaging to the musculoskeletal assessment process enhances surgical preparedness and diagnostic accuracy, making it a vital component in managing patients. Besides their role in diagnosis, CT scans contribute to the therapeutic roles of musculoskeletal disorders through image-guided interventions. In CT-guided aspirations or injections of joints, risks are minimized and treatment effectiveness increases with procedures such as corticosteroid injection for arthritis or joint effusion aspiration. With these focused treatments supported by accurate imaging, patients have improved outcomes and increased rates of procedural success. Also, the ability of CT to provide real-time imaging intra-procedure allows for immediate assessment of needle placement and, therefore, reduces the risk of complications. Such accuracy, made possible by CT-guided procedures, further supports the role of this imaging modality in modern musculoskeletal medicine, an indication of its dual role of diagnosis and therapy. For these advantages, their incorporation into routine clinical practice is their weight in gold in terms of optimizing therapeutic regimens for musculoskeletal disorders. CT scanning is, however, not without limitations, such as possible radiation exposure. Patients who receive repeated scans or serial imaging can accumulate a significant dose of radiation and create possible long-term health risks. Consequently, clinicians must duly weigh the merits and demerits of CT scanning in musculoskeletal evaluation. Emphasizing a wise approach, the use of appropriate protocols and guidelines becomes indispensable to prevent excess radiation exposure while still taking advantage of the strengths of CT scans as diagnostic aids. Also, technological innovation in imaging technology and technique, including low-dose CT protocols, attempts to reduce radiation without compromising image quality. With ongoing research advancements, the application of CT scans in musculoskeletal imaging remains essential, with ongoing assessment and optimization necessary to ensure optimum patient care while minimizing potential harms associated with exposure to radiation (Focal Spot, 1999; Chi et al., 2014) (Figure 13.15).

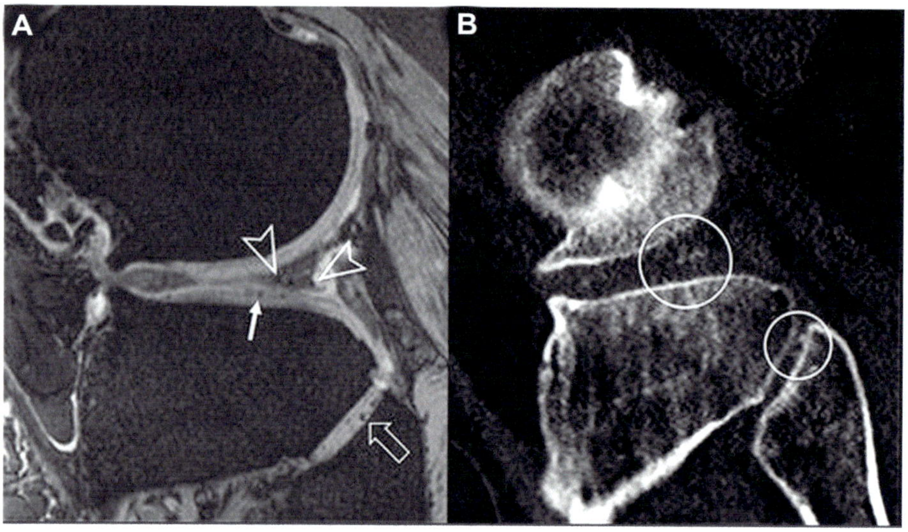

Figure 13.15. CT scans and their role in musculoskeletal imaging.

Source: https://pubs.rsna.org/cms/10.1148/radiol.220634/asset/images/medium/radiol.220634.fig6.gif.

13.5.3. X-Rays and Their Limitations in Soft Tissue Evaluation

For musculoskeletal imaging, X-rays have served as a first-line imaging method for evaluating osseous pathology for decades. Although their use in depicting osseous anatomy is well established, their limitations become apparent when soft tissue evaluation is paramount. X-rays are basically reliant upon the existence of dissimilarities within mineralized structures relative to surrounding structures, typically rendering them inadequate for depicting the details of muscles, tendons, ligaments, and other soft tissues. Thus, conditions such as soft tissue tumors, inflammation, and small tears remain undiagnosed, and there is a requirement for adjunct imaging modalities for definitive diagnosis. This deficiency was instrumental in highlighting the urgent need for better modalities with better contrast in soft tissue examination, ultimately leading to ultrasound as an essential adjunct in musculoskeletal assessment. Even though they are used on a regular basis, X-rays often lead to misdiagnosis when assessing complicated musculoskeletal disease, particularly that of mostly soft tissues. Osteomyelitis, for example, poses a challenge to diagnose, often requiring modalities beyond basic radiography to diagnose associated soft tissue inflammation or injury. In such cases, the X-ray sensitivity is below the needs, as they may fail to note important alterations, especially during the initial stages of the disease progression. Worth noting is that, based on literature, while plain films may initially exhibit osteolytic changes, follow-up imaging with MRI or ultrasound is commonly indicated for confirmation and soft tissue evaluation appropriately (Buchanan et al., 2016). Thus, physicians are compelled to adopt a multimodal imaging approach in hopes of accomplishing a correct diagnosis and effective treatment planning. In addition, recent technologies have taken over the diagnostic niche created by X-rays in evaluating soft tissues, particularly in the orthopedic environment. Ultrasound is one such example, as it has gained popularity due to the fact that it can assess soft tissue structures in real time, providing dynamic images vastly better than static X-ray images. The application of ultrasound during musculoskeletal exams has been extremely useful, particularly in the detection of conditions such as tendon ruptures or muscle sprains, where X-rays are not very helpful. Additionally, advances in the technology of ultrasound, such as computer-assisted orthopedic surgical systems, provide promising avenues for enhanced diagnostic precision (Kalová et al., 2019). With medicine shifting towards integrative diagnostic systems, it is necessary to take note of the shortfalls of standard X-rays in guaranteeing that the correct imaging techniques are employed in comprehensive musculoskeletal assessments.

13.6. Future Directions in MSK Ultrasound

The future of musculoskeletal (MSK) ultrasound holds revolutionary changes that could redesign the diagnosis and management of musculoskeletal disorders. With the increasing need for low-cost, non-invasive imaging strategies, technological advancements are arriving in full swing. On one promising front, artificial intelligence (AI) is being embedded in ultrasound machines to enhance image interpretation and analysis. Machine learning can be utilized to provide more accurate assessments of musculoskeletal conditions, such as tendinopathy and muscle tears, by identifying patterns that are not necessarily detectable with the naked eye. The integration of AI could not only make the diagnosis more streamlined but also improve clinical results by having the ability to identify pathologies earlier on and with more customized treatment strategies. Another significant advance is observed in the development of new ultrasound techniques and treatments, notably with MRI-guided focused ultrasound surgery (MRgFUS). The minimally invasive procedure utilizes sophisticated imaging apparatus to effectively treat various musculoskeletal conditions.

As noted in recent research, opportunities for MRgFUS include the treatment of pain as well as disease treatment in the form of tendinopathy and bursitis, where conventional treatments fail. Having the capability of providing both imaging and therapeutic capabilities, MRgFUS constitutes a paradigm shift in the way the clinician treats the patient within the MSK environment. As developing such technologies continues, they will tend to enhance treatment specificity and efficacy as well as provide faster recovery for the patient. Additionally, the future direction of MSK ultrasound is most likely to emphasize incorporating imaging modalities and biomarker identification for more powerful diagnostic capabilities. Based on recent studies, early diagnosis using advanced imaging technology is essential to minimize musculoskeletal diseases prevalent in aged populations and intense athletes. The synergistic impact of ultrasound and biomarkers can enhance knowledge about disease progression and treatment efficacy, and provide a better overview of a patient's condition. Through leveraging such technologies, such as 3D printing of custom-made implants and sophisticated imaging modalities, the musculoskeletal ultrasound's role can significantly improve patient outcomes and increase the accuracy of diagnoses in a number of clinical circumstances (Albisinni et al., 2015; Adamczyk et al., 2025) (Figure 13.16).

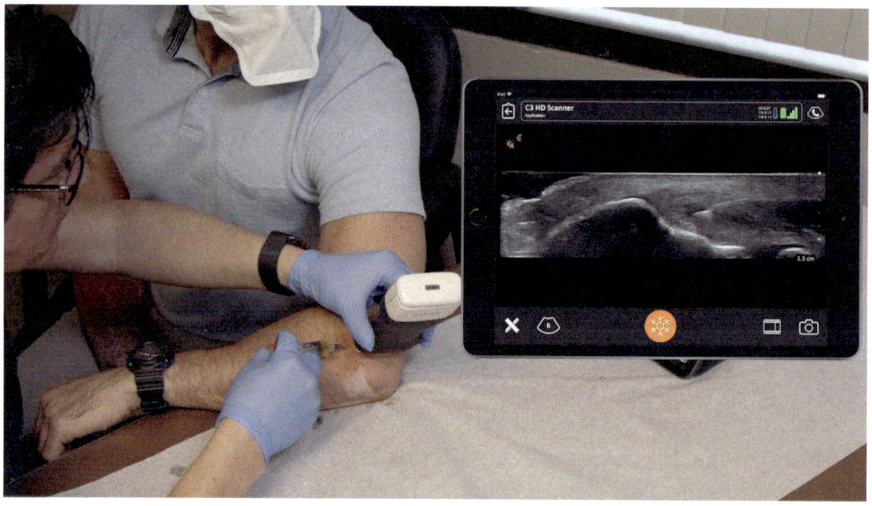

Figure 13.16. Future directions in MSK ultrasound.

Source: clarius.com. https://external-content.duckduckgo.com/iu/?u=https%3A%2F%2Fclarius.com%2Fwp-content%2Fuploads%2F2021%2F08%2Fhirahara-12.jpg&f=1&nofb=1&ipt=27d72d5f7ea0661c3023aa74b568d64697e4b822ecad694c106b2972b5f57e01.

13.6.1. Technological Advancements in Ultrasound Equipment

In the last few years, the technology of ultrasound machines has enormously broadened the capability of musculoskeletal (MSK) imaging. Transducer developments with higher frequencies and in advanced algorithms for imaging have improved the spatial resolution and the quality of ultrasound images. These advances provide clinicians with a greater ability to diagnose and delineate a number of musculoskeletal conditions, from ruptures of tendons to fluid collections. In addition, bedside ultrasound machines are now available, with the capability to perform bedside evaluation and expand the practice of ultrasound diagnosis to remote regions. This development not only makes timely intervention possible but also enhances the growing trend of point-of-care ultrasound, as rapid evaluation facilitates better outcomes for patients. The incorporation of these technologies into widespread practice has enabled more efficient and tailored treatment regimens, ultimately leading to enhanced quality of care provided in the MSK specialty. Moreover, advancements in Doppler ultrasound technology have been a boon to understanding the dynamics of blood flow through musculoskeletal tissues. By using Doppler imaging, doctors can assess vascularity in pathological tissue, giving them feedback regarding a range of diseases such as tumors or inflammation. It allows advanced examination of the underlying anatomy that is indispensable for correct diagnosis and treatment planning. Besides, the integration of ultrasound with image fusion technology, whereby ultrasound images are correlated with computed tomography (CT) or magnetic resonance imaging (MRI) data, has facilitated anatomical contexting. This intersection of multimodal methods assists healthcare practitioners in developing integrated evaluations of musculoskeletal disorders, structural and functional. With developments in ultrasonography technology, it is an excellent tool in the clinicians' toolkit for MSK health. Aside from the ongoing evolution of ultrasonography technology, there is increased demand for education and training of healthcare professionals. Advanced imaging technologies require professionals not only to be knowledgeable about the equipment but also to acquire expertise in image interpretation that is generated. Therefore, more literature and training programs aimed at improving MSK ultrasound skills among radiologists, orthopedic surgeons, and physiotherapists are being published. Continuing professional development in this area is necessary because adequate training ensures advances in technology are translated into improved clinical practice. Just as in the field of veterinary medicine, where imaging technology like computed tomography (CT) has transformed diagnostic capability, so also are these advances found on the human health front (Keane et al., 2017). As healthcare providers become increasingly skilled at utilizing these technologies, their impact on patient care and outcomes will be progressively important (Focal Spot, 1983).

13.6.2. Artificial Intelligence Incorporation in Image Analysis

The use of artificial intelligence (AI) for imaging analysis is revolutionizing the image of musculoskeletal (MSK) ultrasound, enhancing diagnostic accuracy and patient outcomes. Through the use of advanced algorithms, AI allows for improved interpretation of high-resolution ultrasound images, allowing practitioners to identify pathologies that the human eye might otherwise fail to detect. These algorithms tend to utilize large datasets to train on a variety of musculoskeletal conditions in order to offer good performance in actual use. The ability of AI to scan lots of data at high velocity brings a new standardization and precision to the method of ultrasound diagnostics that is particularly precious in sectors that need fine attention to detail, such as orthopedics and rheumatology. Hence, AI integration is not a technological advancement; it is a revolutionary aspect in MSK condition diagnosis and treatment. Based on the advancement achieved in AI technology and deep learning architectures such as convolutional neural networks (CNNs), they are state-of-the-art image analysis techniques in MSK ultrasound. Such sophisticated networks are also proficient at tasks like image classification, segmentation, and object detection to facilitate comprehensive analysis of ultrasound images (Bejnordi et al., 2017). With such models, investigators and doctors can develop models that not only indicate anomalies but also classify tissue types more accurately. This feature enhances diagnosis, as AI makes differentiation between malignant and benign lesions or assessment of the severity of conditions such as arthritis possible. Ongoing refinement of these algorithms serves to keep the rising interpretability of AI in check, thereby contributing significantly to early diagnosis and planning for the treatment of patients with musculoskeletal diseases. Additionally, the development of computer-assisted orthopedic surgery (CAOS) systems demonstrates the utility of AI in combination with ultrasound imaging (Kalová et al., 2019). The systems use volumetric images derived from ultrasound combined with sophisticated navigation technologies, enabling accurate interventions that were previously considered impossible. The integration of ultrasound with AI-based CAOS platforms significantly increases the precision of procedures, minimizing complications and maximizing patient recovery time. Through real-time analysis of ultrasound data in real-time during surgery, AI can assist surgeons in meeting desired anatomical targets as well as enhance overall procedural efficacy. Such a combination of technologies not only demonstrates the ability of AI in image interpretation but also emphasizes its usefulness in complementing surgical techniques, ultimately leading to improved outcomes in the treatment of musculoskeletal conditions.

13.6.3. Expanding Applications in Sports Medicine and Rehabilitation

Integration of musculoskeletal (MSK) ultrasound into sports medicine and rehabilitation is a milestone in the diagnosis and treatment of sports injuries. The modality augments other imaging technologies by providing real-time visualization of soft tissues, allowing clinicians to assess conditions such as tendon injury, muscle tear, and joint effusions with image clarity superior to ever before. For instance, recent studies indicate that sonoelastography, one technique for measuring tissue elasticity, is able to identify tendon abnormalities not visible with conventional ultrasound. By exhibiting pathological characteristics in patients initially presenting with normal results on standard imaging, sonoelastography offers a valuable adjunctive tool, adding to the diagnostic roles of sports medicine clinicians (Abate et al., 2015). Such accuracy in diagnosis ultimately enables more specific treatment plans, thereby optimising the rehabilitation process and enabling faster return to sport.

In addition to improved diagnostics, the application of MSK ultrasound enables new types of therapy, such as in the case of chronic musculoskeletal pathologies. Perhaps one of the most promising methods is that of platelet-rich plasma (PRP) for the treatment of such injuries as rotator cuff tears. As highlighted in more recent literature, PRP is appealing because it has the capability to exploit the body's own natural mechanisms for healing, something especially crucial in athletes whose careers hang in the balance with quick recovery. Ultrasound-assisted PRP injections have the ability to maximize the accuracy of therapy, with growth factors being directly delivered to the site of pathology. The mounting evidence supporting the application of PRP for the rehabilitation of rotator cuff injuries not only suggests the improvement of patient outcomes but also minimizes the need for invasive surgical interventions (Loccisano, 2016). Thus, MSK ultrasound facilitates the integration of such biologic interventions into practice, ushering in paradigm change in sports rehabilitation. The expanding role of MSK ultrasound in sports medicine is best illustrated by its use in follow-through of the healing process following injury. Regular ultrasound scanning allows clinicians to follow the course of injuries and change rehabilitation protocols as necessary. This real-time feedback loop enables healthcare experts to make informed decisions regarding when an athlete is ready for return to sport and thereby enhance performance and safety. Of relevance to the situation is the capability to detect minute differences in tissue dynamics and hence prevent recurrences. Sonoelastography also contributes to this monitoring capacity by establishing stiffness changes of the tissues, which inform healing phases. As sports medicine professionals increasingly adopt the application of MSK ultrasound both for diagnosis and monitoring, they can handle common challenges of athletes' rehabilitation more effectively, especially improving the effectiveness of interventions and limiting the risk of re-injury (Abate et al., 2015; Loccisano, 2016).

SUMMARY

The application of musculoskeletal ultrasound (MSK) has transformed rheumatology and orthopedic diagnostic imaging at a very rapid pace. Because of its non-invasive aspect, soft tissues can be optimally evaluated, and this leads to early diagnosis and management of musculoskeletal illnesses. This becomes even more significant because the majority of pathologies may not be evident on routine imaging examinations. As proved by studies, sonoelastography has proven to effectively reveal tendon pathologies where traditional ultrasound findings were lacking, evidencing its additive role to MSK evaluations (Abate et al., 2015). Integration of MSK ultrasound techniques into routine clinical practice enhances diagnostic reliability and offers real-time feedback for patient care. Moreover, the multi-faceted application of MSK ultrasound extends beyond diagnosis. Its role as a point-of-care device allows for precise intra-articular and periarticular assessment, critical in the appropriate management of most rheumatic diseases as reflected in contemporary literature (Iagnocco & Naredo, 2016). In addition, MSK ultrasound helps clinicians perform guided procedures such as aspirations, injections, and biopsies with greater safety and efficacy. Through direct visualization of anatomical structures, it minimizes the risks of blind techniques. Consequently, this imaging modality facilitates an increased level of individualized therapeutic regimen, consistent with the principles of personalized medicine increasingly being underscored within contemporary healthcare. Ultimately, the creation and incorporation of musculoskeletal ultrasound is a paradigm shift in the management of musculoskeletal conditions. As practitioners make more use of the clinical value of this imaging tool, future studies will likely uncover additional uses and methodological innovations, including the coupling of sonographic characteristics with advanced elastography techniques (Abate et al., 2015). The future of MSK ultrasound in the coming years appears promising because it can potentially push diagnostic models forward and increase patient care levels in numerous fields in rheumatology and orthopedics. Continuing education and training of healthcare professionals on the new ultrasound technologies will be essential in assisting in reaching their full potential and in delivering the highest level of care for patients based on current imaging practices.

The significance of musculoskeletal ultrasound (MSK) is that it serves as both a diagnostic and treatment strategy in rheumatology. MSK ultrasound, being non-invasive, has been cited for its ability to provide comprehensive evaluations of intra-articular and periarticular structures that play a vital role in diagnosing various rheumatic and musculoskeletal disorders. This modality enhances the ability of the clinician to assess conditions such as arthritis, thus transforming patient management protocols. By enabling accurate visualization of anatomical structures, MSK ultrasound enables interventions to be completed at the right time, thus potentially improving patient outcomes through early detection and effective planning of treatment. Besides simple assessment, the use of MSK ultrasound also extends to guiding clinical interventions such as aspirations, injections, and biopsies. This capability to allow real-time imaging enhances procedural accuracy, thereby lowering the risk of complications and enhancing therapeutic outcomes. The advancements in this imaging technique mirror its growing significance in clinical practice and research as clinicians increasingly take advantage of MSK ultrasound for overall management of musculoskeletal disorders. As a point-of-care device, its application in a variety of different healthcare situations demonstrates both its use and suitability across many different patient needs and contexts. The biomechanics of foetal movement are an intriguing observation of the development of musculoskeletal structures from early on. Investigations have established that the physical environment of the uterus is of dominant importance in foetal movement for the purpose of normal skeletal development. For instance, reduced or unusual foetal movement has been linked to conditions such as developmental dysplasia of the hip and arthrogryposis, showing the connection between musculoskeletal well-being and movement. Applications of these biomechanical laws not only enhance our understanding of the common paediatric issues but also have potential for application to fetal medicine and musculoskeletal disorder prevention, eventually contributing to the broader discourse on the worth of motion in foetal and postnatal development (Nowlan, 2015).

CLOSER LOOK

ULTRASOUND COMPUTER-ASSISTED ORTHOPEDIC SURGERY (UCAOS)

Ultrasound Computer-Assisted Orthopedic Surgery (UCAOS) is a new technology that combines the real-time imaging capability of ultrasound with the accuracy and data integration capabilities of computer-assisted navigation systems. Traditional orthopedic surgery has long utilized preoperative imaging such as X-rays, CT scans, and intraoperative fluoroscopy as anatomical guidance. However, these modalities lack real-time capability, expose the patient and operative team to ionizing radiation, or provide poor soft-tissue contrast. UCAOS overcomes all these drawbacks through the capability of surgeons to visualize musculoskeletal structures in dynamic, real-time intraoperatively, thus enabling more accurate, safe, and optimal outcomes.

In UCAOS, the ultrasound imaging is utilized during surgery using navigation software that reconstructs the real-time anatomical structures to achieve precise localization of bones, joints, ligaments, and implants. The location of the ultrasound probe is tracked by a navigation system, usually using infrared cameras and markers that projects the probe's position in three-dimensional space. This data is then calculated by high-end software that generates an interactive, real-time map of the operating field. This technology is of specific benefit in minimally invasive surgery where visualization is limited, and in joint arthroplasty, spinal, or trauma surgery where landmarks are obscured or altered. The most significant possible application of UCAOS is in total knee arthroplasty (TKA), where proper alignment and implant placement are critical to long-term success. UCAOS allows radiation-free, intraoperative real-time inspection of bone surfaces and soft tissues, permitting accurate positioning of the prosthetic components. Likewise, in spinal surgery, UCAOS assists in placing pedicle screws and the avoidance of neurovascular structures without fluoroscopy, reducing cumulative radiation dose. In trauma surgery, it makes fracture reduction and implant placement able to evaluate without repeated X-ray imaging. The advantages of UCAOS are numerous. It offers dynamic, radiation-free imaging, which proves particularly beneficial in pediatric or reoperation cases. It enhances intraoperative decision-making, reduces intraoperative use of CT or fluoroscopy, and assists in leading to shorter operating times and decreased complications. Additionally, the added capability of soft-tissue visualization allows for more precise ligament balancing and cartilage assessment in joint procedures—abilities that are not offered by standard systems. Accuracy in implant placement achieved with UCAOS has been proven to be similar or better than that achieved with other navigation systems.

While promising, UCAOS is not without difficulties. Heavy operator dependency, steep learning curves, and the requirement for specialized training hinder its general applicability. Ultrasound image quality is degraded by artifacts, soft-tissue interfaces, and bone-air interfaces, which are to be interpreted by experts. Compatibility with proven operating room practice and expense are also impediments, although continued technological refinement and increased clinical experience are gradually eroding these hurdles. Later models using artificial intelligence, 3D mapping, and robotic assistance are further enhancing the accuracy and applicability of UCAOS.

References

1. Aabenhus, T., Abbott, T., Aitken, A., Akhtar, N., Alehagen, U., et al. (2016). Evidence for models of diagnostic service provision in the community: Literature mapping exercise and focused rapid reviews. https://core.ac.uk/download/78902098.pdf (accessed on 12th July 2025).
2. Abate, M., Frizziero, A., Galletti, R., Galletti, C., et al. (2015). Sonoelastography in the diagnosis of tendinopathies: An added value. https://core.ac.uk/download/53528698.pdf (accessed on 12th July 2025).
3. Abo, A., Bailitz, J., Blaivas, M., Chilstrom, M., et al. (2018). Systemwide clinical ultrasound program development: An expert consensus model. https://core.ac.uk/download/213444194.pdf (accessed on 12th July 2025).
4. Adamczyk, S., Domino, W., Dziewic, J., Dzwonnik, A., et al. (2025). Imaging diagnostics, biomarkers, and emerging trends in orthopedic research and treatment. https://core.ac.uk/download/636385661.pdf (accessed on 12th July 2025).
5. Albisinni, U., Battista, G., Bazzocchi, A., Catalano, C., et al. (2015). MRI-guided focused ultrasound surgery in musculoskeletal diseases: The hot topics. https://core.ac.uk/download/98341478.pdf (accessed on 12th July 2025).
6. Andre, M., Byra, M., Chang, E., Du, J., et al. (2019). Quantitative ultrasound and B-mode image texture features correlate with collagen and myelin content in human ulnar nerve fascicles. https://core.ac.uk/download/231896728.pdf (accessed on 12th July 2025).
7. Auckland University of Technology, Forrest, G., Jedrzejczak, D., Leech, M., McKiernan, H., Ministry of Health, New Zealand Medical Radiation Technologists Board, et al. (2018). Exploring the clinical use of ultrasound imaging: A survey of physiotherapists in New Zealand. https://core.ac.uk/download/155776972.pdf (accessed on 12th July 2025).
8. Barbulescu, A. L., Chisalau, B. A., Ciurea, P. L., Criveanu, M., et al. (2019). The effect of glucosamine, chondroitin and *Harpagophytum procumbens* on femoral hyaline cartilage thickness in patients with knee osteoarthritis–An MRI versus ultrasonography study. https://core.ac.uk/download/216811083.pdf (accessed on 12th July 2025).
9. Beckers, S. K., Carow, J. B., Ghassemi, A., Knobe, M., et al. (2012). Arthroscopy or ultrasound in undergraduate anatomy education: A randomized cross-over controlled trial. https://core.ac.uk/download/14526068.pdf (accessed on 12th July 2025).
10. Bejnordi, B. E., Ciompi, F., Ghafoorian, M., Kooi, T., et al. (2017). A survey on deep learning in medical image analysis. http://arxiv.org/abs/1702.05747 (accessed on 12th July 2025).
11. Bergman, E. H. J., Declercq, J., Hauspie, S., Martens, A., et al. (2011). Anatomy and imaging of the equine metacarpophalangeal/metatarsophalangeal joint. https://core.ac.uk/download/55889827.pdf (accessed on 12th July 2025).
12. Buchanan, M. D., Grant, S., Shuler, F. D., et al. (2016). A comparison of imaging modalities for the diagnosis of osteomyelitis. https://core.ac.uk/download/232729304.pdf (accessed on 12th July 2025).
13. Chi, Z. G., Huang, Q. H., Lu, M. H., Zheng, Y., et al. (2014). Development of a portable 3D ultrasound imaging system for musculoskeletal tissues. https://core.ac.uk/download/61012682.pdf (accessed on 12th July 2025).

14. Cox, B. F., Fatahi, M., Fernandez-Gutierrez, F., French, J., et al. (2015). Comparative ergonomic workflow and user experience analysis of MRI versus fluoroscopy-guided vascular interventions: An iliac angioplasty exemplar case study. https://core.ac.uk/download/228177186.pdf (accessed on 12th July 2025).

15. Delaney, L. J., Eisenbrey, J. R., Fang, T., Fitzgerald, R., et al. (2019). Ultrasound-triggered antibiotic release from PEEK clips to prevent spinal fusion infection: Initial evaluations. https://core.ac.uk/download/213449826.pdf (accessed on 12th July 2025).

16. Derrington, S. M., Greis, A. C., & McAuliffe, M. (2015). Evaluation and nonsurgical management of rotator cuff calcific tendinopathy. https://core.ac.uk/download/46974922.pdf (accessed on 12th July 2025).

17. Finucci, A., Iagnocco, A., Rutigliano, I. M., Scirocco, C., et al. (2015). Musculoskeletal ultrasonography in gout. https://core.ac.uk/download/74318651.pdf (accessed on 12th July 2025).

18. Iagnocco, A., & Naredo, E. (2016). One year in review: Ultrasound in arthritis. https://core.ac.uk/download/74318648.pdf (accessed on 12th July 2025).

19. Kalová, M., Kubíček, J., Oczka, D., Tomanec, F., et al. (2019). Recent trends, technical concepts and components of computer-assisted orthopedic surgery systems: A comprehensive review. https://core.ac.uk/download/287649034.pdf (accessed on 12th July 2025).

20. Keane, M., Paul, E., Rauch, C., Rutland, C., et al. (2017). Computed tomography in veterinary medicine: Currently published and tomorrow's vision. https://core.ac.uk/download/80784172.pdf (accessed on 12th July 2025).

21. Kim, J., Maranna, S., Parange, N., Watson, D., et al. (2025). A scoping review on the integration of artificial intelligence in point-of-care ultrasound: Current clinical applications. https://core.ac.uk/download/656889328.pdf (accessed on 12th July 2025).

22. Lento, P. H., & Primack, S. (2007). Advances and utility of diagnostic ultrasound in musculoskeletal medicine. https://core.ac.uk/download/pdf/8288298.pdf (accessed on 12th July 2025).

23. Loccisano, A. (2016). Platelet-rich plasma for the treatment of partial rotator cuff tears. https://open.bu.edu/bitstream/2144/14355/9/Loccisano_bu_0017N_10415.pdf (accessed on 12th July 2025).

24. Maliborski, A., & Serafin-Król, M. (2017). Diagnostic errors in musculoskeletal ultrasound imaging and how to avoid them. https://core.ac.uk/download/pdf/144875396.pdf (accessed on 12th July 2025).

25. Manske, R., Voight, M. L., Wolfe, C., & Page, P. (2024). Diagnostic musculoskeletal ultrasound for medial collateral ligament injuries: Applications in rehabilitation. *International Journal of Sports Physical Therapy, 19*, 1166–1171. https://www.semanticscholar.org/paper/c4e11a835b0467f1f0a1cd50bea368d48c16d7ff (accessed on 12th July 2025).

26. *Focal Spot, Fall 1979*. Bernard Becker Medical Library Archives. Washington University School of Medicine. https://core.ac.uk/download/129069226.pdf (accessed on 12th July 2025).

27. *Focal Spot, Fall/Winter 1980*. Bernard Becker Medical Library Archives. Washington University School of Medicine. https://core.ac.uk/download/129069886.pdf (accessed on 12th July 2025).

28. . *Focal Spot, Spring/Summer 1983.* Bernard Becker Medical Library Archives. Washington University School of Medicine. https://core.ac.uk/download/129069238.pdf (accessed on 12th July 2025).

29. *Focal Spot, Winter 1983.* Bernard Becker Medical Library Archives. Washington University School of Medicine. https://core.ac.uk/download/129069236.pdf (accessed on 12th July 2025).

30. *Focal Spot, Spring 1997.* Bernard Becker Medical Library Archives. Washington University School of Medicine. https://core.ac.uk/download/129069307.pdf (accessed on 12th July 2025).

31. *Focal Spot, Fall/Winter 1999.* Bernard Becker Medical Library Archives. Washington University School of Medicine. https://core.ac.uk/download/129069316.pdf (accessed on 12th July 2025).

32. Sommerich CM, Lavender SA, Evans K, Sanders E, Joines S, Lamar S, Radin Umar RZ, Yen WT, Li J, Nagavarapu S, Dickerson JA. (2016) Collaborating with cardiac sonographers to develop work-related musculoskeletal disorder interventions. Ergonomics. 59(9):1193-204. doi: 10.1080/00140139.2015.111661 https://core.ac.uk/download/144159074.pdf (accessed on 12th July 2025).

33. Nowlan, N. C. (2015). Biomechanics of fetal movement. https://core.ac.uk/download/76995826.pdf (accessed on 12th July 2025).

34. Patience, A., Speed, C. A., Bowen, C. J., Miller, D. L., Hendry, G. J., Siddle, H. J., et al. (2018). Survey of ultrasound practice amongst podiatrists in the UK. https://core.ac.uk/download/293885607.pdf (accessed on 12th July 2025).

35. Vanden Bossche, L., & Vanderstraeten, G. (2015). A multi-center, double-blind, randomized, placebo-controlled trial protocol to assess Traumeel injection vs dexamethasone injection in rotator cuff syndrome: The TRAumeel in ROtator cuff syndrome (TRARO) study protocol. https://core.ac.uk/download/55799136.pdf (accessed on 12th July 2025).

36. Wolfe, C., Voight, M., Page, P., & Manske, R. C. (2023). Musculoskeletal ultrasound: An essential tool in diagnosing patellar tendon injuries. https://core.ac.uk/download/573884619.pdf (accessed on 12th July 2025).

37. Zhang, M., & Xie, K. (2025). Advances in musculoskeletal ultrasound for assistive diagnosis in pain clinics. *Pain and Therapy, 14*, 791–801. https://www.semanticscholar.org/paper/84b48f15229fd6c6a81f139df6b0085f3a4b8b96 (accessed on 12th July 2025).

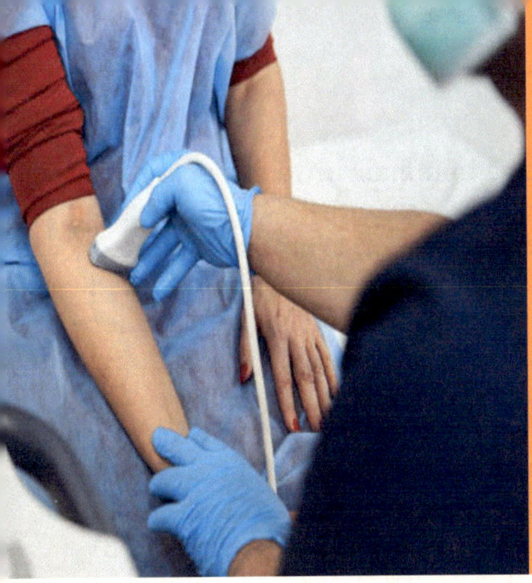

Chapter 14

VASCULAR ACCESS AND SOFT TISSUE IMAGING ULTRASOUND

Contents

Introduction

The coming of vascular access and soft tissue imaging ultrasound is a breakthrough in modern medical practice, where technology utilization and clinical practice optimize patient advantage. As medicine advances, the requirement for reliable vascular access methods becomes more important, particularly in emergencies and surgery. Effective visualization of vascular structures and soft tissues through the use of ultrasound technology has enabled the significant alteration of the methodology of procedures requiring intravenous access or assessment of vascular integrity. Not only does this approach of imaging and procedural intervention assist in more accuracy, but it also lessens the risks associated with standard access methods. It is crucial that healthcare professionals learn about the nuances of these techniques to be able to deliver care founded on the latest technological advances. Moreover, the evolution of ultrasound technology has significantly changed medical imaging practice, more precisely, vascular access. Traditional imaging modalities are generally labor-intensive and carry the risks of radiation exposure. On the other hand, ultrasound provides a minimally invasive approach that allows real-time imaging of blood vessels and adjacent structures. Advantages of employing ultrasound for vascular access include improved localization accuracy, reduced complication rates, and improved patient comfort. As observed in recent studies, the use of ultrasound-assisted modality has been found to have a much greater success rate than conventional techniques, further establishing its clinical significance. The continuous innovation of ultrasound technologies not only continues to improve the ability to navigate vascular networks but also the overall experience for both practitioners and patients. Beyond enabling vascular access, the use of ultrasound is also used for characterization of soft tissue, a growing concern in clinical diagnostics. The ability to diagnose illness on the basis of imaging of soft tissues can be best utilized in the evaluation of soft tissue masses, tendon injuries, and fluid collections. Techniques such as Shear Wave Elastography (SWE) have also been identified as possible tools to assess the mechanical properties of soft tissues that can yield valuable information regarding pathology without the need for invasive testing. This new approach allows practitioners to monitor changes in tissue stiffness and vascularization, as seen in recent research. By integrating vascular assessment with imaging of soft tissues, health practitioners can adopt a more holistic view of patient well-being, leading to improved diagnostic accuracy and tailored treatment strategies, emphasizing the important place of ultrasound in contemporary medical practices (Baeumlin et al., 2016; Dizier et al., 2018) (Figure 14.1).

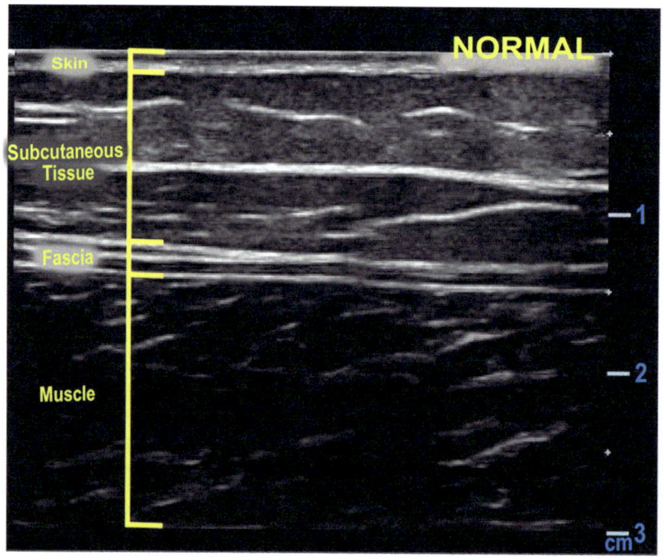

Figure 14.1. Soft tissue ultrasound.

Source: Brian D. Euerle (2020). Soft Tissue Ultrasound. www.acep.org/sonoguide/basic/soft-tissue-ultrasound. https://www.acep.org/siteassets/sites/sonoguide/media/images/soft-tissue-msk-images/figure-2.-normal-skin-subcutaneous-tissue-and-fascia.png.

Definition of Vascular Access

Vascular access is an important medical term that describes the creation of a route for intravenous access to the vascular system, most notably for the infusion of fluids, medication, or to draw blood. This is the most critical procedure in most healthcare settings, including hospitals and outpatient clinics, because it facilitates many clinical interventions ranging from minor medications to complicated therapies such as dialysis and chemotherapy. Vascular access depends on various factors, including the anatomical location of access placement, the access device type used, and the individual physiological properties of the patient. Thus, a proper understanding of vascular access is essential to ensure optimum patient benefits and minimize the chances of complications, such as infection or thrombosis. To better understand the importance of vascular access, it is pertinent to know in which manner it is associated with imaging modalities such as ultrasound. Ultrasound has been increasingly utilized in order to better visualize and assess vascular structures in an effort to enhance the success rates of vascular access procedures. Ultrasound allows for real-time imaging, which makes it easier for practitioners to spot suitable veins or arteries and guide the placement of catheters and other equipment with greater accuracy. Not only does this technology enhance the precision of vascular access, but it also reduces the number of failed punctures, which are painful and distressing for the patients. Therefore, the application of ultrasound in vascular access procedures is an important addition to the overall quality of care. Further, studies on the mechanical properties of blood vessels, such as vessel stiffness and wall thickness, have been gaining momentum in recent years due to the implications for cardiovascular health understanding. Techniques such as arterial shear wave elastography (SWE) have turned into non-invasive techniques for the measurement of these properties, which could contribute to early detection of cardiovascular disease. The importance of vascular access transcends even the immediate therapeutic control and leads ultimately to the advantage of perpetuating vascular disease and health management. In this context, the scrupulous balancing of both anatomical and physiological factors, complemented by advanced imaging techniques, highlights the central role that vascular access plays in supporting effective treatment modalities. With developments in the field, the integration of vascular access, ultrasound, and emerging diagnostic technologies promises to disclose additional improvements in patient care and health outcomes (Figure 14.2).

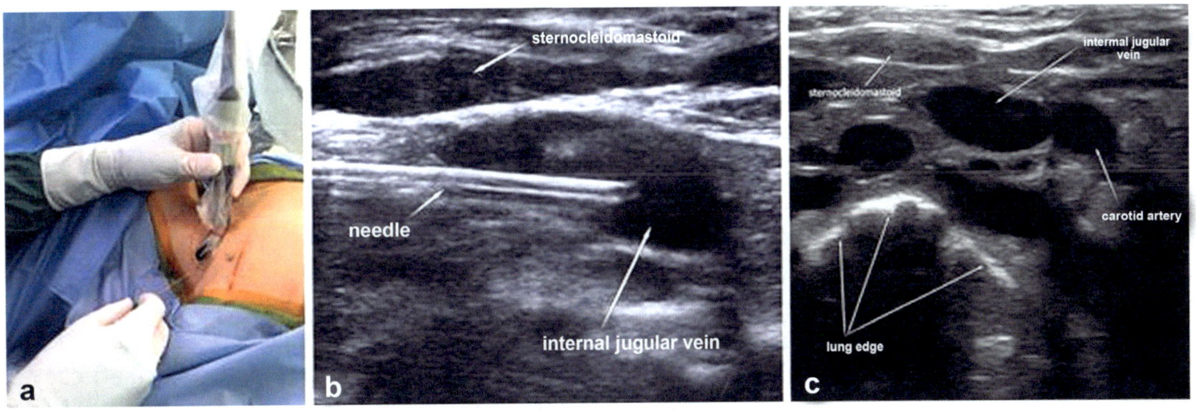

Figure 14.2. Vascular access ultrasound.

Source: https://radiologykey.com/wp-content/uploads/2016/04/A324411_1_En_18_Fig3_HTML.jpg.

Importance of Ultrasound in Medical Imaging

The application of ultrasound in medicine has grown more significant, particularly in vascular access and the evaluation of soft tissue. In contrast to other imaging techniques, ultrasound is non-invasive, provides real-time images, and doesn't employ ionizing radiation, positioning it as a necessary tool in the clinical setting. Visualization of vascular structures and analysis of blood flow dynamics enhances diagnosis and enables minimally invasive interventions. Ultrasound is of immense value in the guidance of interventions such as central venous catheter placements or peripheral intravenous access, which are increasingly becoming emergently needed for patient care in a wide variety of medical conditions. The fact that ultrasound provides immediate feedback during a procedure greatly reduces the risk of complications and enhances overall patient safety, again highlighting its vitally indispensable nature in modern medical practice. Furthermore, studies have highlighted the extensive applications of ultrasound beyond routine vascular treatment, specifically in specialized medicine. As an instance, in podiatric medicine, utilization of ultrasound in the assessment of musculoskeletal conditions has been highlighted as important, with approximately 49% of podiatrists utilizing ultrasound in musculoskeletal conditions and 46% in vascular tests (Patience et al., 2018). As physicians increasingly see the utility of tailored imaging examinations, ultrasound becomes an essential adjunct to standard methods of assessment. Not just used for disease diagnosis, ultrasound also steers therapeutic maneuvers through facilitating treatments. This versatility yet again illustrates how ultrasound enhances decision-making mechanisms in the clinic, in turn leading to improved patient outcomes across every medical discipline. Furthermore, ongoing developments in ultrasound technology and practice training have continued to advance applications of the use of ultrasound in medical imaging. Contrast agent development, including that of eXIA 160, has allowed for the unobstructed visualization of vascular networks, as seen in studies on wall shear stress and its relevance to the atherosclerosis condition (de Wilde et al., 2016). These innovations not only provide more specific images but also provide for exact analyses critical to the diagnosis and treatment of vascular disease. Furthermore, the requirement for special training in ultrasound application defines a growing area of professional expertise in medical specialties. Even as ultrasound becomes more and more an integral part of clinical practice, establishing competency standards and developing broad-based training programs remains vital to ensure proper use of this imaging modality in a safe and effective manner by healthcare professionals. The importance of ultrasound as a pillar of medical imaging will therefore keep expanding further, enhancing its use in patient management and overall medical care.

14.1. Types of Vascular Access

In the health sector, there should be stable vascular access, particularly when imaging soft tissues by ultrasound. There are various modes of vascular access, with peripheral intravenous (PIV) and central venous catheters (CVC) being the most prevalent. Peripheral intravenous access is typically applied in short-term management as it is not difficult to insert and results in limited complications. However, it is challenging in patients with complex venous anatomy or in the case of extended treatment. In such cases, central access has priority, which allows for the infusion of drugs, fluids, and blood products directly into larger veins that receive larger volumes. A correct perception of these modes of access ensures procedural efficacy and patient safety under imaging, particularly where accurate visualization of vascular structures is critical. Further complications are introduced when intra-arterial access is considered, especially in the context of contrast-enhanced imaging. This method is particularly useful for localized scanning of isolated soft tissue structures as it allows for more targeted delivery of contrast agents, enhancing the diagnostic yield of ultrasound imaging. In a comparative study comparing intra-arterial versus intravenous contrast enhancement in equine patients, significant enhancements in imaging of anatomical structures were reported via intra-arterial techniques, demonstrating the impact that vascular access can have upon imaging outcomes (Baeumlin et al., 2016). The ability of the intra-arterial technique to provide the examination of lesions, which are equivalent to high levels of blood supply, demonstrates its worth within clinical practice, and it demonstrates its importance within all-round diagnostic approaches. Apart from differences in types of access, catheter design and care considerations are also important. New technologies, such as ultrasound-guided placement, are revolutionizing the extent of vascular access with better visualization and fewer procedural complications. These advances also contribute to the creation of successful vascular access in challenging cases, further improving the success rates of peripheral and central lines. Moreover, awareness of each vascular access type's potential complications—for example, infection, thrombosis, and misplacement—enables clinicians to undertake preventive measures, ensuring maximal outcomes in the treatment of patients. The dynamic development of vascular access technologies also maximizes the overall effectiveness of soft tissue imaging techniques, like ultrasound, by providing physicians with greater confidence in establishing timely and accurate diagnoses (Figure 14.3).

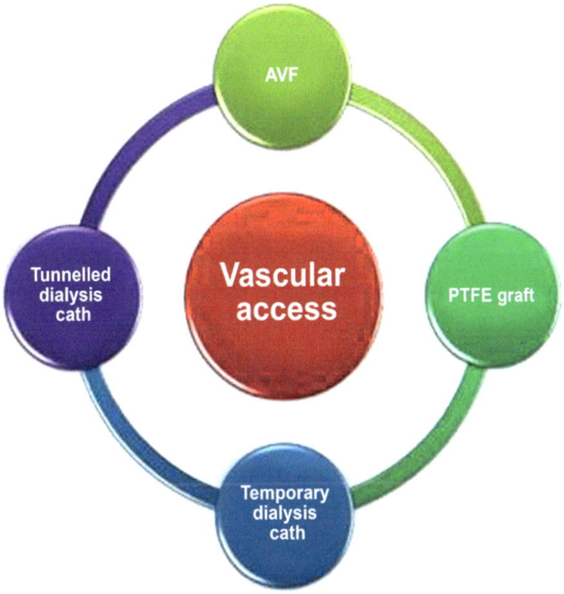

Figure 14.3. Types of vascular access.

Source: https://kidnecare.com/wp-content/uploads/2016/09/vascular-access.jpg.

14.1.1. Peripheral Venous Access

The peripheral venous access clinical practice is the cornerstone of modern medical practice, particularly in cases that require intravenous therapy, administration of drugs, or blood withdrawal. The process involves inserting a catheter into a peripheral vein, usually of the forearm or hand, and it offers instant and effective entry into the vascular system. With advances in ultrasound technology, peripheral venous access guidance is far more efficient, enhancing cannulation success, particularly in obese patients with difficult venous access due to edema or vascular disease.

Ultrasound-guided procedure not only makes the process more effective but also lessens the possibility of complications such as hematomas or arterial punctures and thus is a resource both in emergency and elective practice. The addition of soft tissue imaging ultrasound in peripheral venous access underscores the advancement in vascular access techniques. By providing real-time visualization of the veins, ultrasound allows for measurement of target vessel size, depth, and likely anatomy to ensure precision in catheter placements. Ultrasound is particularly helpful in pediatric and geriatric patients, where venous anatomy is challenging to work with. The non-invasive property of ultrasound also facilitates continuous monitoring of procedures with adjustment accordingly, without introducing patients to additional risk. Advanced techniques, such as the development of conformal ultrasound devices that can remain stable in the presence of dynamic motion, illustrate the advances in imaging technology to provide safer and more efficient vascular access procedures (Acosta et al., 2020).

There is new evidence that newer ultrasound technologies can be used for other purposes as a diagnostic tool. Specifically, wearables' technology for capturing blood pressure waveforms from deeply implanted vessels has the potential to revolutionize clinicians' approach to vascular access and monitoring (Bhaskaran et al., 2018). The technologies have the capacity to augment patient outcomes by utilizing prolonged cardiovascular monitoring and reducing the number of repeated invasive procedures. Incorporation of these non-invasive devices into routine practice could enhance patient safety and satisfaction as more research advances. Lastly, the creation of peripheral venous access technologies and soft tissue imaging ultrasound leads to a more comprehensive patient care practice that bridges the gap between short-term clinical needs and long-term health tracking (Figure 14.4).

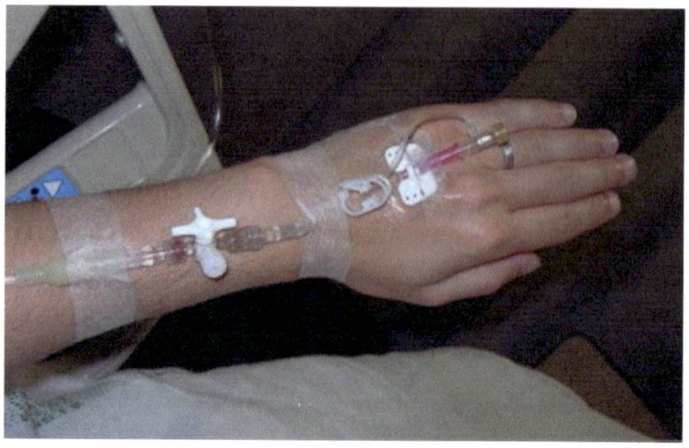

Figure 14.4. Peripheral venous access.

Source: https://www.sharinginhealth.ca/images/IV_hand.jpg.

14.1.2. Central Venous Access

The insertion of central venous access is a life-saving intervention in today's medical field, giving medical practitioners direct access to the central venous system. The capacity to do so is essential for the administration of drugs, fluids, and nutritional therapy, as well as for the measurement of central venous pressure. Central venous catheters (CVCs) are typically inserted into large veins such as the internal jugular, subclavian, or femoral veins, where healthcare providers can successfully bypass peripheral vascular resistance. CVC insertion is more frequently performed under ultrasound guidance, with real-time visualization of vascular anatomy, thereby reducing the risk of incorrect placement and complications. Notably, the incorporation of ultrasound not only decreases complications of blind punctures but also helps in the identification of perfect anatomical landmarks, thus leading to improved cannulation success. Ultrasound-guided central venous catheter insertion has revolutionized the catheter placement procedure, particularly in patients with challenging vascular anatomy. Conventional methods, although effective, often utilize anatomical landmarks subject to potential distortion by obesity, edema, or anatomical discrepancies. On the other hand, ultrasound imaging provides a real-time image of the target vessel in which clinicians can assess venous patency and size and avoid nearby structures such as nerves and arteries. Moreover, intra-procedure real-time ultrasound guidance can lead to immediate feedback, which avoids complications such as accidental arterial puncture or pneumothorax. The newer technology of ultrasound has also enhanced these techniques further, with ultrasound devices that can fit against the skin and ease blood flow to make it easier to manipulate and monitor from heavily implanted vessels, enhancing clinical outcomes in general (Bhaskaran et al., 2018).

In addition to aiding catheter placement, ultrasound is also crucial in post-insertion management of central venous access. It is also a key factor in determining the catheter tip position, most essential for optimal position within the central venous system to prevent complications such as thrombosis or catheter infection. Evidence shows that the use of ultrasound can accurately confirm correct catheter placement in real time without subsequent imaging studies, enhancing patient safety. Moreover, ultrasound use is not only confined to initial placement but also beneficial for complications assessment, such as thrombus formation within the vessel or catheter-related infections. This broadened view of central venous access lends support to the addition of imaging modalities to vascular access protocols, with a positive effect on patient outcomes and evidence-based practice advice (Baeumlin et al., 2016) (Figure 14.5).

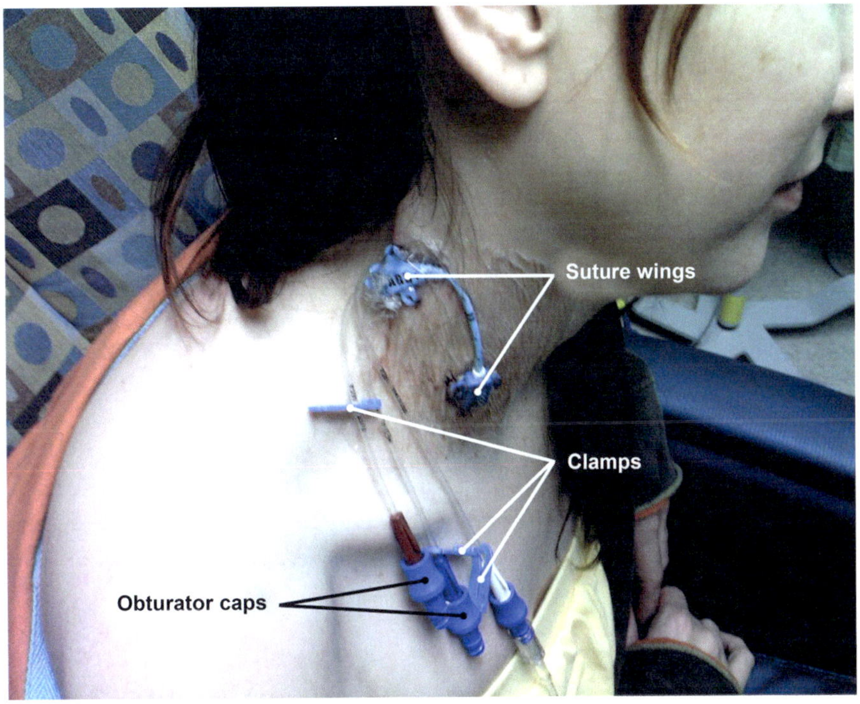

Figure 14.5. Central venous access.

Source: *Zipdoc/www.wikem.org.* https://media-us.amboss.com/media/views/62fc92d8d35002.93843441.jpg.

14.1.3. Arterial Access

Arterial access is a key feature in the technique of vascular access and soft tissue imaging ultrasound, its function in the evolution of diagnostic potential. Arterial access provides direct access to the arterial system, facilitating the possibility of a variety of procedures, including angiography, fluid sampling, and targeted therapy. Precision of arterial access is of primary concern; it possesses certain advantages over venous access, such as enhanced observation of blood flow kinetics and the ability to more precisely administer contrast agents. Arterial access is rendered safer and more efficient through the utilization of ultrasound imaging. By making use of real-time imaging, clinicians can more specifically direct vascular structures, reducing the likelihood of complications such as hematoma or thrombosis.

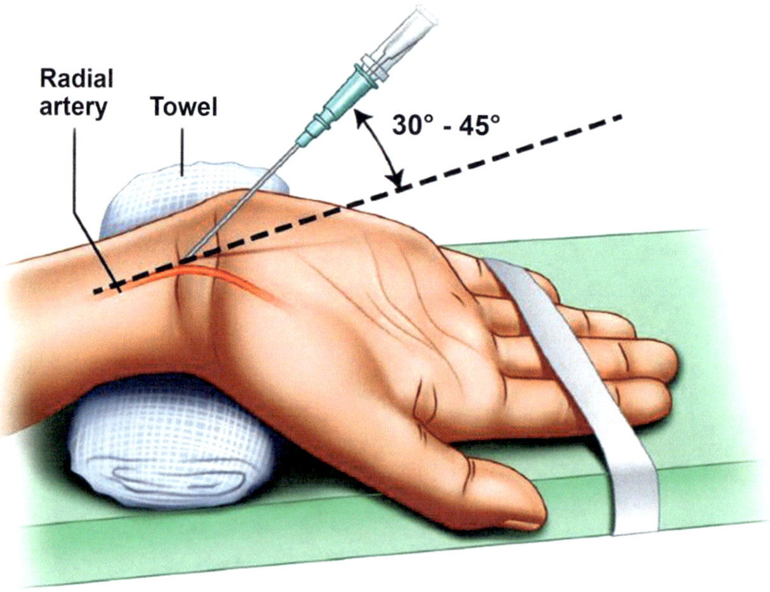

Figure 14.6. Arterial access.

Source: Abide, A.M., Meissen, H.H. (2021). Arterial Line Access and Monitoring. Interventional Critical Care. Springer, Cham. https://doi.org/10.1007/978-3-030-64661-5_11. https://media.springernature.com/lw685/springer-static/image/chp%3A10.1007%2F978-3-030-64661-5_11/MediaObjects/323414_2_En_11_Fig6_HTML.png.

14.2. Ultrasound Technology in Vascular Access

Ultrasound technology has emerged as a valuable asset in the realm of vascular access, enhancing the safety and efficiency of venous and arterial catheterization procedures. With its provision of real-time imaging, ultrasound facilitates the visualization of vascular anatomy and enables healthcare workers to determine the optimal access site. This technology minimizes reliance on anatomical landmarks, whose patient-to-patient variability may be large, thus a reduction in risk of such complications as arterial puncture or hematoma development. Furthermore, dynamic imaging ability gives practitioners the capability to observe blood flow and vessel patency during catheter placement, eventually leading to improved outcomes and patient satisfaction. The use of ultrasound in vascular access procedures is a revolution in clinical practice, reflecting the importance of precision in interventions to meet critical patient needs adequately. The use of ultrasound technology for vascular access has also brought some incredible successes in procedural training and skill development among medical professionals. Conventional training paradigms rely heavily on observation and simulation, which may fail to equip the trainees for the nuances of true-life clinical practice. Under ultrasound guidance, trainees can acquire practical experience while directly engaging with real-time images, improving their vascular anatomy knowledge and technical skills. This modality not only provides greater confidence among providers but also encourages the use of evidence-based procedures that can potentially standardize care in a wide range of clinical settings. Additionally, continuing education programs are increasingly incorporating ultrasound-assisted methodology, reaffirming the place of this technology in the continuing evolution of healthcare professionals dedicated to patient-centered care. Furthermore, the expanded applications of ultrasound technology extend beyond classical vascular access interventions to more complex interventional procedures. As exemplified in new treatment methods, for example, MRI-guided focused ultrasound surgery (MRgFUS), the integration of imaging and intervention can provide significant benefits to patients with varied pathologies, including musculoskeletal conditions. This new approach takes advantage of both imaging uses and therapeutic applications of ultrasound, demonstrating the technology's flexibility within a clinical environment. The cross-talk between imaging and treatment modalities offers the possibility of less invasive therapy, further reducing patients' convalescence time and associated healthcare costs. Finally, the employment of ultrasound in vascular access and related applications is an important development in medical practice, enhancing both therapeutic efficacy and diagnostic precision (Focal Spot, 2007; Albisinni et al., 2015) (Figure 14.7).

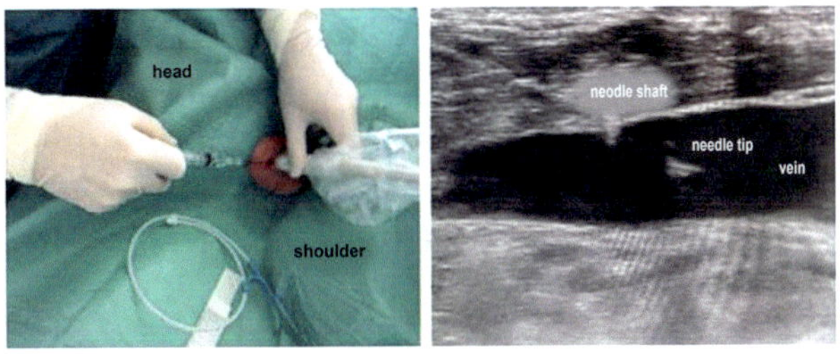

Figure 14.7. Ultrasound technology in vascular access.

Source: Wastl D, Dietrich CF, Morf S, Crossey F, Blaivas M, et al. (2023) Ultrasound Guided Vascular Access Practical Issues (Pictorial Essay). Arch Emerg Med Crit Care 7(2): 1061. https://www.jscimedcentral.com/public/assets/images/uploads/image-1704706727-1.PNG.

14.2.1. Principles of Ultrasound Imaging

Ultrasound imaging is based on sound wave propagation and reflection and uses high-frequency sound waves to produce real-time images of inner structures. When ultrasound waves are emitted from a transducer, they propagate in the body and reach various tissues, which reflect waves back. The degree of reflection, or echogenicity, varies in various tissues based on their density and composition. For example, soft tissues will return sound waves differently than bone or fluid-filled structures. Differential reflection is important to distinguish between various types of tissues in applications for vascular access and soft tissue imaging. Last but not least, the transducer receives echoes that reflect back and converts them into digital signals, which form images that aid healthcare professionals in diagnosing and successfully guiding treatments. One of the primary applications of ultrasound imaging is in the use of vascular examination. Surprisingly, studies indicate that a high proportion of practitioners, particularly podiatrists, employ ultrasound in practice, and this is primarily for vascular examination and planning treatment (Patience et al., 2018). Handheld Doppler ultrasound allows for the investigation of blood flow patterns, surveillance for pathology, and surveillance of interventions in real-time. The natural benefits of ultrasound, such as not being invasive, not using ionizing radiation, and the ability to provide immediate feedback, make it more beneficial in vascular testing. Physicians are now better recognizing these advantages, which translate into improved patient outcomes, timely intervention, and overall better healthcare delivery. Moreover, the integration of ultrasound modalities can be extended to advanced therapeutic applications, such as MRI-guided focused ultrasound surgery (MRgFUS), which shows the convergence point of imaging and treatment modalities. This sophisticated approach utilizes the principles of ultrasound by employing MRI for targeting precise tissues, particularly in musculoskeletal ailments (Albisinni et al., 2015). The non-invasive nature of MRgFUS is a paradigm change towards the treatment of aggressive pathologies with the highest regard for patient safety. Utilization of the strength of ultrasound imaging enables practitioners to not only visualize but to intervene optimally, thereby extending the application of ultrasound in clinical practice. This merging of imaging modality and therapeutic intervention underscores the importance of excellence in principles of ultrasound by practitioners who perform the treatment of vascular and soft tissue (Figure 14.8).

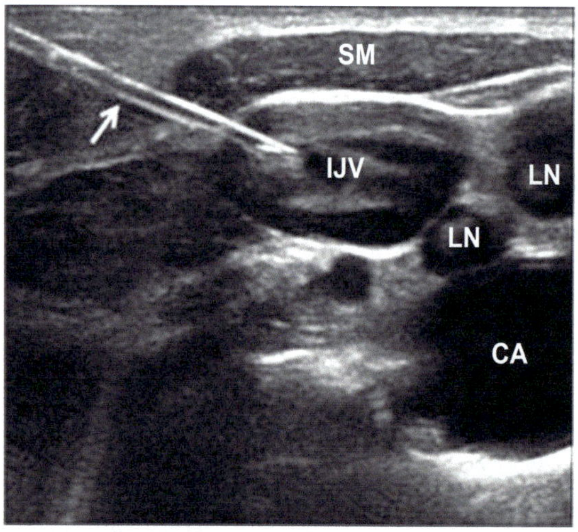

Figure 14.8. Principles of ultrasound imaging in vascular access.

Source: https://cdnintech.com/media/chapter/62354/1512345123/media/F11.png.

14.2.2. Equipment Used in Ultrasound-Guided Procedures

In soft tissue and vascular access imaging, ultrasound-guided procedures tap into a broad array of highly advanced equipment designed to enhance accuracy and performance. Central to these procedures is the ultrasound machine equipped with transducers that emit high-frequency sound waves. The sound waves travel through tissue in such a way that soft tissues and vascular structures surrounding them can be visualized in real time. The resolution and quality of the image of the ultrasound are significant because they have a direct effect on the clinician's ability to accurately identify anatomy and pathology. In addition, advances in technology have introduced portable and point-of-care ultrasound platforms that allow for bedside or emergency procedure ease of performance, which enhances patient outcomes through enabling faster interventions. In addition, the integration of needle guidance systems in ultrasound devices has considerably transformed the practice of minimally invasive interventions. By means of advanced algorithms, the systems provide real-time feedback of needle position, enabling practitioners to achieve directed access to a blood vessel or other soft tissue structures with high accuracy. This accuracy is extremely beneficial in complicated cases where anatomic irregularities may pose difficulties. Furthermore, improvements in needle technology, such as echogenic needles, allow for better visualization under ultrasound scanning and more accurate visualization of the trajectory of the needle by operators, minimizing the risks of complications. Such an advanced line of equipment not only boosts clinician confidence but also enhances patient safety for the procedures that are otherwise required to be more invasive and risky. Moreover, the application of complementary technologies such as elastography adds additional information related to tissue properties that are critical in guiding ultrasound interventions. Elastography quantifies tissue stiffness and is useful in distinguishing between malignant and benign lesions or evaluating vascular wall condition. This technology development is reflective of the global trend towards increased examination completeness during ultrasound-guided interventions. Also, next-generation ultrasound machines can have artificial intelligence to improve image analysis and interpretation. Their integration is part of a broader mission towards increasing diagnostic accuracy and optimizing procedural outcomes in vascular access and soft tissue imaging, a trend facilitated by developing technologies like MRI-guided focused ultrasound surgery as reported in the literature today, a showcase of interventional refinement in contemporary medicine (Albisinni et al., 2015; Focal Spot, 2007) (Figure 14.9).

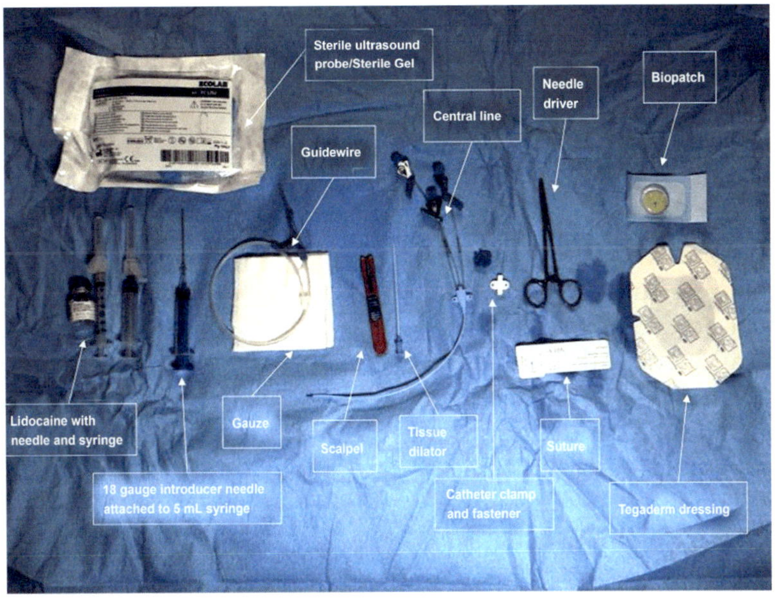

Figure 14.9. Equipment used in ultrasound-guided procedures for vascular access.

Source: S. Genobaga and J. Cleek. Ultrasound-Guided Central Line. https://pocus101.b-cdn.net/wp-content/uploads/2023/03/Ultrasound-Guided-Central-Line-CVL-Materials-Complete-Setup.png.

14.2.3. Advantages of Ultrasound Over Traditional Methods

Ultrasound technology has many benefits over conventional imaging techniques, especially in the case of vascular access and soft tissue imaging. One of the main advantages is that it is non-invasive, which minimizes patient risk tremendously. Contrary to magnetic resonance imaging (MRI) or computed tomography (CT), both of which may subject patients to ionizing radiation or require the administration of contrast agents, ultrasound utilizes high-frequency sound waves to produce real-time images of soft tissues. This facet makes it safer for patients, especially in such sensitive populations as children and pregnant women. Furthermore, its absence of ionizing radiation eliminates concerns regarding long-term exposure hazards, further emphasizing ultrasound's beneficial profile in practice. Another important advantage of ultrasound is its ability to depict real-time images, aiding in rapid clinical decision-making in a number of circumstances, like vascular access procedures. This real-time imaging allows medical professionals to visualize blood vessels and surrounding structures during the procedure itself, minimizing opportunities for complications such as hematoma or misplacement of the catheter. As opposed to established imaging technologies, while efficient, they come with the requirement of repositioning or moving the patient, which means time lag and increased risk during life-critical procedures. The ability to guide needles or catheters with ultrasound visualization supports its place as an essential device in gaining proper vascular access, thus enhancing overall procedural efficacy and patient quality. In addition, advances in ultrasound technology, such as the development of portable machines, further support its superiority over traditional methods. Portable ultrasound machines enable clinicians to perform imaging at the bedside, enhancing access and reducing patient transfers. This availability is particularly useful in emergency departments where speed is critical and immediate information can be life-saving. Furthermore, the cost-effectiveness of ultrasound compared to MRI and CT imaging contributes to widespread use in numerous clinical environments. With progressively advanced healthcare, embracing technologies with improved efficiency and patient safety, ultrasound becomes an essential modality that belongs to these agendas, further amplifying its advantages over traditional imaging.

14.3. Indications for Ultrasound-Guided Vascular Access

Use of ultrasound-guided vascular access has gained significant traction in the last decade of medical practice on the basis of its usefulness for enhancing the accuracy and safety of the procedure. It is particularly indicated in patients with difficult vascular access, such as the obese, a history of vascular surgeries, or occult vascular anatomy. These challenges could significantly complicate traditional access methods, leading to increased patient discomfort, longer procedure time, and increased complications. Through the assistance of ultrasound imaging of vascular landmarks in real-time, professionals gain improved skills to conduct navigation of the complexities of individual anatomies, thereby increasing the rate of successful first-attempt cannulation and reducing the risk of complications associated with multiple punctures. In critical and emergency situations, the immediate establishment of vascular access is needed for the administration of blood products, fluid, or a drug. Ultrasound guidance is advisable in situations where an immediate intervention is necessary, particularly in emergency conditions where other ways are not possible because visibility is lacking or there are anatomical challenges. Within such a risky environment, the ultrasound can expedite the process, allowing for quicker opening at the same time that it minimizes risks from less precise or blind methods. Ultrasound not only aids in the detection of vessels but is also a valuable resource in determining catheter size and length decision-making and, ultimately, better patient outcomes in both acute and chronic environments. Also, ultrasound-guided vascular access is equally important in outpatient and elective procedures where accuracy and patient comfort are paramount. The procedure is not only utilized in routine placements, for example, central venous catheters and peripherally inserted central catheters (PICC lines), which need accurate placement to avoid complications such as thrombosis or infection. By visualizing the position of the vessel and surrounding structures, ultrasound eliminates complications related to malpositioning. Besides, patients become less nervous when a procedure is performed with the assistance of ultrasound because they are convinced that their safety and comfort become the priority. This extra care is in keeping with other imaging modalities, such as MRI-guided procedures, where an effort is being made to fuse accuracy with minimal invasive technique (Albisinni et al., 2015; Andrani et al., 2017) (Figure 14.10).

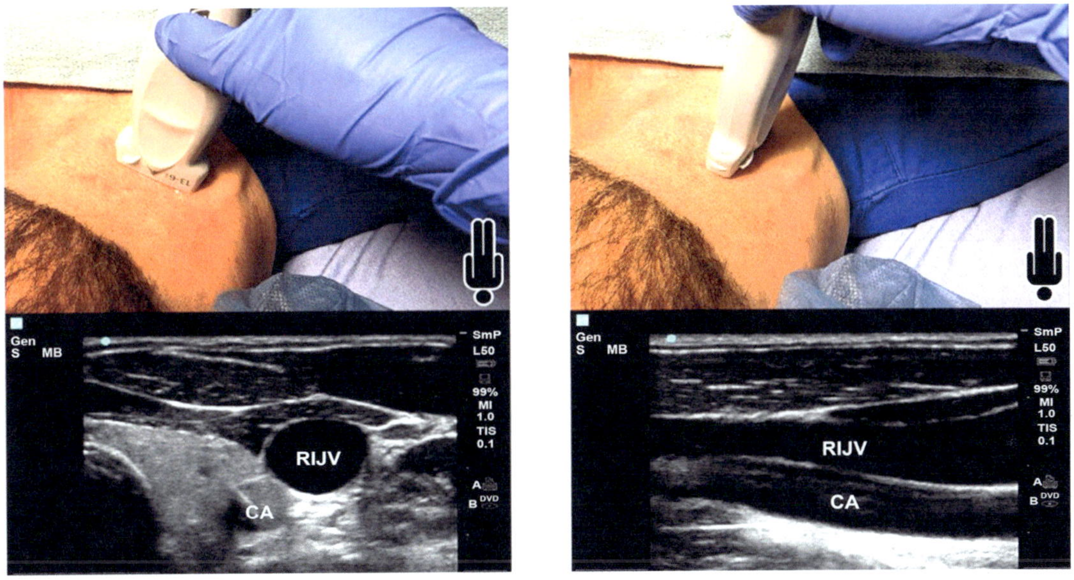

Figure 14.10. Indications for ultrasound-guided vascular access.

Source: Annette V. et.al.(2025). Guidelines for Performing Ultrasound-Guided Vascular Cannulation. ASE. https://onlinejase.com/article/S0894-7317(24)00632-1/fulltext

14.3.1. Patient-Specific Factors

In balancing the success of ultrasound-guided vascular access and soft tissue imaging, patient-specific factors are key in determining procedural achievement as well as patient outcomes. These encompass a wide variety of patient factors, including age, body habitus, comorbidities, as well as the specific target anatomical sites for access. For instance, the obese patient experiences challenges in vascular structure visualization owing to the increased thickness of tissues, leading to challenges in placing needles and accessing them. The structure of variations in skin and tissue also has an effect on the ultrasound's clarity and diagnostic quality of the images and therefore directly impacts the precision of guiding interventions. It is essential to comprehend these nuances for clinicians because they can modify ultrasound techniques to meet the precise needs of their patients and hence enhance the overall effectiveness of vascular interventions. Patient background and individual pathology also have an important role in selecting ultrasound modalities and approaches. Certain conditions, such as prior surgeries, vascular anomalies, or the presence of a tumor, may necessitate certain imaging modalities to visualize involved vessels or soft tissue elements appropriately. For instance, patients who have had prior venous intervention may possess altered anatomy, where accurate evaluation in the form of ultrasound is necessary to strategize new access points properly. Patient-specific imaging techniques also lead to fewer complications and greater patient satisfaction, finally resulting in quicker recovery times and greater total success. Clinicians must hence be adept at utilizing patient-specific information in their procedural planning for optimal outcomes in vascular access and soft tissue imaging. Patient-specific factors' interaction with ultrasound technology is also revealed through advanced imaging modalities such as MRI-guided focused ultrasound surgery (MRgFUS). This minimally invasive procedure utilizes non-ionizing imaging technologies tailored to the specific requirements of individual patients and anatomical structures, creating new possibilities for treating musculoskeletal disorders (Albisinni et al., 2015). The development and implementation of the new technology helps to accentuate the need for tailoring ultrasound use to offset patient-specific dynamics. Besides, due to the progress in medical technology, the role of personalized medicine in vascular access and soft tissue imaging will play an even greater role, making the therapeutic interventions more specific. Through the keeping of patient-specific factors at the core of clinical practice, the quality of ultrasound applications and related interventions could be significantly improved by healthcare practitioners (Focal Spot, 2005) (Figure 14.11).

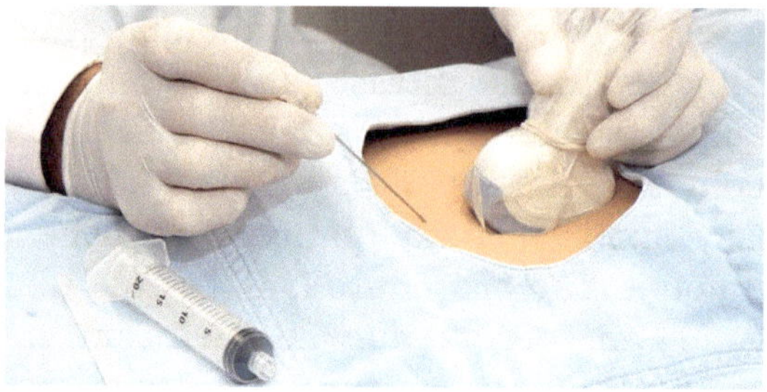

Figure 14.11. Patient-specific factors for ultrasound-guided vascular access.

Source: us.edm-imaging.com. https://us.edm-imaging.com/cdn/shop/articles/Why_should_ultrasound_be_used_for_vascular_access_procedures_600x600_crop_center.jpg?v=1689856387.

14.3.2. Clinical Scenarios Requiring Ultrasound Guidance

In clinical practice, ultrasound guidance plays a crucial role in cases that require precise vascular access, for example, the insertion of central venous catheters. The traditional methods cause complications like arterial puncture and incidental hematoma formation. Ultrasound enables real-time visualization of structures and significantly enhances the precision of needle placement. This technology not only assists with vein location but also allows assessment of nearby tissues, which is important in preventing complications. As shown in studies on ultrasound-assisted procedures, there is a marked reduction in puncture attempts and associated complications. Furthermore, the learning curve for practitioners using ultrasound is dramatically lower compared to standard procedures, highlighting the importance of integrating this technology into standard procedures. Thus, its employment is a breakthrough measure in improving patient safety and procedural success in vascular access situations. Apart from vascular access, ultrasound guidance plays an imperative role in soft tissue imaging for intervention, such as drainage of abscesses. In the management of soft tissue lesions, accurate localization plays an important role in making therapeutic interventions effective and minimizing patient discomfort. Ultrasound application enhances the clinician's ability to identify the size, shape, and exact location of abscesses or other fluid collections. This is achieved through the evaluation of lesion characteristics in real time, which is crucial in determining the best approach to drainage. The effectiveness of ultrasound for this clinical condition not only reduces the need for more invasive surgical procedures but also enables outpatient management of disorders that would otherwise require hospitalization. As shown in more current studies, the incorporation of ultrasound-guided procedures in clinical workflows has led to improved patient outcomes and satisfaction, attesting to its usefulness in modern medical practice. Emerging technologies and techniques further refine ultrasound's use in multidimensional clinical contexts. As an illustration, MRI-guided ultrasound therapies are being used more and more to treat musculoskeletal conditions since they are non-surgical and yet efficient. As explained in recent literature, such methods allow real-time monitoring and guiding through interventional procedures, to conduct streamlined operations with potentially improved outcomes. The assessment of such cases, particularly with peripheral interventions, is that inclusion of advanced imaging devices has the prospect of diminishing procedure times while maintaining high accuracy. From comparisons of routine fluoroscopy protocols and MRI-guided procedures, studies have demonstrated outstanding improvements in efficiency as well as patient protection. Lastly, these advancements also reflect a broader trend towards multimensional imaging modalities that will dramatically change intervention methods in vascular access and soft tissue imaging, ushering in the avenues of enhanced clinical education and training paradigms within the medical field (Albisinni et al., 2015; Cox et al., 2015).

14.3.3. Complications Related to Non-Ultrasound-Guided Access

The achievement of vascular access by non-ultrasound-guided techniques may have a myriad of complications that have an immediate impact on patient outcome. Among the significant risks of such techniques is accidental puncture of adjacent anatomical structures, that is, nerves and arteries. Such mistakes have immediate effects in the shape of hematomas, which, apart from causing pain, also have potential for long-term sequelae like chronic pain and impairment of function. Also, a lack of real-time visualization during the procedure will lead to redundant cannulation, increasing the risk of infection through increased exposure for longer periods at the puncture site. The implications of such an occurrence emphasize the need for critical consideration of alternative methods that can be used in an effort to enhance the safety and efficacy of vascular access procedures. Apart from procedural mistakes, non-ultrasound-guided vascular access may also result in delayed complications, such as thrombosis or catheter infection. Without imaging guidance, the identification of proper venous targets is delayed, resulting in suboptimal positioning that compromises blood flow and thrombus formation. This not only complicates initial treatment but may lead to additional intervention, thus extending patient morbidity. Catheter-associated bloodstream infections (CRBSIs) are induced particularly by unmonitored catheterization practices, where poor technique or incorrect care might go unnoticed. The resulting excessive complication burden would flatten healthcare systems by causing unnecessary hospitalization and additional healthcare costs, triggering ultimately raising questions about the cost-effectiveness of non-guided approaches to access. Moreover, ultrasound use during vascular access procedures has been shown to decrease complications of non-guided approaches considerably. Ultrasound guidance enables clinicians to have an actual-time picture of vascular structures, thus enhancing needle placement precision and reducing risks of complications. Examples are studies that have reported a considerable decline in the incidence of hematoma formation and CRBSIs with the use of ultrasound guidance compared to traditional techniques. In addition, the changing landscape of ultrasound technology continues to present developments like portable devices that could be used to increase bedside availability and facilitate emergency treatment. With the underlying healthcare demands and needs for proper interventions, the advantage provided by ultrasound-guided access point to a critical shift towards improved vascular access solutions, ultimately culminating in better patient safety and outcomes, especially in the wake of newly arising public health challenges, such as those experienced during the COVID-19 pandemic (Cui et al., 2020) (Figure 14.12).

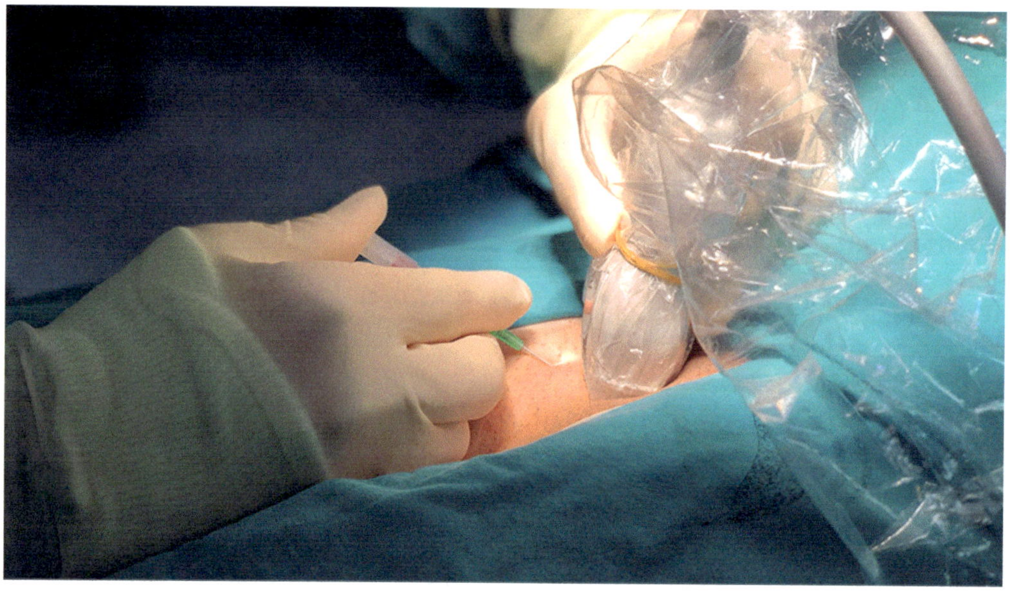

Figure 14.12. Complications associated with non-ultrasound-guided access.

Source: https://d14d5nk8lue86f.cloudfront.net/s3fs-public/2023-10/Ultrasound%20Cuts%20Vascular%20Complications%2C%20Bleeds%20in%20Transfemoral%20Access.jpg.

14.4. Soft Tissue Imaging with Ultrasound

Ultrasound imaging of soft tissues has been a valuable asset in both research and clinical settings. As the one imaging modality that provides real-time imaging, ultrasound enables clinicians to assess soft tissues such as fascia, tendons, muscles, and ligaments with precision. It is best utilized in vascular access, where anatomy identification by precise standards is essential for successful catheter placement and prevention of complications. Moreover, ultrasound's capability to quantify blood flow makes it even more valuable in vascular abnormality and disease evaluation. Through the use of sound waves to generate images, the technology offers a non-invasive method that does not require the ionizing radiation present in X-rays and CT scans. In comparison to other imaging technologies, soft tissue ultrasound provides an enhanced level of safety, real-time feedback, and portability, and as such, it is an unreserved preference for clinicians and patients. Soft tissue imaging capability of ultrasound is further enhanced by technological advancements, such as the development of high-frequency transducers and contrast-enhanced ultrasound. These developments significantly increase resolution to the point of permitting focused examination of complex anatomical structures that can be inadequately visualized with standard methods. Additionally, ultrasound-guided procedures can improve accuracy in interventions, like aspirations or injections that are most frequently performed on an outpatient basis. It decreases the possibility of damage to surrounding tissues and improves efficacy in therapeutic intervention. By providing real-time feedback, ultrasound, in addition to assisting in diagnosis, also guides therapeutic intervention. It is critical to translate these advancements to clinical practice in order to best use the potential of ultrasound in vascular access and soft tissue imaging. In addition, ultrasound imaging of soft tissues has opened new frontiers in the field of interventional radiology. For example, MRI-guided focused ultrasound surgery (MRgFUS) is a prime example of how advanced imaging methods are being merged with treatment options, providing a minimally invasive technique for the management of several musculoskeletal disease states (Albisinni et al., 2015). This hybrid technique exploits ultrasound's precision to perform thermal ablation and monitor therapy, offering promising outcomes without the dangers of standard surgery. These advancements signal a shift toward more patient-centered care in which precision is prioritized for surgery. Its applications to enhanced imaging capabilities have far-reaching implications reaching beyond treatment into diagnostic accuracy and spurring interdisciplinary practice in medicine. Lastly, as there are continued developments in technology, the future of vascular access and soft tissue imaging will likely be increasingly dynamic and lay emphasis on the central role of ultrasound in modern medical practice (Focal Spot, 2007) (Figure 14.13).

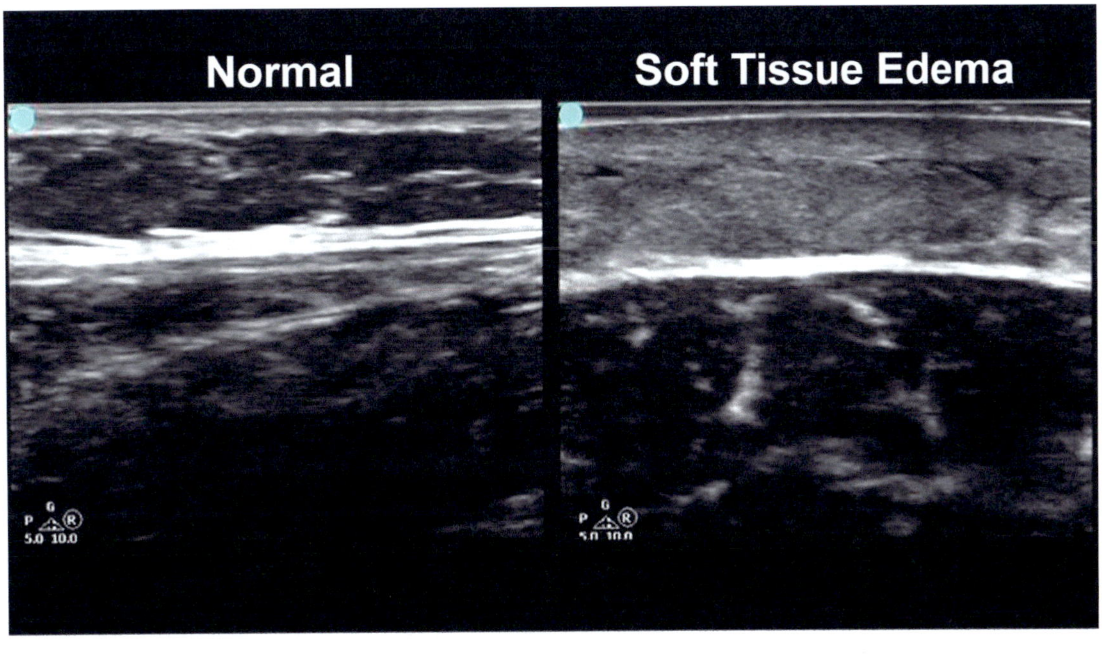

Figure 14.13. Soft tissue imaging with ultrasound.

Source: POCUS - Soft Tissue Ultrasound - Subcutaneous Air. www.youtube.com/@POCUSGeek.

14.4.1. Role of Ultrasound in Soft Tissue Evaluation

The use of ultrasound in the assessment of soft tissue has been highly considered due to its non-invasive method and real-time imaging. Ultrasound has gained specific use in assessing most soft tissues, such as muscles, tendons, and ligaments. With the dynamic visualization of such soft tissues, ultrasound allows for the detection of abnormalities such as tears, cysts, and inflammation. It is especially valuable in sports medicine, where rapid imaging can facilitate diagnosis and the management of immediate treatment. Their portability also enhances the value of ultrasound machines in clinical and outpatient settings, improving patient outcomes. Relative to other imaging modalities with more preparation and possibly radiation, ultrasound represents a safer alternative, which allows reliable evaluation of soft tissues without causing much distress to the patient. Moreover, the application of ultrasound in vascular access procedures has revolutionized the way medical practitioners have conducted catheter placements ever since. The resolution images that ultrasound offers enable blood vessels and overlying soft tissues to be visualized, thereby reducing risks of such complications as hematomas or misplacements. The method enhances procedural success rates, especially in the case of patients with difficult anatomy or obesity, where standard landmarks may be obscured. In addition, ultrasound-guided vascular access minimizes the attempts needed, thereby cutting short the duration it takes to perform the procedure and improving the quality of patient experience. With the incorporation of ultrasound in daily practice, healthcare professionals are able to provide more accurate placements, thus enhancing patient safety and satisfaction when undergoing vascular procedures. In recent years, technological advancements such as increased image resolution and the development of targeted probes have further expanded its application in the evaluation of soft tissues. Research indicates that techniques such as MRgFUS are a potential future for the treatment of most musculoskeletal pathologies with precise monitoring and minimal invasiveness. This technology relies on sophisticated ultrasound applications to comfortably navigate therapeutic interventions (Albisinni et al., 2015). With improvements yet to come for ultrasound imaging, its role in the evaluation of soft tissue will be increasingly vast, offering novel pathways for less-invasive treatment. These advances make it increasingly clear that continuous education and training of healthcare professionals in using ultrasound would be essential so that they continue to become skilled at harnessing this potent instrument for both diagnosis and treatment.

14.4.2. Ultrasound-Diagnosed Conditions of Common Soft Tissues

The use of ultrasound imaging has increasingly taken center stage in the diagnosis of most soft tissue disorders, more so those related to the musculoskeletal system. The non-invasive method provides real-time imaging of soft tissues and allows clinicians to assess such structures as muscles, tendons, ligaments, and bursae. Many conditions diagnosed by ultrasound include rotator cuff tears, tendinitis, and bursitis. For instance, diagnosing rotator cuff tears, which may be caused by trauma or by degenerative changes, can be adequately assessed with the assistance of ultrasound since it can yield proof of the integrity of the rotator cuff tendon and its surrounding structures. As noted, age-related tears in the rotator cuff rise impressively with increasing years, and hence it is both diagnostic and management-relevant. The reliability of ultrasound, therefore, becomes a critical element in the earlier diagnosis of such injuries early in time, enabling early intervention that can enhance patient outcomes as well as minimize recovery times. Ultrasound is also very useful in the diagnosis of tendinitis, which is an inflammatory reaction of tendons, typically secondary to repetitive stress injuries. Tendinitis can affect numerous tendons of the lower body, the most prevalent being the Achilles and patellar tendons. Ultrasound allows for cautious assessment of tendon morphology, with details about thickening, rupture, or echogenic alterations characteristic of tendinitis. Imaging of tendon architecture and identification of overlying inflammatory alterations are precious features in accurate diagnosis and individual management protocols. Injections under ultrasound guidance also represent a precious therapeutic intervention for tendinitis, facilitating accurate delivery of corticosteroid or platelet-rich plasma (PRP) to the affected area. This technique not only alleviates symptoms but has the ability to heal as well, recognizing ultrasound's dual use in diagnosis and healing (Baeumlin et al., 2016).

Bursitis, another common soft tissue affliction, can also be easily diagnosed using ultrasound imaging. Bursae, small fluid-filled sacs that reduce friction between moving tissues, may become swollen due to overuse, trauma, or systemic inflammatory illnesses. On ultrasonography, bursitis is characterized by the accumulation of fluid within the bursa, which is hypoechoic compared to adjacent tissue. Imaging of associated soft tissue abnormalities, such as edema or degeneration of tendons, is also helpful for making a diagnosis. Early diagnosis by ultrasonography is crucial because untreated bursitis can advance to chronic pain and loss of function. With its ease of use as well as ability to offer instant results, ultrasound is a focal tool in the diagnostic process for patients who have soft tissue pathologies, making it a very important resource in today's clinical environment (Baeumlin et al., 2016) (Figure 14.14).

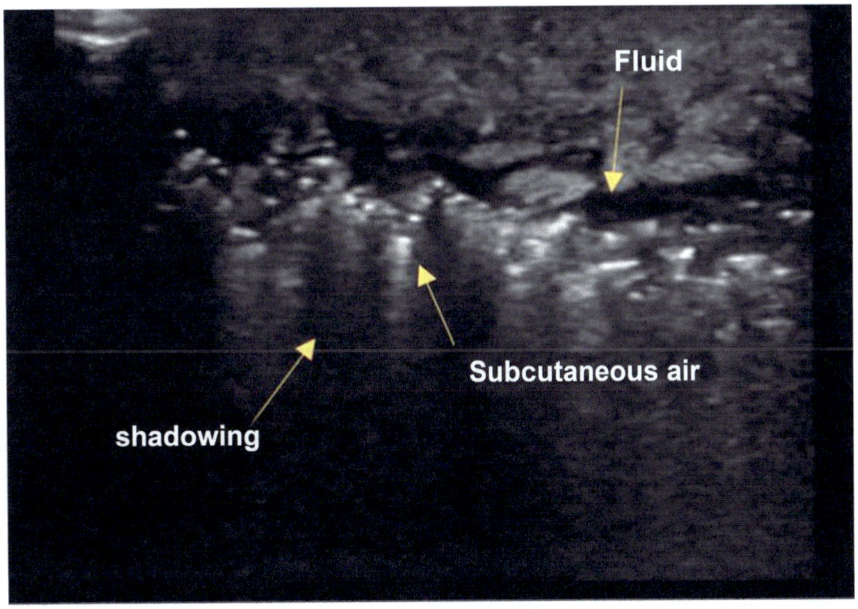

Figure 14.14. Common soft tissue conditions diagnosed with ultrasound.

Source: Keaton Cameron-Burr (2022). Soft Tissue Infection: Diagnosis by Ultrasound. https://brownemblog.com/blogposts/2022/7/1/soft-tissue-infection

14.4.3. Comparison of Ultrasound with Other Imaging Modalities

If vascular access and soft tissue imaging are to be considered, ultrasound is a unique and versatile imaging modality relative to other alternatives, such as magnetic resonance imaging (MRI) and computed tomography (CT). MRI and CT can provide exquisite cross-sectional images of internal structure, but are generally lacking in the real-time visualization abilities that are an integral part of ultrasound technology. This difference is extremely significant in vascular access procedures where precision and timing are crucial. Ultrasound makes it possible for clinicians to visualize blood vessels in real-time, enabling guided interventions. Furthermore, comparative safety and cost-effectiveness highlight its advantages; as compared to MRI and CT, ultrasound does not utilize ionizing radiation and hence is a safer option for various applications in clinical practice, particularly in susceptible individuals and children. Except for safety and cost considerations, everyday applications of ultrasound in tissue imaging and vascular access are also made convenient by its mobility. Portable ultrasound machines revolutionized clinical practice, particularly in emergency and outpatient wards. This portability provides bedside examination and immediate decision-making, which contrasts with the less mobile settings of MRI and CT scanners that require patients to be transferred to specialized imaging rooms. College of Podiatrys' findings underscore the increased application of handheld Doppler ultrasound in various medical practices, with 93% of podiatrists using it for vascular assessment, indicating its adoption into routine screening and treatment practices (Patience et al., 2018). Through this hands-on approach, several interventions are greatly eased through placing diagnostic instruments in the hands of practicing clinicians. In addition, although ultrasound has many benefits, its disadvantages must not be ignored. As an instance, the efficacy of ultrasound may be affected by patient-dependent factors like obesity or marked tissue edema that may impede visualization. In these situations, MRI or CT can offer superior resolution and penetration depth to evaluate deeper structures or difficult pathologies not well evaluated by ultrasound. Although ultrasound is primarily utilized for superficial soft tissue and vascular evaluation, it is often complemented with other modalities in a synergistic strategy to enhance overall diagnostic accuracy. The synergistic imaging strategy is most sharply highlighted in advanced medical treatments such as stem cell therapy, where imaging plays an important front-line role when tracking interventions and outcomes (Jokerst & Wang, 2016). Lastly, understanding the distinct roles and limitations of these imaging modalities informs an integrative model of patient treatment and effectiveness.

14.5. Techniques for Ultrasound-Guided Procedures

Ultrasound-guided procedures have transformed vascular access and soft tissue imaging using real-time imaging techniques that boost precision and reduce the risk of complications. The real-time visualization of anatomical structures guides medical professionals to navigate complex vascular systems and surrounding tissues more effectively. This is most evident in interventions such as central venous catheter placements, in which ultrasound can allow visualization of the intended vessel and surrounding anatomy and reduce trauma and increase success rates. The addition of Doppler ultrasound enhances this practice even more by giving hemodynamic information and assisting in locating near arteries, thus reducing accidental arterial puncture risks. This shows how sonography is an essential tool in most modern-day medical procedures and has come a long way from being only a diagnostic procedure. The best practice and results with ultrasound-guided procedures are achieved through hands-on experience and application of the evidence-based method. It is encouraged that practitioners conduct simulation-based education, which boosts the skill and confidence of clinicians in the performance of such complex procedures. Improvements in ultrasound technology, including high-resolution imaging and the availability of hand-held machines, can now be used to train in a variety of clinical settings so that the practitioner becomes both familiar with anatomical landmarks and with the ultrasound equipment itself. Compliance with proven protocols, for example, concerning the definition of needle angles and depth of insertion, is also very crucial for the prevention of complications associated with vascular access. With improvements to techniques, increased importance has been put on continuous education and optimization of skills, which underscores the commitment to procedural safety and patient safety in ultrasound-guided procedures. In addition, ongoing research on ultrasound-guided interventions looks for novel ways to maximize the applications of this modality. Your use of MR-guided focused ultrasound (MRgFUS) is a good example, since it marries imagery and therapeutic potential, particularly for diseases of soft tissue and bone. This approach not only enhances lesion targeting but also monitors treatment response in real time. As an example, studies have highlighted the utility of using T2-based thermometry in tracking temperature changes within bone marrow during ablation therapy so that practitioners can properly assess tissue response and adjust treatment plans based on that. This synergy of technologies shows how ultrasound-guided therapeutics are advancing, holding great promise for medical therapy in vascular access and other areas (Albisinni et al., 2015; Bucknor et al., 2016) (Figure 14.15).

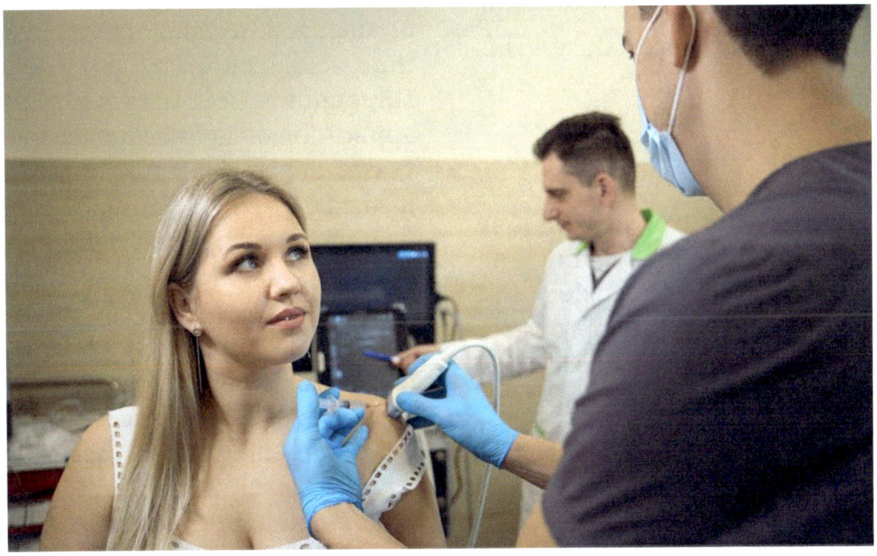

Figure 14.15. Techniques for ultrasound-guided procedures soft tissue conditions.

Source: Svitlana Hulko/istockphoto.com. https://media.istockphoto.com/id/2152452852/photo/medical-doctors-performing-ultrasound-guided-glenohumeral-joint-puncture-on-lady.jpg?s=612x612&w=0&k=20&c=LMvxov9iyTX7VZRKtQifn__oSBKpO9sxxpV2-dkaJR8=

14.5.1. Preparation and Positioning of the Patient

Patient positioning and preparation are critical factors in the successful performance of vascular access and soft tissue imaging ultrasound examinations. Successful patient positioning enhances the visibility of the anatomical structures and provides easier access to the target area for operators. This not only involves placing the patient in a convenient position but also ensuring adequate support so that there is minimal movement during the examination. For instance, supine patient positioning can be convenient for vascular access as it facilitates gravity to distend the vessels and makes it more comfortable to manipulate ultrasound transducers. Also, apt draping techniques can enhance patient comfort and maintain a sterile field, which is critical in cases that may compromise the skin barrier. Apart from physical positioning, extensive preparatory measures need to be carried out to make the patient suitable for the procedure. This includes thorough pre-procedure assessments to identify any condition that will impact vascular access success, for example, previous surgery or obesity. Education of the patient about the procedure, its purpose, and any preparatory requirements, such as fasting and hydration, is essential in relieving anxiety and ensuring cooperation. Moreover, the appropriate imaging modalities, such as MRgFUS, can also be employed to aid in pre-procedure evaluation. As well as providing high-resolution anatomical data, the mentioned imaging modalities aid in planning the most effective path for vascular access, resulting in enhanced procedure effectiveness and patient safety (Albisinni et al., 2015). In vascular access planning, the choice of ultrasound unit and compatible transducer is also important since patient positioning might influence the effectiveness of these devices. Advanced technology, for example, computer-guided systems, can also facilitate more precise positioning and orientation during ultrasound-guided procedures. These robotic aid devices can maximize the accuracy of needle placement, reduce operator fatigue, and ultimately lead to better patient outcomes (Troccaz, 2009). Though this changing health care environment encompasses such technology, patient preparation and positioning remain focal points, retaining the human element of care while capitalizing on technological progress to advance the quality of soft tissue imaging ultrasound practice in general.

14.5.2. Step-by-Step Approach to Ultrasound-Guided Access

The step-by-step sonographic technique of vascular access is an evolving practice with far-reaching implications on procedure success and patient safety. Initially, healthcare providers must conduct a precise analysis of patients' anatomy to establish target vessels accurately. This procedure begins with the utilization of ultrasound imaging, through which real-time visualization of vascular structures and surrounding soft tissue is possible. With the application of high-frequency linear transducers, vessel depth, diameter, and direction can be measured by clinicians while keeping in mind anatomical variations. This first step not only enhances accuracy in needle placement but also minimizes the risk for hematomas and accidental arterial puncture, emphasizing the pivotal function played by ultrasound in rendering vascular access techniques fruitful. Following anatomical assessment, the next step in the ultrasound-guided access protocol is to emphasize meticulous preparation of the technique. Physicians must establish a sterile field and use appropriate ultrasound gel to provide optimal quality images. While the ultrasound probe is still in place, practitioners must conduct a dynamic assessment, observing the target vessel against its anatomical context during various respirations. This dynamic imaging is crucial as it will indicate any potential movement of the surrounding structures, and the operator can then modify their strategy based on that. Furthermore, combined ultrasound imaging with procedural maneuvers will provide accurate visualization of the needle traversing through the skin and soft tissue planes to finally enable vascular access safely and effectively. Finally, following successful access, the employment of a follow-up assessment is required to preserve the patency of the vascular access site. The clinician must monitor for symptoms of complications such as thrombosis or infection, and employ ultrasound to non-invasively check the integrity of the intervention. Current studies highlight the benefit of novel ultrasound tools, including Shear Wave Elastography (SWE) that may be able to show information about vascular access risks and arterial stiffness (Dizier et al., 2018). This aspect of treatment is valuable because it informs clinical decision-making related to the management of vascular devices and potential interventions to maintain venous patency. Moreover, measuring soft tissue interactions with improved imaging methods will put us in a position to enhance the understanding of how variations in anatomy influence ultrasound-guided access in an attempt to achieve better patient outcomes and procedural innovation (Bini et al., 2017).

14.5.3. Post-Procedure Care and Monitoring

Effective post-procedure care and monitoring are critical components in ensuring the safety and efficacy of vascular access and soft tissue imaging ultrasound interventions. Following the procedure, it is paramount to carefully assess the insertion site for signs of complications such as hematoma, infection, or thrombosis. Continuous monitoring of vital signs, along with specific assessments of limb perfusion, can provide essential insights into the patient's recovery process. Vigilant observation for abnormalities enables prompt intervention, thereby reducing the risk of serious complications. Additionally, providers should educate patients about warning signs that necessitate immediate medical attention, ensuring that patients remain informed participants in their own care and recovery. Patient comfort and education are central elements in post-procedural care following vascular access procedures. Providers should offer clear instructions regarding activity restrictions and care for the access site, which can include keeping the site clean, dry, and protected. Patients should also be instructed on how to manage pain or discomfort and when to follow up with their healthcare provider. Supporting the patients' understanding of their care helps foster adherence to post-procedure protocols, which can significantly improve outcomes. An informed patient is more likely to recognize unusual symptoms and initiate timely responses, thereby enhancing the overall effectiveness of the treatment plan and promoting a smoother recovery process. Furthermore, the role of follow-up appointments cannot be understated in the context of post-procedure care and monitoring. These appointments provide an opportunity for healthcare providers to review the patient's recovery and assess the functionality of the vascular access site. During these encounters, practitioners can also address any physical or emotional concerns that may arise post-procedure, thereby contributing to a holistic approach to patient care. Notably, structured follow-up can facilitate early detection of complications, which is essential in ensuring long-term success in vascular interventions. As emphasized in the literature, establishing robust post-procedure monitoring protocols significantly mitigates potential risks and promotes optimal patient outcomes, which aligns with contemporary best practices in vascular access management (Acosta et al., 2020; Kitsiou et al., 2013) (Figure 14.16).

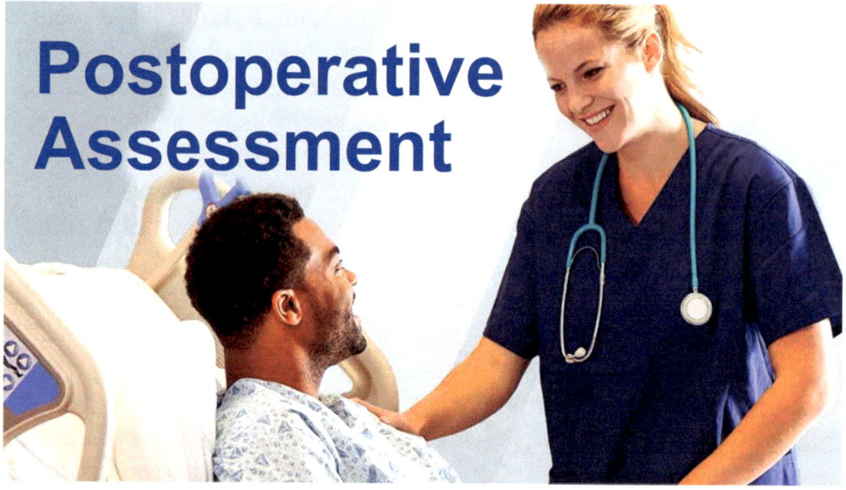

Figure 14.16. Postoperative assessment and monitoring.

Source: Ausmed. (2022). *Postoperative Assessment and Monitoring. https://cdn-images.ausmed.com/ausmed-course/COURSE124v1.1.jpg*

14.6. Challenges and Limitations of Ultrasound

In vascular access and soft tissue imaging, ultrasound has some restrictions and challenges that can discourage its reliability and efficacy. Operator dependency is one such prevalent issue wherein the precision of ultrasound images may largely be based on the experience and ability of clinicians. Inconsistent results can lead to variable outcomes, finally affecting patient outcomes. Further, the skill to learn requires extensive practice and training, which can potentially be a limiting factor in healthcare settings where ultrasound is used infrequently or by less proficient practitioners. Expertise required to use ultrasound underscores the natural constraint on how best to utilize the potential of ultrasound for vascular and soft tissue applications. Yet another restricting severe aspect of ultrasound pertains to its acoustic properties, which tend to be rather divergent depending on the patient's body habitus and the particular structures under examination. In patients with increased body mass index, the ultrasound waves tend to be subject to greater attenuation, leading to suboptimal quality images and an inability to visualize deeper vessels or tissue. Furthermore, tissues like bony structures and air-containing organs have the ability to scatter ultrasound waves, making it difficult to correctly identify vascular landmarks. Such inherent physical limitations may markedly restrict the diagnostic application of ultrasound, frequently requiring adjunct imaging modalities such as MRI or CT scans, especially in complicated scenarios where exact anatomical definition is needed (Albisinni et al., 2015). Additionally, the evolving context of ultrasound technology itself presents opportunities as well as obstacles to its application in vascular access and soft tissue imaging. Though technological advances such as MRI-guided focused ultrasound surgery have shown promise in various clinical contexts, incorporating these technologies into current practice is problematic. This contrast highlights the need for continuous education and innovation among practitioners and investment in advanced equipment that may not be conveniently placed in every healthcare setting. Additionally, disparity in access to healthcare facilities can limit the use of these technologies on a large scale, particularly in poorly funded systems. Hence, while ultrasound offers an innocent and dynamic imaging technique, these limitations demand a careful examination of its role and capability in contemporary medicine (Boss et al., 2019) (Figure 14.17).

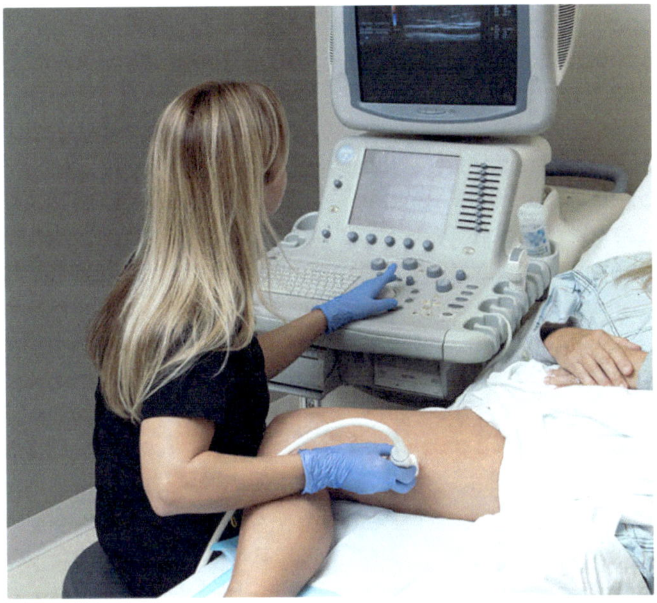

Figure 14.17. Challenges and limitations of ultrasound of vascular access and soft tissue imaging.

Source: https://tinsleysurgical.com/services/vascular-ultrasound/

14.6.1. Operator Dependency and Skill Level

The operator's skill level does play a vital role in the successful performance of vascular access and soft tissue imaging ultrasound procedures. Improvements in ultrasound technology have definitely aided better imaging, but the achievement of optimal results is solely dependent on the skill level of the operators. Inexperienced operators may struggle to interpret ultrasound images and hence increase the chances for misdiagnosis or procedural complications. Research evidence gives hints that experienced practitioners always provide better clinical results since they have superior methods and better decision-making abilities. In the opinion of the American Institute of Ultrasound in Medicine, a strict demand for good training courses is of utmost importance to develop the skills of future sonographers in vascular access protocols to reduce variability linked to operator dependence (Krige et al., 2009). Dependence on the operator is particularly observed during the performance and interpretation of ultrasounds in challenging-to-image anatomical regions. In vascular access, for example, the ability of operators influences the number of successful cannulation procedures. Long practice and exposure allow operators to recognize anatomical variation and vessel condition that render a procedure successful. Interestingly, continuous updation and real-world experience are necessary to develop their skills, as attested by evidence demonstrating a significant reduction in complication rates with increased experience among operators. Further, standardization of procedures through formal training is likely to lead to improvement in variability seen among operators and create more uniform patient outcomes across the board. Enhancement of operator competency is a critical component in ensuring patient safety and procedural efficacy in vascular access and soft tissue imaging. Workshops, simulations, and peer-reviewed assessments are key vehicles for ongoing professional development to guarantee the acquisition of expertise in such domains. Furthermore, learning communities may facilitate knowledge transfer and improve best practices among practitioners. Institutions and healthcare centers must place utmost importance on such educational courses to bridge the gaps in key areas relating to operator dependency. With an environment of competency and ongoing learning, practitioners can not only upgrade their skill sets but also the overall dependability of ultrasound as a diagnostic tool. Emphasis on operator education is needed to close any gaps in know-how and create effective and safe imaging protocols (Krige et al., 2009).

14.6.2. Limitations in Certain Patient Groups

In the case of ultrasound imaging of soft tissue and vascular access, it is necessary to recognize constraints that exist in specific populations of patients to optimize clinical outcomes. Patients with rheumatoid arthritis (RA) pose significant challenges to effective vascular access acquisition. RA patients have altered vascular anatomy along with inflammatory changes in soft tissues, which complicate the identification of optimal access sites. In addition, these patients are also at increased risk for cardiovascular morbidity that may further reduce the reliability of ultrasound measurements. Endothelial dysfunction in RA patients with anti-carbamylated protein antibodies (anti-CarP) has been proven to exist, suggesting that inflammation may influence not only vascular structure but also the efficacy of ultrasound-guided interventions and thus require specialized procedures in such a population (Alessandri et al., 2017). Furthermore, the comorbidities and age of the patients predominantly characterize the efficiency of vascular access and imaging ultrasound. Older patients possess anatomical changes related to age, for example, arterial stiffness and calcification that undermine traditional ultrasound techniques. Even more so, morbidities like obesity conceal anatomical landmarks, making the quality of images acquired poor. Patients with comorbidities pose an unusual challenge, as the combination of different medical conditions may lead to both vascular access and other imaging procedure complications. For instance, monitoring in real time of cardiovascular risk factors in such patients becomes essential, given the established links between other autoantibodies and vascular function in RA patients as markers of tiered complexity in managing these individuals' health (Alessandri et al., 2017). Finally, the psychological and cognitive variables of certain patient populations also determine the success of ultrasound procedures. Cognitive-impaired patients might not be capable of adhering to the pre-procedure instructions required, which affects the success rate in imaging and intervention. Anxiety and fear associated with ultrasound procedures also lead to movement during scanning, which can impair image quality. With each of these restrictions resolved, healthcare professionals must be proficient in applying a patient-specific approach. Tailoring communication and procedural techniques to fulfill specific patient needs—particularly for individuals with higher cardiovascular risk, such as RA patients—can significantly help maximize the overall efficacy of vascular access and imaging ultrasound practice. This emphasis on individual care emphasizes the importance of adapting strategies to reduce current barriers among different patient groups (Alessandri et al., 2017).

14.6.3. Technological Advancements and Future Directions

The union of vascular access and imaging ultrasound of the soft tissue technology is a giant leap in medical diagnosis and therapeutic procedures. Advances such as micro-robotic platforms designed to navigate the human body offer a revolution in accessing challenging anatomical locations, particularly in previously unexploited vasculature. These microrobots can be deployed through natural lumina, giving rise to less invasive procedures that are more convenient for patients and reduce recovery time. Furthermore, the remote control of these devices obviates current limitations with systemic therapy, offering new avenues for treatment success. As research continues to advance in this field, efforts need to be directed towards developing robust engineering tools and biological compatibility to improve the safety and effectiveness of these robotic interventions (Ahmed et al., 2024).

Artificial intelligence (AI) is becoming more and more a reference point in vascular access and soft tissue imaging. By automating image capture and interpretation processes, AI elevates diagnostic accuracy and workflow efficiency with very little burden on medical professionals. New technologies such as photon-counting computed tomography (CT) scanners and ultra-high-field magnetic resonance imaging (MRI) devices are available, enabling high-resolution images with lower radiation exposure. These technologies not only improve the potential for diagnosis but also help in reducing environmental burden from conventional imaging modalities. With the use of biodegradable contrast agents and energy-efficient systems, the application of AI in imaging also talks about a concentration on being sustainable in medical practice. This change highlights the need for constant research and sharing to ensure that technological advancements are made at par with the requirements of the modern medical practice (Adadzi et al., 2024). Looking ahead, imaging technologies integration with genomics and telemedicine is capable of transforming soft tissue imaging, ultrasound, as well as vascular access. With real-time data and predictive analytics, clinicians can develop patient-specific treatment plans. Further, gap-filling between accessibility to existing imaging technologies remains a persistent challenge. Efforts must be directed towards making these cost-effective solutions more universally accessible in order to expand access to these nascent technologies, particularly in underserved communities. Lastly, the convergence of imaging, AI, and other emerging technologies promises to revolutionize diagnostic approaches, improve patient care, and sustain more equitable health systems. With these fields advancing further, interdisciplinary integration will play a crucial role in ensuring that the advances of these innovations reach maximum utility for patients as well as healthcare professionals (Adadzi et al., 2024).

SUMMARY

In general, integration of vascular access techniques and ultrasound scanning of soft tissues significantly enhances clinical evaluation accuracy. The use of advanced imaging modalities, such as Shear Wave Elastography (SWE), allows non-invasive quantification that provides informative data about arterial stiffness and vascular function. As demonstrated through recent research, SWE can quantitatively monitor shear wave speed changes in relation to invasive blood pressure changes efficiently, highlighting its potential for application in real-time arterial condition monitoring (Dizier et al., 2018). This is a long-awaited advancement toward improved patient outcomes as it aids in early detection of vascular abnormalities and cardiovascular condition management. Furthermore, the relative effectiveness of intravenous and intra-arterial techniques in contrast-enhanced imaging points out the optimal approach in evaluating complex anatomies such as those of the equine head. The intra-arterial method yields an extreme contrast enhancement with a low amount of contrast medium, contributing to a more accurate diagnosis for pathologies with increased blood flow (Baeumlin et al., 2016). This efficiency validates the necessity for practitioners to adopt evidence-based practice, such that imaging technologies enhance diagnostic capability but also enhance patient safety and comfort. Lastly, the convergence of advanced imaging technologies and vascular access technologies necessitates continuing research and development in clinical practice. As clinical practitioners increasingly use ultrasound imaging to assess vascular and soft tissue disease, it is necessary to stay current regarding the newest methods and their related benefits. By offering an interactive environment that combines clinical expertise and technological expertise, clinical practitioners are able to build improved diagnostic streams, thereby enhancing patient care quality in vascular and ultrasound medicine.

While exploring the universe of vascular access and soft tissue imaging ultrasound, it is of utmost importance to recognize the role of accurate diagnosis and effective treatment modalities. The use of ultrasound technology in vascular access intervention not only optimizes visualization but also provides improved patient outcomes by minimizing complications. Ultrasound-guided techniques of inserting central venous catheters have been highlighted in newer research to have decreased insertion-related complication rates, including hematoma and pneumothorax. Also, newer ultrasound technology is improving the accurate visualization of the vascular anatomy, allowing for easier access with fewer punctures. Thus, the use of ultrasound during vascular access is essential in achieving optimized patient safety and procedural success. Another fundamental aspect of the discussion on the imaging of soft tissues via ultrasound is emphasizing a multidisciplinary process of diagnosis and management. Of note, in a symposium consensus, is collaboration among radiologists, surgeons, and physiotherapists because it encourages a comprehensive understanding of sports like Sportsman's groin—now named 'inguinal disruption'—and its management. The recognition that there is no such hernia in those cases emphasizes the need for clinicians to modify their diagnostic models with a focus on unusual tissue tension and related findings. This model of collaboration enhances the evaluation process to allow for customized treatment alternatives to have far-reaching benefits for patients. Through the synthesis of perspectives from multiple specialties, practitioners are able to align their approaches with existing best practices, ultimately leading to improved healthcare provision. Lastly, the role of ultrasound also entails the treatment and diagnosis of conditions such as rotator cuff calcific tendinopathy, a prevalent condition in patients presenting with shoulder pain. Diagnostic evaluation of the condition by means of radiography, MRI, or ultrasound facilitates an adequate understanding of the underlying pathogenesis that subsequently translates into more effective management regimens. Conservative management approaches, including ultrasound-guided methods and physical therapy, have been proven to be effective without the need for surgery. This demonstrates the potential of ultrasound not only in diagnosis but as a therapeutic agent, thus firmly establishing its place in medical practice. In general, the combination of diagnostic imaging and effective treatment methods allows clinicians to offer complete care, facilitating the key function of ultrasound in vascular access and for imaging soft tissue (de Beaux et al., 2013; Derrington et al., 2015).

CLOSER LOOK

SHEAR WAVE ELASTOGRAPHY (SWE)

Shear Wave Elastography (SWE) is a cutting-edge, non-invasive imaging technology that quantifies tissue stiffness by measuring the propagation of shear waves in soft tissue. As compared to traditional ultrasound, where anatomical structures are imaged using acoustic reflection, SWE provides functional information on tissue elasticity—providing important clinical information, especially in the detection and staging of diseases involving fibrosis or abnormal tissue hardness. The underlying principle of SWE is the generation of low-frequency shear waves with acoustic radiation force pulses from an ultrasound probe. Shear waves travel orthogonally in tissue, and speed is monitored in real time. Since stiffer tissue transmits shear waves at a higher rate than more compliant tissue, the resulting speed information can be converted to a stiffness measurement, typically in meters per second (m/s) or kilopascals (kPa).

SWE has also found growing significance in hepatology for the staging of liver fibrosis in chronic liver disease patients, like hepatitis B, hepatitis C, alcoholic liver disease, and NAFLD. Through the provision of a reproducible, non-invasive, and dependable alternative to liver biopsy, SWE allows doctors to stage liver fibrosis, track disease progression, and assess response to treatment. It facilitates the discrimination between fibrosis stages—ranging from F0 (no fibrosis) to F4 (cirrhosis)—relevant to clinical decision-making and prognostication. Furthermore, SWE is feasible at the bedside or outpatient clinic and is cost-effective and convenient.

Outside of the liver, SWE is used more and more in thyroid nodules, prostate disease, and musculoskeletal disorders evaluation. In breast imaging, SWE enhances diagnostic specificity by differentiating between benign and malignant masses since malignant tumors are significantly stiffer due to dense cellular structure and desmoplastic reaction. In thyroid imaging, SWE may help identify nodules at higher risk for malignancy, and this can impact the decision of whether to biopsy. In prostate and kidney exams, SWE is emerging as a useful tool for locally stiff lesions that will probably be tumors. Within the musculoskeletal domain, SWE is used to quantify the stiffness of tendons, muscles, and ligaments in such conditions as tendinopathy, fibrosis, or muscle strain and provides information not obtainable from traditional imaging.

SWE has certain definite advantages. SWE is noninvasive, involves no ionizing radiation, and provides instantaneous, real-time quantitative data. The elastograms of stiffness maps are overlaid on conventional B-mode images, with intuitive visual correlation between structure and function. It also reduces sampling variability compared to strain elastography, in that no manual compression is required, and is thereby less operator-dependent. SWE is not, however, entirely without limitation. Accuracy of measurement can be affected by variables such as patient obesity, ascites, excessive motion, and near-vessel or bony exposure. Inflammation, congestion, or other non-fibrotic conditions can also alter tissue stiffness and need to be properly correlated in the clinic.

References

1. Acosta, S., Azuma, N., Bastos Gonçalves, F., Björck, M., et al. (2020). Editor's choice: European Society for Vascular Surgery (ESVS) 2020 clinical practice guidelines on the management of acute limb ischemia.
2. Adadzi, J., Anderson II, J., Azi, C. I., Carsrud, J., et al. (2024). Transformative advancements in diagnostic imaging: Reducing risks, enhancing accuracy, and promoting sustainability. EurJ Med Health Res; 2(5):153-72. https://core.ac.uk/download/621451782.pdf (accessed on 12th July 2025).
3. Ahmed, D., Diller, E., Iacovacci, V., Menciassi, A., et al. (2024). Medical microrobots. https://core.ac.uk/download/621390309.pdf (accessed on 12th July 2025).
4. Albisinni, U., Battista, G., Bazzocchi, A., Catalano, C., et al. (2015). MRI-guided focused ultrasound surgery in musculoskeletal diseases: The hot topics. https://core.ac.uk/download/98341478.pdf (accessed on 12th July 2025).
5. Alessandri, C., Ciciarello, F. L., Colasanti, T., Conti, L., et al. (2017). Association between antibodies to carbamylated proteins and subclinical atherosclerosis in rheumatoid arthritis patients. https://core.ac.uk/download/98347599.pdf (accessed on 12th July 2025).
6. Andrani, F., Anzidei, M., Bezzi, M., Catalano, R., et al. (2017). Imaging-guided chest biopsies: Techniques and clinical results. https://core.ac.uk/download/127588220.pdf (accessed on 12th July 2025).
7. Ansari, N. A., Buonocore, V., Gigli, S., Maccioni, F., et al. (2015). Role of magnetic resonance imaging in the detection and characterization of solid pancreatic nodules: An update. https://core.ac.uk/download/154949520.pdf (accessed on 12th July 2025).
8. Baeumlin, Y., Bergman, E. H. J., Broeckx, B., Crijns, M., et al. (2016). Intra-arterial versus intravenous contrast-enhanced computed tomography of the equine head. https://core.ac.uk/download/55743201.pdf (accessed on 12th July 2025).
9. Bhaskaran, S., Chen, Y., Chen, Z., Gong, X., et al. (2018). Monitoring of the central blood pressure waveform via a conformal ultrasonic device. https://core.ac.uk/download/323064840.pdf (accessed on 12th July 2025).
10. Bini, F., Blasi, G., Fiorentini, S., Larsson, H., et al. (2017). Influence of wall thickness and diameter on arterial shear wave elastography: A phantom and finite element study. https://core.ac.uk/download/98337803.pdf (accessed on 12th July 2025).
11. Boss, M. K., Kent, M. S., & Nolan, M. W. (2019). Emerging translational opportunities in comparative oncology with companion canine cancers: Radiation oncology. https://core.ac.uk/download/323068226.pdf (accessed on 12th July 2025).
12. Brennan, P., Galvin, P. L., Grech, R., Grech, T., et al. (2014). Imaging of adult ocular and orbital pathology: A pictorial review. https://core.ac.uk/download/323186424.pdf (accessed on 12th July 2025).
13. Bucknor, M., Han, M., Krug, R., Ozhinsky, R., et al. (2016). T2-based temperature monitoring in bone marrow for MR-guided focused ultrasound. https://core.ac.uk/download/323074239.pdf (accessed on 12th July 2025).

14. Cox, B. F., Fatahi, M., Fernandez-Gutierrez, F., French, L., et al. (2015). Comparative ergonomic workflow and user experience analysis of MRI versus fluoroscopy-guided vascular interventions: An iliac angioplasty exemplar case study. https://core.ac.uk/download/228177186.pdf (accessed on 12th July 2025).
15. Cui, M. D., Huang, L., Jia, Y., et al. (2020). Chinese expert consensus on critical care ultrasound applications during the COVID-19 pandemic. https://core.ac.uk/download/322850186.pdf (accessed on 12th July 2025).
16. de Beaux, A., Kingsnorth, A., Sheen, A. J., Akermark, B. M., Stephenson, B., Beatty, B., Brennan, R., et al. (2013). *Treatment of the sportsman's groin*: British Hernia Society's 2014 position statement based on the Manchester Consensus Conference. https://core.ac.uk/download/9362135.pdf (accessed on 12th July 2025).
17. De Wilde, D., Gijsen, F. J. H., McCann, G., Ridwan, H., et al. (2016). Contrast-enhanced micro-CT imaging in murine carotid arteries: A new protocol for computing wall shear stress. https://core.ac.uk/download/91389700.pdf (accessed on 12th July 2025).
18. Derrington, S. M., Greis, A. C., & McAuliffe, M. (2015). Evaluation and nonsurgical management of rotator cuff calcific tendinopathy. https://core.ac.uk/download/46974922.pdf (accessed on 12th July 2025).
19. Dizier, B., Messas, E., Mirault, T., Papadacci, F., et al. (2018). Non-invasive evaluation of aortic stiffness dependence with aortic blood pressure and internal radius by shear wave elastography and ultrafast imaging. https://core.ac.uk/download/217845686.pdf (accessed on 12th July 2025).
20. Jokerst, J. V., & Wang, J. (2016). Stem cell imaging: Tools to improve cell delivery and viability. https://core.ac.uk/download/323064235.pdf (accessed on 12th July 2025).
21. Kitsiou, A., Caforio, A. L. P., Porta-Sanchez, A., Vahanian, A., Iung, B., Carrera, C., Szymanski, C., et al. (2013). ESC core curriculum for the general cardiologist (2013). https://core.ac.uk/download/55756305.pdf (accessed on 12th July 2025).
22. Krige, J. E. J. (2009). Modern imaging in patients with obstructive jaundice. https://core.ac.uk/download/478413915.pdf (accessed on 12th July 2025).
23. Loccisano, A. (2016). Platelet-rich plasma for the treatment of partial rotator cuff tears. https://open.bu.edu/bitstream/2144/14355/9/Loccisano_bu_0017N_10415.pdf (accessed on 12th July 2025).
24. *Focal Spot, Spring 2005.* Bernard Becker Medical Library Archives. Washington University School of Medicine. https://core.ac.uk/download/129069341.pdf (accessed on 12th July 2025).
25. *Focal Spot, Winter 2006/2007.* Bernard Becker Medical Library Archives. Washington University School of Medicine. https://core.ac.uk/download/129069354.pdf (accessed on 12th July 2025).
26. NASA. (1977). *Aerospace Medicine and Biology: A Continuing Bibliography with Indexes, Supplement 172.* https://core.ac.uk/download/pdf/42876149.pdf (accessed on 12th July 2025).
27. Patience, A., Speed, C. A., Bowen, C. J., Bowen, C. J., Miller, D. L., Hendry, G. J., Siddle, H. J., et al. (2018). Survey of ultrasound practice amongst podiatrists in the UK. https://core.ac.uk/download/293885607.pdf (accessed on 12th July 2025).

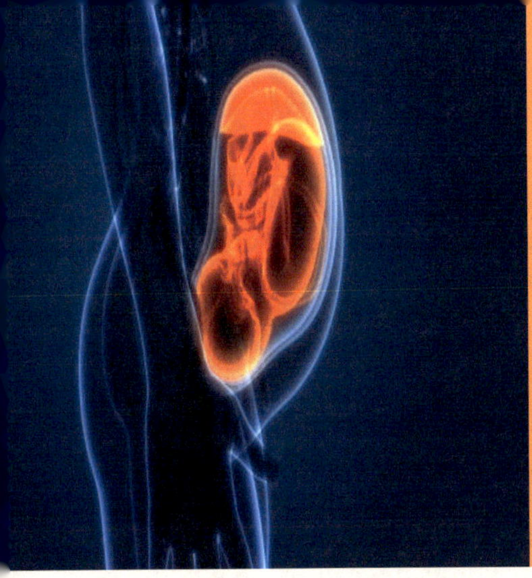

Chapter 15

ULTRASOUND IN EMERGENCY AND CRITICAL CARE

Contents

Introduction

The integration of ultrasound technology into critical care and emergency medicine has been a proven game-changer in modern medicine. Ultrasound, particularly its point-of-care applications, provides rapid assessment and diagnosis at the bedside, filling a critical need in emergencies. As doctors strive to get the most out of patients during emergencies, the application of ultrasound has become increasingly apparent, particularly considering how quick it is, how mobile, and how it provides real-time pictures. Furthermore, advancements in teleultrasound technologies such as FaceTime and Google Glass enable experienced clinicians to remotely guide and educate less skilled health workers, broadening learning potential and access to basic skills in ultrasonography (Austin et al., 2019). The increased body of evidence underscores the importance of training in ultrasound and its application in high-stakes environments, positioning it as an essential tool in clinical practice. For the acute care setting, point-of-care ultrasound (POCUS) has been invaluable in various diagnostic assessments, especially in acute illnesses such as transient ischemic attacks (TIAs) and strokes. Traditional imaging, including computed tomography angiography (CTA), typically entails patient transport, leading to time delay, thereby increasing the risk of adverse effects. Studies indicate that carotid POCUS is able to determine significant stenosis accurately, offering a time-saving approach that may aid prompt decision-making in the emergency department. Findings indicate good sensitivity and specificity in detecting over 50% stenosis, which justifies the clinical use of ultrasound for rapid assessment during life-threatening health emergencies (Nemnom et al., 2020). As these technologies continue to improve, they provide emergency care professionals with the knowledge to make informed decisions, ultimately generating safer patients and treatment results. Furthermore, the employment of ultrasound is not reserved for diagnostics alone; it has a paramount role to play in guiding therapeutic interventions in emergency medicine. The consequences of having the ability to visualize anatomy and pathology in real-time are that clinicians can make evidence-based decisions, from trauma fluid management to aiding invasive procedures like central line placement. The level of skill required to conduct these exams and have this information available is increasingly being recognized within emergency and critical care educational programs. As highlighted through recent pilot studies, health professionals who are not medically trained but are supervised by experts can be instructed to perform acute care POCUS scans effectively and demonstrate that with adequate training and support, the implementation of ultrasound devices may be extended (Austin et al., 2019). Overall, continued progress and integration of ultrasound technology into emergency and critical care settings reflect a commitment to improving patient care through education and innovation (Figure 15.1).

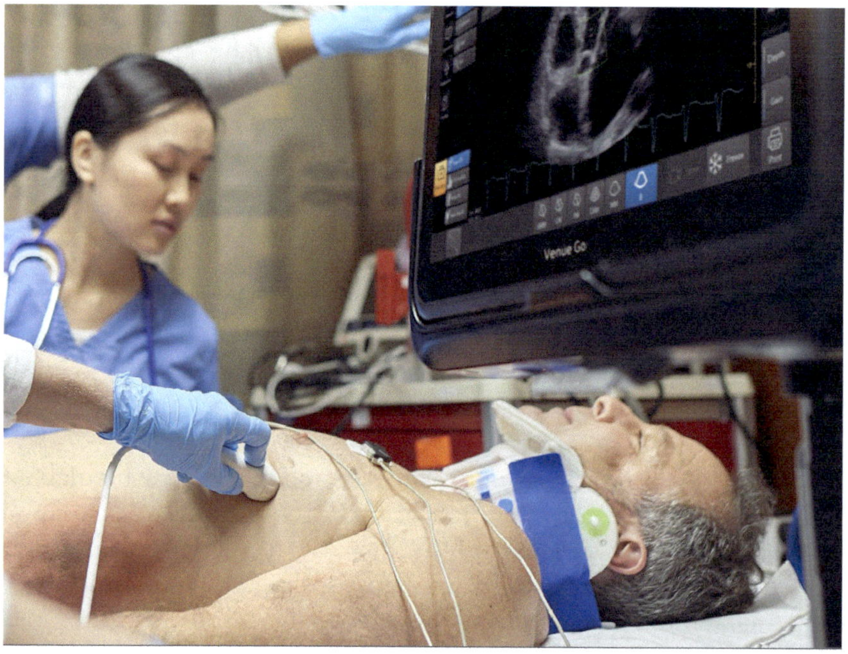

Figure 15.1. Ultrasound in emergency and critical care.

Source: GE Health Care. www.gehealthcare.com

Definition of Ultrasound Technology

Ultrasound technology, the backbone of modern medical imaging, employs high-frequency sound waves to produce images of the body's internal structures. It is a principle based on echolocation, where sound waves emitted by a transducer travel through body tissues and return to provide valuable information about organ shape, size, and function. This non-invasive technology is particularly valuable in emergency and critical care scenarios to enable rapid diagnosis and treatment planning without exposing patients to ionizing radiation. Ultrasound's capability to image soft tissues in real time makes it an invaluable tool in assessing conditions such as trauma, cardiopulmonary distress, and abdominal emergencies, and therefore an invaluable asset for healthcare practitioners working under time pressure. Physicians are finding more uses for ultrasound technology beyond the conventional imaging use. The use of ultrasound in point-of-care procedures is a prime example of its versatility, making not only diagnostic evaluation but also directed therapeutic interventions possible. This trend towards bedside ultrasound provides quick access to imaging, which improves critical decision-making in acute care scenarios. Moreover, advancements in portable ultrasonics have made the service of conducting studies in diverse settings, from rural hospitals to emergency departments, readily available. As such, a systematic approach to delivering these ultrasound services is now needed to ensure the highest outcomes, as deemed in foundational recommendations that address priorities for leadership, training, and quality assurance in healthcare systems (Abo et al., 2018). In addition, the development of ultrasound technology has increased its scope of application, especially in telemedicine and eHealth projects, which improve the access to patient care in rural areas. Integrated healthcare project developments fuse ultrasound technology with telecommunication systems in order to provide teleconsultation and collaborative care among healthcare professionals divided by geographical distances. Such systems facilitate the delivery of ultrasound images and vital biosignals over various communication networks, thereby broadening access to expert medical skills beyond geographical locations (Androulidakis et al., 2011). As a result, ultrasound technology not only facilitates real-time care in emergency conditions but also facilitates the development of innovative solutions that address disparities in health, ultimately improving patient outcomes in critical care conditions.

Importance of Ultrasound in Critical and Emergency Care

The application of ultrasound technology in emergency and critical care medicine provides potential for revolutionary enhancement in patient outcomes. Point-of-care ultrasound (POCUS) allows real-time visualization of internal structures, facilitating expedited diagnostic decision-making in high-acuity situations. Such an ability to conduct real-time examination is particularly valuable in emergency environments, where prompt interventions are potentially dramatic in their effects on survival rates. Studies have shown that POCUS can reduce the time to diagnose life-threatening conditions such as cardiac tamponade, hemothorax, or abdominal aortic aneurysm, making the management of the patient more effective and potentially eliminating the need for invasive procedures. As discussed in recent articles, the real-time feedback provided by the use of ultrasound enhances the process of diagnosis, enabling the medical practitioners to respond promptly on the basis of clear visual evidence, as discussed in Choi et al. (2023). Thus, the utilization of ultrasound technology in emergencies is becoming the standard fast enough to change the landscape of acute patient treatment. Training and proficiency in using ultrasound are critical for clinicians in emergency and critical care settings. To utilize the full potential of POCUS, clinicians must receive extensive education not only in technical proficiency but also in the critical thinking necessary for appropriate interpretation of ultrasound findings. Continuous education is essential to maintain practitioners' competency in the emerging and evolving techniques and practices of ultrasound, as flawed interpretation carries high clinical risks. Moreover, collaboration among multi-professional teams like radiologists and emergency medicine doctors is crucial in building a culture of ultrasound competence. By adhering to well-delineated guidelines and protocols, as advised by institutions like the International Society of Ultrasound in Obstetrics and Gynecology (ISUOG), health systems can foster the optimal and appropriate use of ultrasound, as elucidated in Lees et al. (2020). Also, ultrasound has been a critical component in patient monitoring in critical care environments, with its potential to enhance diagnostic and therapeutic functions. It provides a non-invasive means to monitor a variety of physiological parameters, including cardiac function, fluid status, and organ perfusion, which are especially critical in the management of critically ill patients. This enables dynamic adjustments in the patient's treatment plan to be made after real-time data, enabling personalized medicine practices. For instance, interventions such as central line placement and paracentesis with ultrasound guidance can significantly reduce complications and optimize procedural success rates without compromising patient safety. As such, ultrasound not only enables primary diagnosis but also continues to be a part of patient management ongoingly, thus proving irreplaceable within the critical care continuum. This interdisciplinary application underscores the necessity of integrating ultrasound training into emergency and critical care practice to optimize patient outcomes in the most appropriate manner (Figure 15.2).

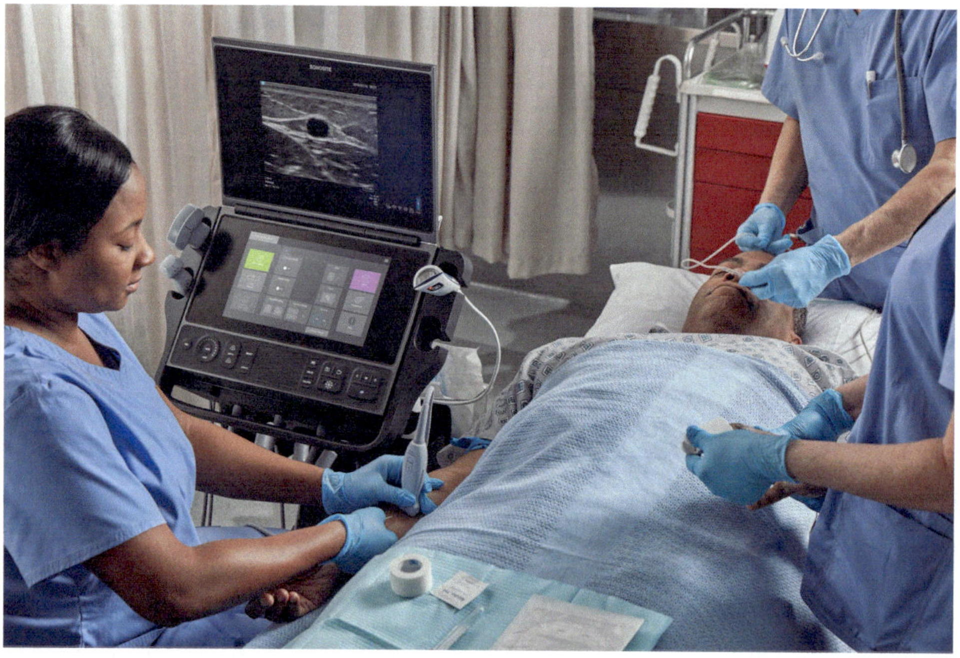

Figure 15.2. Ultrasound in emergency and critical care.

Source: Jeremy Boyd (2023). epmonthly.com. https://epmonthly.com/article/getting-a-line-on-ultrasound-guided-peripheral-intravenous-placement/

15.1. Historical Background of Ultrasound

The origins of ultrasound technology date back to the early 20th century, with ultrasonic waves being developed for multiple purposes. Initially used in the sonar technology of World War I, ultrasound initially functioned as a submarine detection device. Soon after, its use in the field of medicine was realized when scientists began testing whether sound waves could be used to image internal body structures. By the 1950s, the introduction of commercial ultrasound equipment was a significant breakthrough. Physicians subsequently began to utilize ultrasound for prenatal diagnosis, providing a noninvasive way of viewing the developing fetus, thus providing the basis for its application today in emergency and critical care settings. Ultrasound technology has evolved to provide more sophisticated imaging capabilities, significantly improving diagnostic accuracy and patient outcomes. The introduction of ultrasound in emergency and critical care medicine is a paradigm shift in clinical practice. It was realized by early users that ultrasound can be employed for rapid diagnosis and assessment in situations of potentially fatal emergencies, such as trauma or acute abdominal pain.

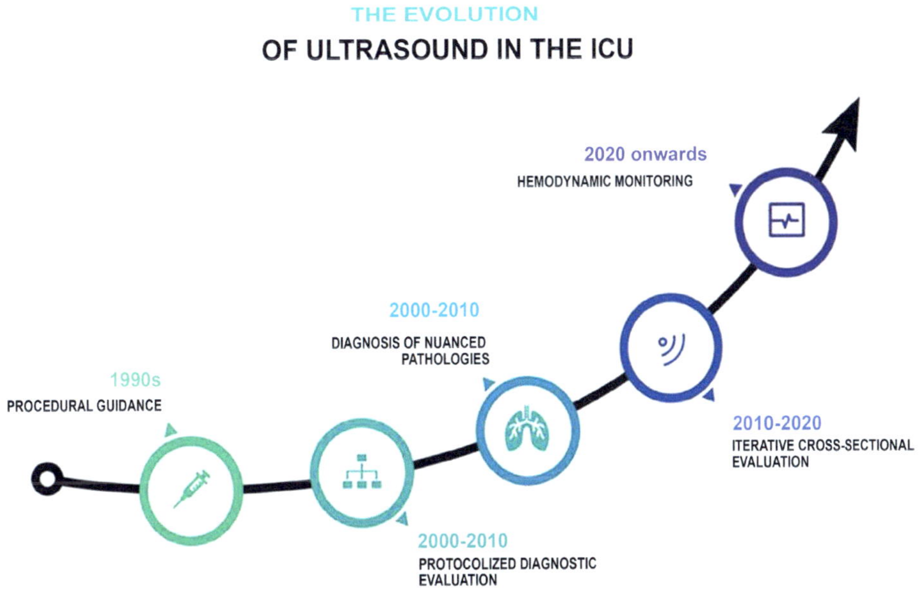

Figure 15.3. The evolution of ultrasound in critical care.

Source: Barjaktarevic I, Kenny JS, Berlin D, Cannesson M. (2021). The Evolution of Ultrasound in Critical Care: From Procedural Guidance to Hemodynamic Monitor. Journal of Ultrasound in Medicine: Official Journal of the American Institute of Ultrasound in Medicine. 40(2):401-405. DOI: 10.1002/jum.15403. PMID: 32750199; PMCID: PMC7855649.

The mobility of the ultrasound technology and its immediacy allowed medical professionals to make timely decisions with the lack of the need for lengthy patient transfer. Scientific innovations, such as the introduction of Doppler ultrasound and real-time scanning, further added to its diagnostic capability. Not only did this innovation change clinicians' approach to emergencies, but it also fortified the role of ultrasound in guiding procedures, such as central line placement or drainage of abscesses. With hospitals embracing this technological advancement, ultrasound proved crucial, giving a face-lift to the life of care delivered in critical situations. The consequences of embracing ultrasound technology in clinical practice reach beyond immediate care to the research and educational fields as well.

Development of databases like MIMIC-IV has made electronic health record data accessible in such a manner that extensive amounts of it are accessible for research on the use and effectiveness of ultrasound in various clinical settings. This data is of paramount value to grasping ultrasound's effect on patient care pathways and outcomes. The ability to analyze de-identified patient data from emergency and critical care cases allows researchers to study the richness of ultrasound use, identifying trends and establishing protocols to generalize practice. This evidence-based approach not only improves professional knowledge but also attempts to maximize training techniques in healthcare professionals to guarantee competent and effective application of ultrasound in high-stakes environments (Jhnson et al., 2023; Nornan et al., 2017) (Figure 15.3).

15.1.1. Development of Ultrasound Technology

The development of ultrasound technology has undergone a remarkable transformation since its inception, significantly impacting emergency and critical care. Initially, ultrasound was limited to specialized settings, predominantly employed by trained professionals in hospitals. However, advancements in technology have led to innovations such as high-definition imaging, portable machines, and handheld devices, making ultrasound accessible in a variety of clinical environments. These developments have democratized ultrasound imaging, allowing for its application in remote and resource-limited areas. Portable ultrasound systems, in particular, enable healthcare providers to quickly assess patients at the point of care, facilitating timely interventions and enhancing decision-making in critical situations. Such shifts not only expand the reach of diagnostic capabilities but also improve patient outcomes, underscoring the importance of continuously evolving ultrasound technology in the field of emergency medicine (Kaffas et al., 2024). In emergency and critical care settings, the significance of ultrasound has magnified due to its capacity for rapid, non-invasive diagnosis. Regular imaging modalities such as X-ray or computed tomography (CT) have typically required patient transport and longer processing times, which can delay critical treatments. In contrast, ultrasound allows for immediate evaluation of life-threatening conditions such as trauma, pulmonary edema, and intra-abdominal bleeding. The integration of point-of-care ultrasound (POCUS) is particularly notable in emergency departments, where clinicians can conduct evaluations directly at the bedside. This immediacy in diagnosis makes a substantial difference in clinical management, as timely identification of conditions supports quicker responses to life-threatening emergencies. The technical advancements in ultrasound equipment have streamlined its use in various scenarios, demonstrating its vital role in enhancing patient care (Muhmmed et al., 2024). Furthermore, the evolution of ultrasound technology has been complemented by the incorporation of artificial intelligence (AI), which has the potential to revolutionize how imaging is utilized in emergency care. AI algorithms can assist in image acquisition, interpretation, and diagnostic accuracy, effectively supporting clinicians' decision-making processes. This evolution is particularly relevant in high-stakes environments where every second can affect patient outcomes. As the technology advances, training programs are evolving to emphasize familiarization with both ultrasound technique and AI integration, ensuring that healthcare providers are well-equipped to utilize these innovations. The future of ultrasound in emergency and critical care not only hinges on the technological advancements themselves but also on the dissemination of knowledge and the training of healthcare personnel to maximize the benefits of these innovations. As ultrasound technology continues to develop, it holds the promise of becoming an indispensable tool in emergency medicine (Kaffas et al., 2024) (Figure 15.4).

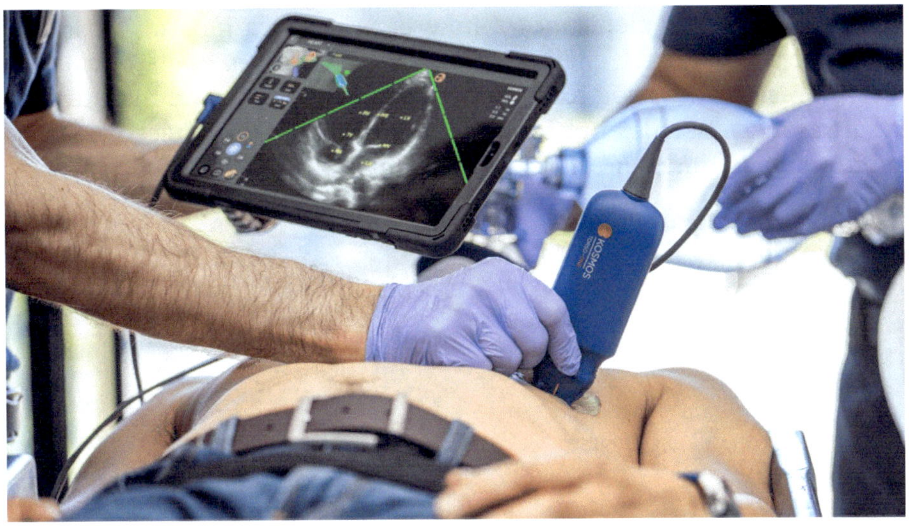

Figure 15.4. The development of ultrasound technology.

Source: EchoNous. Emergency Medicine. https://echonous.com/specialty/emergency-medicine/

15.1.2. Early Applications in Medicine

Use of the ultrasound technology in medicine has progressed a great distance from its beginnings, and early utilization was applied mostly for diagnostics. The earliest location to find out about ultrasound was obstetrics, where the tech's capacity to render images of fetal development revolutionized prenatal medicine. The first use was due to a need for non-invasive diagnostic equipment that could provide essential information without subjecting the patient to harmful radiation. As more was learned about the technology, it also became apparent that its application overlapped into other sections of medicine, including emergency care. Emergency physicians then recognized the speed and convenience with which ultrasound enabled rapid examinations of trauma patients and paved the way for its common use in critical care settings. The history of ultrasounds clinical application in critical and emergency care has been characterized by a sudden and sharp boost in its ability to make a diagnosis. Most research that has been conducted over the last 10 years has shown that bedside ultrasound has served to enhance patient evaluation by emergency doctors and critical care practitioners. This is particularly important for critically ill patients whose instability bars them from utilizing traditional imaging modalities. The convenience of ultrasound in handheld form allows for real-time evaluation in dynamically changing environments and significantly impacts patient management. The initial applications now extend to include diverse analyses ranging from evaluating the function of the heart to the diagnosis of fluid accumulation and enabling invasive intervention, such as paracentesis and thoracentesis. The versatility of ultrasound has thus enabled a paradigm shift in the provision of emergency care, with opportunities for interventions earlier and more effectively (Masoumi et al., 2020). Moreover, technological advancement in ultrasound over recent years has further highlighted its use in telemedicine and disaster medicine as well as value in urgent care scenarios. With advancement in mobile health applications and point-of-care ultrasound, clinicians are able to offer quick assessment in low-resource settings. Telemedicine technologies enhance communication and coordination among emergency units, and ultrasound enables real-time diagnostic capability, transforming the disaster response paradigm. The advancement shows how early applications of ultrasound created the foundation for current sophisticated medical practice based on patient-centric care, particularly in times of crisis. Addressing the need for effective medical response to disasters underscores the central role that ultrasound assumes not only in everyday clinical practice but also in augmenting emergency response during times of crisis (Abualenain, 2024) (Figure 15.5).

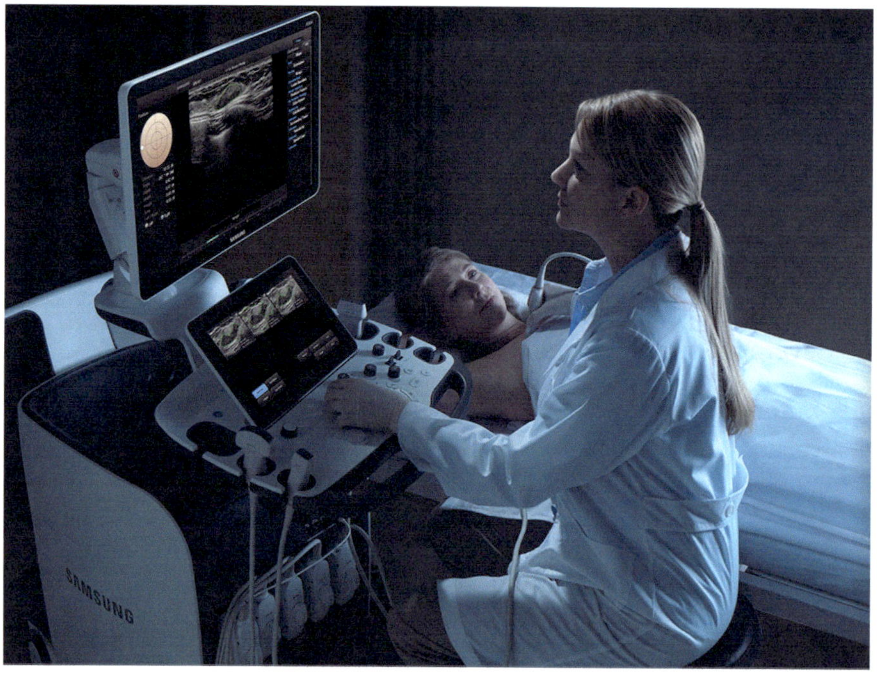

Figure 15.5. The integration of ultrasound technology.

Source:Avante Health Solutions. https://avantehs.com/learn/expert-advice/Revolutionizing_Ultrasound_Technology

15.1.3. Evolution of Ultrasound in Emergency Settings

The evolution of ultrasound technology in the setting of emergency has transformed the practice of clinical medicine, enabling rapid and accurate diagnosis. In the past, the use of ultrasound was confined to specialized units, which limited its access and applicability within acute care settings. With modern advancements in portable ultrasound machines and point-of-care ultrasound (POCUS) education, access to this valuable diagnostic modality within the setting of emergency has become democratized. Emergency physicians can now perform bedside examinations to make timely decisions in critically ill patients. Ultrasound use in emergency practice has proven to be required for the diagnosis of conditions such as cardiac tamponade, pneumothorax, and abdominal free fluid, and its value and capability in time-sensitive situations are now apparent. This change is part of an overall paradigm shift toward immediate, evidence-based practice that positions ultrasound at the core of modern emergency medicine. New data has also established the viability of remotely guiding ultrasound exams in emergency departments, marking an interesting new direction in telemedicine. To illustrate, a study demonstrated that nonmedically trained personnel were able to conduct ultrasound exams efficiently with the guidance of a POCUS-trained anesthesiologist utilizing teleultrasound technology. This approach not only enhances training for new providers but also maximizes the use of resources in emergency departments by closing skill gaps (Austin et al., 2019). Teleultrasound facilitates immediate advice, and less-experienced personnel can perform essential evaluations as well as acquire crucial skills in ultrasound imaging. As emergency rooms continue to grapple with overcrowding and diminishing personnel resources, the use of such telehealth practices will become more widespread, highlighting the contributions of education and communication in enhanced patient care.

"The improvements in ultrasound use in the emergency setting have spilled over into other categories, including pediatric and geriatric medicine, to meet the unique needs of various populations." Evolution of targeted ultrasound protocols, such as those specifically for frail older patients, is a more individualized route to emergency medicine (Agarwal et al., 2019). Ultrasound-based Comprehensive Geriatric Assessment for frailty screening has been encouraging to maximize outcomes among older adults with acute health concerns. By optimizing ultrasound techniques and protocols to be applicable across various populations, emergency medicine is evolving to meet the demands of an aging population and enhance the quality of care provided. Ultimately, the ongoing advances in adaptability and technology will continue to make ultrasound a valuable resource to emergency and critical care practice for the future.

15.2. Types of Ultrasound in Emergency Care

Overall, different types of ultrasound use are applied in emergency care to encourage timely and effective diagnosis and treatment of patients. A major one of these areas is the use of point-of-care ultrasound (POCUS), especially bedside evaluation. POCUS can evaluate serious conditions like trauma, cardiac issues, and abdominal issues, hence becoming a valuable tool in emergency care. The ability to perform rapid evaluations not only facilitates immediate decision-making but also maximizes patient outcomes by allowing timely interventions. Moreover, as indicated in current research, hospitalists have reported the utility of POCUS to aid in diagnostic and therapeutic management, while there is a problem in training and availability, which may limit its effectiveness in practice (Graham et al., 2019). Another important application of ultrasound used in emergency medicine is the FAST (Focused Assessment with Sonography for Trauma) exam. The specific application is essential to detect effusions and hemorrhages in trauma patients, particularly in the context of blunt abdominal trauma. The FAST exam offers a pain-free means to assess for internal injury quickly, thus guiding subsequent treatment, which is the need for exploratory surgery. In addition, practitioner training to conduct FAST exams efficiently can be planned into structured programs for enhancing ultrasound competencies among emergency personnel. Such education programs could potentially accelerate knowledge gaps and the rate at which efficient assessments are attained, thereby realizing enhanced patient outcomes in acute care situations (Graham et al., 2019). Moreover, technology developments have led to the development of telemedicine technologies that integrate ultrasound capabilities into emergency response systems. Remote systems can enable it to become possible for medical professionals to collaborate and consult specialists through tele-ultrasound and thus disseminate the application of ultrasound diagnostics to underserved populations or distant locations. It has been a promising technique for enhancing emergency medical treatment so that in-the-field units can receive real-time feedback on ultrasound results and decision-making. The technology developed for this purpose not only improves effective data transfer but also involves continuous education for physicians, where experts remain skilled in utilizing ultrasound in emergency medicine. Effectiveness in the use of such technologies can revolutionize emergency care so that patients everywhere can be provided with timely and appropriate interventions (Figure 15.6).

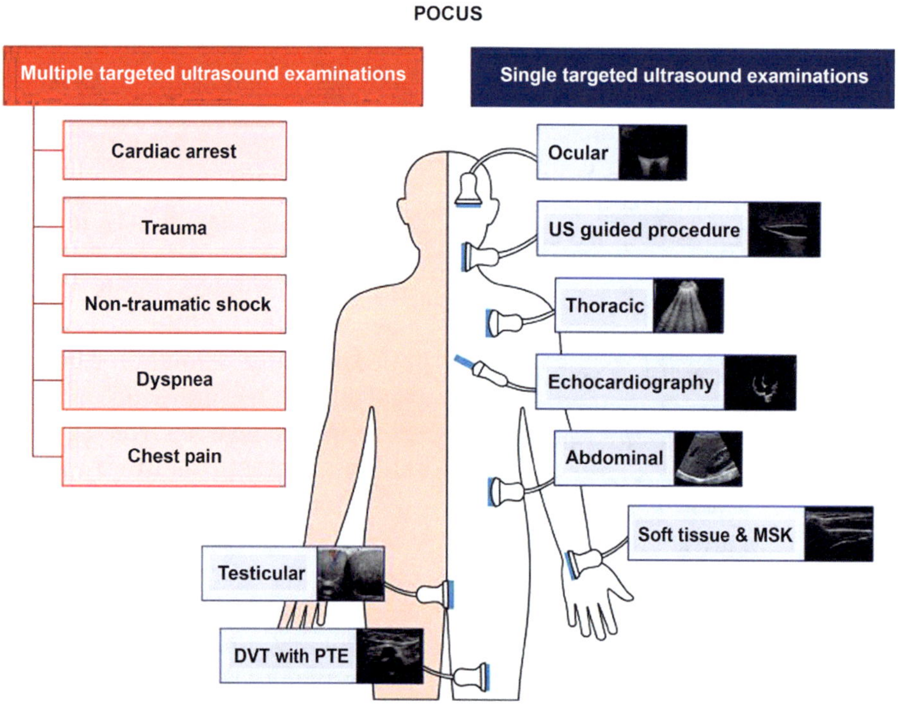

Figure 15.6. Types of ultrasound used in emergency care.

Source: Choi WJ, Ha YR, Oh JH, et.al. (2020). Clinical Guidance for Point-of-Care Ultrasound in the Emergency and Critical Care Areas after Implementing Insurance Coverage in Korea. J Korean Med Sci. 2020 Jan; 35(7):e54. https://doi.org/10.3346/jkms.2020.35.e54

15.2.1. Bedside Ultrasound

Integration of bedside ultrasound in critical and emergency care significantly enhances the diagnostic role of medical practitioners. Internal structures can be imaged in real-time using this imaging technique, allowing for timely intervention. Point-of-care ultrasound (POCUS) enables physicians to quickly examine for trauma, cardiac issues, and pulmonary conditions and thereby improve patient outcomes. Recent studies of remote ultrasound guidance through tools like video conferencing have produced promising results, enabling novice practitioners, such as first-year undergraduate students new to this practice, to conduct proficient acute care ultrasound scans under the guidance of an experienced expert. This new technique not only opens up the horizon of ultrasound utilization in emergency situations but also bridges the gap of competence and accessibility, ultimately providing a more efficient healthcare workforce (Austin et al., 2019). In the field of geriatrics, the use of bedside ultrasound extends beyond mere diagnosis, positioning itself as an important tool in managing complex conditions typical among elderly patients. Studies have shown that ultrasound can perform better than standard imaging methods, particularly in cases of acute dyspnea, pneumonia, and heart failure, thereby being most successful in older populations where the patients may have mobility issues.

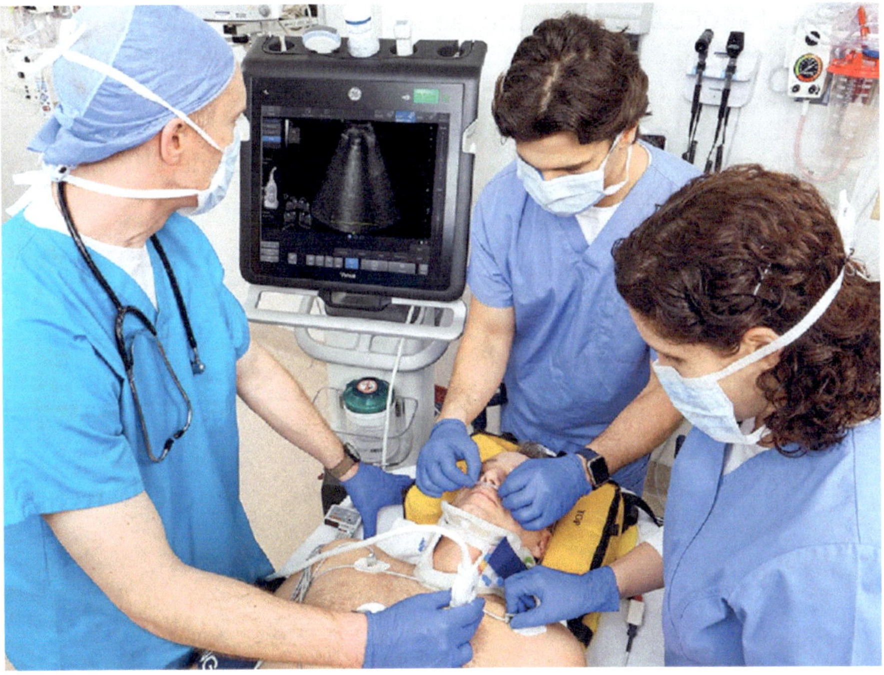

Figure 15.7. Bedside ultrasound.

Source: https://external-content.duckduckgo.com/iu/?u=https%3A%2F%2Fimages-cdn.welcomesoftware.com%2FZz01NGRmMDliMGE0ZGQxMWVkYTE2MWFhMWQxMDQ5NTMwOA%3D%3D%2Ffeature-auto-b-lines-desktop.jpg&f=1&nofb=1&ipt=700ad236af21c386ad71c09e6dfcdfb3327db98ac739294a53b4e8b4a2dc2f1e.

The study points out the potential of ultrasound for the diagnosis of conditions that were earlier demonstrated to pose considerable diagnostic challenges. In addition, diaphragm ultrasound is also emerging as a suitable technique to manage weaning from mechanical ventilation, highlighting its significance in optimizing patient care in life-threatening respiratory incidents. These advances call for the urgent necessity of specific research into the geriatric population in order to fully utilize the advantage of bedside ultrasound in this group (Incalzi et al., 2020). As bedside ultrasound comes of age throughout emergency and critical care specialties, its use is poised to revolutionize clinical practice. The ability to conduct rapid, bedside ultrasounds facilitates enhanced triage and management of acute illness, ultimately enhancing patient safety and efficiency within the emergency department environment. As training methodology enhances and expands, so too does the potential for POCUS to be utilized appropriately by non-specialist providers. The confluence of medical education and technology means that the future holds even greater promise to extend those capabilities further, with bedside ultrasound incorporated into the practice of acute care. By investing in education and technology in support of bedside ultrasound practice, the healthcare community can observe that this powerful diagnostic tool will be utilized in the best possible manner, working to improve patient care in all medical settings (Figure 15.7).

15.2.2. Point-of-Care Ultrasound (POCUS)

Point-of-care ultrasound (POCUS) is becoming an indispensable tool to be utilized in the field of emergency and critical care due to its capability of providing real-time and immediate imaging from the bedside of a patient. This simple access to such diagnostic data significantly enhances clinical decision-making as well as patients' outcomes. Unlike other conventional imaging machines that may require patients to be transported and long waiting periods, POCUS allows clinicians to simply see the anatomy as well as assess pathologies.

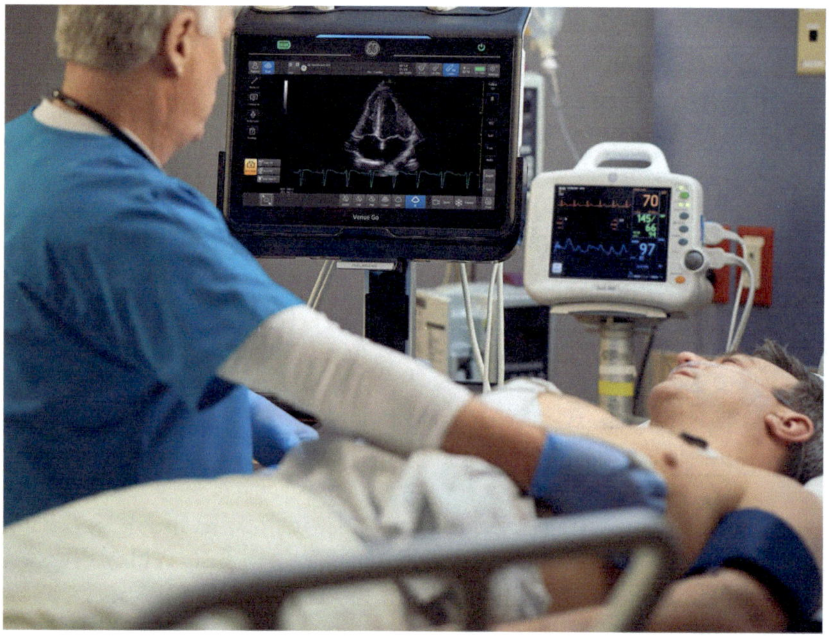

Figure 15.8. Point-of-care ultrasound.

Source: GE Healthcare. https://www.gehealthcare.com/insights/article/point-of-care-ultrasound-vs-traditional-ultrasound-what%27s-the-difference?srsltid=AfmBOopKgCIKaA6l7U0EdT0hss0ICqBUuTM8TJa7282LlJxsXIVzJ54g

Its applications range from trauma patient assessment to the guiding of procedures such as central line placement and thoracentesis. This versatility echoes the capacity of POCUS to bridge the gap between diagnostic accuracy and timely intervention, particularly in emergent scenarios where seconds count and hence brings it to the forefront of current-day emergency and critical care. Despite growing appreciation for POCUS in the clinical environment, among the main challenges still faced is inadequate training and education for the practitioners. Healthcare practitioners express high confidence levels for their ultrasound competencies following completion of training courses, as evidenced by dramatic improvement in pre- and post-course knowledge assessment (Graham et al., 2019). However, this confidence is progressively lost over time unless there is frequent practice and exposure to ultrasound machines, leading to a loss in competence as well as utilization (Graham et al., 2019). The deficit between the potential advantage of POCUS and hospitalists' actual ability, therefore, indicates an immediate need for more frequent education, resource access, and support systems to maintain practitioner competency in this valuable skill set. Besides, the application of ultrasound training in medical schools is questionable, with varying levels of evidence to determine its utility. A systematic review found inconsistencies in the utility of POCUS in anatomy and physical examination teaching, but gains in diagnostic accuracy for some pathologies. This challenges the need for inclusion of POCUS training in curricula based on costs and time taken. Besides, while many proponents believe that patient care quality can be enhanced by ultrasound training, the existing evidence remains inconclusive. Therefore, medical educators need to balance the requirement for ultrasound skill among future health professionals against the requirement for solid, evidence-based curricula to justify its inclusion in undergraduate medical schools (Figure 15.8).

15.2.3. Transesophageal Echocardiography (TEE)

Transesophageal echocardiography (TEE) has increasingly found its place in the limelight of emergency medicine as an essential tool, providing important information regarding cardiac function during resuscitation attacks. With TEE, there is direct visualization of cardiac structures and function without the interference of the transthoracic, which is usually experienced. This aspect is beneficial in acute cases, where rapid diagnosis of cardiac conditions such as cardiac arrest and shock becomes the priority. Recent studies indicate that the application of TEE in ED has grown extensively, with EM TEE literature going up from a single paper in 1991 to 20 papers in 2023, evidence of growing interest in its application (Chu et al., 2025). Emergency care physicians are now more aware of TEE's function in enabling emergency procedures, thereby solidifying its place in the rapidly evolving practice of emergency care. The TEE training innovations emphasize the importance of simulation-based training among doctors. Effective training enhances the level of expertise among emergency doctors, which allows them to achieve TEE during stressful situations. Simulators employed in echocardiography offer invaluable hands-on experience with the capacity to practice interpreting and acquiring images in a mock setting. Integration of low-cost cardiac phantoms that are printed in 3D into training modules has emerged as a new measure for improving learning. Research indicates that image quality and phantom usability are comparable with established commercial trainers and that the phantoms can be utilized as an efficient tool for learning at a low cost (Meineri, 2021). These teaching innovations are most important in equipping emergency care professionals with the skills needed to conduct TEE competently when the situation demands it. With TEE on the rise in the application of emergency settings, its indications have illuminated the diverse cardiac conditions that emergency practitioners face. Specifically, TEE has proven invaluable for the identification of cardiac arrest-related conditions, with evidence indicating that it is utilized in approximately 72.7% of instances of such conditions, and as a valuable tool employed during shock evaluations and procedural facilitation (Chu et al., 2025). These applications emphasize the sharpness of TEE in acute clinical practice and its merit for inclusion as a routine emergency procedure. With emergency medicine increasingly embracing this technology, it not only competes to improve outcomes for patients but also elevates the quality of care being provided within high-stress settings. Systematic application of TEE is thus on the verge of becoming an intrinsic component of critical care, actively responding to the challenges brought about by rapidly changing patient status (Figure 15.9).

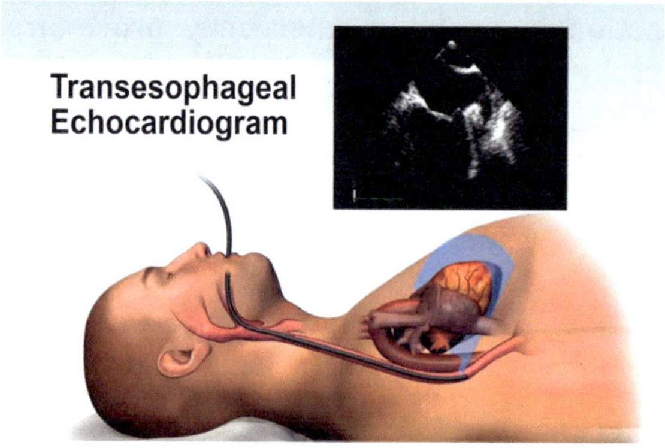

Figure 15.9. Transesophageal echocardiography (TEE).

Source: oneheartcardiology.com.au https://i.vimeocdn.com/video/566965180-91d344b83946710939fc5295951af8599707dd3aa0a166449c16c9de4a5d770b-d?f=webp.

15.3. Benefits of Ultrasound in Emergency Situations

Use of ultrasound technology in acute environments has transformed diagnostic roles, enabling clinicians to respond quickly and effectively to make decisions on patient management. Among the strengths of point-of-care ultrasound (POCUS) is its ability to provide real-time, instantaneous imaging, enabling rapid assessment of critical conditions such as trauma, cardiac arrest, and intestinal emergencies. By allowing physicians to visualize anatomical structures and detect abnormalities within minutes, ultrasound accelerates the pace of emergency procedures, with the ultimate outcome being improved patient outcomes. Principles of effective use of clinical ultrasound (CUS) emphasize the role that ultrasound plays in improving workflow optimization to enable required diagnostic capabilities to be at the core of emergency medicine practice in healthcare systems (Abo et al., 2018). This skill is most crucial in pressure-cooker environments like emergency departments, where time-sensitive cases must be quickly and accurately evaluated. In addition, the integration of POCUS in the practice of emergency medicine not only streamlines diagnosis but also therapeutic patient management. For instance, ultrasound can guide interventions like fluid drainage, nerve blocks, and vascular access, reducing risks of complications and enhancing patient safety. The growing role of hospitalists in the promotion of POCUS signals a shift toward greater hands-on, skill-based practice in inpatient care. Current evidence suggests that practical education significantly raises practitioners' skills and confidence with ultrasound, demonstrating the tool value in resolving real-time clinical dilemmas. However, ongoing education and access to ultrasound machines are required to maintain proficiency and guarantee that this technology still delivers value in the context of enhancing patient care in emergencies (Graham et al., 2019). Through the accomplishment of these challenges, the healthcare system can maximize the potential benefits of POCUS in critical care environments. Briefly stated, the advantages of ultrasound in emergency practice extend beyond immediate imaging to encompass overall patient management and care as well. Greater availability of ultrasound machines allows emergency practitioners to more effectively treat acute clinical situations, reducing time to diagnosis and the possibility of mistakes. Apart from that, the application of robust training programs strengthens the competence of healthcare professionals in the use of ultrasound as a diagnostic imaging tool, besides improving overall confidence in image interpretation. By alleviating barriers associated with training and availability of equipment during emergency conditions, the health fraternity can optimize the utilization of ultrasound to create a significant impact on enhanced outcomes in urgent and critical care conditions (Abo et al., 2018; Graham et al., 2019). Thus, continued advocacy and innovation of ultrasound technology in emergency care continue to make it necessary for patient safety improvement and quality of care.

15.3.1. Non-Invasive Nature of Ultrasound

The non-invasive nature of ultrasound technology renders it a valuable resource in emergency and critical care settings. Because it employs sound waves to generate instant images of internal anatomy, ultrasound eliminates the danger of invasive treatments, such as infection and problems related to anesthesia. This characteristic proves especially valuable in acute settings where speedy diagnosis can play a critical role in influencing patient outcomes.

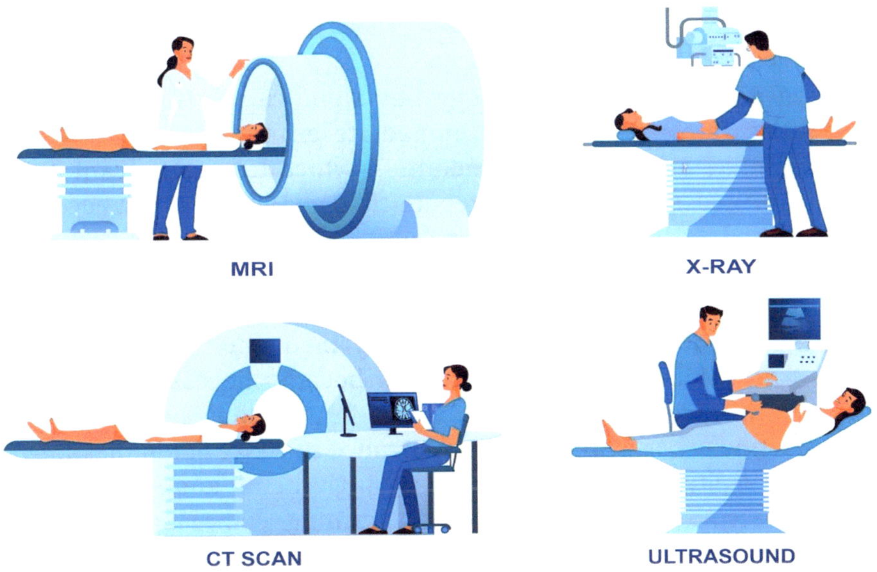

Figure 15.10. Role of non-invasive imaging in diagnostics.

Source: Inspiring.team/shutterstock.com

In acute heart failure, for instance, ultrasound can assess cardiac function and fluid status without the discomfort of invasive monitoring techniques. Non-invasive assessment enables physicians to quickly make appropriate patient management decisions, thus optimizing care in time-sensitive environments where seconds are critical. The importance of POCUS in airway management also underscores the significant advantages of non-invasive imaging. Traditional methods of determining airway anatomy can often produce inconclusive results, creating doubt in the middle of high-risk, time-sensitive procedures. POCUS, on the other hand, produces dynamic real-time images that can clearly define upper airway structures and therefore enhance the clinician's ability to predict difficult intubation conditions. Such capability is particularly critical in emergency and critical care, where airway obstruction or respiratory failure needs to be addressed immediately. By confirming accurate endotracheal placement through the aid of ultrasound, healthcare providers can be certain that they are accurately taking care of such critical situations, greatly reducing the potential for complications arising due to misplacement or improper therapy (Bellinger et al., 2023).In addition, that ultrasound is not invasive means that it is receptive to inclusion in existing management protocols without enormous procedural imposition. For instance, the use of ultrasound to evaluate cardiac conditions or diagnose pleural effusion can be done at the bedside, facilitating streamlined diagnosis and treatment. Direct access of this nature reduces the need for patient transportation to imaging units, hence lessening delay in care delivery. The easy incorporation of ultrasound into routine clinical practice, aside from ensuring higher diagnostic precision, also ensures a better workflow for intensive care and emergency departments. Lastly, the lack of invasiveness of ultrasound technology aligns well with its role in enhancing patient safety, maximizing management policies, and bettering overall clinical performance in emergency and critical care (Bueno et al., 2017) (Figure 15.10).

15.3.2. Real-Time Imaging Capabilities

The real-time imaging of ultrasound technology has significantly transformed the practices of emergency and critical care by providing for immediate examination and diagnosis of virtually all medical disorders. Unlike other imaging modalities, which take significant amounts of time in processing, ultrasound provides instantaneous feedback to clinicians, which accordingly helps them formulate speedy, informed decisions pivotal to patient outcomes. The ability to visualize dynamic physiology in real-time as it occurs, that is, organ movement and blood flow, provides the potential for rapid intervention at the time of requirement, for example, cardiac arrest or trauma. As ultrasound becomes more and more ubiquitous within emergency medicine, integration of these real-time imaging capabilities into clinical work processes has become necessary to enhance the overall effectiveness of care within high-stress environments. In addition, the application of ultrasound in the emergency department has brought the importance of strict guidelines into focus to ensure optimal usage. As clinical ultrasound (CUS) is increasingly being adopted by various specialties, it is important to have accurate protocols regarding training, competency, and quality assurance (Abo et al., 2018). By creating standardized practices, health facilities can provide consistency in ultrasound usage and thus maximize its advantage. Through guidelines, practice variability can be minimized and real-time diagnoses can be more accurate, leading to improved patient care in the case of emergency and critical care. By way of demarcating necessary elements of ultrasound equipment and competency needs, health systems are well placed to utilize the advantages of real-time imaging technology. Moreover, the incorporation of advanced technologies, such as autonomous systems, further reinforces the real-time imaging capability of ultrasound in critical care. Such sophisticated machines may improve surgical precision through robot-assisted surgery that utilizes real-time biosignals and imaging information (Das et al., 2017). Not only does the use of robotic systems improve the precision of procedures, but it also introduces new possibilities for interventions that can better or even exceed human capabilities or skills. When autonomous surgery is paired with ultrasound technology, clinicians are presented with revolutionary tools that not only improve the effectiveness of care but also enhance patient safety. The convergence of real-time imaging and robotic autonomy promises future innovations to potentially reshape the future of emergency and critical care medicine, underscoring the necessity of continuous technological progress within healthcare settings.

15.3.3. Rapid Decision-Making Support

In critical and emergency care, the ability to make rapid decisions is crucial as clinicians are faced with unpredictable and risky situations. Ultrasound technology has emerged as a valuable tool that aids medical professionals in making informed and timely decisions when evaluating patients. By providing real-time images, ultrasound allows the rapid assessment of such conditions as cardiac disease or internal bleeding, without the delays generally entailed by traditional imaging techniques. This is particularly important in emergent situations where timing is of the essence; mistakes or delays can have serious consequences for patients. Because ultrasound's capacity to deliver real-time information, it enhances the more responsive decision-making cycle and increases the overall efficacy of care being provided within acute settings. The use of ultrasound in expedited decision-making algorithms is more extensive than its application in the emergency department. In tactical missions, for instance, ultrasound was identified as a valuable resource for tactical emergency medical services (TEMS) where timely intervention and triage are of utmost priority. Application of ultrasound technology in these high-pressure environments not only supports real-time evaluation but also has an impact on stabilization and transportation planning for critically ill patients.

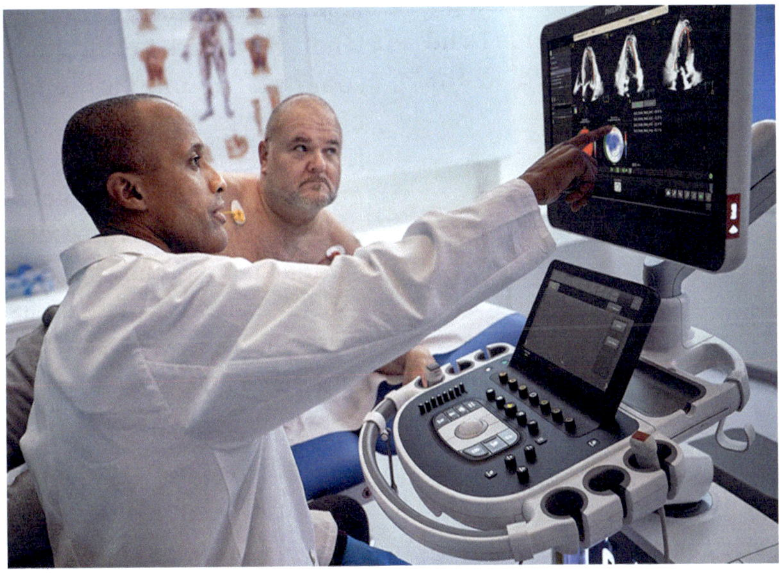

Figure 15.11. Rapid decision-making support of ultrasound.

Source: https://www.philips.com/c-dam/corporate/newscenter/global/standard/resources/healthcare/2024/AI-in-cardiovascular-ultrasound/EPIQ-X5-1c-Echolab-Autostrain-header.jpp.jpg.

As shown by the report, ultrasound can properly inform triage processes and direct associated care pathways in a way that maximizes the use of resources. The utility of ultrasound in the facilitation of effective, rapid triage and clinical decision-making justifies its worth in both conventional and specific emergency scenarios, further solidifying its place as an integral component of modern emergency care. In addition, the use of ultrasound technology brings about a paradigm change in how medical professionals deal with patient care and decision-making. Because it is easy to use and has minimal training needs, healthcare workers can learn to use ultrasound in a short while, and hence its utility extends even in resource-poor environments. Democratization of ultrasound enhances its utility as a decision-aiding tool, facilitating quick evaluation and treatment in most environments, from the urban emergency department to the remote or austere setting. The concept of ultrasound as an accelerated decision-making process underscores the need for ongoing education and training in its use by clinicians. Consequently, as emergency and critical care expand and mature, utilization of ultrasound to achieve timely and accurate decision-making becomes increasingly significant to improving patient outcomes and adding quality to care being provided in the acute setting (Figure 15.11).

15.4. Common Applications of Ultrasound in Emergency Medicine

The application of ultrasound technology in emergency medicine has revolutionized the rapid assessment of critically ill patients. Point-of-care ultrasound (POCUS) allows clinicians to perform bedside imaging, significantly reducing time from assessment to diagnosis. This capability is particularly useful in acute scenarios where seconds count, such as in trauma assessments. For instance, POCUS will detect free intraperitoneal fluid or cardiac effusions quickly, which can guide instantaneous decision-making, like surgical intervention in extreme cases. Also, that ultrasound is not invasive decreases discomfort for patients and eliminates radiation dangers, making it less dangerous than other imaging techniques. As such, POCUS is an essential tool in emergency departments, enhancing diagnostic capability and patient results overall with immediate intervention (Abualenain, 2024).

The second most prevalent application of ultrasound in emergency medicine is with procedural guidance intervention. Emergency practitioners are regularly forced to perform procedures such as central venous catheterization, thoracentesis, or joint injection under suboptimal circumstances. Ultrasound provides real-time visual feedback, enhancing the accuracy and safety of such interventions. Using this imaging modality, anatomical structures can be localized accurately, which is particularly useful in critically ill patients or when landmark techniques cannot be used in some cases. Complications have been found to be less with ultrasound-guided interventions, first-attempt success is higher, and the providers' confidence levels are also higher. Consequently, the integration of ultrasound in standard emergency practice not only improved procedural efficiency but also enhanced patient trust in medical practitioners (Androulidakis et al., 2011).

Finally, the use of ultrasound is not limited to observing and evaluating various emergency presentations, primarily cardiovascular and respiratory emergencies. In suspected cardiac tamponade or congestive heart failure, ultrasound can quickly scan cardiac function and make assumptions regarding hemodynamic stability. In addition, in presentations of respiratory distress, ultrasound can differentiate between obstructive and compressive etiologies, thus directing treatment regimens more effectively than physical examination. Through real-time monitoring, ultrasound allows dynamic assessment of patient status, enabling the clinician to make immediate interventions and therapeutic plan adjustments. With the ongoing growth of emergency medicine, the use of ultrasound technology is still a core component of it to ensure better diagnostic accuracy, procedural competency, and improved patient care strategies in every kind of emergency case (Abualenain, 2024) (Figure 15.12).

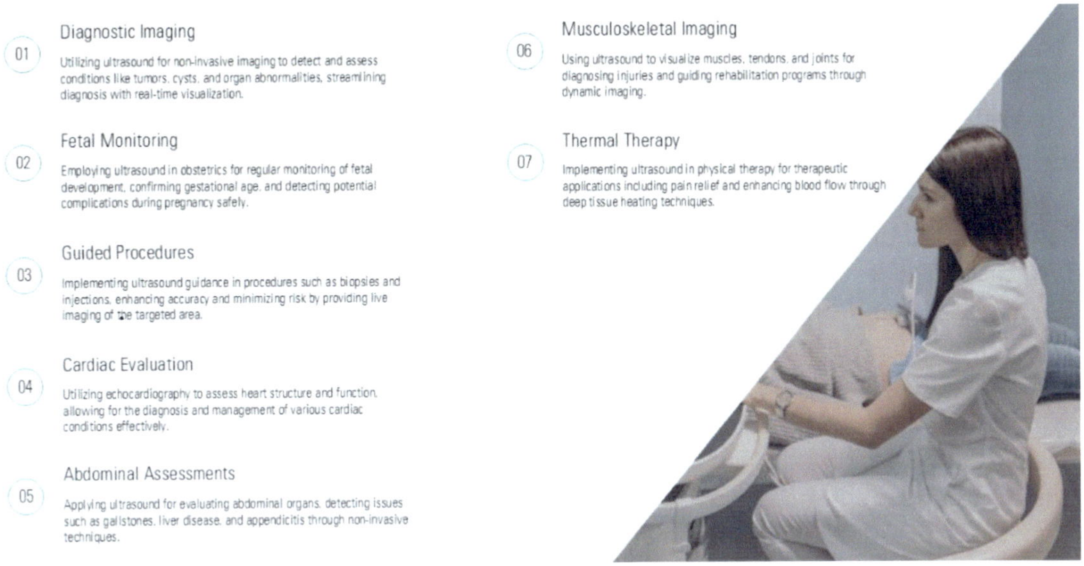

Figure 15.12. Common applications of ultrasound in emergency medicine.

Source: https://www.slideteam.net/media/catalog/product/cache/1280x720/a/p/applications_of_ultrasound_in_medicine_ppt_presentation_st_ai_ss_slide01.jpg.

15.4.1. Assessment of Trauma Patients

Care of trauma patients' demands urgent and correct evaluation to guide emergency decisions. Point-of-care ultrasonography (POCUS) is now a significant modality in this context, with non-invasive imaging of intracorporeal organs to detect pathology in the form of free fluid and organ injury. Its plus point is that bedside emergency evaluations can be conducted, thereby expediting the process of diagnosis. It has been shown through studies that even non-medically trained individuals can successfully apply POCUS with telemedicine expert input. For example, a study showed that a POCUS-trained anesthesiologist successfully instructed non-medically trained subjects to perform cardiac, pulmonary, and abdominal exams to high image quality ratings. This emphasizes the significance of POCUS in the case of trauma, in which early diagnosis is paramount, attesting to its role as a low-cost, revolutionary tool in the field of emergency medicine (Austin et al., 2019).

In the realm of trauma care, Assessment of Trauma utilizing ultrasound technology is focused on detecting life-threatening injuries such as pneumothorax and hemorrhagic shock. An official approach using the Extended Focused Assessment Sonography for Trauma (eFAST) protocol is able to diagnose free intraperitoneal fluid and chest trauma. The benefit of focused training in ultrasound cannot be overstated; recent evaluations revealed that emergency medicine residents who underwent formal, proctored training enhanced their performance to conduct these critical examinations with competence. Registrars reported greater self-confidence in the use of ultrasound following training, which equates to a higher level of practical application within clinical practice. This sustained confidence is paramount in acute fields of practice since practitioners must be able to rapidly interpret sonographic results to allocate priorities to management and greatly improve patient outcomes (Fear et al., 2015).

Furthermore, the use of teleultrasound technology adds to the improvement of trauma patient assessment in emergency cases. The capability to connect remote experts with local providers enables an entire evaluation even in settings where direct mentorship may not be offered. This kind of innovation provides precious help in diagnosing complex cases, easing skill uptake among fresh users. Interestingly, it was demonstrated in a pilot study that non-clinical attendees could perform important ultrasound scans with mentoring, achieving high satisfaction scores and effective learning outcomes. As telemedicine increases, its use in emergency medicine can be extended to ultrasound training, allowing more practitioners to take part in trauma examinations. It is this convergence of POCUS, formal training, and remote specialist review that transforms the landscape of emergency and critical care and enhances trauma patient care in various clinical environments (Austin et al., 2019; Fear et al., 2015).

15.4.2. Evaluation of Cardiac Conditions

The evaluation of cardiac illness is a critical component of emergency and critical care, in which rapid and correct assessment can significantly determine the outcome of the patient. Ultrasound, and particularly point-of-care ultrasound (POCUS), has emerged as a vital tool for this purpose. Its ability to provide real-time imaging of cardiac anatomy and function allows clinicians to make instant decisions regarding diagnosis and treatment. Recent studies revealed that teleultrasound technologies can be effectively utilized by trained clinicians, and that they can train novice clinicians to conduct important cardiac exams remotely. It is particularly beneficial in high-stakes conditions where specialist services might not always be available. Integrating these technologies into routine practice enhances the availability and promptness of cardiac evaluations, and patients receive appropriate care on time when needed the most (Austin et al., 2019). In addition, the ability to perform ultrasound scans for cardiac disease has been especially pertinent in the COVID-19 climate. With healthcare systems experiencing unprecedented pressures, ultrasonography became more favored since it does not require invasive intervention and is transportable. It can be performed bedside, thus decreasing patient transportation and airborne infection exposure. In addition, remote consultation through advanced networks, such as 4G or 5G, facilitates the delivery of specialist advice while practicing physical distancing. This versatility of ultrasound in addressing emergent needs reflects its evolving role in cardiac care, in which continuity of care must be maintained. By adopting ultrasound as a standard procedure in emergency settings, health care providers can enhance their diagnostic capabilities, leading to enhanced patient management interventions for acutely presenting cardiac conditions (Cui et al., 2020).

The effectiveness of ultrasound in evaluating cardiac conditions extends beyond mere visualization; it has also been demonstrated to yield diagnostic accuracy. Evidence shows that untrained individuals, too, can be successfully guided to perform appropriate cardiac exams, having satisfactory image quality, and performed in minutes. Pilot test results indicate that untrained operators successfully carry out complex cardiac imaging tests under supervision, achieving competence on par with experienced physicians. This would imply a promising model for training and deploying ultrasound techniques in all healthcare settings, particularly in resource-poor settings. With continuing advances in the technology of ultrasound, the use of ultrasound in assessing cardiac disease in the critical and emergency care environment will become more prevalent, offering more paths to better patient outcomes and more efficient clinical operations (Austin et al., 2019).

15.4.3. Diagnosis of Abdominal Emergencies

Diagnosis of abdominal emergencies needs to be a meticulous and systematic process, since these pathologies range from non-specific to life-threatening. Clinicians should be able to distinguish between a few causes of abdominal pain, which include appendicitis, pancreatitis, bowel obstruction, and ruptured abdominal aortic aneurysm. History and physical examination are still the foundation of conventional diagnosis, but their inclusion of ultrasound technology has greatly augmented diagnostic processes in emergencies and intensive care. Ultrasound enables real-time imaging and visualization of various abdominal organs, facilitating rapid diagnoses that can practically determine outcomes in care. With increased accessibility and affordability, emergency departments are now more qualified than ever to utilize ultrasound in abdominal emergency management, indicating a trend towards faster and less invasive diagnostic methods. In abdominal emergencies, ultrasound has some inherent benefits that can accelerate abdominal emergency management. Its use is most obvious in trauma cases, in which immediate assessment of intra-abdominal hemorrhage is critical. For instance, FAST scan has become a standard diagnostic test for detecting free fluid in the abdomen. By enabling real-time visualization of potential organ injury, ultrasound is a vital adjunct to surgical decision-making in order to reduce time to intervention. In addition, because of portability, bedside assessment can be achieved, which is critical in situations where patient transport could be hazardous or impractical. Its utility in the evolving context of prehospital use, especially within Tactical Emergency Medical Services (TEMS), reflects its importance in complex cases where timely evaluation directly influences results (Dixon et al., 2012).

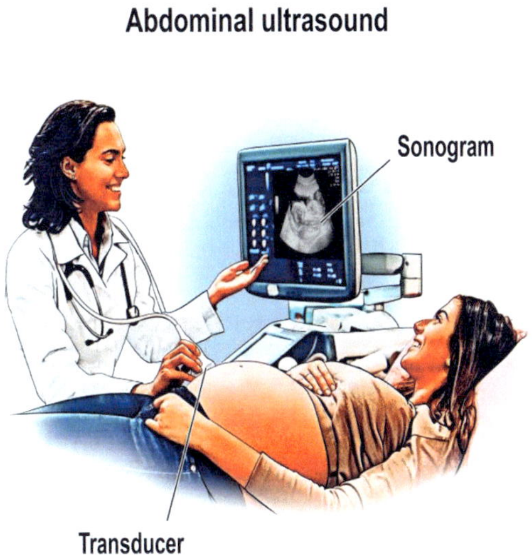

Figure 15.13. Diagnosis of abdominal emergencies of ultrasound.

Source: Cleveland Clinic (2023). https://my.clevelandclinic.org/-/scassets/images/org/health/articles/4994-abdominal-ultrasound.

The versatility of ultrasound in the diagnosis of abdominal emergencies likewise applies to counseling on the following interventions as necessary. For example, in suspected appendicitis or biliary obstruction, not only ultrasound diagnose the disease, but it also facilitates therapeutic procedures like aspiration or drainage under guidance. This dual function creates an active attitude toward the care of the patient, minimizing time loss due to traditional imaging modalities. In addition, ultrasound avoids the ionizing radiation of CT scans and hence is a safer alternative for certain categories of patients, that is, children and pregnant women. With technological advances in ultrasound, the growing role of ultrasound in the diagnostic arsenal against abdominal emergencies mirrors the necessity for training and expertise among medical professionals. The growing application of ultrasound for such acute diagnoses is a significant departure from emergency medicine practice (Kitsiou et al., 2013) (Figure 15.13).

15.5. Challenges and Limitations of Ultrasound

The use of ultrasound technology in emergency and critical care settings has undoubtedly changed the diagnostic process, but there are some in-built challenges and limitations that must be addressed. Included among them is the depth and breadth of training required for healthcare providers to become proficient in ultrasound techniques. The sophistication of calibrating machine settings, identifying anatomical nuances, and interpreting results accurately makes it crucial to have extensive training programs. Despite the existence of proctored education and training programs, inconsistencies in the quality of training can result in inconsistent ultrasound skills among providers. This is particularly evident in the emergency department, where time does not typically permit extensive education, which has the potential to compromise patient care. In order to limit such challenges, standardized training curricula and systematic evaluation mechanisms must be established to ensure that clinicians achieve and maintain competencies necessary for the optimal use of ultrasound (Fear et al., 2015). Furthermore, reliability and accuracy in ultrasound imaging can also be compromised by various factors, which further constrain the efficacy of the use of ultrasound in emergency settings. Patient factors, such as obesity or increased abdominal gas, can potentially significantly hamper image definition, leading to misinterpretation and inappropriate clinical management. The degree of experience and skill of the operators is also a potential deterrent towards the achievability of high-quality images. In scenarios where timely assessment is a matter of life and death, the use of ultrasound has the adverse effect of delaying emergency procedures whenever the result is uncertain or suboptimal. It is, therefore, important that emergency practitioners balance the use of ultrasound with other modalities of diagnosis to provide comprehensive care. By means of ongoing education and quality improvement schemes, these variability problems can be addressed so that patient outcomes and safety are enhanced in critical care (Colella et al., 2020). The incorporation of ultrasound in emergency and critical care medicine has also raised issues regarding accreditation and regulation. There is no standardized protocol for the application of ultrasound at present, which can mean inconsistency of practice and potential issues of liability. The most critical thing is to make high accreditation available to practitioners and adhere to best practice guidelines to achieve trust in the application of ultrasound as a diagnostic tool. In addition, the rapid progress of ultrasound technology requires ongoing medical education to stay current with new methods and technology. This continuous learning process, along with institutional encouragement of single-minded training in ultrasound, can alleviate some of the challenges of introducing ultrasound into emergency care. Surmounting these regulatory hurdles will be critical in encouraging the safe and effective use of ultrasound in emergency situations (Fear et al., 2015) (Figure 15.14).

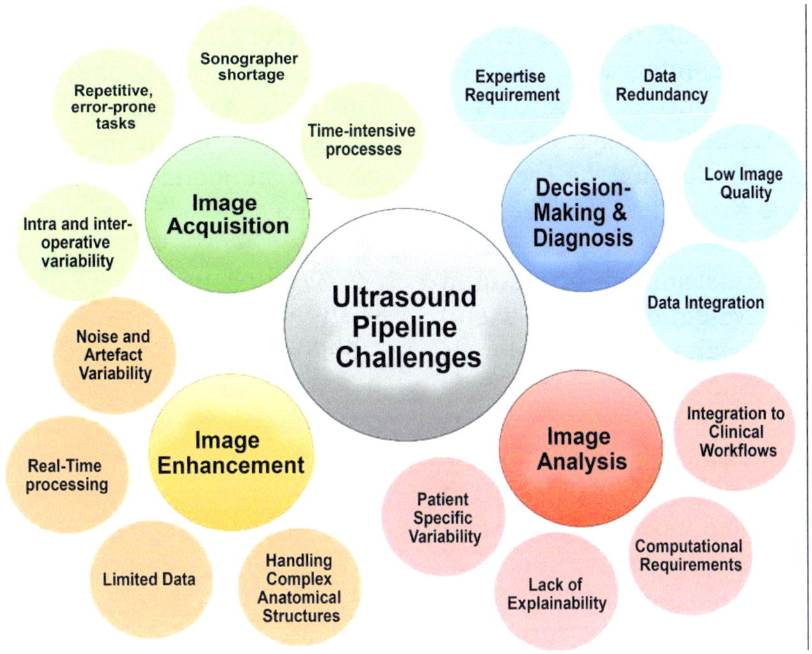

Figure 15.14. Challenges of ultrasound.

Source: Elmekki, H., Islam, S., Alagha, A. et al. (2025) Comprehensive review of reinforcement learning for medical ultrasound imaging. Artif Intell Rev 58, 284. https://doi.org/10.1007/s10462-025-11268-w. https://link.springer.com/article/10.1007/s10462-025-11268-w/figures/24

15.5.1. Operator Dependency and Skill Level

Operator skill and training level are critical to the success of ultrasound in emergency and critical care. Point-of-care ultrasound (POCUS) requires not just technical training, but also an important knowledge component about the principles involved clinically. Better training and acquisition of skills are necessary, as whether or not the operator can take good images directly affects diagnostic correctness. For instance, novice users may be challenged with carrying out the ultrasound probe properly or interpreting the resulting images, potentially leading to incorrect diagnoses. This dependence on operator proficiency highlights the need for extensive education and practice guidelines appropriate for the varying levels of experience of healthcare providers. As technology evolves, it is important that training devices keep up to provide all users with the skills they need to implement POCUS in high-risk settings where speed of decision is of utmost importance. It is also with the incorporation of artificial intelligence (AI) into ultrasound imaging that come the opportunities and challenges in terms of operator dependence. AI has the capability to standardize image acquisition and interpretation, for which it can strengthen the skills of less skilled operators. For instance, automated functions can assist in the measurement of critical parameters, such as the Left Ventricular Ejection Fraction or the Inferior Vena Cava Collapsibility Index, to assist in clinical decision-making in the acute care setting. AI software, however, cannot replace the nuanced perception developed from extensive clinical experience. Constraints such as image degradation, patient-specific problems, and the inability of AI to appreciate some clinical scenarios make it necessary for operators to maintain a firm basic skill set. Therefore, even as AI can be used to expand access, integration must be complemented with disciplined training to make sure providers possess basic analysis skills in emergency settings. Additionally, the aspect of operator dependence highlights the need for continuous assessment and feedback systems to facilitate skill acquisition in ultrasound practice. Continuous evaluation can be useful in determining where healthcare professionals might need further training, thus creating a culture of improvement and learning. This is especially important in emergency and critical care, which are environments with high patient turnover rates and mixed levels of case complexity. Developing an effective feedback loop can both enhance individual practitioners' performance and the team's overall performance. With the rising application of POCUS, and particularly in low-resource environments, training programs must adapt so that they are more equipped to manage operator variability. The implementation of technologies such as peer review and simulation-based training can be very beneficial to practitioners in refining their skills while seeing their strengths and weaknesses. Ultimately, an ongoing training and testing plan will ensure that ultrasound applications in emergency care continue to develop.

15.5.2. Limitations in Imaging Quality

In critical and emergency imaging, the quality of imaging is a critical aspect of decision-making and delivering optimal care to the patient. While ultrasound, with its advantage of portability and real-time imaging, has its own limitations as well, which may affect image quality. Operator experience, the physiology of the patient, and patient habitus are critical variables that determine how successful the use of ultrasound will be. These situations can lead to suboptimal quality images, with the possibility of limiting proper diagnosis or satisfactory control of severe conditions. For instance, imaging in obesity patients or patients with extensive subcutaneous tissue becomes extremely challenging, resulting in decreased cardiac, pulmonary, or abdominal examination accuracy.

Another factor that impacts image quality is the inherent consistency within ultrasound equipment and technology. Imaging performance has actually been improved by technology on ultrasound machines, but performance inconsistency is still present between the different machines and situations. Reckoning on the expertise of the operator is contributing to this issue; the less competent operators can be completely unable to manipulate the ultrasound probe or interpret the images. Studies have shown that even with advanced guidance, such as through remote teleultrasound technologies, the quality of images produced by non-clinical operators can lag behind images produced by clinically trained staff. Thus, the diagnostic risk of errors underscores the significance of strict training and standardization in ultrasound practice to mitigate such constraints (Austin et al., 2019). Moreover, the incorporation of ultrasound in emergency and critical care environments has also revealed a long-standing problem of interpretive mistakes, which have been attributed to both image quality and to the environment wherein ultrasound is being utilized. With emergency rooms growing more dependent on ultrasound for rapid bedside diagnosis, variations in patient acuity and clinical presentation can create layers of complexity. For instance, while some emergency practitioners get good-quality images in uncomplicated cases, they are not so fortunate in complicated ones involving critically ill patients and dynamic conditions that may alter the ultrasound appearance. Short time for examination and the clinical urgency that is always present tend to exaggerate these difficulties. Thus, despite the growing role of ultrasounds in emergency medicine, it is crucial to detect and bridge these imaging quality limitations in order to enhance diagnostic sensitivity and enhance patient care (Baker et al., 2020) (Figure 15.15).

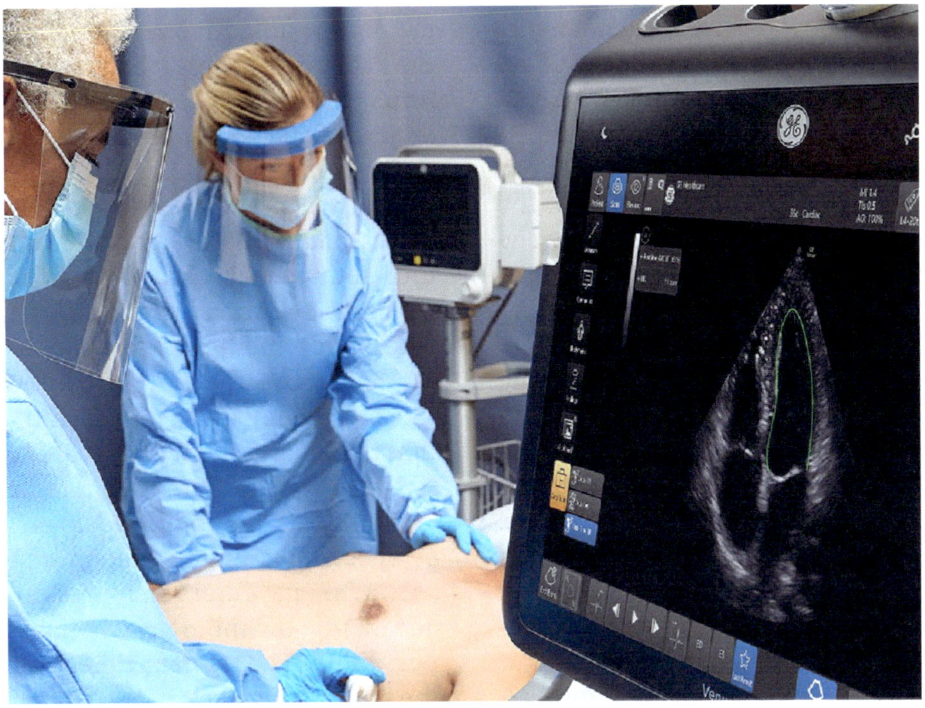

Figure 15.15. Limitations in ultrasound imaging quality of emergency and critical care.

Source: GE Healthcare (2022.) Critical Care Ultrasound: Benefits, Challenges, and Best Practices. https://images-cdn.welcomesoftware.com/Zz02ZGM3M2VlZTUzYjAxMWVkYjkyYmRlODhjZWY2OTFkOQ==/real-time-desktop.webp.

15.5.3. Situational Constraints in Emergency Environments

In emergency and critical care settings, situational constraints profoundly impact the efficacy of medical intervention, particularly the use of ultrasound diagnostics. Circumstances involving restricted access to resources, time-constrained situations, and high-stress settings are likely to compromise practitioners' ability to utilize ultrasound effectively. For instance, when there is a need for instant decision-making, the practitioners are compelled to perform scans under non-ideal circumstances, like crowded emergency rooms or pre-hospital areas. These limitations in the situation not only complicate the process but also increase the potential for diagnostic and therapeutic errors. For this reason, it is essential to make sense of these factors, which make it possible to determine the use of ultrasound technology as well as the success rate of patients with critical status. Situational limitations in emergency situations are also frequently multiplied by the medical staff's insufficient training and experience in the use of ultrasound. While advances have promoted wider access to ultrasound technology, the need for proper training remains paramount. Emergency medical care workers should be proficient in interpreting ultrasound images quickly and correctly. However, time limitations and the sheer intensity of emergency care restrict training sessions in most instances, establishing a gap that can have adverse effects on patient treatment. A lack of knowledge of ultrasound protocols and emergency procedures can lead to underutilization of this valuable diagnostic tool, hence decreasing its potential for enhancing patient management and outcome in the acute environment. In addition to this, external factors such as communication breakdown and environmental distractions also pose additional challenges in the effective use of the ultrasound in the emergency environment. The application of e-health technologies can alleviate some of these constraints by streamlining communication and data exchange among health care teams and consequently increasing workflow and coordination. For instance, the application of wireless systems may enhance access to patient data and imaging reports and facilitate timelier decision-making in real time. As e-Health solutions continue to evolve, their integration with traditional medical practice will be key to overcoming situational constraints and maximizing the utilization of ultrasound in emergency care settings, leading to improved patient safety and medical outcomes. Adapting to these dynamics is required for ongoing emergency medical services development and integration of new technologies like ultrasound in critical care management (Champion et al., 2013;Mihaylova & Zvikhacheskaya, 2011).

15.6. Future Trends in Ultrasound Technology

The promise of the future of ultrasound technology in emergency and critical care is to revolutionize the modality of diagnosis and management of patients with urgent conditions. Among the key advancements is the integration of telemedicine with point-of-care ultrasound (POCUS). Real-time ultrasound imaging transmission is likely to enhance the process of decision-making, especially in resource-limited or remote settings where specialty health care is either not accessible or delayed. By remote specialists' capacity for providing real-time advice, teleultrasound not only enhances training but also enhances diagnostic effectiveness and patient care in times of crisis. This technology can significantly impact outcomes by encouraging timely intervention and effective resource allocation, as reported by studies highlighting telemedicine's strength in supporting disaster response efforts (Abualenain, 2024). Furthermore, wearable ultrasounds are also increasingly becoming a potential future direction of ultrasound in emergency medicine. As tiny as they can be carried inside the pocket or strapped against the body, they offer quick and easy imaging that is also critical in acute care. With advances in battery life and miniaturization, these systems may be employed by first responders or specially trained personnel at the accident scene or in emergency room triage. With advancing technologies, it has the ability to potentially enable real-time diagnosis outside the boundaries of clinical environments and can be part of a proactive patient care culture to potentially streamline the workflows of critical care and emergency response to deliver care to patients as quickly as possible. Finally, the synthesis of machine learning and artificial intelligence into ultrasound technology is ready to shape the future of diagnosis in emergency and critical care. These algorithms can not only interpret ultrasound images, identify patterns, but also provide preliminary interpretations that will lead clinicians to make rapid decisions. Early studies indicate that AI can support non-specialists in the performance of ultrasound scans, as has been shown in a study where a POCUS-expert instructed lay people to carry out ultrasound scans through telemedicine technology. Such innovative integration of human and AI capabilities could lead to more precise and quicker assessments, thus decreasing the chances of missing elements during critical evaluation (Austin et al., 2019). Where these technologies overlap, they can redefine the standard and improve patient safety, constituting an enormous revolution in the utilization of ultrasound in high-stakes environments.

15.6.1. Advancements in Portable Ultrasound Devices

The emergence of handheld and portable ultrasound machines has transformed emergency and critical care medicine significantly. Once confined to the hospital setting, such imaging modalities are accessible in various settings, such as remote and resource-poor environments. Handheld and portable ultrasound technology has increased accessibility of diagnostic imaging through real-time bedside diagnosis by emergency care providers without the need for traditional large machines. Notably, enhanced image quality and user-friendly interfaces enhance the efficacy of these tools, enabling practitioners to make timely decisions. Implementation of point-of-care ultrasound as a part of routine practice is a shift towards embracing technology that supports clinical needs, ultimately leading to improved patient outcomes and acceleration of care delivery in life-threatening emergencies (Kaffas et al., 2024). A key aspect of handheld ultrasound technology is its capability to enable point-of-care ultrasound (POCUS) utilization. These devices enable one to perform full assessments within different clinical environments, including trauma, cardiac disease, and procedural guidance. Their hand-held nature allows for quick and effective assessment of patients and significantly decreases treatment initiation time. In addition, the training and education of healthcare workers in the use of such technology make them more confident and competent, which is essential in emergency settings. With advancements, the ultrasound systems have become part of indispensable components of modern-day emergency practice, displacing the use of diagnostic methods and supporting a more effective healthcare system. The continuous push for innovation in the field emphasizes the importance of leveraging technology for better clinical decision-making (Kaffas et al., 2024).

With growing technology, the integration of digitalization strategies like artificial intelligence (AI) and the Metaverse into portable ultrasound machines shows other groundbreaking potential. These innovations not only contribute to imaging capability but also support remote consultations and training for healthcare workers, especially in challenging environments. With the implementation of AI, handheld ultrasound devices can further automate image interpretation and support diagnostic accuracy, allowing practitioners to allocate their time and skills to valuable patient interactions. Besides, the convergence of enabling technologies facilitates immersive experiences for patient education and real-time interaction between medical teams. Such developments open the way for a more interconnected healthcare system that ultimately spans the gap between care providers and recipients of care, thus enabling more personalized care in emergencies and critical care (Figure 15.16).

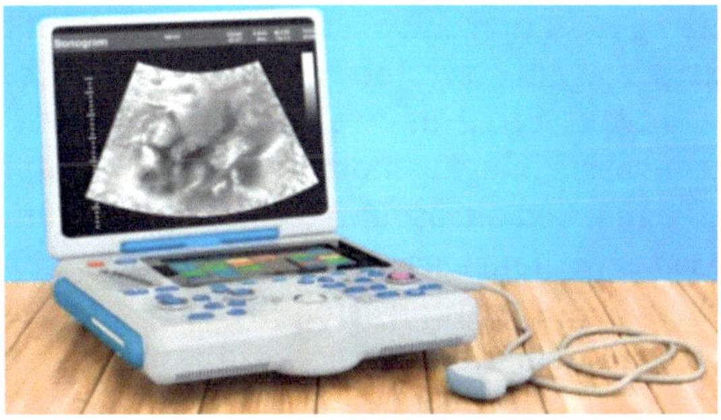

Figure 15.16. Advancements in portable ultrasound devices.

Source: Kristina (2025). ehealthcommunity.org. https://ehealthcommunity.org/wp-content/uploads/2025/03/advancements-in-portable-ultrasound-devices-400x225.webp.

15.6.2. Integration with Artificial Intelligence

The integration of artificial intelligence (AI) in ultrasound has introduced revolutionary advancements in emergency and critical care. With the application of machine learning algorithms, AI accelerates real-time image analysis to enable healthcare professionals to provide more timely and accurate diagnoses. For instance, algorithms are now capable of assisting in detecting diseases such as fluid accumulation or organ damage by analyzing ultrasound images with a level of accuracy as good as experienced radiologists. This innovation not only increases diagnostic accuracy but also reduces the cognitive burden of practitioners under high-pressure situations, ultimately allowing for more effective patient management. In workflow process automation, AI-based applications ensure prompt intervention in emergency departments, which is crucial for improving patient outcomes in critical situations. Further, improved efficiency created through AI in ultrasound technology overcomes the key challenges with conventional imaging technologies. The traditional methods are riddled with risks, such as excessive use of ionizing radiation and possible side effects of the contrast agent described in recent overviews. The advent of AI allows the development of non-invasive imaging modalities, which, coupled with enhanced ultrasound technology, eliminate the risks without sacrificing superior diagnostic accuracy. Elastography, for instance, provides critical information on the hardness of tissues without the drawbacks of the traditional method. Also, AI-based technologies will enhance the utilization of biodegradable contrast media and be in accordance with new principles of sustainable healthcare practice. This alliance between patient protection and environmental conservation shows the manner in which AI integration in emergency and critical care units' results in better holistic management of patients. The financial implications of integrating AI into ultrasound technology also warrant close scrutiny as healthcare providers look for cost-effectiveness alongside the necessity of quality care. As existing research shows, AI-augmented ultrasound imaging can produce substantial long-term savings by reducing follow-up procedures and hospital stay needs. More precise diagnostics allow for better-equipped treatment plans and forego unnecessary health expenses. Nevertheless, inequities in access to advanced AI technologies are an issue because not every health system is able to deploy these innovations uniformly. It is thus vital to address these economic issues to deliver the benefits of AI for ultrasound evenly among different patient populations. Continued collaboration between technology developers, clinicians, and policymakers is required to build systems that foster innovation and accessibility to this emerging field.

15.6.3. Potential for Expanded Training and Education

The evolving nature of critical and emergency care medicine emphasizes the utmost significance of graduate education and training in ultrasound technology. With clinical ultrasound (CUS) becoming a central field in several medical specialties, the enforcement of strict guidelines is presently of utmost importance. The guidelines need to encompass prime issues such as leadership, training, competency, credentialing, and quality assurance, with the objective of achieving uniform CUS practices within health systems. Through addressing these areas, healthcare institutions will be in a position to foster an ongoing professional learning culture and prioritize effective utilization of ultrasound. Additionally, the creation of effective training models can contribute significantly to enhancing the workforce's ability to offer timely and correct patient assessment in emergency situations, enhance care processes, and promote patient outcomes, in alignment with systematic development recommendations advocated in existing literature (Abo et al., 2018). In addition, the integration of teleultrasound technologies provides a unique chance of expansion and capability for point-of-care ultrasound (POCUS) accessibility and competency. Recent studies demonstrate the potential for remote mentoring to aid novice users, allowing them to perform complex ultrasound exams under the mentorship of an expert user. This approach not only democratizes access to ultrasound training but also broadens the skill base of health care professionals, allowing them to provide critical evaluations in life-threatening situations. Through technology such as video conferencing, instructors are able to reach more learners, including those who do not have formal medical training, which can change the sharpness of care in diverse settings. As evidenced through studies, healthcare professionals who are not medically trained have successfully conducted proper ultrasound scans with the guidance of specialists, and this proves to be the success of this new teaching method (Austin et al., 2019).

Lastly, the contributions of greater ultrasound training and education are not restricted to actual clinical application; they are also significant for healthcare systems as a whole. Training courses that equip practitioners with ultrasound competence can equate to more efficient resource use, as medical professionals who are capable of performing on-the-spot evaluations can reduce the requirement for additional imaging studies. This can equate to substantial cost savings as well as improved workflow productivity in emergency departments. Further, facilitating a culture of ongoing learning in ultrasound can foster a pattern of interdisciplinary collaboration so that differing categories of medical professionals can advance their skill sets as a team. Lastly, prioritizing rapid-track training in ultrasound best optimizes patient care while providing the healthcare system with the preparedness to meet the changing medical technologies and patient demand in critical care scenarios.

SUMMARY

The use of ultrasound in emergency and critical care has demonstrated significant promise for the enhancement of patient outcomes. The ability to perform point-of-care ultrasound (POCUS) allows clinicians to make immediate decisions within the acute environment, thus permitting interventions that can prove lifesaving. Repetitive imaging obtained from POCUS, as observed in studies of carotid artery stenosis detection, indicates the usefulness of the technique in rapid assessment programs. With specificity at 86.7% and sensitivity at 70.0%, carotid POCUS is a wonderful complement to standard diagnostic methods, especially where time-limited access to advanced imaging equipment is limited (Nemnom et al., 2020). However, its fair correlation with standard imaging deserves further evaluation before general utilization can be advocated for. POCUS has also emerged as a valuable tool for the management of the airway in emergency departments and intensive care units. Traditional testing methods are generally not effective in accurately assessing difficult airways, presenting a significant challenge for emergency practitioners. The utility of ultrasound in visualizing upper airway anatomy provides decision-making potential, enabling practitioners to anticipate complications related to intubation and other airway intervention-related complications. Evidence shows that POCUS is able to effectively predict post-extubation laryngeal edema and guide emergency cricothyrotomy procedures, hence improving the overall safety of airway management protocols (Bellinger et al., 2023). With technology advancing, the integration of ultrasound into everyday practice is most likely to benefit in patient care greatly.

Lastly, although the use of POCUS in emergency and critical care environments isencouraging, hurdles remain in advancing towards broader utilization. Variability in training, competence maintenance, and resource distribution, particularly in rural communities, are inhibitory factors that must be addressed to ensure their optimal use. Successful utilization of POCUS requires systematic training initiatives and ongoing education for standardization among healthcare providers. Additional research emphasizing the effectiveness and cost-effectiveness of ultrasound across various clinical scenarios will help enable its integration as an expected practice in the emergency department. By understanding and addressing these drivers, we can optimize the function of ultrasound and ultimately result in better patient outcomes across all healthcare landscapes.

In emergency and critical care, ultrasound technology has become a vital instrument employed by healthcare providers. The modality is not invasive and is able to rapidly assess numerous medical pathologies, thus being particularly valuable in settings where time is limited. Ultrasound, for instance, assists in assessing patients who have trauma, enabling clinicians to identify free fluid or organ injury rapidly. Furthermore, the versatility of ultrasound extends as far as the insertion of various procedures, such as central lines and thoracentesis, thereby enhancing procedural effectiveness as well as patient safety. Real-time image visualization has come a long way in revolutionizing clinical decision-making, eventually culminating in improved patient outcomes and reduced time to diagnosis in critical situations, thereby demonstrating its central role in today's emergency care process. The integration of ultrasound in emergency and critical care management necessitates reevaluation of traditional diagnostic procedures. CT or MRI, in the past, was a hallmark technique in the diagnosis of emergencies; however, the ready availability and ease of use of ultrasound have altered clinical agendas. This shift is particularly noted in resource-limited environments, where ultrasound can provide real-time diagnostic data without the logistical inconvenience of transporting patients for more complex imaging. Ultrasound has been found to considerably reduce lengths of hospital stay and increase patient throughput within emergency departments in trials. As the technology continues to advance and the practice of training becomes increasingly prevalent, ultrasound is anticipated to play an increasingly pivotal role in the normalization of emergency medicine care procedures, as exemplified in Androulidakis et al. (2011).

Furthermore, the successful implementation of ultrasound technology in emergency and critical care relies on adequate training and education of health professionals. Equipment and physical infrastructure are less important than making sure that the medical personnel have the skills to perform and interpret ultrasound tests. These skills should be developed through continuous education programs that not only enhance the individual skill level but also develop a culture of collaboration within healthcare settings, enabling members of the team to utilize this technology in real settings effectively. The creation of integrated platforms, as specified in Androulidakis et al. (2011), places importance on the provision of advanced education and telehealth care, which can facilitate remote consultation and collaboration among clinicians. Through ongoing investment in education, ultrasound can realize its full potential as a premier diagnostic tool, ultimately leading to enhanced patient management and outcomes of care within emergency and critical care settings.

CLOSER LOOK

TELEULTRASOUND TECHNOLOGIES

Teleultrasound is an emerging and innovative technology that combines ultrasound imaging and telecommunication equipment to enable remote acquisition, interpretation, and consultation of sonographic images over distance. This integration allows the clinicians and sonographers in one location to perform or enable an ultrasound exam while real-time images are transmitted over to specialists or radiologists at another facility for interpretation and guidance. Teleultrasound technology has profound impacts in resource-limited, rural, and underprivileged areas where access to trained personnel or high-capacity imaging facilities is limited. By bridging geographical and logistical gaps, teleultrasound augments diagnostic capability, supports timely decision-making, and enhances patient outcomes in distant areas.

The two primary teleultrasound modalities are store-and-forward and real-time interactive systems. Store-and-forward systems consist of the acquisition of ultrasound images or video clips, digital storage, and transmission later for expert review. It is useful in asynchronous processes and areas of poor internet connectivity. In comparison, teleultrasound in real-time provides concurrent video and audio interaction during the scan, enabling remote specialists to direct the examination, offer suggestions for probe placement, and provide concurrent image interpretation. Real-time interaction significantly enhances diagnostic accuracy and is of invaluable advantage in critical care, obstetrics, emergency medicine, and trauma.Technological advancements have played a key role in the development of teleultrasound. Portable and handheld ultrasound equipment now interfaces with smartphones, tablets, or cloud platforms, allowing images to be sent over secure internet links. Some platforms use AI-based algorithms for assisting inexperienced operators with placing probes or acquiring images, such that ultrasound becomes more accessible to physicians with little training. Improvements in wireless probes, smartphone software, and cloud-based storage have also made it possible to send and interpret ultrasound images faster, more reliably, and more scalable. Teleultrasound platforms are also being integrated into telemedicine networks and electronic health records, promoting seamless clinical communication and documentation.

Teleultrasound has a wide range of applications. In global health, it allows for prenatal screening, trauma assessment, and infection surveillance in the developing world and rural areas. In urban hospitals, teleultrasound allows for triage and monitoring of pandemics or disaster relief, reducing unnecessary hospital transfers. It is gaining popularity in space medicine, military medicine, and off-shore or sea-based health care where access to radiological consultation is radically limited. Further, teleultrasound supports medical education and training by offering trainees and learners remote expert supervision and feedback during live scanning. While promising, teleultrasound technologies are plagued by various challenges. These include issues of data privacy, inconsistent image quality due to operator inexperience, bandwidth limitations, and the need for standardized protocols. Further, legal and regulatory frameworks governing remote diagnostics are still evolving, particularly concerning cross-border licensure and liability. Nevertheless, ongoing improvements in internet infrastructure, user training, and device affordability continue to overcome these limitations.

REFERENCES

1. Abo, A., Bailitz, J., Blaivas, M., Chilstrom, J., et al. (2018). Systemwide clinical ultrasound program development: An expert consensus model. https://core.ac.uk/download/213444194.pdf (accessed on 12th July 2025).
2. Abualenain, J. (2024). Use of technology in disaster medicine. https://core.ac.uk/download/629950511.pdf (accessed on 12th July 2025).
3. Adadzi, J., Anderson II, J., Azi, C. I., Carsrud, J., et al. (2024). Transformative advancements in diagnostic imaging: Reducing risks, enhancing accuracy, and promoting sustainability. https://core.ac.uk/download/621451782.pdf (accessed on 12th July 2025).
4. Agarwal, S., Bankart, J., Bannerjee, J., Bell, P., et al. (2019). East Midlands Research into Ageing Network (EMRAN) discussion paper series. https://core.ac.uk/download/228199189.pdf (accessed on 12th July 2025).
5. Agodokpessi, G., Alovokpinhou, F., Beye, S. A., Boillat-Blanco, N., et al. (2022). Point-of-care ultrasound for tuberculosis management in sub-Saharan Africa: A balanced SWOT analysis. https://core.ac.uk/download/527938301.pdf (accessed on 12th July 2025).
6. Androulidakis, A., Bracale, U., Konnis, G., Koutsouris, D., et al. (2011). A feasibility study for the provision of electronic healthcare tools and services in areas of Greece, Cyprus, and Italy. https://core.ac.uk/download/16664902.pdf (accessed on 12th July 2025).
7. Austin, B., Davis, W., Le, D. Q., Ma, L., et al. (2019). Feasibility evaluation of commercially available video conferencing devices to technically direct untrained nonmedical personnel to perform a rapid trauma ultrasound examination. https://core.ac.uk/download/323310769.pdf (accessed on 12th July 2025).
8. Baker, O., Chou, S. C., & Schuur, J. D. (2020). Changes in emergency department care intensity from 2007-16: Analysis of the National Hospital Ambulatory Medical Care Survey. https://core.ac.uk/download/287622017.pdf (accessed on 12th July 2025).
9. Bellinger, R., Chao, K., Chou, E. H., Healy, D., et al. (2023). Point-of-care ultrasound in airway evaluation and management: A comprehensive review. https://core.ac.uk/download/619410115.pdf (accessed on 12th July 2025).
10. Bueno, H., Christ, M., Cowie, M., Cullen, L., et al. (2017). Indications and practical approach to non-invasive ventilation in acute heart failure. https://core.ac.uk/download/144473095.pdf (accessed on 12th July 2025).
11. Champion, P., Clayton, J., de Winton, M., Edwards, M., et al. (2013). Review of best management practices for aquatic vegetation control in stormwater ponds, wetlands, and lakes. https://core.ac.uk/download/29201681.pdf (accessed on 12th July 2025).
12. Chengoden, R., Victor, N., Huynh-The, T., Yenduri, G., Jhaveri, R. H., Alazab, M., Bhattacharya, S., et al. (2023). Metaverse for healthcare: A survey on potential applications, challenges, and future directions. *IEEE Access, 11*, 12765–12795. https://doi.org/10.1109/access.2023.3241628 (accessed on 12th July 2025).
13. Choi, W., Cho, Y. S., Ha, Y. R., Oh, J. H., Lee, H., Kang, B. S., Kim, Y. W., et al. (2023). Role of point-of-care ultrasound in critical care and emergency medicine: Update and future perspective. *Clinical and Experimental Emergency Medicine, 10*, 363–381. https://doi.org/10.15441/ceem.23.101 (accessed on 12th July 2025).

14. Chu, S. E., Hsieh, Y. L., Lee, C. W., Lee, C. H., et al. (2025). Trends in studies on transesophageal echocardiography in emergency medicine: A scoping review. https://core.ac.uk/download/655768777.pdf (accessed on 12th July 2025).
15. Colella, M. R., Gaither, J., Schulz, K., Smith, D., et al. (2020). Innovative approaches to emergency medical services fellowship challenges. https://core.ac.uk/download/287621995.pdf (accessed on 12th July 2025).
16. Cui, M. D., Huang, L., Jia, Y., et al. (2020). Chinese expert consensus on critical care ultrasound applications during the COVID-19 pandemic. https://core.ac.uk/download/322850186.pdf (accessed on 12th July 2025).
17. Das, N., & Yip, M. (2017). Robot autonomy for surgery. http://arxiv.org/abs/1707.03080 (accessed on 12th July 2025).
18. Dixon, J. D., Goodloe, J. M., Whelan, L., Thomas, S. H., & Justice, W. (2012). Trauma ultrasound in civilian tactical medicine. https://core.ac.uk/download/26353223.pdf (accessed on 12th July 2025).
19. Dornan, T., Feilchenfeld, Z., Kuper, A., Whitehead, C., et al. (2017). Ultrasound in undergraduate medical education: A systematic and critical review. https://core.ac.uk/download/74405617.pdf (accessed on 12th July 2025).
20. Fear, M., Hird, K., & Sweetman, G. (2015). Experience of a tutor-centric model for sonography training of emergency department registrars in an Australian urban emergency department, 2009–2012. https://core.ac.uk/download/213607033.pdf (accessed on 12th July 2025).
21. Graham, W. C., Cochard, E., & Fulkerson, Z. (2019). Implementation of a point-of-care ultrasound skills practicum for hospitalists. https://core.ac.uk/download/187423815.pdf (accessed on 12th July 2025).
22. Incalzi, R. A., Lauretani, F., Nouvenne, A., Scarlata, S., et al. (2020). The geriatric patient: The ideal one for chest ultrasonography? A review from the chest ultrasound in the elderly study group (GRETA) of the Italian Society of Gerontology and Geriatrics (SIGG). https://core.ac.uk/download/227572191.pdf (accessed on 12th July 2025).
23. Johnson, A. E. W., Bulgarelli, L., Shen, L., Gayles, A., Shammout, A., Horng, S., Pollard, T., et al. (2023). MIMIC-IV, a freely accessible electronic health record dataset. *Scientific Data, 10*. https://doi.org/10.1038/s41597-022-01899-x (accessed on 12th July 2025).
24. Kaffas, A. E., Vo-Phamhi, J. M., Griffin, J. F., & Hoyt, K. (2024). Critical advances for democratizing ultrasound diagnostics in human and veterinary medicine. *Annual Review of Biomedical Engineering, 26*, 49–65. https://doi.org/10.1146/annurev-bioeng-110222-095229 (accessed on 12th July 2025).
25. Kim, J., Maranna, S., Parange, N., Watson, D., et al. (2025). A scoping review on the integration of artificial intelligence in point-of-care ultrasound: Current clinical applications. https://core.ac.uk/download/656889328.pdf (accessed on 12th July 2025).
26. Kitsiou, A., Caforio, A. L. P., Porta-Sanchez, A., Vahanian, A., Iung, B., Carrera, C., & Szymanski, C. (2013). ESC core curriculum for the general cardiologist (2013). https://core.ac.uk/download/55756305.pdf (accessed on 12th July 2025).

27. Lees, C., Stampalija, T., Baschat, A., da Silva Costa, F., Ferrazzi, E., Figueras, F., Hecher, K., et al. (2020). ISUOG practice guidelines: Diagnosis and management of small-for-gestational-age fetus and fetal growth restriction. *Ultrasound in Obstetrics and Gynecology, 56*, 298–312. https://doi.org/10.1002/uog.22134 (accessed on 12th July 2025).

28. Masoumi, G., Mohammadi, F., Mosaddegh, R., Rezai, H., et al. (2020). The promising applications of ultrasound in emergency medicine and critical care related to cancer: A review. https://core.ac.uk/download/429339577.pdf (accessed on 12th July 2025).

29. Meineri, M. (2021). Evaluation of a patient-specific, low-cost, 3-dimensional printed transesophageal echocardiography human heart phantom. https://core.ac.uk/download/482717641.pdf (accessed on 12th July 2025).

30. Mihaylova, L., & Zvikhachevskaya, A. (2011). Novel wireless communication protocol for e-health applications. https://core.ac.uk/download/67556.pdf (accessed on 12th July 2025).

31. Muhmmed, B., Muhmmed, A., Mohammed, D., Alsaeedi, S., Salem, A., Mohammed, Y., Alotibi, F. O., et al. (2024). Radiology in emergency medicine: Life-saving imaging. *Power System Technology*. https://www.semanticscholar.org/paper/64f1ceaad160e745a4b22e0bb715d7cee391faa6 (accessed on 12th July 2025).

32. N/A. (1997). *Focal Spot, Fall/Winter 1997.* https://core.ac.uk/download/129069309.pdf (accessed on 12th July 2025).

33. N/A. (2002). *Focal Spot, Spring 2002.* https://core.ac.uk/download/129069323.pdf (accessed on 12th July 2025).

34. Nemnom, M. J., Park, L., Perry, J. J., Stotts, S., et al. (2020). Can emergency physicians perform carotid artery point-of-care ultrasound to detect stenosis in patients with TIA and stroke? A pilot study. https://core.ac.uk/download/305124073.pdf (accessed on 12th July 2025).

35. Practice Bulletin No. 183. (2017). Postpartum hemorrhage. *Obstetrics and Gynecology, 130*, e168-e186. https://doi.org/10.1097/aog.0000000000002351 (accessed on 12th July 2025).

INDEX

C

D

E

F

G

H

I

J

K

L

M

N

O

P

Q

R

S

T

U

V

W